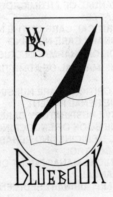

SAUNDERS BLUE BOOKS™ SERIES

Published

Adler et al.: MEDICAL EVALUATION OF THE SURGICAL PATIENT
Boden & Capone: CORONARY CARE
Chung & Lam: ESSENTIALS OF ANESTHESIOLOGY
Copass & Eisenberg: THE PARAMEDIC MANUAL
Eisenberg & Copass: EMERGENCY MEDICAL THERAPY
Eisenberg et al.: MANUAL OF ANTIMICROBIAL THERAPY AND
    INFECTIOUS DISEASES
Hodson & Truog: CRITICAL CARE OF THE NEWBORN
Huang et al.: CORONARY CARE NURSING
Johnson: BLUE BOOK OF PHARMACOLOGIC THERAPEUTICS
Larson & Eisenberg: MANUAL OF ADMITTING ORDERS AND
    THERAPEUTICS
Larson & Vazquez: CRITICAL CARE NURSING
Levine: CARE OF THE RENAL PATIENT
Luce et al.: INTENSIVE RESPIRATORY CARE
Metz & Larson: BLUE BOOK OF ENDOCRINOLOGY
Okamoto: PHYSICAL MEDICINE AND REHABILITATION
Palmer: INFECTION CONTROL
Solomon et al.: CLINICAL MANAGEMENT OF SEIZURES
Soper et al.: EMT MANUAL
Stamey & Kindrachuck: URINARY SEDIMENT AND URINALYSIS

Forthcoming

Bernard et al.: NUTRITIONAL AND METABOLIC SUPPORT FOR
    HOSPITALIZED PATIENTS
Lamberg & Lamberg: DERMATOLOGY IN PRIMARY CARE
Nelson et al.: ENVIRONMENTAL EMERGENCIES
Rosenstock & Cullen: CLINICAL OCCUPATIONAL MEDICINE

BLUE BOOK
OF
MEDICAL
DIAGNOSIS

RICHARD O. CUMMINS, M.D., M.P.H., M.Sc.

Associate Professor of Medicine,
University Hospital, University of Washington,
Seattle, Washington

MICKEY S. EISENBERG, M.D., Ph.D.

Associate Professor, Department of Medicine;
Director, Emergency Medical Service,
University Hospital, University of Washington,
Seattle, Washington

1986
W. B. SAUNDERS COMPANY

Philadelphia, London, Toronto, Mexico City,
Rio de Janeiro, Sydney, Tokyo, Hong Kong

W. B. Saunders Company: West Washington Square
Philadelphia, PA 19105

Library of Congress Cataloging in Publication Data

Cummins, Richard O.

Blue book of medical diagnosis.

(Saunders blue books series)

1. Diagnosis—Handbooks, manuals, etc.   I.
   Eisenberg, Mickey S.   II. Title. [DNLM: 1.
   Diagnosis. WB 141 C971b]

RC71.C88 1986   616.07′5′0202   85–2181

ISBN 0–7216–1218–0

Acquisition Editor: John Dyson

Production Manager: Frank Polizzano

Blue Book of Medical Diagnosis   ISBN   0-7216-1218-0

Last digit is the print number: 9   8   7   6   5   4   3   2   1

INTRODUCTORY NOTE

The Saunders Blue Books™ Series is intended to provide in a handy, convenient format, up-to-date information about therapy and patient care across a wide range of clinical fields. These books are designed to help practicing physicians, nurses, emergency personnel, other health care professionals, and students in the health sciences to deliver quality patient care. Our series derives its title from the very first W.B. Saunders publication (Hare: *Essentials of Physiology*, 1888). That book was part of a famous list of 24-question compends known as the "Blue Series." The purpose of that Series was to sort out important scientific and clinical facts so that students could review and assess their knowledge. The name of the present Series reflects its heritage from that pioneering venture. Today, when scientific information is growing exponentially, health professionals recognize an increasing obligation both to remain current and to select from this sea of data and clinical experiences those that add significantly to that foundation upon which sound clinical practice is based. The volumes in Saunders Blue Books™ Series should be regarded as portable clinical tools—as vital to quality patient care as a stethoscope or blood pressure cuff.

MICKEY S. EISENBERG, M.D., PH.D.
Consulting Editor, SAUNDERS BLUE BOOKS SERIES

CONTRIBUTORS

RICHARD K. ALBERT, M.D.

Associate Professor of Medicine, University of Washington School
of Medicine, Seattle, Washington. Assistant Chief, Pulmonary and
Critical Care Section; Director, MICU, Seattle Veterans Administration Medical Center, Seattle, Washington.

Tuberculosis

SCOTT BARNHART, M.D.

Acting Assistant Professor, Department of Medicine, University of
Washington School of Medicine, Seattle, Washington. Harborview
Medical Center, Seattle, Washington.

*Acute Respiratory Failure; Cough; Hemoptysis; Pleural Effusions;
Shortness of Breath*

EDWARD A. BENSON, M.D.

Section of Endocrinology and Metabolism, Mason Clinic. Clinical
Instructor, University of Washington School of Medicine, Seattle
Washington.

Hypoglycemia

DAVID H. BOLDT, M.D.

Associate Professor of Medicine and Chief, Division of Hematology,
University of Texas Health Science Center at San Antonio. Chief,
Hematology Section, Audie L. Murphy Memorial Veterans Administration Hospital, San Antonio, Texas.

Leukemias; Lymphomas

STUART L. BURSTEN, M.D.

Senior Research Fellow in Nephrology, University of Washington
School of Medicine, Seattle, Washington.

*Electrolyte Disorders: Hyponatremia, Hypernatremia, Hypokalemia,
and Hyperkalemia; Acute Renal Failure; Chronic Renal Failure*

PETER COGGAN, M.D.

Assistant Professor of Family Medicine, University of Washington
School of Medicine, Seattle, Washington.

Alcoholism

MILES CRAMER, B.S., R.V.T.

Manager, Peripheral Vascular Laboratory, University of Washington Hospital, Seattle, Washington.

Diagnosis of Acute Venous Thrombosis

RICHARD O. CUMMINS, M.D., M.P.H., M.Sc.

Associate Professor of Medicine, University of Washington School of Medicine, Seattle, Washington. Attending Physician, University Hospital Emergency Medical Services, Seattle, Washington.

Acid-Base Disorders; Infectious Mononucleosis; Anemia; Arthritis Associated with Spondylitis; Progressive Systemic Sclerosis (Scleroderma); Mixed Connective Tissue Disease and the CREST Syndrome; Systemic Lupus Erythematosus; Dementia

RICHARD A. DEYO, M.D., M.P.H.

Assistant Professor, Department of Medicine, University of Texas Health Science Center at San Antonio. Attending Physician, Medical Center Hospital and Audie L. Murphy Memorial Veterans Administration Hospital, San Antonio, Texas.

Arthralgias and Myalgias

ANDREW K. DIEHL, M.D., M.Sc.

Associate Professor and Chief, Division of General Medicine, University of Texas Health Science Center at San Antonio. Attending Physician, Medical Center Hospital and Audie L. Murphy Memorial Veterans Hospital, San Antonio, Texas.

Gallbladder Disease

ROBERT DREISIN, M.D.

Pulmonary Consultant, The Thoracic Clinic, Providence Medical Center, Portland, Oregon.

Interstitial Lung Disease

MICKEY S. EISENBERG, M.D., Ph.D.

Associate Professor, Department of Medicine, University of Washington School of Medicine, Seattle, Washington. Director, Emergency Medicine Service, University Hospital, Seattle, Washington.

Congestive Heart Failure; Electrocardiographic Diagnosis; Sexually Transmitted Disease; Diabetes Mellitus

WILFRED Y. FUJIMOTO, M.D.

Professor of Medicine, University of Washington School of Medicine, Seattle, Washington. Attending Physician, University Hospital; Associate Medical Staff, Harborview Medical Center, Seattle, Washington.

Adrenal Gland Diseases: Cortisol Excess; Adrenal Gland Diseases: Glucocorticoid Deficiency

MARY T. HO, M.D.

Acting Assistant Professor of Medicine, University of Washington School of Medicine, Seattle, Washington. Attending Physician, University Hospital Emergency Medicine Services, Seattle, Washington.

Chest Pain

STEPHEN K. HOLLAND, M.D., M.P.H.

Robert Wood Johnson Clinical Scholars Program, Veterans Administration Clinical Scholar, University of Washington School of Medicine, Seattle, Washington.

The Solitary Pulmonary Nodule; Proteinuria; Breast Nodule

EDWARD W. HOOK, III, M.D.

Assistant Professor of Medicine, University of Washington School of Medicine, Seattle, Washington. Associate Director, STD Clinic, Harborview Medical Center, Seattle, Washington.

Infective Endocarditis

MITCHELL A. KARTON, M.D.

Acting Instructor in Medicine, Attending Physician, Emergency Medical Service; Senior Research Fellow, Division of Endocrinology, Metabolism, and Clinical Nutrition, University of Washington Hospitals, Seattle, Washington.

Cardiomyopathy; Amenorrhea; Hypercalcemia; Hypocalcemia; Thyroid Disease; Valvular Heart Disease

ARTHUR KELLERMANN, M.D., M.P.H.

Acting Instructor of Medicine, University of Washington School of Medicine, Seattle, Washington. Research Fellow, Harborview Medical Center, Seattle, Washington.

Coma; Delirium

MICHAEL B. KIMMEY, M.D.

Senior Fellow in Gastroenterology, Acting Instructor of Medicine, University of Washington School of Medicine, Seattle, Washington.

Abdominal Pain; Hepatomegaly; Nephrolithiasis; Cirrhosis; Malabsorption; Pancreatitis

BARBARA DOLE KIRBY, M.D.

Formerly Associate Professor of Medicine, University of Washington School of Medicine, Seattle, Washington. Attending Physician, Emergency Medicine Service, University Hospital, Seattle, Washington. Director, Division of Infectious Disease, Chicago Medical School, Chicago, Illinois.

Acquired Immunodeficiency Syndrome (AIDS); Meningitis and Encephalitis; Toxic Shock Syndrome; Pneumonia; Urinary Tract Infections

THOMAS D. KOEPSELL, M.D., M.P.H.

Associate Professor, Department of Epidemiology; Adjunct Associate Professor, Department of Medicine; University of Washington School of Medicine, Seattle, Washington. Physician, Seattle Veterans Administration Medical Center, Seattle, Washington.

Polyarthritis; Degenerative Joint Disease

JEFFREY B. KOPP, M.D.

Nephrology Fellow, University of Washington School of Medicine, Seattle, Washington.

Acute Glomerulonephritis and the Nephritic Syndrome

SHOBA KRISHNAMURTHY, M.D., M.B.B.S.

Assistant Professor, University of Washington School of Medicine, Seattle, Washington. Gastroenterologist, Pacific Medical Center, Seattle, Washington.

Constipation

THOMAS R. MARTIN, M.D.

Associate Professor of Medicine, University of Washington School of Medicine, Seattle, Washington. Pulmonary Section, Seattle Veterans Administration Medical Center, Seattle, Washington.

Chronic Obstructive Pulmonary Disease

RICHARD J. MAUNDER, M.D.

Assistant Professor of Medicine, Division of Respiratory Diseases, University of Washington School of Medicine. Respiratory Diseases, Harborview Medical Center, Seattle, Washington.

The Adult Respiratory Distress Syndrome

RUSSELL McMULLEN, M.D.

Instructor, Department of Medicine, University of Washington School of Medicine, Seattle, Washington. Attending Physician, Emergency Medicine Service, University Hospital, Seattle, Washington.

Viral Hepatitis

OLIVER W. PRESS, M.D., Ph.D.

Acting Instructor in Medicine, Division of Oncology, University of Washington School of Medicine, Seattle, Washington. Associate in Clinical Research, Fred Hutchinson Cancer Research Center, University of Washington, Seattle, Washington.

Fever in the Immunocompromised Host; Fever of Unknown Origin; Lymphadenopathy; Septic Shock; Opportunistic Infections

DAVID O. RALPH, M.D.

Assistant Professor, Respiratory Disease Critical Care Medicine, University of Washington School of Medicine, Seattle, Washington. Associate Director, Intensive Care Unit, University Hospital, Seattle, Washington.

Cor Pulmonale

PAUL G. RAMSEY, M.D.

Assistant Professor, University of Washington School of Medicine, Seattle, Washington. Attending Physician, University Hospital, Seattle, Washington.

Intestinal Infections; Otitis, Pharyngitis, and Sinusitis; Septic Arthritis and Osteomyelitis; Skin Infections

PATRICIA SATO, M.D.

Instructor, Department of Medicine, Division of Respiratory Diseases, University of Washington School of Medicine. Respiratory Diseases, Harborview Medical Center, Seattle, Washington.

Pleuritic Chest Pain; Asthma; Pulmonary Embolism; Sarcoidosis

CHRISTINA M. SURAWICZ, M.D.

Assistant Professor of Medicine, University of Washington School of Medicine, Seattle, Washington. Gastroenterologist and Head of GI Endoscopy, Harborview Medical Center, Seattle, Washington.

Chronic Diarrhea; Idiopathic Inflammatory Bowel Disease

JAMES TALCOTT, M.D.

Acting Instructor in Medicine, University of Washington School of Medicine, Seattle, Washington. Clinical Fellow in Medical Oncology, Dana Farber Cancer Institute, Boston, Massachusetts.

The Solitary Pulmonary Nodule; Ascites

HASI M. VENKATACHALAM, M.B., D.S., M.P.H.

Clinical Associate Professor, Division of General Medicine, University of Texas Health Science Center at San Antonio, San Antonio, Texas.

Headache

ALAN J. WATSON, M.B., M.R.C.P.I.

Instructor of Medicine, Johns Hopkins University School of Medicine, Baltimore, Maryland. Instructor of Medicine, Assistant Director of Dialysis, Johns Hopkins Hospital, Baltimore, Maryland.

Nephrotic Syndrome

ACKNOWLEDGMENTS

We greatly appreciate the editorial guiding light provided by John Dyson and the design assistance of Lorraine Kilmer of W. B. Saunders Company.

We thank Sheila Huang, R.N., R.S., for permission to use portions of chapters on congestive heart failure and cardiac rhythm disturbances from CORONARY CARE NURSING (W. B. Saunders Company, 1983).

Judy Prentice and Joyce Hendrickson painstakingly and without complaints typed the manuscripts.

PREFACE

> *Diagnosis:* the process of making adequate decisions with inadequate information.
>
> *Anonymous*

How do doctors go about making a diagnosis? Research in this area suggests that good diagnosticians follow an almost stereotyped sequence of reasoning.

Step One: Clinical information is gathered. This can be a chief complaint, a temperature, the age, sex, or appearance of a patient, laboratory results, radiographs, and many other items.

Step Two: Possible diagnoses come to mind. This occurs almost simultaneously with step one. Good clinicians do not wait until they gather all the information but begin to think of diagnoses upon entering the examining room and seeing the patient. (This is called "cue acquisition" and "hypothesis activation" in the jargon of decision-making.) Many, perhaps most, medical problems—the compound fracture, the middle cerebral artery occlusion, Graves' disease, and lacerations—are diagnosed almost at a glance, and the diagnostic process stops. A loose analogy would be to say that step two has stimulated a number of diagnoses (usually four to seven) to be written on an imaginary mental slate.[1]

Step Three: Possible diagnoses are evaluated and refined. In this step the diagnoses on the imaginary slate are erased, added to, or underlined for emphasis.

Clinicians evaluate the possible diagnoses primarily by asking further questions. There is an enduring clinical axiom that most diagnoses are made during the history-taking. Laboratory tests and radiographs may also be used. Research into clinical problem-solving suggests that the central strategy clinicians use is "feature-matching" or family resemblance.[2–4] Clinicians possess knowledge about various diagnoses. They attempt to match the features of the patient's problems with their prior knowledge of the diagnoses they consider possible. They catalog features from the patient's history, physical examination, or laboratory tests that might match a mental picture of various diagnoses.

There is great richness and complexity in this apparently simple step. An expert clinician mentally can build a case for and against several diagnoses at the same time. Questions may branch out to confirm, eliminate, or discriminate between various diagnoses. The clinician may refine a diagnostic possibility by exploratory questions and search for complications or related conditions. Similarly, another clinician may inquire about temporal relationships, the need for action, or the possibility of effective therapy.[2]

Step Four: A tentative diagnosis is selected.   The best match or closest resemblance between the diagnoses considered in step two and the information gathered in steps one and three is selected as the diagnosis. With surprising frequency this entire process is completed minutes after the doctor has entered the examining room.[1] Often tests and radiographs are requested only to confirm or rule out the final diagnosis. The clinician then directs attention to therapeutic issues, and the diagnostic process becomes less active, although it never stops.

In the writing of the *Blue Book of Medical Diagnosis,* we have been acutely aware of these diagnostic steps. At the very center of medical problem-solving is the clinician's knowledge of medical diagnoses and problems.[2-3] Consequently, we present a concise distillation of basic textbook and review article descriptions of common medical problems and diseases. We follow a time-honored approach and outline the most frequent signs, symptoms, and laboratory findings. For each problem and diagnosis we have gathered, whenever possible, consensus statements of diagnostic criteria. Today many task forces, quality assurance committees, and consensus panels have attempted to define the essential criteria for making selected diagnoses. Similarly, they often recommend specific laboratory and radiographic evaluations for problems. We have researched and presented these recommendations for as many problems and diseases as possible.

But we have attempted something more. We have supplied additional information to assist the clinician in the crucial third step of the diagnostic process, the evaluation of possible diagnoses. We have provided expected incidences and prevalences, quantitative differential diagnoses, and a critical appraisal of laboratory and radiologic information.[5-7]

The clinician must not only know the classic description of diseases and problems, which we present, but must also consider competing explanations. This requires knowledge of possible diagnoses. Unfortunately, most books on differential diagnosis fail to supply information on the expected frequencies of the diseases contained within a differential diagnosis. Whenever possible, our contributors have supplied quantitative information about differential diagnoses. Often this takes the form of a simple statement of disease incidence, which is valuable information for diagnostic decision-making.

We also emphasize critical appraisal of both clinical and laboratory evidence. The editors and several of the contributors are trained clinical epidemiologists. We bring to this work the perspective of clinical epidemiology.[7] Instead of including a simple list of recommended laboratory evaluations, we try to appraise tests by presenting their reliability, accuracy, predictive values, sensitivity, and specificity. Unfortunately, many data for this task are not available. Perhaps this handbook will encourage others to perform needed evaluations of diagnostic technology.

We hope this book will assist physicians in problem-solving and help them to arrive at more discriminating diagnoses.

RICHARD O. CUMMINS, M.D.
MICKEY S. EISENBERG, M.D., PH.D.

REFERENCES

1. DeGowin EL, DeGowin RL: Diagnostic reasoning. *In* DeGowin EL, DeGowin RL (eds.): Bedside Diagnostic Examination. 4th ed. New York, Macmillan Publishing Company, Inc., 1981, pp. 1–9.
2. Kassirer JP, Gorry GA: Clinical problem solving: A behavorial analysis. Ann Intern Med 89:245–255, 1978.
3. Elstein AS, Shulman LS, Sprafka SA: Medical Problem Solving: An Analysis of Clinical Reasoning. Cambridge, Harvard University Press, 1978.
4. Eddy DM, Clanton CH: The art of diagnosis: Solving the clinicopathological exercise. N Engl J Med 306:1263–1268, 1982.
5. Cutler PI (ed.): Problem Solving in Clinical Medicine: From Data to Diagnosis. Baltimore, Williams & Wilkins, 1979.
6. Feinstein AR: Clinical Judgment. Baltimore, Williams & Wilkins, 1967.
7. Sackett DL: Clinical disagreement I: How often it occurs and why. Clinical disagreement II: How to avoid it and how to learn from one's mistakes. Can Med Assoc J 123:499–504, 613–617, 1980.
8. Wulff HR: Rational Diagnosis and Treatment. Oxford, Blackwell Scientific Publications, 1976.
9. Murphy EA: The Logic of Medicine. Baltimore, Johns Hopkins University Press, 1976.

CONTENTS

NEPHROLOGY

Symptoms and Signs

Diseases

INFECTIOUS DISEASE

Signs, Symptoms, and Syndromes

Diseases

ENDOCRINOLOGY

Symptoms and Signs

Diseases

GASTROENTEROLOGY

Symptoms and Signs

Processes

Diseases

HEMATOLOGY

Symptoms and Signs

Diseases

RHEUMATOLOGY

Symptoms and Signs

Diseases

NEUROLOGY

Symptoms and Signs

Diseases

CARDIOLOGY

---1---

CHEST PAIN

By MARY HO, M.D.

EPIDEMIOLOGY

A. Chest pain is the initial complaint of 4 to 7 per cent of all patients seeking medical attention at emergency departments and walk-in clinics.

B. Acute ischemic heart disease, including acute myocardial infarction, unstable angina, and new onset angina, is by far the most common life-threatening cause of chest pain.

C. Over 1.5 million patients with suspected acute ischemic heart disease are admitted to coronary care units in the United States annually. Only 30 to 50 per cent of these patients have confirmation of acute disease. Because of the lack of a rapid and accurate method of differentiating between true acute myocardial ischemia and conditions that simulate it, the physician's judgment is the most crucial element determining the final disposition of patients with chest pain.

DIFFERENTIAL DIAGNOSIS

A. The causes of chest pain are numerous and range from harmless to life-threatening (Table 1–1).

B. The frequency of occurrence of diseases causing chest pain varies depending on the institution and the patient population. In the outpatient setting, however, the most common diagnoses are chest wall pain and chest pain of unknown origin, presumably innocuous.

C. Among patients with chest pain suggestive of ischemic heart disease who are referred for coronary arteriography, up to 30 per cent have no detectable major vessel disease.

D. Of patients with anginalike chest pain (but no evidence of coronary disease) who are referred for gastrointestinal evaluation, up to 50 per cent have an esophageal etiology.

EVALUATION OF THE PATIENT WITH CHEST PAIN

For diagnostic and management purposes it is most useful to separate patients with chest pain into two categories: those with abnormal hemodynamics and those with normal hemodynamics.

TABLE 1–1. CAUSES OF CHEST PAIN

Cardiovascular disorders
  Angina pectoris
  Myocardial infarction
  Tachyarrhythmia
  Bradyarrhythmia
  Aortic stenosis and insufficiency
  Mitral valve prolapse
  Mitral stenosis
  Hypertrophic cardiomyopathy (idiopathic hypertrophic subaortic stenosis)
  Pericarditis
  Postmyocardial infarction syndrome
  Aortic dissection
  Aortic aneurysm, leaking
  Superficial thrombophlebitis (Mondor's syndrome)

Pulmonary disorders
  Pneumothorax
  Pneumomediastinum
  Pleurisy and pleurodynia
  Pulmonary embolus, infarction
  Pulmonary hypertension
  Pneumonia

Gastrointestinal disorders
  Esophageal disorders (esophageal spasm, esophagitis, hiatal hernia)
  Perforated esophagus, stomach, or duodenum
  Peptic ulcer disease
  Pancreatitis
  Cholecystitis
  Splenic flexure syndrome

Musculoskeletal disorders
  Costochondrodynia
  Cervical and thoracic disc or joint disease
  Tietze's syndrome
  Thoracic outlet syndrome
  Muscle spasm and fibrositis
  Chest wall tenderness (nonspecific)

Miscellaneous disorders
  Anxiety states (hyperventilation syndrome)
  Herpes zoster
  Intrathoracic neoplasm

While the etiologies of the two categories overlap, the differential diagnosis for chest pain with abnormal hemodynamics is relatively limited. (Causes of chest pain with abnormal hemodynamics and their distinguishing features are listed in Table 1–2.)

A. Abnormal Hemodynamics

  1. Abnormal hemodynamics exist when either or both of the following conditions are present:

   a. Shock. Signs of shock include arterial hypotension, altered sensorium, oliguria or anuria, cool and clammy skin, and, frequently, rapid respiration. Milder degrees of shock may only be detected by postural blood pressure determinations.

b. **Central Venous Pressure Elevation.** This is manifested initially by distended, superficial neck veins and dyspnea and can progress to pulmonary edema with the appearance of rales and frothy sputum. Peripheral edema, ascites, and hepatomegaly are usually absent when central venous engorgement is of acute onset. Pulmonary edema is usually not present in conditions causing primary obstruction to venous return, such as pulmonary embolism and tension pneumothorax.

2. An accurate and rapid assessment to determine the definitive therapy is especially crucial in the evaluation of patients with chest pain and abnormal hemodynamics. *Diagnosis and therapy must proceed simultaneously.*

3. In addition to the conditions listed in Table 1–2, shock from any cause is a major stress that can precipitate myocardial ischemia or infarction. This is especially true in the elderly and in patients with coronary vascular lesions that do not normally cause symptoms. Acute blood loss, sepsis, drug overdose, and less commonly anaphylaxis must be considered in the initial evaluation.

B. Normal Hemodynamics

(Table 1–3 lists the most common causes of chest pain and their distinguishing features.)

Patients with chest pain and normal hemodynamics present a diagnostic challenge. Initial evaluation should focus primarily on differentiating between causes that are potentially life-threatening and those that are more benign.

The following discussion outlines a systematic approach to the evaluation of patients with chest pain who are not in severe distress, with emphasis on the diagnosis of ischemic heart disease.

HISTORY

A carefully elicited thorough history is the most useful step in diagnosing the cause of chest pain. Physical examination and routine laboratory tests are often nonspecific or useful mainly to confirm the diagnosis already suspected from the history.

A. Quality of Pain

1. The typical pain of ischemic heart disease is often described as squeezing, strangling, crushing, a tightness, pressure, heaviness, or more vaguely as a "funny feeling." The discomfort of angina or myocardial infarction may not be perceived as pain by many patients. Thus, it is important to ask the patient not only about chest pain but also about the presence of any chest discomfort not usually present.

2. The classic gesture, the "Levine sign," is a clenched fist held over the sternum. This is highly suggestive of myocardial ischemia.

3. A sharp, knifelike pain is not typical of myocardial ischemia

Text continued on page 10.

TABLE 1-2. DIAGNOSTIC FEATURES OF CONDITIONS CAUSING CHEST PAIN WITH ABNORMAL HEMODYNAMICS

HEMODYNAMIC STATE	DIAGNOSIS	SIGNS AND SYMPTOMS
Shock without central venous pressure elevation	Aortic dissection	Severe tearing chest pain, often radiating to back; history of hypertension or Marfan's syndrome; pulse deficits, especially if transient; widened mediastinum occasionally present on chest x-ray; angiogram or CT scan diagnostic.
	Leaking abdominal aneurysm	Abdominal or back pain also present; usually elderly with a history of hypertension; pulsatile abdominal mass; cross-table lateral or ultrasound (more sensitive) diagnostic; surgical emergency.
	Myocardial infarction with excess vagal tone	Squeezing, retrosternal chest pain; nausea, vomiting, diaphoresis; bradycardia; ECG usually diagnostic.
	Gastrointestinal blood loss	Nausea, vomiting, abdominal pain; stigmata of liver disease or history of heavy ethanol abuse often present; hematemesis, melena, or maroon stools diagnostic; in early upper intestinal bleeding, stool guaiac may be negative and hematocrit normal; gastric lavage is diagnostic if positive.
Shock with central venous pressure elevation	Tension pneumothorax	Pleuritic chest pain; respiratory distress; deviated trachea with hyperresonant hemithorax and absent or decreased breath sounds; pulmonary edema absent; chest x-ray diagnostic.

Severe bradycardia or tachycardia

ECG shows ventricular rate <50 or >160 and ischemic pattern; pulmonary edema often present; usually necessary to rule out myocardial infarction.

Cardiac tamponade

Dyspnea; faint heart sounds, narrow pulse pressure, elevated pulsus paradox; diffuse low voltage on ECG, electrical alternans; pulmonary edema often absent; globular heart on chest x-ray (absent if acute onset); echocardiogram diagnostic.

Cardiogenic shock (myocardial pump failure)

Severe dyspnea; marked pulmonary edema and often new murmur of mitral regurgitation or ventricular septal defect; bronchospasm due to cardiac asthma; ECG usually diagnostic of infarction.

Massive pulmonary embolus

Severe dyspnea with sharp pleuritic chest pain; predisposing conditions of peripheral venous disease, period of immobility or decreased activity, recent surgery, pregnancy, oral contraceptive use, malignancy, systemic infection; right heart strain on physical examination, ECG, or chest x-ray; pleural rub; chest x-ray with pleural effusion, consolidation, or truncated pulmonary vasculature; ventilation perfusion scan suggestive and pulmonary angiogram diagnostic.

TABLE 1–3. DIAGNOSTIC CLUES TO CAUSES OF CHEST PAIN*

| | | HISTORY | | | | | | | |
| | Previous Attacks of Similar Pain | Pain | | | | Common Associated Findings | SIGNS | OTHER ABNORMALITIES | OTHER COMMENTS |
CAUSE		Location	Character	Onset	Duration				
Angina	Usually	Retrosternal, radiating to left arm	Squeezing, oppressive	With stress or exercise	2–10 minutes up to 20–30 minutes	Occasionally dyspnea; dizziness and syncope rare	Often none; S_4 occasionally	ECG often normal between attacks	Relieved by nitroglycerin.
Acute myocardial infarction	In some cases	Retrosternal, radiating to left arm, neck; rarely in back	Squeezing, oppressive, increases with time	No precipitating factor necessary	>30 minutes	Nausea and vomiting, diaphoresis, dyspnea	Heart failure, restlessness, shock; cardiac examination often normal	ECG may be diagnostic or normal.	Elevated CK, AST, or CK MB isoenzymes. Normal isoenzyme levels on one determination do not exclude diagnosis.
Mitral valve prolapse	Usually	Variable	Variable	Variable	Variable; usually hours	Dyspnea, dizziness common; syncope in some	Midsystolic click or murmur in most cases	ECG may show inverted T waves on leads II, III, and aVF. Echocardiogram is diagnostic.	Arrhythmia or sudden death may occur. Usually seen in young women. High-arched palate or chest or spine deformities may be present.
Aortic stenosis	May have occurred	Like angina	Like angina	Like angina	Like angina	Syncope, dyspnea	Systolic ejection murmur transmitted to carotid arteries;	ECG usually shows left ventricular hypertrophy.	More common in older men.

Aortic insufficiency	May have occurred	Like angina	Like angina	Like angina	May be prolonged	Dyspnea	Diastolic murmur transmitted to carotid arteries; water-hammer and Quincke's pulse; wide arterial pressure; delayed carotid pulse	ECG may be normal or may show left ventricular hypertrophy. Echocardiography and angiocardiography are diagnostic.	History of rheumatic heart disease, connective tissue disease, or syphilis.
Pericarditis	May have occurred	Retrosternal	Variable; often pleuritic and relieved by sitting	Variable	Hours to days	Variable	Pericardial friction rub in many	ECG may be diagnostic, nonspecific, or normal.	Relieved by sitting. Perform echocardiography to detect fluid.
Aortic dissection	No	Retrosternal and back	Tearing, maximal at onset	Sudden	Variable	Myocardial infarction, stroke, limb ischemia, syncope	Stroke, absent pulses, hematuria, shock	Chest x-ray shows widened mediastinum. ECG may show acute myocardial infarction. Pulsatile abdominal mass.	Angiography or CT scan is definitive. Hypertension or connective tissue disease may be present.
Pleurisy	No	Variable; usually lateral thorax	Pleuritic	Usually sudden	Variable	Subjective dyspnea	Often none; occasionally friction rub, low-grade fever	Occasionally pleural effusion.	Negative lung scan or pulmonary angiogram.

Table 1–3. Continued on following page

TABLE 1–3. DIAGNOSTIC CLUES TO CAUSES OF CHEST PAIN* *Continued*

	Previous Attacks of Similar Pain	HISTORY Pain — Location	HISTORY Pain — Character	HISTORY Pain — Onset	Duration	Common Associated Findings	SIGNS	OTHER ABNORMALITIES	OTHER COMMENTS
CAUSE									
Pneumothorax	May have occurred	Variable	Variable; often pleuritic	Usually sudden	Variable	Dyspnea and cough; shock if tension pneumothorax is present	Tachycardia, lung collapse with or without mediastinal shift	Chest x-ray is diagnostic but needs careful examination.	
Pneumomediastinum	No	Retrosternal	Variable; often pleuritic	Usually sudden	Variable	Dyspnea	Mediastinal crunch	Chest x-ray is diagnostic.	Usually associated with pneumothorax.
Pulmonary hypertension	Usually	Retrosternal	Like angina	Like angina	Variable	Dyspnea, fatigue, exercise syncope	Loud P_2, right ventricular lift	ECG shows right heart strain. Chest x-ray shows signs of pulmonary hypertension.	
Pulmonary embolism	May have occurred	Variable; usually lateral thorax	Usually strong pleuritic component	Usually sudden	Minutes to hours	Dyspnea, cough, and tachypnea; hemoptysis sometimes	Friction rub or splinting in some	Hypoxia and hypocapnia. Chest x-ray usually abnormal, but findings are not specific.	Abnormal lung scan or pulmonary angiogram.
Pneumonia	Rare	Over affected lobe	Pleuritic	Variable	Variable	Fever and chills, cough, dyspnea, sputum production	Fever, rales with or without consolidation, friction rub	Infiltrates on chest x-ray; purulent sputum.	

Esophagitis, esophageal spasm, hiatal hernia	Usually	Retrosternal or epigastrium	Changes with eating	Usually gradual	Variable	Gastrointestinal symptoms; flushing, sweating	None	Positive barium swallow and Goldstein (acid perfusion) test.	Relieved by antacids or topical anesthesia.
Perforated duodenal ulcer	No, or milder pain of ulcer	Retrosternal to epigastrium	Severe	Variable	Variable	Variable	Epigastric pain	Free air in peritoneum; elevated amylase.	Rare as cause of chest pain.
Pancreatitis	May have occurred	Retrosternal to epigastrium	Variable	Variable	Hours to days	Vomiting, anorexia	Epigastric or upper quadrant tenderness	Markedly elevated urine or serum amylase.	Rare as cause of chest pain.
Cholecystitis	Usually	Right upper quadrant; occasionally epigastrium or retrosternal	Variable	Usually sudden	Hours to days	Vomiting, anorexia	Epigastric or right upper quadrant tenderness	Abnormal liver function tests. Sonography is diagnostic.	Rare as cause of chest pain.
Musculoskeletal disorder (Tietze's syndrome, stitch, etc), rib fracture	Variable	Costochondral junctions; retrosternal and lateral	Pleuritic ache, "sticking" sensation	Gradual to sudden	Variable; fleeting for stitch	Splinting	Tender costosternal junctions, especially first and second ribs, or over affected ribs; rarely swelling over joints	None.	Relieved by lidocaine corticosteroid injection.

*Reprinted with permission of the authors and publisher, from Mills J, Ho MT: Chest pain. Chap. 5. *In* Mills J, Ho MT, Trunkey DD (eds.): Current Emergency Diagnosis and Treatment. Los Altos, Lange Medical Publishing, 1983, pp. 57–72.

but must be interpreted with caution, since patients may be referring to the severity rather than the quality of pain.

B. Location of Pain

1. Discomfort related to myocardial ischemia is most commonly centered in the retrosternal region. The pain may radiate up the neck to the maxilla, down the arms (more often the left), or to the back. Less commonly the pain may be confined to one of the areas in the usual path of radiation.

2. Pain of myocardial infarction is also retrosternal, although up to 35 per cent of patients may have pain located elsewhere, especially in the epigastric region. Nevertheless, in patients with myocardial infarction who have a history of angina, 94 per cent experience the myocardial pain in the same location as the angina pain, even if the site of angina pain is atypical.

3. Esophageal dysfunction is the most common cause of central chest pain that is confused with myocardial ischemia. Fifty per cent of patients with esophageal dysfunction have central chest pain, and one third have "anginalike" chest pain.

C. Duration of Pain

1. Pain caused by angina usually lasts 2 to 10 minutes but can last up to 20 to 30 minutes, especially when it is precipitated by emotional stress.

2. Pain of myocardial infarction usually lasts more than 30 minutes.

3. Pain caused by mitral valve prolapse often lasts for hours but frequently is associated with other features that are atypical of myocardial ischemia.

4. Pain lasting a few seconds or less is not caused by myocardial ischemia.

D. Provocation of Pain

1. Angina is often precipitated by exertion, emotional stress, or cold weather, food, or drink. Pain begins *during* the stress as opposed to *after* the event. Prinzmetal's or variant angina is caused by coronary artery spasm and usually occurs at rest, often at the same time each day.

2. In contrast to angina, pain of myocardial infarction often occurs without any identifiable precipitating event and begins during rest or sleep in 20 to 40 per cent of patients.

3. Pain on swallowing, eating, or lying down is more frequently caused by esophageal dysfunction but may also occur with pericarditis or, less commonly, with angina. On the other hand, 70 per cent of patients with documented esophageal disease have effort-related chest pain.

4. Pleuritic pain or pain with movement usually suggests pulmonary, musculoskeletal, or mediastinal involvement. Pain of pericarditis may be pleuritic. However, pain of myocardial ischemia is rarely pleuritic.

E. Relief of Pain

1. Pain caused by angina usually subsides within 1 to 15 minutes of the patient's cessation of the activity provoking the pain. Esophageal spasm, however, can be similarily relieved.

2. Patients with pericarditis or esophageal dysfunction usually

report improvement or relief of symptoms upon assuming the sitting position. This relief must be interpreted carefully, since patients with dyspnea related to myocardial ischemia or pulmonary disease also feel better in a more upright position. Occasionally angina may be associated with transient left ventricular dysfunction, producing mild pulmonary congestion that causes the patient to have orthopnea.

3. Nitroglycerin usually relieves chest pain caused by angina within 5 to 10 minutes. Unfortunately, nitroglycerin is also very effective in relieving pain related to esophageal spasm within the same time period. Moreover, almost a fifth of patients with myocardial infarction also experience pain relief. Thus, in the situation in which a physician highly suspects myocardial ischemia as the cause of a patient's chest pain, nitroglycerin may reinforce that belief. However, if the physician is uncertain of the origin of a patient's chest pain, relief of pain with nitroglycerin is not helpful in determining the diagnosis.

4. Rapid relief with antacids is reported by only a quarter of patients with reflux esophagitis. Conversely, up to 4 per cent of patients with myocardial ischemia may experience relief. Therefore, like nitroglycerin, antacid only helps to strengthen the case for an already strongly suspected diagnosis but should not be used as a diagnostic test.

5. Complaints of nausea, vomiting, diaphoresis, or dyspnea are commonly associated with chest pain caused by myocardial ischemia. Unfortunately, these symptoms are nonspecific and occur frequently in patients with other conditions. Moreover, absence of these associated symptoms does not exclude ischemic heart disease.

F. **Risk Factors.** (See Table 1–4.)

1. The presence of risk factors does not in itself imply that an

TABLE 1–4. RISK FACTORS FOR CORONARY ARTERY DISEASE

Sex (male > female)
Age
Family history of coronary artery disease
Cigarette smoking
Hypertension
Elevated serum cholesterol level
   (low high-density lipoprotein:low-density lipoprotein ratio)
Diabetes mellitus
Oral contraceptive drugs, estrogen, or menopause
Personality type (Type A)
Obesity
Elevated serum triglyceride level
Hyperuricemia or gout
Sedentary lifestyle
Excess alcohol consumption
Electrocardiographic evidence of left ventricular hypertrophy
Mediastinal radiation
Coffee (controversial)

individual patient's chest pain is caused by ischemic heart disease; more importantly, the absence of risk factors does not exclude ischemic heart disease.

2. When two or more risk factors are present in one individual, their effects are additive.

3. Cigarette smoking, hypertension, and elevated serum cholesterol are all strong independent risk factors for coronary vascular disease.

PHYSICAL EXAMINATION

Special attention should be paid to features of the physical examination that can rule in or exclude certain diagnoses. Occasionally, more than one disease process may be present. For example, the stress of pneumonia may precipitate angina in a patient with aortic stenosis.

A. Patients with angina, unstable angina, uncomplicated acute myocardial infarction, esophageal disorders, pulmonary embolus, or psychogenic chest pain usually have no diagnostic abnormalities detectable by physical examination.

B. Vital signs should include blood pressure and pulse, taken in the supine and sitting positions, presence and degree of pulsus paradox, respiratory rate, and temperature (rectal if oral temperature is unreliable).

C. Examine the fundus for diabetic or hypertensive changes and the pharynx for the high-arched palate often seen in patients with Marfan's syndrome and occasionally in mitral valve prolapse.

D. Examine the chest wall carefully by inspection and palpation.

1. The rash of herpes zoster (cluster of vesicles in a dermatome distribution) or Tietze's syndrome (erythematous nodules over the costochondral junction) are diagnostic.

2. Pain on palpation of the chest wall may indicate musculoskeletal disorders such as costochondritis, rib fracture or contusion, thoracic outlet syndrome, or cervical or thoracic radicular syndrome.

CAUTION: Care must be taken to ascertain that the pain elicited by palpation of the chest wall is identical to that of the patient's chief complaint.

E. Percuss and auscultate over both the anterior and posterior lung fields and mediastinum, while listening for any abnormal sounds.

F. **Cardiovascular System**

1. Assess central venous pressure with the patient's upper body elevated 30 degrees. The distance in centimeters between the sternal angle and a horizontal line extending from the uppermost part of pulsation of the *internal* jugular vein, when added to 5 cm (estimated distance from the sternal angle vertically to the heart), is an approximation of the jugular or central venous pressure.

2. Inspect and palpate for heaves, lifts, or thrills.
3. Auscultate for any abnormality in S1 or S2 and for any abnormal sounds such as S3, S4, click, murmur, or rub.
4. Determine the intensity and amplitude of carotid, femoral, and other peripheral pulses.

G. Examine the abdomen carefully, looking especially for bruits, abnormal aortic pulse, or any evidence of intra-abdominal disease. A gently performed rectal examination to check for stool guaiac involves little risk for patients with acute myocardial infarctions and is indicated when gastrointestinal bleeding is a possibility.

H. Examine the patients' legs for evidence of thrombophlebitis (see Chapter 2): swelling, redness, tenderness, increased warmth, and presence of cords.

LABORATORY STUDIES

Laboratory tests should be tailored to the individual situation. Limitations in the interpretation of test results must be recognized. The validity of a test is defined by its sensitivity and specificity. However, the interpretation of a test result also depends on the probability that a given disease is present in the individual to be tested (pretest probability of disease). Thus, a test with known sensitivity and specificity when applied to patients with different probability of disease can yield results with quite different interpretations. For example, a test with sensitivity of 80 per cent and specificity of 80 per cent when applied to a population with 90 per cent probability of disease has a 97 per cent posttest likelihood of disease when the test is positive but only a 31 per cent probability that the disease is absent when the test is negative. (See inside of back cover.) On the other hand, when this test is applied to a population with a 10 per cent probability of disease, the posttest likelihood of disease with a positive test result is only 31 per cent, whereas a negative test result yields a 97 per cent probability that the disease is absent. In general, a positive test result is useful in a population with a high prevalence of a disease, and a negative test result is useful in a population with a low prevalence of disease. The converse of both situations at best is useless but may cause misinterpretation of the test result or increase the uncertainty of a diagnosis. The following discussion primarily emphasizes those laboratory tests that are commonly used in the diagnosis of ischemic heart disease.

A. The pretest likelihood (prevalence of the disease in the population tested) of coronary artery disease in patients with chest pain is shown in Table 1–5.

B. *Electrocardiographic (ECG)* changes consistent with acute myocardial infarction are new Q waves (in leads I, AVL, or in two diaphragmatic or precordial leads), ≥ 1 mm ST segment elevation or depression in the same lead combinations, or new complete left bundle branch blocks.

1. In one study in a patient population with high pretest likeli-

TABLE 1–5. PRETEST LIKELIHOOD OF CORONARY ARTERY DISEASE IN SYMPTOMATIC PATIENTS ACCORDING TO AGE AND SEX*†

AGE (YR)	NONANGINAL CHEST PAIN		ATYPICAL ANGINA		TYPICAL ANGINA	
	Men	Women	Men	Women	Men	Women
30–39	5.2 ± 0.8	0.8 ± 0.3	21.8 ± 2.4	4.2 ± 1.3	69.7 ± 3.2	25.8 ± 6.5
40–49	14.1 ± 1.3	2.8 ± 0.7	46.1 ± 1.8	13.3 ± 2.9	87.3 ± 1.0	55.2 ± 6.5
50–59	21.5 ± 1.7	8.4 ± 1.2	58.9 ± 1.5	32.4 ± 3.0	92.0 ± 0.6	79.4 ± 2.4
60–69	28.1 ± 1.9	18.6 ± 1.9	67.1 ± 1.3	54.4 ± 2.4	94.3 ± 0.4	90.6 ± 1.0

*Reprinted with permission of the author and publisher, from Diamond GA, Forrester JS: Analysis of probability as an aid in the clinical diagnosis of coronary artery disease. N Engl J Med 300:1350–1358, 1979.

†Each value represents the per cent ±1 standard error of the per cent.

hood of myocardial infarction and ECG changes consistent with acute myocardial infarction, *sensitivity* was 80 per cent, *specificity* was 69 per cent, predictive value was 72 per cent, false positive rate was 28 per cent, and false negative rate was 21 per cent.

2. However, in another study of patients referred to an emergency room with presumed acute myocardial infarction who actually had infarctions, only 64 per cent had ECG changes of acute ischemia or infarction, 30 per cent had nonspecific changes, and 6 per cent were normal.

3. Because of the high risk of morbidity and mortality in patients with acute myocardial infarctions, the presence of an infarct pattern on ECG is helpful in spite of the high false-positive rate. Nonspecific changes or a normal ECG neither confirm nor exclude myocardial infarction in patients who have a high pretest likelihood of ischemic heart disease because their posttest likelihood remains high (negative test result with high prevalence of disease).

4. In patients with very low pretest likelihood of disease as determined by the history and physical examination, an ECG may not be useful, since the presence of nonspecific changes only introduces diagnostic confusion (positive test result with low prevalence of disease).

5. A chronic left bundle branch block pattern obscures the ECG changes of an acute anterior infarction.

C. **Serum Enzyme Analysis.** Because of the time course of serum enzyme concentration changes (Fig. 1–1), serial evaluations are necessary. The result of a single value is not useful. *A single serum enzyme value should not be used as a screening test to determine whether a patient is to be admitted to or discharged from the hospital.* If the patient's pretest likelihood of disease is high enough to warrant serum enzyme analysis, the patient should be admitted.

1. *Aspartate Aminotransferase (AST) (Previously Known as SGOT).* Sensitivity is 83 to 97 per cent when measured one

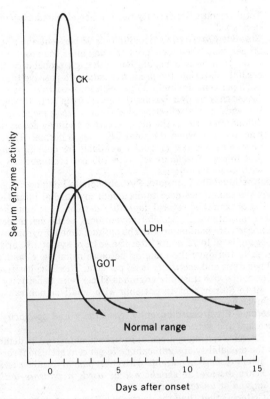

Figure 1–1. The time course of serum enzyme concentration changes following a typical myocardial infarction. CK = creatine phosphokinase; LDH = lactic dehydrogenase; GOT = glutamic oxaloacetic transaminase. (Reprinted with permission of authors and publisher, from Braunwald E, Alpert JS: Acute myocardial infarction. Chap. 261. *In* Petersdorf RG, Adams RD, et al. (eds.): Harrison's Principles of Internal Medicine. 10th ed. New York, McGraw-Hill, 1983, pp. 1432–1443.)

day following the onset of symptoms. *Specificity* is poor, since AST is found in many organs. AST may be falsely elevated in patients taking erythromycin when the colorimetric assay is used.

2. *Lactic Dehydrogenase (LDH).* *Sensitivity* is 86 to 87 per cent when measured three days after the onset of symptoms. Like AST, LDH elevation is nonspecific. LDH determination is especially useful if the patient is admitted several days after possible infarction, since the creatine kinase (CK) level and AST may have returned to normal.

3. *LDH Isoenzyme (LDH₁/LDH₂>1).* *Sensitivity* is 80 to 95 per cent when measured within 48 hours of myocardial infarction.

Total serum LDH activity need not be elevated. *Specificity* is very good.

4. *Creatine Kinase (CK).* *Sensitivity* is 96 per cent and *specificity* 65 per cent when measured one day after the onset of symptoms. In a patient population with high probability of myocardial infarction, the *predictive value* of a positive test result is 75 per cent, giving a 25 per cent false-positive rate.

5. *CK Isoenzyme (MB Fraction).* *Sensitivity* is 70 to 100 per cent, the wide range reflecting the various assay techniques. Radioimmunoassay is the most sensitive and may detect the MB fraction even when the total CK level is normal. This is the most sensitive test currently available for detecting myocardial injury. *Specificity* is 77 to 100 per cent, again varying with assay techniques.

D. **Technetium-99m Stannous Pyrophosphate Imaging.** This technique is sometimes used to document myocardial infarctions in patients examined several days after developing symptoms or in other situations in which conventional tests for myocardial infarction are nondiagnostic. The optimal time for pyrophosphate imaging is 36 to 72 hours after the onset of symptoms, and after seven to ten days the imaging becomes negative. *Sensitivity* is 89 per cent, and *specificity* is 86 per cent. The false-positive rate in patients with unstable angina is 41 per cent. Sensitivity drops to 40 to 50 per cent in patients with small or nontransmural infarctions.

E. **Exercise Electrocardiography.** *Sensitivity* and *specificity* vary with age and sex.

1. Exercise testing is a useful initial screening test to determine the probability of significant (≥75 per cent occlusion) coronary artery disease in patients with chest pain atypical for ischemic heart disease. *It should not be used in patients with rest angina or unstable angina.*

2. Criteria other than the degree of ST segment depression must also be considered. For example, a drop in systolic blood pressure, attainment of a heart rate lower than expected, and shorter duration of exercise before developing ST segment depression are all associated with a higher likelihood of significant coronary artery disease.

3. In one study the false-positive test rate was 8 per cent in men and 67 per cent in women (average age 50 years). Conversely, the false-negative rate was 37 per cent in men and 12 per cent in women. Thus, a positive test result is useful to predict the presence of disease in men, and a negative test result is useful to exclude disease in women with low pretest probability of disease.

F. **Exercise Thallium-201 Imaging**

1. *Sensitivity* is 82 per cent and *specificity* is 91 per cent.

2. Suboptimal exercise end-point and administration of beta-adrenergic blockers increase the false-negative rate.

3. This is the initial test of choice in patients who have abnormal ST elevation or depression on the resting electrocardiogram that make interpretation of a simple exercise electrocardiogram difficult.

4. The presence or absence of significant coronary artery disease can be determined with more confidence when the postexercise electrocardiographic determination of probability of disease is used as the pretest probability for exercise thallium imaging. Combining the serial likelihood of two independent tests can yield a more useful posttest likelihood of disease and may obviate further more expensive or invasive tests.

G. Radionuclide Angiocardiography
   1. *Sensitivity* is 82 per cent and *specificity* is 84 per cent.
   2. This test is useful mainly in patients with an indeterminate probability of having coronary artery disease after both exercise electrocardiography and exercise thallium imaging have already been performed and the patient is not a candidate for coronary angiography.
   3. An exercise radionuclide angiocardiogram is somewhat more sensitive than an exercise thallium scan and can provide quantitative measurements of ejection fraction. However, radionuclide imaging is difficult to interpret in patients with arrhythmias, high sympathetic tone (augmented left ventricular performance at rest), valvular heart disease, or primary myocardial disease.

H. Coronary Angiography with Ergot Stimulation. This is currently the "gold standard" for the determination of the presence or absence of coronary artery disease. Coronary angiography is the initial test of choice in patients with anginalike chest pain at rest or in patients with an unstable chest pain pattern who are unresponsive to usual medical therapy.

I. Echocardiography
   1. This test may be used to confirm the presence of valvular abnormalities, hypertrophic cardiomyopathy, pericardial effusion, or prior myocardial infarctions already suspected on completion of the history and physical examination.
   2. Echocardiography may be obtained concurrently with any of the above noninvasive tests, since it primarily identifies noncoronary cardiac causes of chest pain.
   3. Except in assessing wall motion and estimating ejection fraction, echocardiography does not determine the presence or absence of coronary artery disease. It should not be used as the sole test in the evaluation of patients suspected of having ischemic heart disease, especially since coronary artery disease can be present concomitantly with noncoronary heart disease.

J. Laboratory Test for Assessment of Noncardiac Causes of Chest Pain
   1. *Ventilation Perfusion Scan.* Perfusion scans alone are highly sensitive for detecting pulmonary embolism and are reliable in excluding disease when it is normal. However, specificity is low. The probability of pulmonary embolus in a patient with multiple perfusion defects is 81 per cent when mainly lobar, 58 per cent when segmental, and 7 per cent when subsegmental. When these defects are associated with ventilation mismatches, the probability of pulmonary embolism

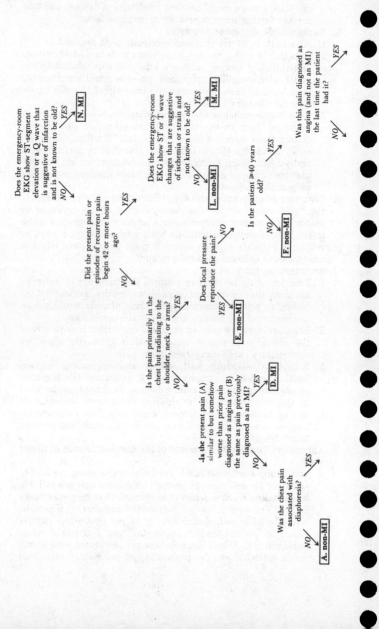

Does the emergency-room EKG show ST-segment elevation or a Q wave that is suggestive of infarction and is not known to be old?

YES → **N. MI**

NO

Did the present pain or episodes of recurrent pain begin 42 or more hours ago?

YES

NO

Does the emergency-room EKG show ST or T wave changes that are suggestive of ischemia or strain and not known to be old?

YES → **M. MI**

NO → **L. non-MI**

Is the patient ≥40 years old?

YES

NO → **F. non-MI**

Was this pain diagnosed as angina (and not an MI) the last time the patient had it?

YES

NO

Is the pain primarily in the chest but radiating to the shoulder, neck, or arms?

YES

NO

Does local pressure reproduce the pain?

YES → **E. non-MI**

NO

Is the present pain (A) similar to but somehow worse than prior pain diagnosed as angina or (B) the same as pain previously diagnosed as an MI?

YES → **D. MI**

NO

Was the chest pain associated with diaphoresis?

YES

NO → **A. non-MI**

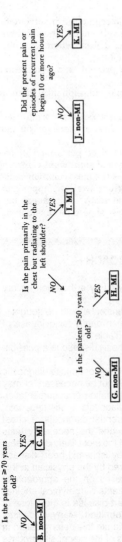

Figure 1-2. Computer-derived decision tree for the classification of patients with chest pain. Each of the 14 letters (A through N) identifies a terminal branch of the tree. For any given patient, start with the first question regarding ST-segment elevation and then trace the patient through the relevant subsequent questions until a terminal branch is reached. In the Yale-New Haven Hospital sample, seven terminal branches (C, D, H, I, K, M, and N) contained all 60 patients with acute myocardial infarction as well as 28 patients with unstable angina and 43 patients with other ultimate diagnoses. EKG = electrocardiogram; MI = myocardial infarction. (Reprinted with permission of authors and publisher, from Goldman L, Weinberg M, et al.: A computer-derived protocol to aid in the diagnosis of emergency room patients with chest pain. N Engl J Med 307:588–596, 1982.)

increases to 97 per cent for lobar and segmental involvement and 25 per cent for subsegmental involvement. Thus, pulmonary angiography is needed to detect disease when:
a. A single defect involves a lobe or lung;
b. Multiple segmental defects are present and ventilation scan is not available;
c. Ventilation matches the multiple subsegmental defects seen on perfusion scan;
d. Perfusion defects correspond to chest x-ray abnormalities;
e. Chronic obstructive pulmonary disease involves 50 per cent or more of the lungs.
2. **Gastrointestinal Studies.** These should be performed in patients with chest pain but no evidence of significant coronary artery disease. Esophageal disorder is the most common cause of chest pain in these patients. Barium swallow, upper gastrointestinal series, upper tract endoscopy, esophageal manometry, and possibly Bernstein's test should be considered.

RECOMMENDED DIAGNOSTIC APPROACH

A. Rapid initial assessment should be followed by a thorough history and physical examination.
   1. Signs of shock or central venous distension should be sought.
   2. Examine the lungs, heart, and abdomen briefly for evidence of life-threatening conditions as listed in Table 1–2.
B. Obtain an electrocardiogram if ischemic heart disease is a possibility.
C. At this point, the physician often has a probable or definite diagnostic opinion. Further laboratory evaluation may not be necessary or may be performed selectively, mainly for confirmation or documentation of the suspected diagnosis. When the diagnosis is still uncertain, each of the disorders listed in the differential diagnosis of chest pain (Table 1–1) should be considered, and the necessary tests should be performed to confirm or rule out the most likely diagnoses. Since differentiating chest pain caused by ischemic heart disease is the most perplexing problem encountered by the physician in this evaluation, the following discussion focuses on the approach to diagnosing ischemic heart disease in patients with atypical angina.
   1. The likelihood that acute ischemic heart disease is the cause of the patient's chest pain must be determined. Many guidelines have been proposed to aid the physician in this determination in order to improve the cost-effectiveness of the diagnostic process and to decrease the number of unnecessary coronary-care unit admissions. Two examples are shown in Figures 1–2 to 1–4.
   2. If acute ischemic heart disease is a reasonable probability, the patient should be admitted to a coronary-care unit and have the diagnosis confirmed or ruled out by serial electrocardiograms and cardiac enzyme measurements.
   3. If acute ischemic heart disease is ruled out by these tests or if the chest pain is not acute, other tests are necessary to establish

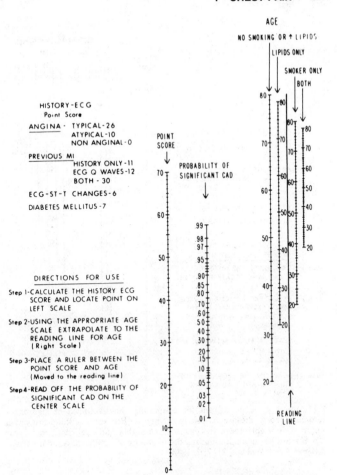

Figure 1–3. A nomogram for estimating the likelihood of significant coronary artery disease (CAD) in men. ECG = electrocardiogram; MI = myocardial infarction. (Reprinted with permission of author and publisher, from Pryor DB, Harrell RE, et al.: Estimating the likelihood of significant coronary artery disease. Am J Med 75:771–780, 1983.)

a diagnosis. Which tests may be useful and cost-effective in determining the presence or absence of significant atherosclerotic coronary disease depends on the individual patient. Cardiology consultation should be obtained in cases in which the diagnostic approach is uncertain. The following is a brief summary of further tests that are available for the evaluation of ischemic heart disease. A more detailed discussion was given earlier under Laboratory Studies.

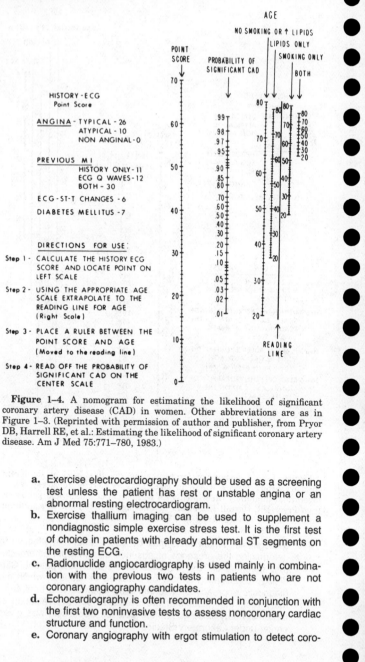

Figure 1–4. A nomogram for estimating the likelihood of significant coronary artery disease (CAD) in women. Other abbreviations are as in Figure 1–3. (Reprinted with permission of author and publisher, from Pryor DB, Harrell RE, et al.: Estimating the likelihood of significant coronary artery disease. Am J Med 75:771–780, 1983.)

a. Exercise electrocardiography should be used as a screening test unless the patient has rest or unstable angina or an abnormal resting electrocardiogram.

b. Exercise thallium imaging can be used to supplement a nondiagnostic simple exercise stress test. It is the first test of choice in patients with already abnormal ST segments on the resting ECG.

c. Radionuclide angiocardiography is used mainly in combination with the previous two tests in patients who are not coronary angiography candidates.

d. Echocardiography is often recommended in conjunction with the first two noninvasive tests to assess noncoronary cardiac structure and function.

e. Coronary angiography with ergot stimulation to detect coronary artery spasm is the definitive test to diagnose chest pain caused by coronary artery disease. It should be performed as the first test of choice in patients with atypical chest pain that is unstable or occurs at rest. It should also be performed in patients with chest pain thought to be caused by significant valvular disease and who are surgical candidates in order to detect associated coronary artery disease.

f. In patients with anginalike chest pain and absence of significant coronary artery disease as determined by these tests, gastrointestinal studies should be performed.

REFERENCES

1. Sox HC: The emergency department evaluation of chest pain. *In* Wolcott BW, Rund DA (eds.): Emergency Medicine Annual. East Norwalk, Appleton-Century-Crofts, 1982, pp. 43–60.

A good review of the evaluation of chest pain related to ischemic heart disease.

2. Mills J, Ho MT: Chest Pain. *In* Mills J, Ho MT, Trunkey DD (eds.): Current Emergency Diagnosis and Treatment. Chap. 5. Los Altos, Lange Medical Publishing, 1983, pp. 55–72.

This chapter offers guidelines for the emergency department evaluation and management of patients with chest pain. Causes of chest pain ranging from the life-threatening to the benign are discussed. An algorithm is included.

3. Levine HJ: Difficult problems in the diagnosis of chest pain. Am Heart J 100:108–118, 1980.

The evaluation of chest pain caused by coronary and noncoronary heart disease and noncardiac conditions is discussed.

4. Goldman L, Weinberg M, Weisberg M, et al.: A computer-derived protocol to aid in the diagnosis of emergency room patients with acute chest pain. N Engl J Med 307:588–596, 1982.

An algorithm is described for differentiating between patients with chest pain caused by acute myocardial infarction and those with chest pain from other causes.

5. Pryor DB, Harrell RE, Lee KL, et al.: Estimating the likelihood of significant coronary artery disease. Am J Med 75:771–780, 1983.

A nomogram is developed for estimating the probability of significant coronary artery disease in patients with chest pain. This probability can then be used as the pretest likelihood of disease.

6. Pozen MW, D'Agostino RB, et al.: A predictive instrument to improve coronary-care unit admission practices in acute ischemic heart disease. N Engl J Med 310:1273–1278, 1984.

Another method is described to help physicians determine the probability that a patient's chest pain is caused by ischemic heart disease.

7. Come PC: Diagnosis of acute myocardial infarction. *In* Eliot RS (ed.): Cardiac Emergencies. 2nd ed. Chap. 2. Mount Kisco, Futura Publications, 1982, pp. 11–62.

This is an excellent review of the diagnosis of acute myocardial infarction. Electrocardiographic changes and serum enzyme analysis are discussed in detail.

8. Berger JH, Zaret BL: Nuclear cardiology. N Engl J Med 305:799–807, 855–865, 1981.

This is a comprehensive review of nuclear cardiology.

9. Diamond GA, Forrester JS: Analysis of probability as an aid in the clinical diagnosis of coronary artery disease. N Engl J Med 300:1350–1358, 1979.

The analysis of serial test results using Bayes' theorem to estimate the probability of angiographic coronary artery disease is discussed.

10. Epstein SE: Implications of probability analysis on the strategy used for noninvasive detection of coronary artery disease: Role of single or combined use of exercise electrocardiographic testing, radionuclide cineangiography and myocardial perfusing imaging. Am J Cardiol 46:491–499, 1980.

Another discussion of the use of probability analysis to estimate the likelihood of significant coronary artery disease using noninvasive tests.

11. Long WB, Cohen S: The digestive tract as a cause of chest pain. Am Heart J 100:567–572, 1980.

This article reviews the gastrointestinal causes of anginalike chest pain and their diagnosis.

2

DIAGNOSIS OF ACUTE VENOUS THROMBOSIS

By MILES CRAMER, B.S., R.V.T.

DEFINITION

Thrombosis (clot) of the venous system usually results from the interactive effects of blood flow stasis, hypercoagulability, and endothelial injury. The precise relationship of these factors is unknown. Venous thrombosis can be superficial or deep, acute or chronic. The term "thrombophlebitis" implies thrombosis resulting from vein wall inflammation and is therefore used to describe thrombosis in the superficial venous system, that is, *superficial thrombophlebitis.* The more correct term for thrombosis of the deep veins is *deep vein thrombosis* (DVT), since the inflammatory component is minimal. DVT most commonly involves the veins located from the knee to the abdomen (proximal veins) or the veins of the calf (distal veins), or both.

PATHOLOGY

Acute DVT frequently begins in the venous sinuses of the calf and valve cusp pockets in the veins of the calf or thigh.* Obstruction

---

*Thrombi may also form in the iliofemoral segment and owing to the compression of the left iliac vein by the right iliac artery, the incidence of left iliofemoral DVT is at least twice that for the right side.

of venous flow results in local inflammation and increased venous pressure distal to the thrombus, which may cause pain, swelling, tenderness, and heat over the involved segment. The thrombus may propagate proximally, distally, embolize, or rarely, spontaneously lyse. If thrombus is not treated,

A. Twenty-eight per cent of general surgery patients develop calf vein thrombi.
B. Eighty per cent of calf vein thrombi spontaneously lyse.
C. As many as 20 per cent of calf thrombi propagate into the popliteal vein.
D. Approximately 50 per cent of popliteal thrombi give rise to clinically significant pulmonary embolism.
   1. Only 30 per cent of patients with pulmonary embolism have symptomatic leg vein thrombi.
   2. Over 80 per cent of patients with pulmonary embolism have lower-extremity thrombosis detected by venography.

Once the thrombus stabilizes, it is eventually covered by endothelium and becomes a permanent venous obstruction. Recanalization may occur in as many as 10 per cent of patients, but there is usually damage to the venous wall with or without valvular damage.

EPIDEMIOLOGY

Deep vein thrombosis accounts for considerable morbidity in both the acute phase when hospitalization is prolonged and in the long-term case as a result of changes from the postthrombotic (postphlebitic) syndrome. In the United States there are 500,000 estimated cases of DVT per year; for every 100 patients who develop DVT, 5 per cent will experience a nonfatal pulmonary embolus and 0.1 per cent will die as a result of pulmonary embolus stemming from DVT. There may be as many as 24 million persons with significant varicose veins, 6 to 7 million with stasis changes in the skin of the legs, and one-half million who have or have had a varicose ulcer.

DIFFERENTIAL DIAGNOSIS

DVT is usually unilateral and rarely occurs spontaneously. It usually develops in the context of a disease or condition that alters venous flow, induces hypercoagulability, or causes injury to the venous lining.

A. Predisposing Factors
   1. *Alteration of Venous Flow (Stasis)*
      a. Postoperative factors (listed in order of significance):*
         Age: for patients with an age differential of 40 years, the older has a 12 times greater risk of DVT.

---

*Approximately 60 per cent of the female population who develop proximal DVT do so in connection with either hormone therapy or childbirth (23 per cent with hormone therapy, 14 per cent after cesarean section, and 23 per cent postpartum).

Varicose veins.
Previous DVT.
Infection.
Severity of operation.
b. Postpartum condition.*
c. Heart failure.
d. Varicose veins.
e. Bed rest.
f. Prolonged travel in a sitting position.
g. Chronic debilitating conditions: Persons with acutely paralyzed limbs (such as after spinal cord injury) seem to have greater susceptibility to DVT than persons with other chronic conditions.

2. *Hypercoagulability*
   a. Malignancy.
   b. Sepsis.
   c. Oral contraceptives:* Increased risk of thromboembolism is 3.5 to 6 times greater for estrogen-therapy patients.
   d. Polycythemia.
   e. Thrombocytosis.

3. *Injury to Vein Lining*
   a. Trauma.
   b. Intravenous catheters or intravenous medications.
   c. Lupus erythematosis.
   d. Septic thrombophlebitis.
   e. Buerger's disease (thromboangiitis obliterans).

B. **Signs and Symptoms.** Clinical assessment of DVT begins by ruling out other causes of unilateral pain, tenderness, swelling, and erythema.

Next, the thrombus should be classified as superficial or deep. If it is deep, whether it is in the proximal or distal venous system must be determined.

1. *Superficial Thrombophlebitis*
   a. This condition is classically located in the greater saphenous vein and its tributaries.
   b. Clinically superficial thrombophlebitis is manifest by an area of localized tenderness, erythema, and induration.
   c. The key clinical sign is a "red line" that follows the path of the superficial vein.

2. *Deep Vein Thrombosis.* Clinical symptoms are highly variable and are inaccurate for diagnostic purposes 50 per cent of the time. Patients with few or no clinical findings may have extensive DVT, and patients with significant findings may

---

*Approximately 60 per cent of the female population who develop proximal DVT do so in connection with either hormone therapy or childbirth (23 per cent with hormone therapy, 14 per cent after cesarean section, and 23 per cent postpartum).

OTHER CAUSES OF UNILATERAL SYMPTOMS

CONDITION	RELATIVE INCIDENCE	CHARACTERISTICS
Cellulitis or lymphedema	Common	a. Edema usually extends onto dorsum of foot (rare in DVT). b. Edema responds poorly to leg elevation. c. Cutaneous erythema and tenderness are usually more pronounced, as in a systemic response. d. Lymphedema is often painless.
Muscle cramps	Occasional	Localized muscular tightness.
Arthritis	Rare	Joint pain; there may be joint effusion.
Ruptured Baker's cyst	Rare	a. Rapid acute swelling of calf, ankle, and foot. b. Initial location of pain in calf and/or popliteal fossa.
Compression from pregnancy	Occasional	a. Partial compression of iliac veins may occur. b. Edema is usually bilateral.
Compression from renal transplant	Rare	a. Patient complains of groin pain. b. Edema may be evident.

have a normal venous system (see other causes). Symptoms of DVT may include:

a. Unilateral lower-extremity pain.
b. Unilateral lower-extremity edema (excluding dorsum of the foot); a circumference greater than 1 cm over the contralateral leg is significant.
c. Tenderness to palpation.
d. Low-grade fever.
e. Hemoptysis (bloody sputum).
f. Inability to fully extend the leg without pain in the calf or popliteal fossa region (positive Homan's sign).
g. Phlegmasia cerulea dolens (blue leg) that is extensive and diffuse. Massive swelling impairs arterial inflow, causing cyanosis.
h. Phlegmasia alba dolens (white leg): massive thrombosis that involves the perivenous lymphatics. The leg turns white as a result of extreme edema.

The determination of proximal or distal DVT is critical to the type of diagnostic test ordered and to subsequent patient management. Isolated calf vein thrombi may be benign and often can be treated with anti-inflammatory drugs, heat, and limb elevation.

Popliteal and proximal vein thrombi require anticoagulant or thrombolytic therapy, or both.

DIAGNOSTIC STUDIES

A. **Invasive Techniques.** The standard objective method of diagnosing DVT is by venography. The most definitive criteria consist of intraluminal filling defects that are consistent in all films and are seen in multiple projections.

VENOGRAPHIC CRITERIA

1. Termination of a column of contrast medium at a constant site with refilling at a site above termination.
2. Nonfilling of a portion of the venous system.
3. Diversion of flow into collaterals.
4. Appearance of contrast medium on either side of a thrombus ("railroad tracking").

1. **Radionuclide Venography**
   a. This technique images only proximal venous thrombosis.
   b. There is a lower risk and less pain to the patient than with standard contrast venography, but it is, overall, less accurate.
2. **Contrast Venography**
   a. This technique images calf vein thrombi and produces more specific images of all veins.
   b. Up to 6 per cent of patients may develop DVT as a result of irritation of venous endothelium by the contrast medium.
3. **Perfusion—Ventilation Lung Scan and/or Pulmonary Arteriogram**
   a. These are used separately or in combination to detect pulmonary embolism.
   b. The pulmonary arteriogram is definitive.

Since venography is invasive and fraught with potential complications, noninvasive tests are frequently substituted because they are faster, less expensive, and painless, and pose no risk to the patient. The diagnostic accuracy of noninvasive tests is generally lower than that of venography.

B. **Noninvasive Techniques**
   1. **Doppler Ultrasound.** High-frequency sound is transmitted transcutaneously through the underlying vessels. The signal is backscattered and shifted in frequency by an amount proportional to the flow velocity. Abnormal characteristics may include the absence of a signal or a continuous high-velocity flow. The test is subjective and fails to detect up to 50 per cent of calf vein thrombi unless the posterior tibial system is involved.

2. *Plethysmography: Strain Gauge (SPG), Impedance (IPG), and Pulse Volume.* These tests measure venous blood volume changes in response to inflation and deflation of a pneumatic thigh cuff. SPG and IPG detect proximal DVT by plotting the venous filling volume (venous capacitance) against the venous emptying rate (venous outflow). Plethysmography fails to detect 80 per cent of calf vein thrombi.

3. *Phleborheography.* This technique works in a manner similar to other plethysmographic techniques except that respiratory variations are used to detect disease. Phleborheography is one of the most accurate plethysmographic tests, but is still quite insensitive to calf vein thrombi.

4. (^{125}I) *Fibrinogen Leg Scanning.* This test is not truly noninvasive, since labeled fibrinogen is injected into the venous system. The tracer is incorporated into a developing thrombus and causes a local "hot spot" that can be detected by external scintillation counting. It is very accurate for detecting calf vein thrombi but only when the tracer can be administered before the risk period. Therefore, it is most accurate as a screening technique.

5. *Thermography.* Intended as a rapid screening technique, thermography provides continuous leg temperature profiles by manually scanning the leg with an infrared radiation transducer. Currently the accuracy of portable units has not been confirmed in the United States.

ACCURACY OF NONINVASIVE TECHNIQUES

	CORRELATION WITH RECENT PROXIMAL DVT (SENSITIVITY)	CORRELATION WITH NORMAL VENOGRAM (SPECIFICITY)	OVERALL ACCURACY
Doppler ultrasound	92%	78%	87%
Plethysmography	91%	87%	89%
Phleborheography	100%	98%	99%
Thermography	95%	50%	82%
(^{125}I) Fibrinogen (symptomatic patients)*	56%	84%	69%
(^{125}I) Fibrinogen (screening)*	90%	96%	93%

*Not useful for detection of proximal DVT.

The accuracy of noninvasive tests may be considerably improved if they are combined. Also, expertise in certain procedures may improve accuracy. For example, in experienced hands Doppler ultrasound may yield a sensitivity of 98 per cent, specificity of 88 per cent, overall accuracy of 96 per cent for proximal DVT.

RECOMMENDED DIAGNOSTIC APPROACH

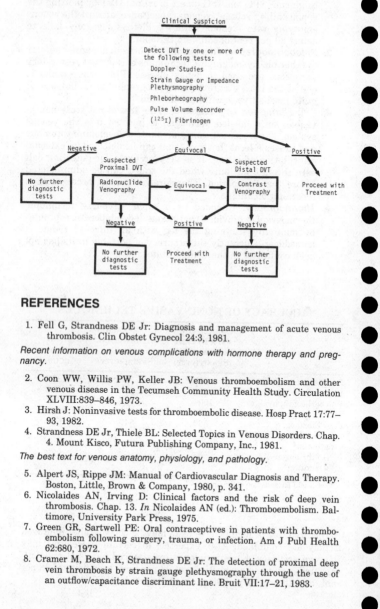

REFERENCES

1. Fell G, Strandness DE Jr: Diagnosis and management of acute venous thrombosis. Clin Obstet Gynecol 24:3, 1981.

Recent information on venous complications with hormone therapy and pregnancy.

2. Coon WW, Willis PW, Keller JB: Venous thromboembolism and other venous disease in the Tecumseh Community Health Study. Circulation XLVIII:839–846, 1973.

3. Hirsh J: Noninvasive tests for thromboembolic disease. Hosp Pract 17:77–93, 1982.

4. Strandness DE Jr, Thiele BL: Selected Topics in Venous Disorders. Chap. 4. Mount Kisco, Futura Publishing Company, Inc., 1981.

The best text for venous anatomy, physiology, and pathology.

5. Alpert JS, Rippe JM: Manual of Cardiovascular Diagnosis and Therapy. Boston, Little, Brown & Company, 1980, p. 341.

6. Nicolaides AN, Irving D: Clinical factors and the risk of deep vein thrombosis. Chap. 13. *In* Nicolaides AN (ed.): Thromboembolism. Baltimore, University Park Press, 1975.

7. Green GR, Sartwell PE: Oral contraceptives in patients with thromboembolism following surgery, trauma, or infection. Am J Publ Health 62:680, 1972.

8. Cramer M, Beach K, Strandness DE Jr: The detection of proximal deep vein thrombosis by strain gauge plethysmography through the use of an outflow/capacitance discriminant line. Bruit VII:17–21, 1983.

This paper is basically research-oriented.

9. Wheeler HB, Anderson FA: Can noninvasive tests be used as the basis for treatment of deep vein thrombosis. *In* Bernstein JJ (ed.): Noninvasive Diagnostic Techniques in Vascular Disease. 2nd ed. St. Louis, CV Mosby Company, 1982.

This text is recommended for concise information on noninvasive tests.

10. Sumner DS: The approach to diagnosis of venous disease. *In* Rutherford RB (ed.): Vascular Surgery. Philadelphia, W. B. Saunders Company, 1977.

___3___

CARDIOMYOPATHY

By MITCHELL KARTON, M.D.

DEFINITION AND CLASSIFICATION

A. The cardiomyopathies make up a diverse group of diseases of cardiac muscle and function not related to atherosclerotic, hypertensive, valvular, pericardial, or congenital disorders.

B. Cardiomyopathies may be classified in several ways. Clinically, the most helpful system of classification describes pathophysiologic categories of cardiac dysfunction: dilated (congestive), hypertrophic, and restrictive (infiltrative) cardiomyopathies.

   1. Dilated (congestive) cardiomyopathy is characterized by a dilated left and/or right heart with impaired systolic function. As the left ventricular ejection fraction decreases, the left ventricle dilates to prevent a decrease in stroke volume and hence in cardiac output. Heart failure, arrhythmias, and emboli often occur.

   2. Hypertrophic cardiomyopathy consists of disproportionate hypertrophy of the left ventricular muscle mass, which typically involves the septum more than the free wall but which is occasionally concentric.

   Previously this disorder had been known by many names, including *idiopathic hypertrophic subaortic stenosis (IHSS), hypertrophic obstructive cardiomyopathy (HOCM),* and *asymmetric septal hypertrophy (ASH).* However, not all patients have dynamic outflow tract obstruction, and systolic function is usually normal. When heart failure occurs it is characterized by diminished diastolic compliance as a consequence of stiff hypertrophied ventricular muscle.

   3. Restrictive (infiltrative) cardiomyopathy is characterized by abnormal diastolic properties without significant compromise of systolic function. Fibrosis or infiltration of the cardiac muscle causes decreased ventricular diastolic compliance. Endomyocardial scarring may also affect either one or both ventricles and restrict filling.

EPIDEMIOLOGY AND GENERAL COMMENTS

Primary cardiomyopathies (whether dilated, hypertrophic, or restrictive) represent 90 per cent of cardiomyopathies. Secondary cardiomyopathies (representing 10 per cent of cardiomyopathies) are part of a systemic disease or the result of a recognizable cause (see Table 3–1).

TABLE 3–1. ETIOLOGIC CLASSIFICATION OF CARDIOMYOPATHIES

Primary (90%)
  A. Idiopathic (D, H, R)*
  B. Familial (L, H)
  C. Eosinophilic endomyocardial disease (R)
  D. Endomyocardial fibrosis (R)

Secondary (10%)
  A. *Infective*
     1. Viral (coxsackievirus)
     2. Rickettsial (*Coxiella*)
     3. Bacterial (staphylococcal)
     4. Fungal (*Aspergillus*)
     5. Protozoal (Chagas' disease)
     6. Metazoal (filarial)
  B. *Metabolic*
     1. Endocrine (D): thyrotoxicosis, hypothyroidism, adrenocortical insufficiency, pheochromocytoma, acromegaly
     2. Familial storage disease and infiltrations (D, R): hemochromatosis, glycogen storage disease, Hurler's syndrome, Refsum's syndrome, Niemann-Pick disease, Hand-Schüller-Christian disease, Fabray-Anderson disease, Morquio-Ullrich disease
     3. Deficiency (D): potassium, magnesium, Kwashiorkor, anemia, beriberi
     4. Amyloid (R) (Primary, secondary, familial): hereditary cardiac amyloidosis, familial Mediterranean fever, senile
  C. *General system diseases*
     1. Connective tissue disorders (D): systemic lupus erythematosus, polyarteritis nodosa, rheumatoid arthritis, progressive systemic sclerosis, dermatomyositis
     2. Infiltrations and granulomas (R, D): sarcoidosis, leukemia, malignancies
  D. *Heredofamilial*
     1. Muscular dystrophies (D): Duchenne's, dystrophia myotonica
     2. Neuromuscular disorders (H, D): Friedreich's ataxia
  E. *Sensitivity and toxic reactions (D)*
     1. Alcohol
     2. Irradiation
     3. Drugs: sulfa, penicillin, anthracyclines, emetine
     4. Metals: cobalt, antimony
  F. *Peripartum heart disease (D)*
  G. *Endocardial fibroelastosis (R)*

*The principal clinical manifestation of each etiologic grouping is denoted by D (dilated), H (hypertrophic), or R (restrictive).

Adapted from Brandenburg RD, et al.: Report on the WHO/ISFC task force on the definition and classification of cardiomyopathies. Circulation 64:437–438, 1981.

DIFFERENTIAL DIAGNOSIS

The differential diagnosis of cardiomyopathy includes pericardial effusion, constrictive pericarditis, coronary artery disease, hypertensive cardiovascular disease, and rheumatic heart disease.

A. **Pericardial Effusion with Tamponade.** The patient with this condition may have symptoms of congestive heart failure. Vital signs are characterized by tachycardia, low systolic blood pressure, and a low pulse pressure with a paradoxic pulse. The neck veins may be elevated but with an absent "y" descent. Heart sounds are often distant without a third or fourth heart sound (S3 or S4). The lungs are usually clear but there may be hepatic congestion and peripheral edema. The chest x-ray may show an enlarged cardiac silhouette but without evidence of pulmonary venous congestion.

B. **Constrictive Pericarditis.** This condition is often difficult to distinguish from restrictive cardiomyopathy. Physical examination may reveal a paradoxic pulse. The neck veins are distended, often Kussmaul's sign (an increase in venous pressure with inspiration) is evident, and the "y" descent is rapid. The lungs are clear, and the heart is not enlarged. There may be a pericardial knock and evidence of hepatomegaly, ascites, and peripheral edema.

Catheterization demonstrates the characteristic "dip and plateau" configuration of ventricular pressures with equal left and right end-diastolic pressure. In restrictive cardiomyopathy this "square root sign" is also present, but usually left ventricular end-diastolic pressure is greater than right ventricular end-diastolic pressure. In both diseases echocardiography demonstrates normal ventricular size and systolic function. Occasionally in a patient with constrictive pericarditis pericardial calcification may be noted on the chest x-ray or echocardiogram.

C. **Coronary Artery Disease.** Ischemic damage from multiple infarctions is often discernible from the history or prior electrocardiograms (ECGs). Chronic angina pectoris is usually absent in dilated cardiomyopathy, but angina-like pain may occur with restrictive and hypertrophic varieties of cardiomyopathy. Occasionally these forms may also express pseudoinfarction q or qs waves on the ECG.

D. **Hypertensive Cardiovascular Disease.** This condition may appear with ischemic, hypertrophic, or congestive changes but usually in the setting of systemic hypertension. In addition, there is sometimes other end organ damage such as renal insufficiency or retinopathy.

E. **Rheumatic Heart Disease.** This condition usually is characterized by significant diastolic murmurs. Valvular calcifications may be seen on chest x-ray or fluoroscopy.

HISTORY

A. **Dilated Cardiomyopathy.** The patient complains of symptoms of congestive heart failure. Light-headedness, weakness, fatigue, and fast heart rates characterize low output failure. Backward failure may engender complaints of dyspnea, orthopnea, ankle swelling, and irregular heart rhythms. The onset of these symptoms is gradual, although occasionally there is sudden evidence of emboli, either systemic or pulmonary.

B. **Hypertrophic Cardiomyopathy.** Many patients are asymptomatic and are relatives of patients with known disease. Others are noted to have characteristic murmurs between adolescence and early middle age. There may be a family history of sudden death (especially in adolescents during or after exercise) or heart failure.

In symptomatic patients, the most common complaint is dyspnea. Chest pain, syncope, fatigue, and palpitations are also common.

C. **Restrictive Cardiomyopathy.** Patients have complaints of exercise limitation and right-sided heart failure such as dyspnea, weakness, and edema. Chest pain is rare. Since restrictive cardiomyopathy is often caused by other specific conditions, the patient may have symptoms in other organ systems that are attributable to diseases such as amyloidosis, hemochromatosis, or sarcoidosis.

SIGNS AND SYMPTOMS

A. **Dilated Cardiomyopathy.** Physical examination may demonstrate cardiomegaly, a narrow pulse pressure with pulsus alternans, an S3 and an S4, regurgitant murmurs (MR/TR), pulmonary hypertension, rales, jugular venous distension, hepatomegaly, and peripheral edema.

B. **Hypertrophic Cardiomyopathy.** Physical examination may demonstrate mild cardiomegaly, an audible S4 and a left ventricular heave or thrill. Often there are a brisk carotid pulse and prominent *a* waves in the jugular venous pulse. The most informative physical finding is the harsh crescendo-decrescendo systolic murmur that increases with the Valsalva maneuver and decreases with squatting.

C. **Restrictive Cardiomyopathy.** Physical examination may demonstrate mild to moderate cardiomegaly, an S3 or an S4, and regurgitant atrioventricular valve murmurs (MR/TR).

In addition, there may be findings mimicking constrictive pericarditis, such as a rapid "y" descent of the jugular venous pulse, Kussmaul's sign, and a paradoxic pulse. Findings of right-sided heart failure, including elevated neck veins, hepatomegaly, and peripheral edema, are often more prominent than those of left-sided failure.

STUDIES

A. **Dilated Cardiomyopathy.** The chest x-ray commonly shows cardiomegaly and congestive heart failure.

The ECG may show sinus tachycardia, atrial and ventricular arrhythmias, an intraventricular conduction defect, nonspecific ST-T wave changes, and q or qs waves with poor R wave progression.

Echocardiography demonstrates chamber dilatation and poor contractile function. Pericardial effusion and mural thrombi may be seen. Radionuclide study shows left ventricular dilatation and dysfunction.

Cardiac catheterization shows left ventricular dilatation and dysfunction, possible regurgitant murmurs (MR/TR), increased left ventricular end-diastolic pressure, possibly increased right ventricular end-diastolic pressure, and decreased cardiac output.

B. Hypertrophic Cardiomyopathy. The chest x-ray may show cardiomegaly and often shows left atrial enlargement.

The ECG often shows ST-T wave changes, left ventricular hypertrophy, and abnormal q waves in inferior and lateral leads. Premature ventricular contraction or ventricular tachycardia may occur frequently; atrial arrhythmias occur, but rarely.

The echocardiogram may show asymmetric septal hypertrophy (a septum to posterior wall thickness ratio of 1.3 to 1.5 or greater), systolic anterior motion of the anterior leaflet of the mitral valve, hypercontractility, enlarged left atrium with a normal or decreased left ventricular end-diastolic dimension, a decreased E to F slope of the mitral valve, and mid-systolic closure or coarse systolic fluttering of the aortic valve.

Radionuclide studies show a small left ventricular cavity with vigorous contraction.

Cardiac catheterization is characterized by elevated right- and left-sided filling pressures, vigorous systolic function with a small or normal left ventricular cavity, and often demonstration of a dynamic left ventricular outflow obstruction. Prominent a waves, asymmetric septal hypertrophy, and a "spike and dome" arterial pressure tracing may also be present.

C. Restrictive Cardiomyopathy. The chest x-ray may show mild cardiomegaly, which is greater on the right than the left.

The ECG may be normal or may demonstrate low voltage, an intraventricular conduction defect, or atrial-ventricular conduction defects.

The echocardiogram may show increased left ventricular wall thickness, small or normal chambers, and a normal or slightly reduced ejection fraction.

Radionuclide studies show normal or small chambers and normal systolic function.

Cardiac catheterization shows normal or small chambers, increased ventricular end-diastolic pressure (left greater than right), a distinctive diastolic "dip and plateau" tracing (also known as the "square root sign"), and preserved systolic function.

RECOMMENDED DIAGNOSTIC APPROACH

A. The history, physical examination, chest x-ray, and ECG are used to accomplish the following:

   1. Determine whether the patient has undiagnosed rheumatic heart disease, coronary artery disease, congenital heart disease, hypertension, or valvular heart disease.

    2. If applicable, clarify whether the patient has signs or symptoms consistent with any of the systemic diseases or etiologies listed in Table 3–1.

    3. To elucidate the patient's key cardiac symptoms and signs.

B. If the evaluation suggests dilated cardiomyopathy, hypertrophic cardiomyopathy, or restrictive cardiomyopathy, the diagnosis can be confirmed in the following ways:

    1. *Dilated Cardiomyopathy.* The diagnosis can be made with echocardiography and radionuclide ejection fraction. Cardiac catheterization is rarely necessary except to rule out hemodynamically significant coronary artery or valvular lesions.

    2. *Hypertrophic Cardiomyopathy.* Echocardiography is the mainstay of diagnosis. Cardiac catheterization defines the degree of diastolic dysfunction and allows a measurement of the systolic gradient, if present.

    3. *Restrictive Cardiomyopathy.* Noninvasive studies are not definitive. Cardiac catheterization reveals the characteristic pressure tracings, and transvenous right ventricular endomyocardial biopsy may identify specific infiltrative causes.

REFERENCES

General

1. Brandenburg RO, Chazov E, Cherian G, et al.: Report on the WHO/ISFC task force on definition and classification of cardiomyopathies. Circulation 64:437–438, 1981.

This is the official international classification system.

2. Hegee JW, Niemann JT, Boman KG, Criley JM: Cardiology for the House Officer. Baltimore, Williams & Wilkins, 1982.

Provides a concise review of clinical evaluation and treatment of the cardiomyopathies.

3. Perloff JK: Cardiomyopathies: Dilated and restrictive. Circulation 63:1189–1198, 1981.

This is a definitive bibliography of all aspects of the dilated and restrictive cardiomyopathies.

Dilated Cardiomyopathy

1. Fuster V, et al.: The natural history of idiopathic dilated cardiomyopathy. Am J Cardiol 47:525–531, 1981.

This is a comprehensive long-term (6 to 20 years) retrospective analysis of 104 patients at the Mayo Clinic who have idiopathic dilated cardiomyopathy. This study discusses the etiology, clinical features, hemodynamics, and clinical course. The severity of the hemodynamic abnormalities at the time of diagnosis correlated with the clinical course.

2. Johnson RA, Palacios I: Dilated cardiomyopathies of the adult. N Engl J Med 307, 17:1051–1058, 18:1119–1126, 1983.

This is a thoughtful review of the causes of dilated cardiomyopathy with a very complete bibliography.

Hypertrophic Cardiomyopathy

1. Canedo M, Canedo MI, Frank MJ: Therapy of hypertrophic cardiomyopathy: Medical or surgical? Clinical and physiologic considerations. Am J Cardiol 48:383–388, 1981.

This is a good short review of the pathophysiology and therapeutics in hypertrophic cardiomyopathy.

2. Criley JM: The bottom line syndrome—hypertrophic cardiomyopathy revisited. West J Med 130:350–353, 1979.

This is an editorial discussion of the controversy surrounding the clinical importance of a dynamic obstruction to outflow in hypertrophic cardiomyopathy.

3. McKenna W, Deanfield J, Faruqui A: Prognosis in hypertrophic cardiomyopathy: Role of age and clinical, electrocardiographic and hemodynamic features. Am J Cardiol 47:532–538, 1981.

The frequency of supraventricular and ventricular arrhythmias in 30 patients with hypertrophic cardiomyopathy was evaluated during submaximal ETT and 48-hour Holter monitoring in an attempt to discover the causes of sudden death in patients with hypertrophic cardiomyopathy.

Restrictive Cardiomyopathy

1. Benotti J, Grossman W, Cohn PF: Clinical profile of restrictive cardiomyopathy. Circulation 61:1206–1212, 1980.

This study reviews the cases of nine patients with idiopathic restrictive cardiomyopathy and finds a good prognosis during a mean follow-up of 22 months. This is in contrast to the evidence that when restrictive cardiomyopathy is associated with a specific infiltrative process, the prognosis is usually poor.

4

CONGESTIVE HEART FAILURE

By MICKEY EISENBERG, M.D., Ph.D.

DEFINITION

Heart failure is defined as the inability of the heart to pump sufficient blood to meet the metabolic requirements of the body. Since inadequate pumping of the heart invariably results in the clinical picture of systemic or pulmonary venous congestion, the term "congestive heart failure" (CHF) is commonly used.

The term "heart failure" is used to describe a set of clinical signs and symptoms such as cardiac enlargement, peripheral edema, and dyspnea on exertion. Usually heart function is abnormal even at rest. Isolated impairment of exercise tolerance as a result of heart disease is generally not described as heart failure.

Pathophysiologically CHF may be classified in several ways. Each system of classification is a different way of conceptualizing the same underlying pathology. These systems are helpful, not only as descriptive classifications, but in terms of treatment. For example, afterload reduction is useful for symptoms of forward failure but not as primary treatment for evidence of backward failure.

A. **Right-Sided versus Left-Sided Failure.** Division into right- and left-sided failure is useful in characterizing predominant symptoms. However, symptoms commonly overlap because of the intimate relationship of the ventricles within the single cardiovascular system. For example, the most common cause of right heart failure is left heart failure.

B. **Forward Failure versus Backward Failure.** The distinction between forward and backward failure is a useful concept for understanding the pathophysiology. Both forward and backward failure are probably present in chronic CHF. Forward failure implies inadequate cardiac output for maintenance of normal metabolism. Backward failure implies that the heart muscle is so impaired that it cannot pump all the blood that it should, so that fluid gradually "backs up" into the lung. See Figure 4–1.

C. **Acute versus Chronic Heart Failure.** An acute event such as myocardial infarction, massive pulmonary embolism, or serious arrhythmia may lead to sudden onset of CHF. CHF may also develop gradually, most commonly in the face of chronic strain on the heart (for example, with hypertension), and lead to chronic symptoms.

D. **Low-Output versus High-Output Failure.** Most heart failure is of the low-output variety. However, sustained increased cardiac output can lead to failure such as thyrotoxicosis, anemia, or pregnancy.

ETIOLOGY

It is convenient to categorize the origins of CHF by conditions causing decreased myocardial contractility and those leading to excess myocardial workload. The most common causes of CHF are hypertension and coronary artery disease.

A. **Decreased Myocardial Contractility**
   1. Coronary artery disease; ischemia, myocardial infarction
   2. Pericardial tamponade
   3. Ventricular aneurysm
   4. Cardiomyopathy
   5. Infiltrative diseases
      a. Myocarditis
      b. Amyloidosis
      c. Hemochromatosis
      d. Sarcoidosis
   6. Collagen disorders
      a. Rheumatoid disorders
      b. Lupus
      c. Scleroderma

B. **Excess Myocardial Workload**
   1. Increased afterload
      a. Hypertension
      b. Aortic or pulmonary stenosis
      c. Obstructive hypertrophic cardiomyopathy
      d. Chronic obstructive pulmonary disease: cor pulmonale
   2. Increased preload
      a. Mitral and tricuspid valve insufficiency

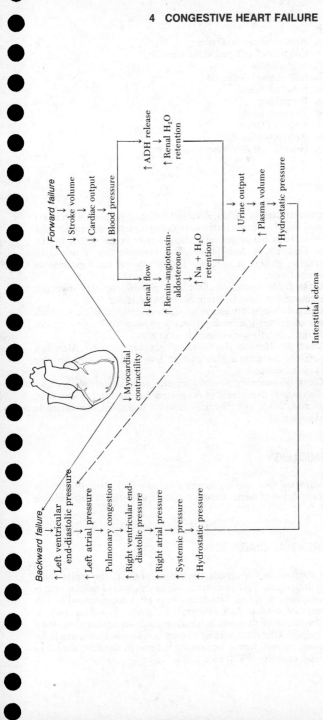

Figure 4–1. Pathophysiology of congestive heart failure. (Reprinted with permission of author and publisher, from Huang SH, Dasher LA, Larson C, et al.: Coronary Care Nursing. Philadelphia, W. B. Saunders Company, 1983, p. 207.)

  b. Aortic valve insufficiency
  c. Congenital left and right shunting
  d. Arrhythmia
3. Increased body demands
  a. Severe anemia
  b. Pregnancy
  c. Thyrotoxicosis
  d. Paget's disease
  e. Arteriovenous fistulas
  f. Nutritional deficiency (beriberi)

SEVERITY

A. Functional Classification. A classification of patients with heart disease based on the relation between symptoms and the amount of effort required to provoke them has been developed by the New York Heart Association. This classification is useful in comparing groups of patients as well as the same patient at different times.
  1. *Class I. No limitation:* Ordinary physical activity does not cause undue fatigue, dyspnea, or palpitation.
  2. *Class II. Slight limitation of physical activity:* Such patients are comfortable at rest. Ordinary physical activity results in fatigue, palpitation, dyspnea, or angina.
  3. *Class III. Marked limitation of physical activity:* Although patients are comfortable at rest, less than ordinary activity leads to symptoms.
  4. *Class IV. Inability to carry on any physical activity without discomfort:* Symptoms of congestive failure are present even at rest. With any physical activity increased discomfort is experienced.

EPIDEMIOLOGY

An estimated four million Americans have CHF. Heart failure is the leading cause of death among hospitalized patients with cardiac disease.

DIFFERENTIAL DIAGNOSIS

Since dyspnea is the cardinal symptom of CHF, the major challenge in diagnosing CHF is distinguishing dyspnea of cardiac origin from pulmonary dyspnea. The difficulty is often compounded by the coexistence of cardiac and pulmonary disease. For situations in which the origin of dyspnea is not clear, pulmonary function tests can be helpful. Obstructive lung disease is diagnosed most easily by a decreased ratio of forced expiratory volume in the first second to forced vital capacity (FEV_1/FVC).

When CHF is considered to be cardiac in origin it is important to identify the precipitating cause.

HISTORY

The history is useful in characterizing the clinical picture, identifying underlying causes, and elucidating precipitating factors.

A. **Characterizing the Clinical Picture.** Answers to the following questions provide useful information regarding the clinical picture:

1. *Is there chest pain, pressure, or discomfort associated with dyspnea?*
2. *Is there dyspnea with exertion or at rest?*
3. *Is there paroxysmal nocturnal dyspnea (PND)?* Are extra pillows or elevation used during sleep? Does the patient sit on the side of the bed to catch his breath? Does the patient need the window open? How long after going to bed does PND develop? (PND is classically said to develop one to two hours after going to bed.)
4. *Is there increased swelling in the ankles or lower legs?*
5. *Is there increased weight gain?*

B. **Underlying Causes.** Often there is a history of underlying cardiovascular disease (myocardial infarction, hypertension, artherosclerotic heart disease, or use of cardiac medications; see under Etiology for other underlying causes).

C. **Precipitating Causes**

1. *Changes in Lifestyle.* Reductions in medication or increased dietary sodium can lead to increased cardiac failure. Alcohol is a cardiac depressant and may exacerbate CHF. Changes in environment such as transition to a hot humid climate can also result in CHF in the presence of underlying heart disease.
2. *Arrhythmias.* Tachyarrhythmia, bradyarrhythmia, and atrioventricular block can all lead to increased CHF.
3. *Pulmonary Embolism.* Patients with underlying CHF have a high risk of developing pulmonary embolism that leads to increased hemodynamic burden on the heart and thus to increased failure.
4. *Infection.* Increased metabolic demands may lead to increased heart failure. Infections of any type—whether systemic, respiratory, genitourinary, related to myocarditis, recurrence of rheumatic fever, or endocarditis—may be responsible.
5. *Iatrogenic.* Use of fluid-retaining drugs (steroids, estrogens, or nonsteroidal anti-inflammatory drugs) or cardiac depressants (beta-blockers, disopyramide, or antineoplastic drugs) can worsen or precipitate CHF.
6. *High-Output States.* Pregnancy, anemia, or thyrotoxicosis alone rarely produces heart failure, but in the presence of underlying heart disease the increased cardiac output can lead to CHF.
7. *Stress (Physical and Emotional).* Prolonged exertion or emotional stress is an identifiable cause of CHF in the presence of underlying heart disease.

SIGNS AND SYMPTOMS

Signs and symptoms of heart failure are multiple because of the intimate relationships of the cardiovascular system to all organ systems. The specific symptoms depend on the ventricle that has failed and the duration of failure. It is important to remember that chronic CHF has elements of right and left failure. Predominant left ventricular failure is manifested with pulmonary congestion. Predominant right ventricular failure is manifested with signs of systemic congestion and peripheral edema.

A. Respiratory Signs and Symptoms
   1. *Dyspnea.* This is a cardinal symptom of left ventricular failure. Although dyspnea is subjective, it may be possible to detect an increased respiratory rate (tachypnea). Patients usually report experiencing dyspnea more rapidly during usual activities or report decreased exercise tolerance from dyspnea on exertion.
   2. *Orthopnea.* Orthopnea is dyspnea that develops in a lying position. Patients may report using extra pillows.
   3. *Paroxysmal Nocturnal Dyspnea (PND).* Usually PND occurs at night and may be considered as exaggerated episodes of orthopnea. Wheezing may accompany PND, giving rise to the term "cardiac asthma." PND is a result of interstitial edema.
   4. *Cough.* This is often an early finding of CHF.
   5. *Pulmonary Edema.* This is the extreme form of pulmonary congestion caused by alveolar edema.
   6. *Hemoptysis.* Severe left ventricular failure can result in rust-colored sputum or pink frothy fluid in pulmonary edema. Frank bloody sputum is not seen.
   7. *Physical Findings.* Depending on the severity of CHF, basilar or diffuse respiratory rales may be heard. Wheezing is not an infrequent finding.

B. Cardiovascular Signs and Symptoms
   1. *Systemic Venous Congestion.* This is a hallmark of right ventricular failure. The following findings may be present:
      a. **Cardiomegaly**
         1). Third heart sound (S3 gallop) occurs early in diastole and is a fairly reliable sign of heart failure in middle-aged or elderly patients. An S3 may be heard normally in children and young adults. Fourth heart sounds (S4 gallop) are also heard but are considered less unique to CHF. With rapid heart rates, S3 and S4 may merge into a "summation gallop."
         2). Pulsus alternans.
         3). Accentuated P_2 (occurs with the development of left ventricular failure and increased pulmonary artery pressure).
         4). Systolic murmurs are common as a result of mild mitral and tricuspid regurgitation as the ventricles dilate.
         5). There may be a precordial heave or thrill.
      b. **Hepatomegaly.** The hepatojugular reflex is usually present.

    c. **Increased Jugular Vein Distension**
    d. **Ankle Edema**
    e. **Weight Gain**
    f. **Ascites**
    g. **Pericardial Effusion**
    h. **Anasarca.** Severe right heart failure can cause excess fluid accumulation everywhere in the body. The face and arms are usually spared because of gravity effects.

C. Central Nervous System Signs and Symptoms
    1. Fatigue, headache, anxiety, and insomnia are common findings.
    2. Severe heart failure is associated with restlessness, irritability, and difficulty in maintaining attention.

D. Renal Signs and Symptoms
    1. Decreased urinary output

E. Gastrointestinal Signs and Symptoms
    1. Right upper quadrant pain, described as an ache or heaviness, occurs secondary to stretching of the hepatic capsule.
    2. Anorexia occurs (nausea, constipation).
    3. Cachexia is seen in severe chronic heart failure.

LABORATORY X-RAY STUDIES

A. Radiographic Findings. Other than the history and physical examination, the chest x-ray is the most important diagnostic test. Findings seen on the chest x-ray are not always synchronous with the clinical findings. There may be a lag of 12 hours for x-ray changes to appear and a delayed resolution of x-ray changes (for up to four days) after clinical improvement of CHF.
    1. *Redistribution of Flow and Venous Congestion.* Blood flow to the lower lung field is reduced, and flow to the upper lung field is increased when the pulmonary capillary wedge pressure is elevated above 18 mm of Hg. Apparent on the chest x-ray is a cephalization of flow that is evidenced as increased vascular markings in the upper portion of the chest x-ray.
    2. *Interstitial Pulmonary Edema.* With increased congestive heart failure fluid accumulates in the interstitial spaces. This may be seen as small lines found in the lower peripheral lung fields and extending to the pleural surface, "Kerley's B lines." Fluid can also accumulate in the lobular septa and may be seen as lines going from the hila outward to the lung parenchyma, "Kerley's A lines." Pulmonary vessels may appear enlarged. Usually pulmonary capillary wedge pressures between 20 and 25 mm Hg are seen in this condition.
    3. *Alveolar Edema.* When pulmonary capillary wedge pressures rise above 25 mm Hg fluid begins to accumulate in the alveolar spaces. This condition is known as pulmonary edema and on chest x-ray appears as a butterfly pattern of bilateral hilar infiltrate.
    4. *Enlarged Cardiac Silhouette.* The cardiac silhouette is often enlarged but may be normal in size (especially with coronary artery disease as the cause of CHF).

B. **ECG.** The cause of CHF may be suggested by various findings. Old myocardial infarction suggests coronary artery disease; left ventricular hypertrophy suggests aortic stenosis or hypertension; persistent ST segment elevation suggests aneurysm; and low limb lead voltage suggests pericardial disease. Low limb lead voltage is a common finding in many cases of CHF, as well as in chronic obstructive pulmonary disease. Pulsus alternans, if present, may be seen on the electrocardiogram.

C. **Echocardiography.** Characteristically a dilated left ventricle is demonstrated. Sometimes ruptured papillary muscles, ventricular hypertrophy, and aortic and mitral valve abnormalities are seen. The echocardiogram is most useful in detecting pericardial effusion. It is also useful in detecting myxomas and hypertrophic cardiomyopathy.

D. **Laboratory.** Electrolytes are usually normal.

E. **Hemodynamic Monitoring.** An early and accurate means of estimating ventricular function is provided by pulmonary artery wedge pressure (PAWP). This parameter is not routinely recommended but should be measured in severely ill patients.

HEMODYNAMIC MONITORING

PAWP	VENTRICULAR FUNCTION
0 to 6 mm Hg	Reduction of circulating volume
6 to 12 mm Hg	Within normal limit
18 to 20 mm Hg	Onset of pulmonary congestion
20 to 25 mm Hg	Moderate pulmonary congestion
25 to 30 mm Hg	Severe pulmonary congestion
>30 mm Hg	Pulmonary edema

Other useful measures are cardiac output and the cardiac index.

RECOMMENDED DIAGNOSTIC APPROACH

History and physical examination plus a chest x-ray and ECG are the essential, initial ingredients in diagnosing CHF. Given the varied presentations and multiple etiologies, it is difficult to recommend a single diagnostic pathway.

REFERENCES

1. Weber KT, Likoff MJ, Janicki JS, et al.: Advances in the evaluation and management of chronic failure. Chest 85:253–259, 1984.
   An up-to-date discussion of heart failure and its management.

2. Rubin SA, Siemienczuk, et al.: Accuracy of cardiac output, oxygen uptake, and arteriovenous oxygen difference at rest, during exercise, and after vasodilated therapy in patients with severe, chronic heart failure. Am J Cardiol 50:973–978, 1982.

A discussion of the exercise physiology and diagnostic tests for diagnosis of heart failure.

3. Goodwin JF: Congestive and hypertrophic cardiomyopathies: A decade of study. Lancet 1:732–739, 1970.

5

COR PULMONALE

By DAVID RALPH, M.D.

DEFINITIONS

Cor pulmonale is defined as cardiac disease caused by dysfunction of the pulmonary system. The cardiac dysfunction results from the effects of pulmonary hypertension on the right ventricle. Although some clinicians restrict the definition of cor pulmonale to situations in which actual right ventricular failure has occurred, it is preferable to also include the earlier states in which the right ventricle is performing adequately but against an increased afterload caused by elevated pulmonary vascular resistance.

The pulmonary dysfunction that causes cor pulmonale can be caused by primary disorders in the pulmonary parenchyma, the pulmonary vasculature, the pleura, the chest wall, the diaphragm and chest muscles, or the respiratory drives. Cor pulmonale may occur acutely or chronically, resulting in right ventricular dilation or dilation with hypertrophy, respectively.

GENERAL COMMENTS AND EPIDEMIOLOGY

A. **Recognition.** At autopsy cor pulmonale accounts for 6 to 7 per cent of adult cardiac disease. Males are most commonly affected, owing to the higher frequency of smoking and chronic obstructive pulmonary disease among males. However, recognition of cor pulmonale is difficult because of the relatively poor sensitivity of clinical, electrocardiographic, and radiographic criteria for its detection. The sensitivity and specificity of echocardiography for detection of cor pulmonale are still under investigation. Invasive catheterization with measurement of pressures in the right heart and pulmonary artery remains the best means to establish the diagnosis. Recognition of cor pulmonale is further complicated by the fact that the symptoms caused by the underlying pulmonary disease are often similar to the symptoms resulting from cor pulmonale. For example, dyspnea and fatigue in a patient with chronic obstructive pulmonary disease may result solely from the ventilation limitation but may also result from superimposed cor pulmonale.

B. **Normal Pulmonary Circulation.** The normal pulmonary circulation is able to accommodate the entire cardiac output at a remarkably low perfusion pressure. The pulmonary vascular resistance may be calculated from the pressure decrement across the circulation divided by the cardiac output:

pulmonary vascular resistance = (mean pulmonary artery pressure − left atrial pressure) ÷ cardiac output

The normal mean pulmonary artery pressure is less than 18 mm Hg. The normal pulmonary vascular resistance is only 10 per cent of the resistance in the systemic circulation. Another remarkable feature of the pulmonary circulation is its ability to continue to operate at low pressures as cardiac output is increased. Even with severe exercise, for example, there is only a mild rise in pulmonary artery pressure because the increased cardiac output is accommodated by opening (recruitment) of previously closed vessels. Recruitment is so effective in modulating pressure that the resting pressure usually does not increase after a pneumonectomy, although the entire cardiac output must be subsequently perfused through one lung.

C. **Mechanisms of Injury.** With simple destruction of lung vasculature the loss of parenchyma must be extensive before pulmonary hypertension supervenes. Although such loss of tissue is one mechanism that may cause pulmonary hypertension, vasospasm is the most common mechanism. Hypoxemia is the most potent stimulus to vasospasm. As the alveolar oxygen partial pressure falls below 60 torr, hypoxic vasoconstriction causes narrowing of small pulmonary arterioles. This response may serve to maintain ventilation-perfusion matching in localized pulmonary processes, but when the hypoxemia is generalized the vasconstriction creates increased resistance and pulmonary hypertension. Acidosis potentiates the vasospasm. Long-term vasoconstriction may lead to the secondary development of muscular hypertrophy, intimal proliferation, and fixed vascular narrowing. In addition to loss of vessels and vasospasm, the other mechanism leading to pulmonary hypertension is obstruction of vessels. With sudden massive obstruction of the majority of the vasculature as a result of acute pulmonary embolism, the normal right ventricle fails, since it cannot generate a pressure over 40 to 50 mm Hg acutely. In contrast, when the pulmonary hypertension occurs progressively over a longer period, the right ventricle may be able to hypertrophy and eventually generate systemic-level pressures before failure supervenes.

DIFFERENTIAL DIAGNOSIS

When right ventricular overload or failure is suspected, the first step is to decide whether the dyfunction is caused by pulmonary or nonpulmonary disorders. The most common cause of pulmonary

TABLE 5–1. MAJOR CAUSES OF
RIGHT VENTRICULAR FAILURE

Left ventricular failure
Mitral valve disease
Constrictive pericarditis
Right ventricular infarction
Cor pulmonale

hypertension and right heart failure is left ventricular myocardial disease with passive transmission of high pressures into the pulmonary circulation. Cardiac valvular disease, left-to-right intracardiac shunts, and primary right ventricular infarction are other causes of right ventricular dysfunction. Diagnosis of these disorders can usually be suspected on the basis of history, physical examination, electrocardiogram (ECG), and radiographic studies. See Table 5–1.

The predominant disorder causing cor pulmonale is chronic obstructive pulmonary disease (chronic bronchitis and emphysema). Chronic obstructive pulmonary disease is the cause of 80 per cent of cor pulmonale in this country. The major mechanism causing pulmonary hypertension in these patients is hypoxemia related to ventilation-perfusion mismatching. Hypoxemia is also the cause of the cor pulmonale that is occasionally observed in other disorders of airflow obstruction (cystic fibrosis, asthma, or bronchiolitis obliterans). Hypoxemia from residence at high altitudes by normal persons may also result in cor pulmonale. Vasospasm from hypoxemia is the basis of pulmonary hypertension and cor pulmonale in the occasional patient who has severe neuromuscular weakness (such as from poliomyelitis or Guillian-Barré syndrome), blunted respiratory drives (primary hypoventilation), upper airway obstruction (tumors, tracheal stenosis, sleep apnea), or chest wall immobility (obesity, kyphoscoliosis). Destruction of vasculature may contribute to exercise-related pulmonary hypertension in emphysema and is the primay cause of cor pulmonale in patients who have pulmonary hypertension caused by a severe restrictive primary pulmonary disorder. The vascular destruction may be related to disorders that destroy the alveoli and interstitium as well as the vessels (sarcoidosis, fibrosing alveolitis, hypersensitivity pneumonitis, pneumoconiosis, or collagen-vascular diseases) or to disorders that primarily involve the vessels only (primary pulmonary hypertension or pulmonary arteritis). See Table 5–2.

HISTORY

A. **Dyspnea.** At first dyspnea appears only on exertion and later at rest as the disease progresses.
B. **Fatigue.** Dyspnea and fatigue, although almost invariably present in cor pulmonale, are not specific, since these symptoms are found in a large number of other cardiac, pulmonary, and metabolic disorders.

TABLE 5–2. CAUSES OF COR PULMONALE

Disorders of reduced airflow (obstructive)
1. Chronic obstructive pulmonary disease (common if hypoxic)
2. Cystic fibrosis (common in the late stage)
3. Asthma, bronchiolitis obliterans (unusual)

Restrictive pulmonary disorders
1. Infiltrative disorders (uncommon): sarcoidosis, collagen-vascular disorders, fibrosing alveolitis, widespread infections
2. Neuromyopathic disorders: polio, myasthenia gravis (rare)
3. Chest wall restriction: kyphoscoliosis (usually only if greater than 100-degree angulation)

Pulmonary vascular disorders
1. Pulmonary embolism
2. Primary pulmonary hypertension
3. Miscellaneous disorders (schistosomiasis, sickle cell disease, intravenous drug abuse)

Disorders of respiratory drives
1. Obesity-hypoventilation syndrome (unusual)
2. Primary hypoventilation (rare)

Obstructive sleep apnea syndrome (only if severe)

C. Other. Other associated conditions include cough, wheezing, sputum production, hemoptysis, and chest pain. The occurrence of these other symptoms depends entirely on the underlying disorder responsible for causing cor pulmonale.

SIGNS AND SYMPTOMS

A. Cardiac. Cardiac signs and symptoms include right ventricular lift, palpable P2 (these signs occur before the onset of failure), elevated neck veins, S3 gallop, murmur of tricuspid insufficiency, edema, and hepatomegaly or hepatojugular reflux (these signs are more common when right ventricular failure supervenes).
B. Extracardiac. Extracardiac signs and symptoms include cyanosis (if hypoxemia is severe), clubbing (with some interstitial lung disorders), increased chest diameter (obstructive airflow diseases), wheezing (obstructive diseases), and crackles (restrictive and obstructive disorders).
  The frequency of cardiac signs in cor pulmonale depends on the etiology of the cor pulmonale. In the presence of chronic obstructive pulmonary disease the cardiac signs are often obscured because of the hyperexpansion of the lungs, which softens the heart sounds and cardiac pulsations. The frequency of the extracardiac findings depends in turn on the disease process causing the cor pulmonale.

DIAGNOSTIC STUDIES

A. Electrocardiogram (ECG). The electrocardiogram shows right ventricular enlargement (dominant R in V_1, associated T wave inversion over right precordium, and right axis deviation) and P-pulmonale.

As with the physical signs, the electrocardiographic signs of right ventricular hypertrophy and P-pulmonale may be difficult to read in the presence of chronic obstructive pulmonary disease because of the associated changes in cardiac axis configuration.

B. **Chest Radiography.** Chest radiograms show right ventricular enlargement, enlargement of the right ventricular outflow tract (these signs are best seen on lateral radiographs), enlargement of central pulmonary arteries (right > 16 mm, left > 18 mm), and attenuation of peripheral branches.

These signs are rather sensitive when present, but false-positive findings also occur; 30 to 40 per cent of patients with chronic obstructive pulmonary disease have some degree of right ventricular hypertrophy at autopsy, whereas the radiographic diagnosis is often not certain in these cases.

C. **Laboratory Findings.** Laboratory findings include hemoglobin evaluation (elevation may reflect chronic hypoxemia; also, hematocrit > 55 is associated with increased blood viscosity, which increases right ventricular work) and serologic studies. Antinuclear antibodies may be examined if collagen vascular disorder is suspected.

D. **Ventilation-Perfusion Lung Scan.** This is essential if pulmonary embolism is suspected.

E. **Echocardiography.** Unfortunately, the right ventricular free wall thickness and the volume of the right ventricle cannot be assessed accurately by echocardiography because of the orientation and complex anatomy of the ventricle and because of the position of the right ventricle under the echogenic sternum. Instead the best signs suggesting cor pulmonale are those that detect effects of pulmonary hypertension. Early systolic closure of the pulmonic valve and retrograde pulmonary artery systolic flow during contrast echocardiography are specific but not sensitive signs of pulmonary hypertension. Echocardiography can nicely evaluate the left atrium for signs of mitral valvular disease or atrial myxoma.

F. **Radionuclide Angiography.** First-pass and equilibrium ventriculography yield estimations of the right ventricular ejection fraction. The accuracy of the first-pass technique is limited by the low number of counts obtained, and thus it is best performed with a multicrystal camera. Equilibrium techniques collect more counts but suffer from interference from counts in the right atrium. Many recent studies have shown that either an ejection fraction of less than 40 to 45 per cent or a decrease in ejection fraction or failure of a normal ejection fraction to rise more than 5 per cent during exercise is predictive of pulmonary hypertension in patients with chronic obstructive pulmonary disease. There is good correlation between pulmonary artery pressures and ejection fraction in groups of patients with chronic obstructive pulmonary disease, but the scatter in the data make a single borderline result difficult to interpret in the individual case.

G. **Right Heart Catheterization.** This procedure is the most accurate means to diagnose cor pulmonale. In addition to providing measurement of the cardiac output, right ventricular pressure, and pulmonary artery pressure, other data that can exclude left ventricular or mitral valve disease (pulmonary artery wedge pressure and trace contour) and that can exclude left-to-right shunts (step-up in oxygen saturation) can be obtained. If indicated, pulmonary arteriography can also be performed. Furthermore, the response of the pulmonary pressure, cardiac output, and vascular resistance to administration of oxygen or vasodilating medications can be assessed.

RECOMMENDED DIAGNOSTIC APPROACH

A. Clinical suspicion is critical to the diagnosis of cor pulmonale at an early stage. The diagnosis of cor pulmonale is considered in the presence of the pulmonary disorders that are frequently complicated by this process.

B. The history is noted for symptoms of pulmonary dysfunction, including the severity of dyspnea (how much exertion is required to cause dyspnea). Since the primary therapy of these disorders includes removal of inciting factors, it is essential to explore the smoking history, history of exposure to allergens or environmental irritants, and history of high-altitude residence.

C. The signs of cor pulmonale should be sought from physical examination.

D. An ECG should be examined next with the knowledge that the signs are specific but not sensitive for cor pulmonale.

E. The chest radiograph should be examined with the knowledge that the signs are neither fully specific nor sensitive.

F. Since signs of cardiac dysfunction are insensitive, a blood gas determination should be obtained for every patient with significant pulmonary disease. If hypoxemia is discovered it must either be reversed by treatment of the underlying disorder or by the administration of supplemental oxygen to attain an arterial Po_2 greater than 55–60 mm Hg to relieve hypoxic vasoconstriction.

G. Pulmonary function testing quantitates the degree of obstruction or restriction. The degree of disease revealed by pulmonary function testing yields an excellent guide to the necessity for further testing, since cor pulmonale usually only complicates disorders that severely limit lung volumes or airflow rates (primary hypoventilation and thromboembolism are important exceptions to this statement).

H. Ventilation-perfusion lung scanning is indicated if thromboembolism is suspected.

I. Examination of the findings obtained by these means generally leads to a diagnosis of the underlying pulmonary disorder and an estimation of its severity. The primary treatment of cor pulmonale is removal of the factors that lead to pulmonary hypertension and excessive afterload rather than inotropic treatment of the right ventricle itself. Accordingly, the underlying disease should first be treated and hypoxemia reversed before invasive catheterization is performed (unless there is still a need to rule out the nonpulmonary causes of pulmonary hypertension discussed earlier). The value of echocardiography or radionuclide angiography depends in large part on the patient's body habitus and on the available equipment and experience of the examiner. Catheterization should be used if the diagnosis remains unclear, if pulmonary arteriography is indicated, or if suspicion of cor pulmonale remains after treatment of hypoxemia. Since the indications for pulmonary vasodilating drugs are still not established and a number of patients have adverse hemodynamic reactions or no benefit with these drugs, it is important to carefully evaluate their hemodynamic effects with catheterization.

REFERENCES

1. Fishman AP: Disorders of pulmonary circulation. Chap. 68–75. *In* AP Fishman (ed.): Pulmonary Diseases and Disorders. New York, McGraw-Hill, 1980.

A textbook discussion of the pathophysiology, etiology, and diagnosis of pulmonary hypertension and cor pulmonale.

2. Harris P, Heath D (eds.): The Human Pulmonary Circulation. London, Churchill Livingstone, 1977.

A superb description of the anatomy, structural and functional relationships, and physiology of the normal and diseased pulmonary circulation.

3. Ross JC: Chronic cor pulmonale. Chap. 53. *In* Hurst JW (ed.): The Heart. New York, McGraw-Hill, 1982.

A brief summary of diagnosis and treatment.

4. Berger HA, Matthay RA: Noninvasive radiographic assessment of cardiovascular function in acute and chronic respiratory failure. Am J Cardiol 47:950–962, 1981.

An extensively referenced review of the value of chest radiography, radionuclide heart imaging, and echocardiography in the assessment of pulmonary hypertension and right heart function.

5. Matthay RA, Harvey J, Berger MD, et al.: Cardiovascular function in cor pulmonale. Clin Chest Med 4:269–295, 1983.

An up-to-date summary.

6

ELECTROCARDIOGRAPHIC DIAGNOSIS

By MICKEY EISENBERG, M.D., Ph.D.

The format followed in this chapter differs from that of other chapters. Instead of a narrative discussion, descriptive characteristics and diagnostic criteria are presented for various clinical conditions in which an electrocardiogram is used. The conditions include normal criteria, arrhythmias, myocardial hypertrophy, myocardial damage, and electrolyte endocrine and drug effects.

NORMAL CRITERIA

A. **PR Interval.** The normal PR interval is 0.12 to 0.20 seconds.
B. **QRS Interval.** The normal QRS interval is less than 0.10 seconds.
C. **QT Interval.** The QT interval is measured from the beginning of the QRS complex to the return of the T wave to baseline. The faster the heart rate, the shorter is the QT interval. The relationship of QT interval to heart rate is determined by the following formula

$$QT \text{ corrected} = QT \text{ measured} \div \sqrt{PR \text{ interval.}}$$

The QT corrected is normally 0.42 seconds. It is easier to consult tables to determine whether the QT interval is prolonged (see later discussion). Another simple rule is to remember that the QT interval should normally be 40 per cent of the measured RR interval. Generally QT intervals are 10 per cent longer in females compared with males. Normally QT intervals for heart rates of 60 to 100 are 0.31 to 0.44 seconds.

QT INTERVALS AND UPPER LIMITS OF NORMAL

	MAXIMUM QT INTERVAL (seconds)	
HEART RATE	Men	Women
40	.49	.53
50	.44	.48
55	.42	.46
60	.40	.44
65	.38	.42
70	.37	.40
75	.36	.39
80	.35	.38
85	.34	.37
90	.33	.36
95	.32	.35
100	.31	.34
110	.30	.33
120	.29	.32
130	.28	.31
150	.26	.29
200	.23	.25

D. **Electrical Axis**
   1. **Normal Axis.** This is −30 to +105 degrees (some cardiologists consider −30 to +90 degrees to be the range of normal).

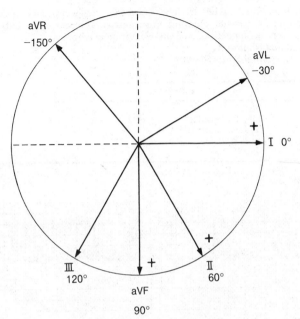

Figure 6–1. Electrocardiographic axes.

    2. *Right Axis Deviation.* This is $\geq$ +105 degrees (commonly seen in cor pulmonale or COPD).
    3. *Left Axis Deviation.* This is $\geq$ −30 degrees (commonly seen in hypertension or aortic stenosis).
Determination of axes can be achieved easily using standard leads (see Fig. 6–1).
E. R Wave Progression. The R wave increases in size from V_1 to V_6 (R wave progression). The R and S waves are normally of equal size in V_3 or V_4. The lead at which the R wave becomes equal to or greater than the S wave is known as the transition zone.

ARRHYTHMIAS

    Diagnosing cardiac rhythm disturbances is important for several reasons: the rhythm may suggest a clinical diagnosis, may require immediate therapy, or may be an indicator of future deterioration. Arrhythmias are commonly classified according to anatomic location of impulse formation (supraventricular or ventricular) and rate (normal, bradycardiac, or tachycardiac). Disturbances in conduction can occur anywhere along the conduction system. This section uses an anatomic classification to categorize rhythm disturbances as sinus rhythms, atrial rhythms, junctional (atrioventricular nodal) rhythms, ventricular rhythms, atrioventricular blocks, intraventricular conduction defects, and pre-excitation syndromes.

A. Sinus Rhythms

1. Normal Sinus Rhythm

DIAGNOSTIC CRITERIA	CAUSES
Rate: 60–100/minute Rhythm: regular P waves: upright in I, II, aVF P:QRS: 1:1	Normal

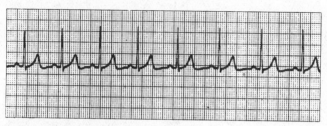

Figure 6–2. Normal sinus rhythm. (Reprinted with permission of publisher, from American Heart Association: Advanced Cardiac Life Support Manual. 1981, pp. VI–6.)

2. Sinus Tachycardia

DIAGNOSTIC CRITERIA	CAUSES
Rate: greater than 100/minute generally less than 160/minute Rhythm: regular P waves: upright in I, II, aVF P:QRS: 1:1	A physiologic response to the need for increased cardiac output, such as in fever, exercise, anxiety, or hypovolemia

3. Sinus Bradycardia

DIAGNOSTIC CRITERIA	CAUSES
Rate: less than 60/minute Rhythm: regular P waves: upright in I, II, aVF P:QRS: 1:1	May be physiologic, as in a well-trained athlete, or secondary to drugs (propranolol) or to sinus node diseases

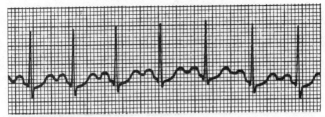

Figure 6–3. Sinus tachycardia. (Reprinted with permission of author and publisher, from Huang SH, Dasher LA, Larson C, et al.: Coronary Care Nursing. Philadelphia, W. B. Saunders Company, 1983, p. 145.)

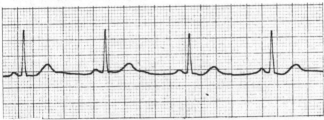

Figure 6–4. Sinus bradycardia. (Reprinted with permission of author and publisher, from Eisenberg M, Copass M: Emergency Medical Therapy. 2nd ed. Philadelphia, W. B. Saunders Company, 1982, p. 5.)

4. Sinus Arrhythmia

DIAGNOSTIC CRITERIA	CAUSES
Rate: a rate of 60–100 is associated with respirations; the rate speeds up during inspiration and slows during exhalation. Rhythm: regular P wave: upright in I, II, aVF P:QRS: 1:1	Normal

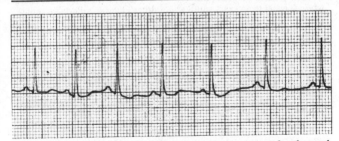

Figure 6–5. Sinus arrhythmia. (Reprinted with permission of author and publisher, from Huang SH, Dasher LA, Larson C, et al.: Coronary Care Nursing. Philadelphia, W. B. Saunders Company, 1983, p. 144.)

5. *Sinus Block.* Sinus block (also called *sinoatrial block*) is classified as first-, second-, or third-degree block.

a. First-Degree Sinus Block. This is characterized by a delay in conduction between sinus node discharge and depolarization of the atria. It is not recognizable in routine electrocardiograms (ECGs).

b. Second-Degree Sinus Block. Two varieties exist:

1). *Type I Sinus Block (Sinus Wenckebach)*

DIAGNOSTIC CRITERIA	CAUSES
Rate: 60–100 Rhythm: regularly irregular; there is a progressive shortening of the sinus cycle followed by a pause. P wave: longest PP interval is less than twice the shortest.	Increase in vagal tone; coronary artery disease involving sinus node; drugs (digoxin, salicylates, quinidine)

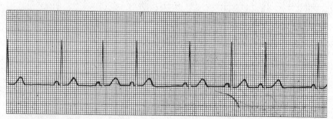

Figure 6–6. Sinus Wenckebach. (Reprinted with permission of author and publisher, from Huang SH, Dasher LA, Larson C, et al.: Coronary Care Nursing. Philadelphia, W. B. Saunders Company, 1983 p. 148.)

2). *Type II Sinus Block*

DIAGNOSTIC CRITERIA	CAUSES
Rate: 60–100 Rhythm: regularly irregular; the pause is equal to an exact multiple of the cycle length (usually 2:1, but may be 3:1, 4:1, etc.).	Increase in vagal tone; coronary artery disease involving sinus node; drugs (digoxin, salicylates, quinidine)

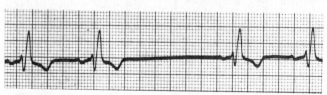

Figure 6–7. Sinus exit block, Type II. (Reprinted with permission of publisher, from Phillips RE, Feeney MK: The Cardiac Rhythms. 2nd ed. Philadelphia, W. B. Saunders Company, 1980, p. 94.)

3). Third-Degree Sinus Block (Sinus Arrest)

DIAGNOSTIC CRITERIA	CAUSES

Rate: 60–100
Rhythm: irregular owing to a pause
P wave: upright in I, II, aVF
P:QRS: 1:1
  If the sinus arrest is long enough,
  escape beats originating in the
  atrioventricular node are likely
  to occur.
	Coronary artery disease involving
	sinus node, increased vagal
	stimulus, inflammatory heart
	disease, or drugs (digitalis,
	quinidine, salicylates)

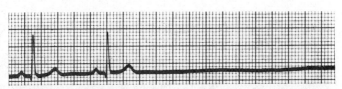

Figure 6–8. Third-degree sinus block. (Reprinted with permission of publisher, from Phillips RE, Feeney MK: The Cardiac Rhythms. 2nd ed. Philadelphia, W. B. Saunders Company, 1980, p. 84.)

6. Sick Sinus Syndrome (Bradycardia-Tachycardia Syndromes)

DIAGNOSTIC CRITERIA	CAUSES
Rate: variable Rhythm: irregularly irregular; often there is a combination of rhythms, including sinus brady- cardia, sinus tachycardia, sinus arrest, atrial fibrillation, atrial flutter, and nodal or ventricular escape beats. P waves: upright in I, II, aVF P:QRS: variable depending on rhythm	Coronary artery disease, degenera- tive fibrosis, inflammatory heart disease

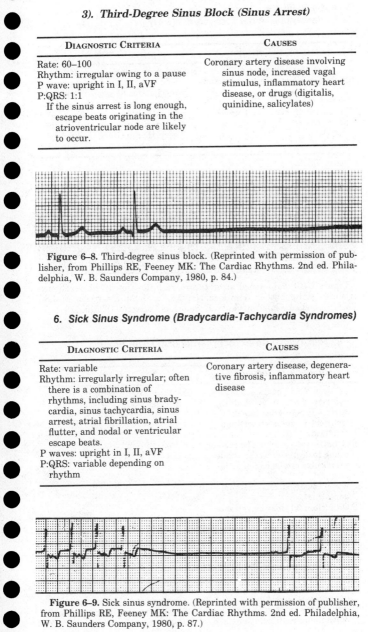

Figure 6–9. Sick sinus syndrome. (Reprinted with permission of publisher, from Phillips RE, Feeney MK: The Cardiac Rhythms. 2nd ed. Philadelphia, W. B. Saunders Company, 1980, p. 87.)

B. Atrial Rhythms

7. Paroxysmal Atrial Tachycardia (PAT)

DIAGNOSTIC CRITERIA	CAUSES
Rate: 150–250 Rhythm: regular; usually starts and stops abruptly P wave: upright in I, II, aVF; may be buried in preceding T wave P:QRS: 1:1	Often seen in individuals with no evidence of heart disease; may be precipitated by sympathetic nervous system stimulation, emotion, fatigue, caffeine, or alcohol; less common causes are cardiac surgery, thyrotoxicosis, and pulmonary embolus

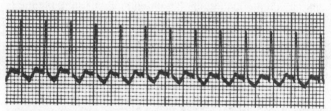

Figure 6–10. Paroxysmal atrial tachycardia. (Reprinted with permission of author and publisher, from Eisenberg M, Copass M: Emergency Medical Therapy. 2nd ed. Philadelphia, W. B. Saunders Company, 1982, p. 11.)

8. Paroxysmal Atrial Tachycardia (PAT) with Block

DIAGNOSTIC CRITERIA	CAUSES
Rate: variable depending on degree of atrioventricular block; atrial rhythm is regular at 150–250; ventricular rate is slower than atrial rate. Rhythm: may or may not be regular owing to degree of block; usually ventricular rate is half of atrial rate. P wave: usually small, abnormal-appearing P:QRS: often 2:1, may be variable	Digitalis toxicity, coronary artery disease

9. Atrial Flutter

DIAGNOSTIC CRITERIA	CAUSES
Rate: variable depending on degree of atrioventricular block Rhythm: atrial is regular at > 300/minute; ventricular rate and	Coronary artery disease, mitral valve disease, pulmonary embolism, hyperthyroidism, after cardiac surgery

rhythm rate may or may not be regular owing to degree of block.

P wave: flutter waves, commonly described as saw-tooth pattern

P:QRS: usually 2 or more P flutter waves to 1 QRS; commonly 2:1, 3:1 or 4:1 but can be variable

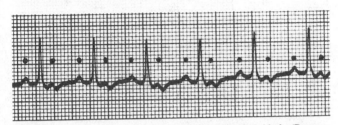

Figure 6–11. Paroxysmal atrial tachycardia (PAT) with block. (P waves are indicated by a dot.) (Reprinted with permission of author and publisher, from Eisenberg M, Copass M: Emergency Medical Therapy. 2nd ed. Philadelphia, W. B. Saunders Company, 1982, p. 13.)

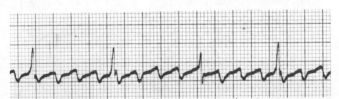

Figure 6–12. Atrial flutter. (Reprinted with permission of author and publisher, from Eisenberg M, Copass M: Emergency Medical Therapy. 2nd ed. Philadelphia, W. B. Saunders Company, 1982, p. 10.)

10. Atrial Fibrillation

Diagnostic Criteria	Causes
Rate: variable; atria are contracting at rate > 350, but only a fraction of the signals fire the atrioventricular node; atrial fibrillation is considered fast if the ventricular rate is > 100/minute and slow if ventricular rate is less than 60. P wave: no discernible P wave; usually there is an irregular undulating baseline. P:QRS: QRS complexes occur at irregularly irregular intervals.	Congestive heart failure, thyrotoxicosis, mitral stenosis, pulmonary embolus, after cardiac surgery, coronary artery disease, cor pulmonale, restrictive pericarditis

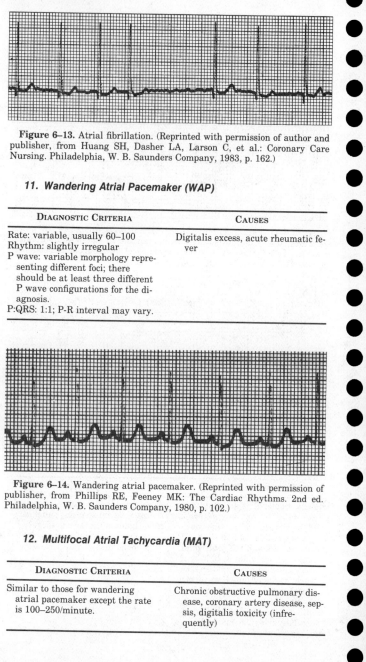

Figure 6–13. Atrial fibrillation. (Reprinted with permission of author and publisher, from Huang SH, Dasher LA, Larson C, et al.: Coronary Care Nursing. Philadelphia, W. B. Saunders Company, 1983, p. 162.)

11. Wandering Atrial Pacemaker (WAP)

DIAGNOSTIC CRITERIA	CAUSES
Rate: variable, usually 60–100 Rhythm: slightly irregular P wave: variable morphology representing different foci; there should be at least three different P wave configurations for the diagnosis. P:QRS: 1:1; P-R interval may vary.	Digitalis excess, acute rheumatic fever

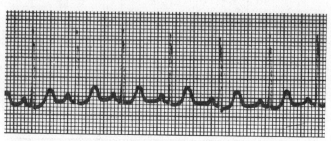

Figure 6–14. Wandering atrial pacemaker. (Reprinted with permission of publisher, from Phillips RE, Feeney MK: The Cardiac Rhythms. 2nd ed. Philadelphia, W. B. Saunders Company, 1980, p. 102.)

12. Multifocal Atrial Tachycardia (MAT)

DIAGNOSTIC CRITERIA	CAUSES
Similar to those for wandering atrial pacemaker except the rate is 100–250/minute.	Chronic obstructive pulmonary disease, coronary artery disease, sepsis, digitalis toxicity (infrequently)

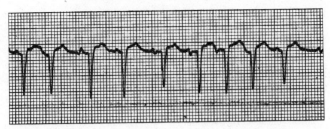

Figure 6–15. Multifocal atrial tachycardia. (Reprinted with permission of author and publisher, from Huang SH, Dasher LA, Larson C, et al.: Coronary Care Nursing. Philadelphia, W. B. Saunders Company, 1983, p. 156.)

13. Premature Atrial Contraction (PAC)

DIAGNOSTIC CRITERIA	CAUSES
Rate: variable depending on amount of PAC Rhythm: irregular; PACs are followed by incomplete compensatory pause. P wave: P wave of PAC typically has a different configuration. P:QRS: 1:1 P wave of PAC may be buried in preceding T wave.	May be seen normally; cardiac stimulants

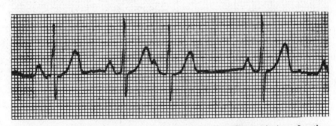

Figure 6–16. Atrial premature beat. (Reprinted with permission of author and publisher, from Huang SH, Dasher LA, Larson C, et al.: Coronary Care Nursing. Philadelphia, W. B. Saunders Company, 1983, p. 153.)

C. Junctional Rhythms (Atrioventricular Nodal Rhythms)
14. Junctional Rhythm (Nodal Rhythm Junctional or Nodal Escape Beats).
Junctional rhythms are usually classified as upper (atrionodal), middle (nodal), or lower (nodal His) as a means to express the relationship of the P wave to the QRS complex.

DIAGNOSTIC CRITERIA	CAUSES
Rate: 40–60 Rhythm: regular P wave: when seen, it is abnormal in configuration and inverted in II, III, and aVF. P:QRS: 1:1, when seen, P wave precedes QRS in upper junctional rhythms; P wave is not seen in middle junctional rhythms, and P wave follows QRS in lower junctional rhythms.	Suppression of the sinoatrial node as may occur in coronary artery disease, digitalis excess, carotid sinus disease, or inflammatory heart disease

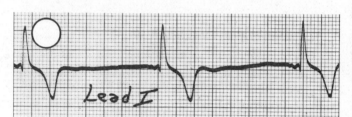

Figure 6–17. Upper junctional rhythm. (Reprinted with permission of publisher, from Phillips RE, Feeney MK: The Cardiac Rhythms. 2nd ed. Philadelphia, W. B. Saunders Company, 1980, p. 209.)

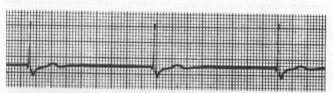

Figure 6–18. Middle junctional rhythm. (Reprinted with permission of publisher, from Phillips RE, Feeney MK: The Cardiac Rhythms. 2nd ed. Philadelphia, W. B. Saunders Company, 1980, p. 209.)

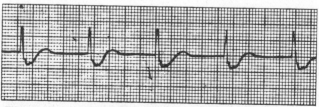

Figure 6–19. Lower junctional rhythm. (Reprinted with permission of publisher, from Phillips RE, Feeney MK: The Cardiac Rhythms. 2nd ed. Philadelphia, W. B. Saunders Company, 1980, p. 209.)

15. Premature Junctional Contraction (PJC) (Premature Nodal Contraction) (PNC)

DIAGNOSTIC CRITERIA	CAUSES
Rate: variable depending on frequency of PJC Rhythm: irregular P wave: when associated with PJC it is abnormal in configuration and may precede or follow PJC. P:QRS: as in junctional rhythm	Coronary artery disease, digitalis excess

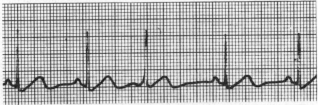

Figure 6–20. Junctional premature beat. (Reprinted with permission of publisher, from Phillips RE, Feeney MK: The Cardiac Rhythms. 2nd ed. Philadelphia, W. B. Saunders Company, 1980, p. 219.)

D. Ventricular Rhythms
16. Premature Ventricular Contraction (PVC)

DIAGNOSTIC CRITERIA	CAUSES
Rate: variable depending on frequency of PVCs Rhythm: irregular P wave: no p wave association with PVC P:QRS: none QRS: > .11 seconds; PVCs may be unifocal, multifocal, and may be isolated or occur in a fixed relationship to the normal QRS.	Coronary artery disease, myocardial infarction, hypoxia, acidosis, hypokalemia, stimulant drugs

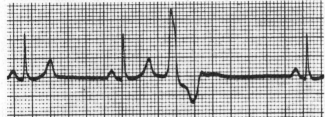

Figure 6–21. Premature ventricular contraction. (Reprinted with permission of author and publisher, from Eisenberg M, Copass M: Emergency Medical Therapy. 2nd ed. Philadelphia, W. B. Saunders Company, 1982, p. 17.)

17. *Ventricular Tachycardia (VT).* VT is defined as three or more PVCs at a rate of > 100 per minute.

Diagnostic Criteria	Causes
Rhythm: sightly irregular P wave: may be noted as atria continue to discharge P:QRS: no relationship QRS: > .11 seconds	Myocardial infarction, coronary artery disease, hypoxia, acidosis

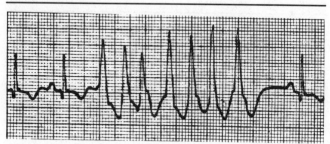

Figure 6–22. Ventricular tachycardia. (Reprinted with permission of author and publisher, from Huang SH, Dasher LA, Larson C, et al.: Coronary Care Nursing. Philadelphia, W. B. Saunders Company, 1983, p. 177.)

18. *Ventricular Flutter*

Diagnostic Criteria	Causes
Rate: 150–300 Rhythm: regular P wave: none P:QRS: none QRS: no distinct QRS complexes; rhythm is a transitional stage between ventricular tachycardia and ventricular fibrillation.	Same as for ventricular tachycardia

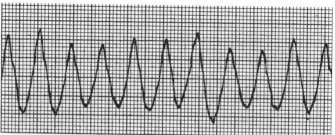

Figure 6–23. Ventricular flutter. (Reprinted with permission of author and publisher, from Huang SH, Dasher LA, Larson C, et al.: Coronary Care Nursing. Philadelphia, W. B. Saunders Company, 1983, p. 179.)

19. Ventricular Fibrillation (VF)

DIAGNOSTIC CRITERIA	CAUSES
Irregular undulations of different shapes No distinct QRS complexes VF may be coarse or fine.	Same as for ventricular tachycardia

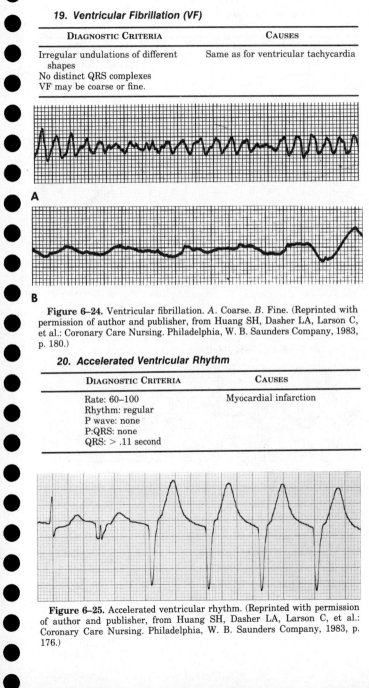

Figure 6–24. Ventricular fibrillation. *A.* Coarse. *B.* Fine. (Reprinted with permission of author and publisher, from Huang SH, Dasher LA, Larson C, et al.: Coronary Care Nursing. Philadelphia, W. B. Saunders Company, 1983, p. 180.)

20. Accelerated Ventricular Rhythm

DIAGNOSTIC CRITERIA	CAUSES
Rate: 60–100 Rhythm: regular P wave: none P:QRS: none QRS: > .11 second	Myocardial infarction

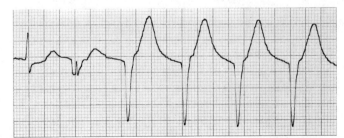

Figure 6–25. Accelerated ventricular rhythm. (Reprinted with permission of author and publisher, from Huang SH, Dasher LA, Larson C, et al.: Coronary Care Nursing. Philadelphia, W. B. Saunders Company, 1983, p. 176.)

21. Idioventricular Rhythm

Diagnostic Criteria	Causes
Rate: 20–40 Rhythm: regular P wave: usually not present P:QRS: no relationship QRS: > .11 second wide, bizarre-appearing	Myocardial infarction, hypoxia, acidosis

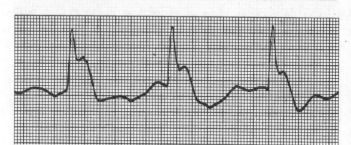

Figure 6–26. Idioventricular rhythm. (Reprinted with permission of author and publisher, from Huang SH, Dasher LA, Larson C, et al.: Coronary Care Nursing. Philadelphia, W. B. Saunders Company, 1983, p. 169.)

22. **Agonal Rhythm.** The rate is very slow with wide irregular slurred QRS complexes. It represents the last remnants of electrical activity in a dying heart.

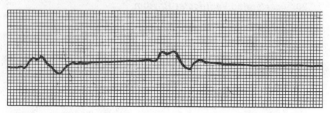

Figure 6–27. Agonal rhythm. (Reprinted with permission of author and publisher, from Huang SH, Dasher LA, Larson C, et al.: Coronary Care Nursing. Philadelphia, W. B. Saunders Company, 1983, p. 182.)

E. Atrioventricular Block
23. First-Degree Atrioventricular Block

Diagnostic Criteria	Causes
Rate: 60–100 Rhythm: regular P wave: normal P:QRS: 1:1; PR interval is > .20 second.	Coronary artery disease, digoxin, rheumatic fever, congenital conditions

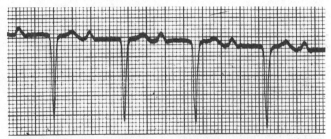

Figure 6–28. First-degree atrioventricular block. (Reprinted with permission of author and publisher, from Eisenberg M, Copass M: Emergency Medical Therapy. 2nd ed. Philadelphia, W. B. Saunders Company, 1982, p. 15.)

24. Second-Degree Atrioventricular Block, Mobitz Type I (Wenckebach)

DIAGNOSTIC CRITERIA	CAUSES
Rate: atrial rate is greater than ventricular rate. Rhythm: atrial rhythm is regular; ventricular rhythm is irregular. P wave: normal P:QRS: PR interval becomes progressively lengthened until a QRS is dropped; RR interval becomes progressively shorter until a QRS is dropped; PP interval remains constant.	Myocardial infarction, rheumatic fever, digitalis toxicity

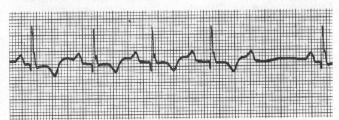

Figure 6–29. Second-degree atrioventricular block, Mobitz Type I. (Reprinted with permission of author and publisher, from Huang SH, Dasher LA, Larson C, et al.: Coronary Care Nursing. Philadelphia, W. B. Saunders Company, 1983, p. 185.)

25. Second-Degree Atrioventricular Block, Mobitz Type II

DIAGNOSTIC CRITERIA	CAUSES
Rate: atrial rate is greater than ventricular rate. Rhythm: atrial rate is regular; ventricular rate may be regular or irregular.	Myocardial infarction, digitalis toxicity

P wave: normal; PR interval is normal, and QRS usually shows bundle branch block.

P:QRS: ratio may be 2:1, 3:1, 4:1, or 3:2; ratio may vary over time; ratios of 2:1 are difficult to distinquish from Mobitz Type I; if in doubt, treat as Type II.

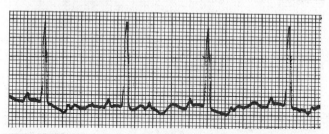

Figure 6–30. Second-degree atrioventricular block, Mobitz Type II. (Reprinted with permission of author and publisher, from Eisenberg M, Copass M: Emergency Medical Therapy. 2nd ed. Philadelphia, W. B. Saunders Company, 1982, p. 186.)

26. Third-Degree Atrioventricular Block, Complete Heart Block

DIAGNOSTIC CRITERIA	CAUSES
Rate: atrial rate is greater than ventricular rate. Rhythm: atrial rate is 60–100; ventricular rate is 40–60 if junctional escape beats occur; ventricular rate is 20–40 if ventricular escape beats occur. P wave: normal P:QRS: no relationship; atria and ventricles are independently contracting. QRS: normal if junction escape beats occur; > .11 second if ventricular escape beats occur.	Coronary heart disease, myocardial infarction, myocarditis, drug toxicity (digitalis, procainamide, quinidine, verapamil)

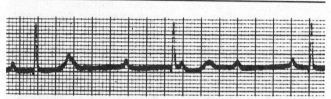

Figure 6–31. Complete heart block. (Reprinted with permission of author and publisher, from Eisenberg M, Copass M: Emergency Medical Therapy. 2nd ed. Philadelphia, W. B. Saunders Company, 1982, p. 16.)

F. Intraventricular Conduction Defects. In all intraventricular conduction defects the rate and rhythm are those of the underlying rhythm. P waves and P:QRS ratio are dependent on the underlying rhythm, for example, sinus versus atrial fibrillation. The QRS is invariably wider than normal because of the alteration in normal conduction.

27. Right Bundle Branch Block (RBBB)

DIAGNOSTIC CRITERIA	CAUSES
QRS: .12–.16 second Wide R or R′ in V_1 and wide S in I, V_5, and F_6 when the QRS is < .12 second; incomplete RBBB is present.	Coronary artery disease, pulmonary embolus, right ventricular hypertrophy

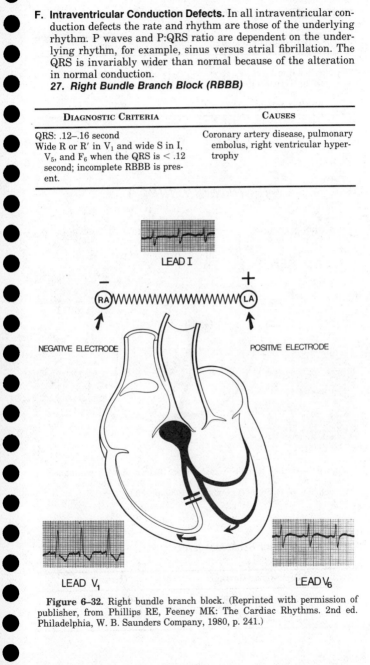

Figure 6–32. Right bundle branch block. (Reprinted with permission of publisher, from Phillips RE, Feeney MK: The Cardiac Rhythms. 2nd ed. Philadelphia, W. B. Saunders Company, 1980, p. 241.)

28. *Left Bundle Branch Block (LBBB)*

Diagnostic Criteria	Causes
QRS: .12 to .16 second Notched R in I aVL, V_6; rS or QS in V1; when the QRS is <.12 second incomplete LBBB is present.	Coronary artery disease, left ventricular hypertrophy

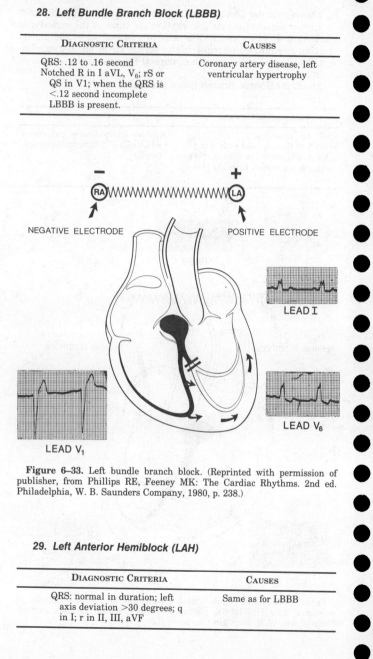

Figure 6–33. Left bundle branch block. (Reprinted with permission of publisher, from Phillips RE, Feeney MK: The Cardiac Rhythms. 2nd ed. Philadelphia, W. B. Saunders Company, 1980, p. 238.)

29. *Left Anterior Hemiblock (LAH)*

Diagnostic Criteria	Causes
QRS: normal in duration; left axis deviation >30 degrees; q in I; r in II, III, aVF	Same as for LBBB

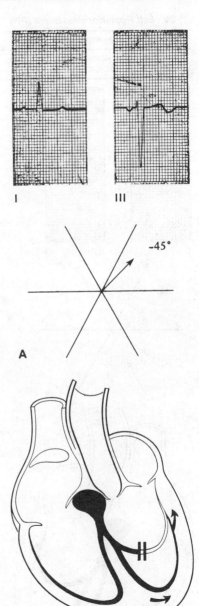

Figure 6–34. Left anterior hemiblock. *A.* ECG changes and axis. *B.* Diagram of heart. (Reprinted with permission of publisher, from Phillips RE, Feeney MK: The Cardiac Rhythms. 2nd ed. Philadelphia, W. B. Saunders Company, 1980, p. 249.)

30. Left Posterior Hemiblock (PH)

DIAGNOSTIC CRITERIA	CAUSES
Right axis deviation >120 degrees; r in I; q in II, III, aVF	Same as for LBBB

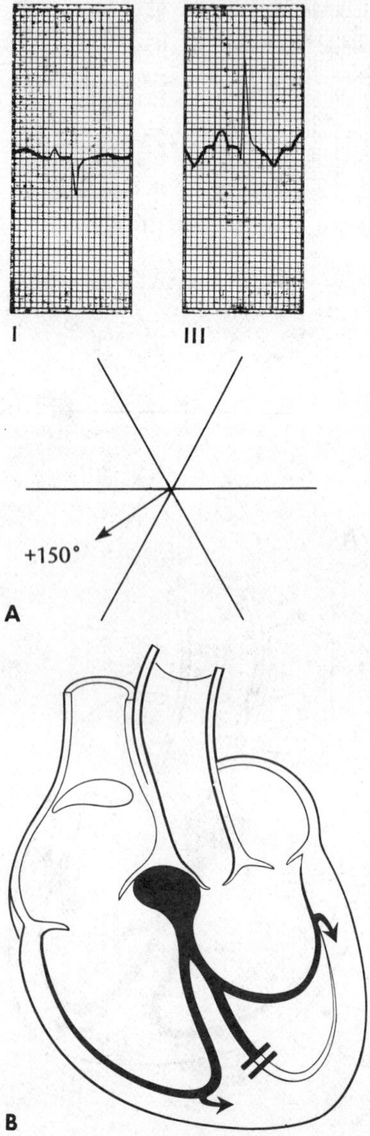

I   III

+150°

A

B

Figure 6–35. Left posterior hemiblock. *A*. ECG changes and axis. *B*. Diagram of heart. (Reprinted with permission of publisher, from Phillips RE, Feeney MK: The Cardiac Rhythms. 2nd ed. Philadelphia, W. B. Saunders Company, 1980, p. 250.)

31. ***Bifascicular Block.*** Bifascicular block occurs when right bundle branch block coexists with either left anterior hemiblock or left posterior hemiblock.

32. ***Trifascicular Block.*** Trifascicular block occurs when right bundle branch block coexists with both left anterior hemiblock and left posterior hemiblock.

33. ***Aberrant Conduction.*** Aberrant conduction is abnormal ventricular conduction of a supraventricular impulse. The result is an abnormally wide deformed QRS complex.

Differentiation of a premature ventricular contraction from a supraventricular impulse with aberrant conduction is often difficult to make, but certain characteristics allow the distinction (See Table 6–1).

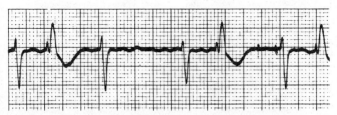

Figure 6–36. Aberrance of RBBB pattern. (Reprinted with permission of publisher, from Phillips RE, Feeney MK: The Cardiac Rhythms. 2nd ed. Philadelphia, W. B. Saunders Company, 1980, p. 245.)

CHARACTERISTICS OF PVC AND ABERRANTLY CONDUCTED BEAT

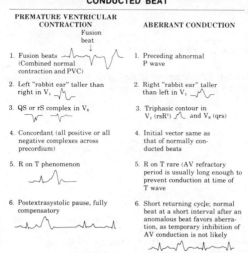

PREMATURE VENTRICULAR CONTRACTION	ABERRANT CONDUCTION
1. Fusion beats (Combined normal contraction and PVC)	1. Preceding abnormal P wave
2. Left "rabbit ear" taller than right in V_1	2. Right "rabbit ear" taller than left in V_1
3. QS or rS complex in V_6	3. Triphasic contour in V_1 (rsR') and V_6 (qrs)
4. Concordant (all positive or all negative complexes across precordium)	4. Initial vector same as that of normally conducted beats
5. R on T phenomenon	5. R on T rare (AV refractory period is usually long enough to prevent conduction at time of T wave
6. Postextrasystolic pause, fully compensatory	6. Short returning cycle; normal beat at a short interval after an anomalous beat favors aberration, as temporary inhibition of AV conduction is not likely

Figure 6–37. (Reprinted with permission of author and publisher, from Eisenberg M, Copass M: Emergency Medical Therapy. 2nd ed. Philadelphia, W. B. Saunders Company, 1982, p. 18.)

G. Preexcitation Syndrome. Preexcitation syndrome occurs when a portion of the ventricle is activated by an accessory pathway. A delta wave is seen on the ECG in the initial portion of the QRS. This is caused by conduction along an accessory pathway. The PR interval is shortened. Clinically preexcitation syndromes are associated with paroxysmal atrial tachycardia and atrial fibrillation.

34. Wolff-Parkinson-White (WPW) Syndrome

DIAGNOSTIC CRITERIA	CAUSES

QRS: >.10 with delta wave
 P:QRS: 1:1
 PR interval: <.12 second WPW is classified into types A and B
     Type A: delta wave positive on V_1, V_2; bundle of Kent is on the left side; the pattern resembles right bundle branch block.
     Type B: delta wave negative on V_1, V_3 and positive on V_4–V_6; bundle of Kent is on the right side; the pattern resembles left bundle branch block.
	Congenital or acquired, associated with mitral valve prolapse, cardiomyopathies, septal defects, Ebstein's anomaly of tricuspid valve

35. Lown-Ganong-Levin (LGL) Syndrome. This is a variant of WPW syndrome except that the QRS duration is less than .10 second.

MYOCARDIAL HYPERTROPHY

A. Right Atrial Enlargement (RAE). The P wave is made up of the right and left atrial components:

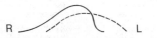

Hypertrophy of the atrium delays inscription of that atrium. Thus in right atrial enlargement the ECG signal from the right side becomes superimposed on the left, and the signal is increased in magnitude. This is called *P-pulmonale.*

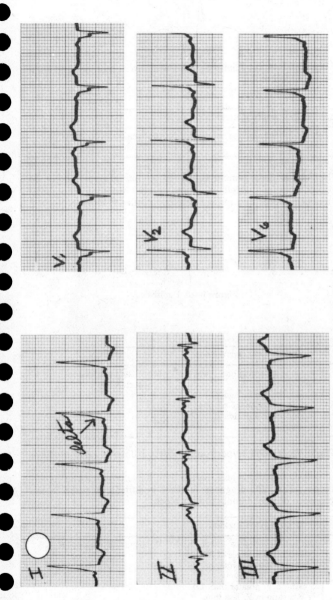

Figure 6-38. WPW syndrome, Type B. (Reprinted with permission of publisher, from Phillips RE, Feeney MK: The Cardiac Rhythms. 2nd ed. Philadelphia, W. B. Saunders Company, 1980, pp. 171, 172.)

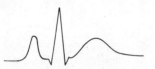

Figure 6–39. P-pulmonale.

DIAGNOSTIC CRITERIA	CAUSES
P wave: ≥.25 minutes in leads II, III, or aVF	Pulmonary hypertension, systemic hypertension

B. Left Atrial Enlargement (LAE). In left atrial hypertrophy the contraction of the left atrium is delayed, causing a prolonged notched appearance in lead II. This is called *P-mitrale.*

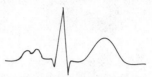

Figure 6–40. P-mitrale.

DIAGNOSTIC CRITERIA	CAUSES
P wave: ≥.12 second and P wave notched in lead II Biphasic P wave in lead VI with terminal component ≥1 mm in depth and duration ≥.04 second	Mitral stenosis, systemic hypertension

C. Right Ventricular Hypertrophy (RVH). Numerous criteria have been proposed for RVH. In general the electrocardiographic diagnosis of RVH is less specific than for left ventricular hypertrophy. The ECG diagnosis of RVH is difficult to make in the presence of right bundle branch block.

DIAGNOSTIC CRITERIA	CAUSES
Right axis deviation > 110 degrees (in the absence of RBBB or anterolateral or inferior myocardial infarction) R/S ratio in V_1 greater than 1.0 or R/S ratio in V_6 less than 1.0	Pulmonary hypertension

D. Left Ventricular Hypertrophy (LVH). Numerous criteria have been proposed for electrocardiographic diagnosis of LVH. The criteria for increased voltage are less valid in young thin individuals and those with thoracic deformity. Conversely, in patients with hyperinflated lungs (emphysema) voltages may be artificially reduced, thus masking LVH. LVH should not be read in the presence of left bundle branch block.

DIAGNOSTIC CRITERIA	CAUSES
LVH is probably present when one of the following criteria is present: *Precordial lead criteria* 1. S in lead V_1 or V_2 + R in V_5 or V_6 >35 mm 2. Sum of maximal pericordial deflection and deepest precordial deflection ≥45 mm 3. R in V5 >25 mm 4. Sum of R in I and S in III >25 mm 5. R in aVL≥11 mm 6. R in aVF≥20 mm	Systemic hypertension, aortic stenosis

These criteria have a sensitivity of 70 to 80 per cent with a false-positive rate of 10 to 15 per cent. Alternative criteria (using a point system) have been proposed by Estes that decrease the false-positive rate to 3 per cent. This improvement is achieved at the expense of lowered sensitivity (54 per cent). The point system is outlined below:

                                                                          Points

1. Amplitude (any of the following):
   a. Largest R wave or S wave in the limb leads
      greater than 20-mm deflection   ⎫
   b. S wave in V_1 or V_2 greater than 30-mm deflection   ⎬   3
   c. R wave in V_5 or V_6 greater than 30-mm deflection   ⎭
2. ST segment and T wave abnormalities
   a. Without digitalis   3
   b. With digitalis   1
3. Left atrial abnormality: Biphasic P wave in V_1 with   3
   terminal component ≥ 1 mm in depth and ≥ .04
   second
4. Left axis deviation: −30 degrees or more   2
5. QRS duration greater than 0.09 second   1
6. Intrinsicoid deflection in V_5 or V_6 ≥ 0.05 second   1

A score of 5 indicates LVH. A score of 4 means that LVH is probable.

E. Combined Ventricular Hypertrophy. Electrocardiographic criteria of both right and left ventricular hypertrophy are seen in only 17 per cent of patients with autopsy-proven biventricular hypertrophy. More common are nonspecific ST-T wave changes. The QRS abnormalities often are balanced out.

MYOCARDIAL INFARCTION (MI)

The diagnosis of myocardial infarction is based on an appropriate history and enzyme and electrocardiographic changes. A definite diagnosis of infarction should not be made solely on the basis of a single ECG. In general, serial ECGs are necessary to document evolutionary changes over time. Furthermore, the initial ECG may be normal or inconclusive in 20 to 50 per cent of cases.

Myocardial infarction may be transmural (with full thickness of the myocardium from endocardium to epicardium) or subendocardial (with partial thickness involving only the subendocardium). Electrocardiographic changes involve abnormal findings in the leads facing the area of damage. Reciprocal changes occur in the leads facing away from the damaged area.

A. **Acute Transmural Myocardial Infarction**
   1. *Electrocardiographic Changes*
      a. **Q Wave.** An abnormal Q wave develops within hours after MI. To be considered abnormal it should be .04 second in duration, and greater than 25 per cent of the R wave in depth, or both, and should be present in more than one lead. The Q wave does not disappear with evolution of the MI. It represents permanent transmural necrosis.
      b. **ST Segment.** Usually the earliest electrocardiographic findings of acute MI are ST elevations (representing the area of injury). The ST segment returns to baseline after hours to days. Other conditions can lead to elevated ST segments. The differential diagnosis of ST segment elevation includes acute transmural myocardial infarction, aneurysm, pericarditis, left bundle branch block, coronary artery spasm, left ventricular hypertrophy with strain, early repolarization, hyperkalemia, cerebral vascular accident, and tricyclic antidepressant use.
      c. **T Wave.** T waves are inverted (representing areas of ischemia). The T wave returns to normal when ischemia passes. Hyperacute changes in T waves sometimes are seen.
      d. **Reciprocal Electrocardiographic Changes.** These changes occur in leads facing the opposite surface of damaged areas. They include (1) ST segment depression and (2) upright T wave.
      e. **Evolution of Electrocardiographic Changes.** The typical evolution of changes is shown in Figure 6–41. The patterns of changes for acute anterolateral, acute inferior, and acute posterior infarctions are shown in Figures 6–42 to 6–48.
      f. **Determination of Location of MI.** Table 6–1 shows changes indicating the locations of myocardial infarctions.
B. **Subendocardial Myocardial Infarction**
   1. *Electrocardiographic Changes.* Q waves do not develop in subendocardial myocardial infarction.

INDICATIVE
CHANGES

RECIPROCAL
CHANGES

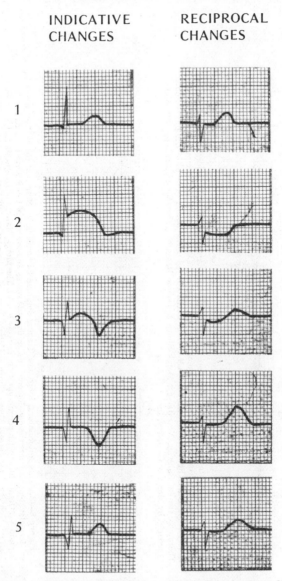

Figure 6–41. Evolutional ECG changes of myocardial infarction. 1. Normal tracing. 2. Hours after infarction. 3. A few days after infarction. 4. Many days to weeks later. 5. Months to years later. (Reprinted with permission of publisher, from Huang SH, Dasher LA, Larson C, et al.: Coronary Care Nursing. Philadelphia, W. B. Saunders Company, 1983, p. 131.)

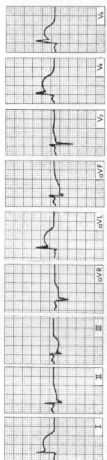

Figure 6-42. Acute anterolateral infarction. This tracing was obtained within a few hours of the onset of illness. There is striking hyperacute S-T segment elevation in leads I, aVL, V₄, and V₆ and reciprocal depression in the other leads. (Reproduced with permission, from Berkow R (ed.): The Merck Manual of Diagnosis and Therapy. 14th ed. Rahway, New Jersey, Merck Sharp & Dohme Research Laboratories, 1982, pp. 498–499. Copyright by Merck & Company, Inc.)

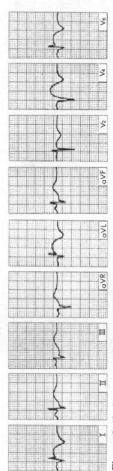

Figure 6-43. Acute anterolateral infarction. Tracing obtained 24 hours later. Note that the S-T segments are less elevated; also note the development of significant Q waves and the loss of the R wave in leads I, aVL, V₄, and V₆. (Reproduced with permission, from Berkow R (ed.): The Merck Manual of Diagnosis and Therapy. 14th ed. Rahway, New Jersey, Merck Sharp & Dohme Research Laboratories, 1982, pp. 498–499. Copyright by Merck & Company, Inc.)

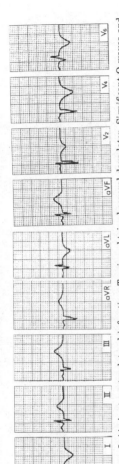

Figure 6–44. Acute anterolateral infarction. Tracing obtained several days later. Significant Q waves and the loss of the R wave voltage persist. S-T segments are now essentially isoelectric. The ECG will probably only slowly change over the next several months. (Reproduced with permission, from Berkow R (ed.): The Merck Manual of Diagnosis and Therapy. 14th ed. Rahway, New Jersey, Merck Sharp & Dohme Research Laboratories, 1982, pp. 498–499. Copyright by Merck & Company, Inc.)

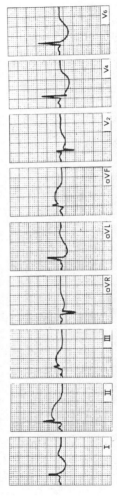

Figure 6–45. Acute inferior diaphragmatic left ventricular infarction. Tracing obtained within a few hours of the onset of illness. Note the hyperacute S-T segment elevation in leads II, III, and aVF and the reciprocal depression in the other leads. (Reproduced with permission, from Berkow R (ed.): The Merck Manual of Diagnosis and Therapy. 14th ed. Rahway, New Jersey, Merck Sharp & Dohme Research Laboratories, 1982, pp. 500–501. Copyright by Merck & Company, Inc.)

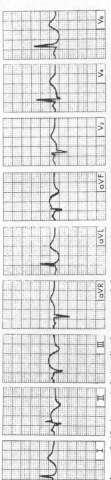

Figure 6–46. Acute inferior diaphragmatic left ventricular infarction. Tracing obtained after the first 24 hours. Note the development of significant Q waves in leads II, III, and aVF and the decreasing S-T segment elevation in the same leads. (Reproduced with permission, from Berkow R (ed.): The Merck Manual of Diagnosis and Therapy. 14th ed. Rahway, New Jersey, Merck Sharp & Dohme Research Laboratories, 1982, pp. 500–501. Copyright by Merck & Company, Inc.)

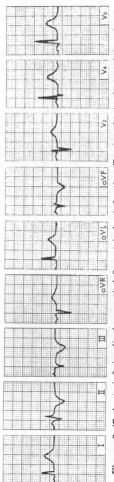

Figure 6–47. Acute inferior diaphragmatic left ventricular infarction. Tracing obtained several days later. S-T segments are now isoelectric. There are abnormal Q waves in leads II, III, and aVF, indicating that myocardial scars persist. (Reproduced with permission, from Berkow R (ed.): The Merck Manual of Diagnosis and Therapy. 14th ed. Rahway, New Jersey, Merck Sharp & Dohme Research Laboratories, 1982, pp. 500–501. Copyright by Merck & Company, Inc.)

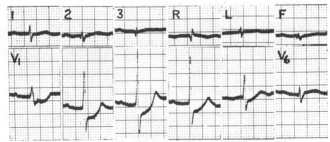

Figure 6–48. Probable acute true posterior infarction. Note prominent and wide R waves in V_1 and other right precordial leads accompanied by reciprocal ST-T changes in the same leads; these features in anterior leads suggest an acute infarction of the opposite, that is, posterior wall. (Reprinted with permission of author and publisher, from Marriott J: Practical Electrocardiography. 6th ed. Baltimore, Williams & Wilkins, 1977, p. 253.)

a. **ST Segment.** Depression of the ST segment of at least 1.0 mm should be present. This represents injury to subendocardial tissue.

b. **T Wave.** There is inversion of the T wave (representing areas of ischemia), which returns to normal when ischemia passes.

c. **ST–T Wave.** ST-T wave changes may occur in other conditions. The differential diagnosis of ST depression and T wave inversion includes subendocardial infarction, bundle branch block, left ventricular hypertrophy with strain, Wolff-Parkinson-White syndrome, cerebrovascular accident, hypokalemia, and cardiomyopathy. Subendocardial injury can occur without electrocardiographic changes.

TABLE 6–1. DETERMINATION OF LOCATION OF MYOCARDIAL INFARCTION

Location	Leads with Indicative Changes (Q, Elevated ST, Inverted T)	Leads with Reciprocal Changes ST Depression (may not always be present)
Inferior (diaphragmatic)	II, III, aVF	I, aVL
Anteroseptal	V_1, V_2, V_3	II, III, aVF
Anterior	V_2, V_3, V_4	II, III, aVF
Anterolateral	I, aVL, V_5, V_6	II, III, aVF
Posterior*	V_1, V_2 (accentuated R waves in these leads)	V_1, V_2

*True posterior myocardial infarction is often difficult to detect. The R:S ratio in V_1 is ≥1. It should not be confused with right ventricular hypertrophy (right axis deviation is not present with true posterior infarction).

ELECTROLYTE AND DRUG EFFECTS

A. Electrolyte Changes

   1. Hypokalemia results in flat T waves and a "prolonged appearing" QT, which is actually caused by T wave flattening and elevation of the U wave giving the appearance of a prolonged QT interval.

   2. Hyperkalemia can result in peaked T waves (best seen in precordial leads). The waves should be 10 mm or greater; 50 per cent of patients have K^+ greater than 7.5 mg per cent. If hyperkalemia is severe, it may cause intraventricular blocks with prolongation of QRS and QT intervals; loss of P wave and "sine wave" pattern may occur.

   3. Hypocalcemia prolongs the QT segment as a result of prolongation of the ST segment. The T wave is usually normal, but inversion occurs in some leads in one third of cases.

   4. Hypercalcemia shortens the QT segment as a result of shortening of the ST segment. The T wave has a sharply sloped upstroke.

B. Drug Effects

   1. Administration of digitalis results in the so-called *digitalis effect*: ST segment depression, which is described as "scooped" with T wave inversions or changes. This condition is often most prominently seen in lateral precordial leads I and aVL. The PR interval may be prolonged.

   2. Quinidine prolongs the QT and QRS intervals. Prolongation of the QT and QRS intervals by greater than 25 per cent suggests toxic levels, and quinidine should be withheld.

   3. Phenothiazines (especially Thorazine and Mellaril) may produce electrocardiographic changes similar to those in hypokalemia. Electrocardiographic changes occur at therapeutic levels in up to 50 per cent of patients taking phenothiazines.

   4. Many other drugs can cause electrocardiographic changes. For example, tricyclics at toxic levels can cause conduction defects, and lithium can cause a variety of changes.

FALSE-POSITIVE ELECTROCARDIOGRAPHIC ABNORMALITIES

This section is included to demonstrate that abnormal electrocardiographic findings may occur in normal individuals. Obviously, the ECG is only one piece of diagnostic information and must be placed in the context of the clinical and laboratory findings before a final diagnosis can be reached.

The following are the most common false-positive electrocardiographic abnormalities.*

---

*A fuller discussion is contained in Fisch C: Abnormal ECG findings in clinically normal individuals. JAMA 250:1321–1323, 1983, from which portions of the above section have been adapted.

A. **P Wave.** Findings of right atrial enlargement (P-pulmonale-Tall P in leads II, III, and aVF) can be seen in tall thin individuals, especially those with a vertically positioned heart.

B. **QRS Complex**
  1. Abnormal Q waves in lead III aVF may be seen in obese patients with elevated diaphragms.
  2. Abnormal Q waves may be seen in leads II, III, and aVF in connection with a tall R wave, usually in thin tall individuals.
  3. A QS complex in V_1–V_3 may be the result of a low-lying diaphragm. Moving electrodes down should reveal R waves.
  4. A tall R wave in V_1 (suggestive of RVH QS complexes with or without inverted T waves in aVL or aVF) may be positional in origin.
  5. Voltage criteria for LVH do not apply for patients under 25 years old or in thin-chested individuals.

C. **T Wave.** T wave inversion in leads V_1–V_4 may be seen in normal individuals, most often healthy young females or in the black population.

D. **Right Bundle Branch Block.** Incomplete right bundle branch block is seen in 2 per cent of the normal population.

E. **Early Repolarization.** An ST segment elevation of 1 to 2 mm may be seen in the anterolateral leads II, III, and V_3–V_6 among normal individuals. Usually a small notch at the end of the R wave is seen.

REFERENCES

1. Alpert MA, Flaker GC: Arrhythmias associated with sinus node dysfunction. JAMA 250:2160–2166, 1983.
An up-to-date summary of recognition and management of sinus node arrhythmias.

2. Fisch C: Abnormal ECG in clinically normal individuals. JAMA 250:1321–1323, 1983.
An interesting discussion of false-positive ECGs from normal individuals.

3. Wo D: Supraventricular tachycardias. JAMA 249:3357–3360, 1983.
A discussion of differential diagnosis among various types of supraventricular tachycardias.

4. Romhilt DW, Estes EH: Point-score system for the ECG diagnosis of left ventricular hypertrophy. Am Heart J 75:752–758, 1968.

5. Chou TC: Electrocardiography: Usefulness and limitations. Cardiovasc Rev Reports 2:192–201, 1981.
A good general discussion.

6. Mills RM, Young E, Gorlin R, et al.: Natural history of ST-segment evaluation after acute myocardial infarction. Am J Cardiol 35:609–614, 1975.

7. Horan LG, Flowers NC, Johnson JC: Significance of diagnostic Q-waves of myocardial infarction. Circulation 43:428, 1971.

7

ELEVATED BLOOD PRESSURE AND HYPERTENSION*

DEFINITION AND CLASSIFICATION

Table 7–1 gives a recommended scheme for categorizing arterial pressure in individuals aged 18 years or older.

The diagnosis of hypertension in adults is confirmed when the average of two or more diastolic measurements on at least two subsequent visits is 90 mm Hg or higher or when the average of multiple systolic measurements on two or more subsequent visits is consistently greater than 140 mm Hg. The patient should be clearly informed that a single elevated reading does not constitute a diagnosis of hypertension but is a sign that further observation is required.

EPIDEMIOLOGY AND GENERAL CONSIDERATIONS

A. More than 60 million individuals in the United States either have been found to have elevated blood pressure (140/90 mm Hg or greater) or have reported being told by a physician that they have hypertension. Prevalence rates increase with age in the United States population, and the rate for black Americans far exceeds the rate for white Americans.
B. Lability of blood pressure has been noted in the literature. To avoid recording an aberrant measurement, individuals should not have their blood pressure measured immediately after a taxing or stressful situation such as walking up several flights of stairs. The average of two or more blood pressure measurements should be obtained with the subject seated comfortably with the arm bared. Upper arm constriction by a rolled sleeve affects the validity of the reading and should be avoided. Systolic and diastolic pressures should be recorded, with the diastolic pressure reported as the disappearance of sound. In addition to the standard-sized cuff, large-sized adult and pediatric-sized cuffs should be available to obtain accurate readings in obese patients and in children. Two or more measurements should be taken at each visit, with the average pressure used as the value for the visit.

Follow-up criteria recommended for asymptomatic individuals are shown in Table 7–2.

---

*This chapter is a slightly modified version of portions from the 1984 Report of the Joint National Committee on Detection, Evaluation and Treatment of High Blood Pressure. Dustan HP, Chairman. NIH Publication, No. 84-1088, June 1984.

TABLE 7–1. BLOOD PRESSURE CLASSIFICATION BASED ON CONFIRMED* DIASTOLIC AND SYSTOLIC PRESSURES IN THE SAME INDIVIDUAL 18 YEARS AND OLDER†

DIASTOLIC BLOOD PRESSURE (MM HG)	SYSTOLIC BLOOD PRESSURE (MM HG)		
	Less than 140	140 to 159	160 or greater
Less than 85	Normal blood pressure	Borderline isolated systolic hypertension	Isolated systolic hypertension
85 to 89	High normal blood pressure		
90 to 104		Mild hypertension	
105 to 114		Moderate hypertension	
115 or greater		Severe hypertension	

*The average of two or more measurements on two or more occasions.
†From the 1984 Report of the Joint National Committee on Detection, Evaluation, and Treatment of High Blood Pressure. Dustan HP, Chairman. NIH Publication, No. 84-1088, June 1984.

TABLE 7–2. FOLLOW-UP CRITERIA BASED ON DIASTOLIC AND SYSTOLIC MEASUREMENTS ON TWO OCCASIONS* IN ASYMPTOMATIC INDIVIDUALS 18 YEARS AND OLDER†

Diastolic Blood Pressure (mm Hg)	Systolic Blood Pressure (mm Hg)		
	Less than 140	140 to 199	200 or greater
Less than 85	Recheck within 2 years‡	*1st occasion:* confirm within 2 months *2nd occasion:* evaluate or refer promptly to a source of care	Evaluate or refer to a source of care within 2 weeks
85 to 89	Recheck within 1 year		
90 to 104		*1st occasion:* confirm within 2 months *2nd occasion:* evaluate or refer promptly to a source of care	
105 to 114	Evaluate or refer to a source of care within 2 weeks		
115 or greater	Evaluate or refer immediately to a source of care		

*Two or more measurements should be taken on each occasion and the average used as the value for that visit.
†From the 1984 Report of the Joint National Committee on Detection, Evaluation, and Treatment of High Blood Pressure. Dustan HP, Chairman. NIH Publication, No. 84-1088, June 1984.
‡Rechecking within one year is recommended for individuals at increased risk (that is, blacks or those with family history, obesity, oral contraceptive use, and high alcohol intake).

DIFFERENTIAL DIAGNOSIS

The prevalence of various forms of hypertension is shown in Table 7–3.

HISTORY

A medical history should include (a) family history of hypertension and cardiovascular disease; (b) patient history of cardiovascular, cerebrovascular, and renal disease or diabetes mellitus; (c) known duration and levels of elevated blood pressure; (d) results and side effects of previous antihypertensive therapy; (e) use of drugs that may influence blood pressure, such as contraceptive pills; (f) history of weight gain, sodium intake, and alcohol use; (g) symptoms suggesting secondary hypertension; (h) psychosocial and environmental factors (emotional stress, cultural food practices, economic status) that may influence blood pressure control; and (i) other cardiovascular risk factors (including obesity, smoking, hyperlipidemia, and carbohydrate intolerance).

A careful history of all prescribed and over-the-counter medications should be obtained from all patients. Several medications may either raise blood pressure or interfere with the effectiveness of antihypertensive drugs. These include, but are not limited to, oral contraceptives, steroidal and nonsteroidal anti-inflammatory agents, nasal decongestants, appetite suppressants, and the tricyclic antidepressants.

TABLE 7–3. PREVALENCE OF VARIOUS FORMS OF HYPERTENSION IN THE GENERAL POPULATION AND IN SPECIALIZED REFERRAL CLINICS*†

DIAGNOSIS	GENERAL POPULATION (%)	SPECIALTY CLINIC (%)
Essential hypertension	92–94	65–85
Renal hypertension		
Parenchymal	2–3	4–5
Renovascular	1–2	4–16
Endocrine hypertension		
Primary aldosteronism	0.3	0.5–12
Cushing's syndrome	<0.1	0.2
Pheochromocytoma	<0.1	0.2
Oral contraceptive–induced	2–4	1–2
Miscellaneous	0.2	1

*Estimates based on a number of reports in the literature.
†Reprinted with permission of publisher, from Williams G, Braunwald E: Hypertensive vascular disease. Chap. 267. In Petersdorf, et al. (eds.): Principles of Internal Medicine. 10th ed. New York, McGraw-Hill, 1983.

SIGNS AND SYMPTOMS

Evaluation of the cardiovascular condition of patients with confirmed hypertension should answer the following three questions:

1. Is target organ involvement present?
2. Are cardiovascular risk factors other than hypertension present?
3. Does the patient have primary or secondary (possibly reversible) hypertension?

Physical examination should include (a) two or more blood pressure measurements with the patient supine or seated and standing; (b) verification in the contralateral arm; (c) height and weight; (d) funduscopic examination for arteriolar narrowing, arteriovenous compression, hemorrhages, exudates, and papilledema; (e) examination of the neck for carotid bruits, distended veins, and enlarged thyroid; (f) examination of the heart for increased rate, size, precordial heave, murmurs, arrhythmias and S3 and S4 heart sounds; (g) examination of the abdomen for bruits, enlarged kidneys, and dilation of the aorta; (h) examination of the extremities for diminished or absent peripheral arterial pulsations and edema; and (i) neurologic assessment.

Physical findings that are suggestive of secondary hypertension include abdominal or flank masses (polycystic kidneys); abdominal bruits, particularly those that lateralize or have a diastolic component (renovascular disease); delayed or absent femoral arterial pulses (aortic coarctation); truncal obesity with pigmented striae (Cushing's syndrome); and tachycardia, sweating, and pallor (pheochromocytoma).

RECOMMENDED DIAGNOSTIC APPROACH

A few simple laboratory tests should be done before initiating therapy. Group I tests are needed for determining severity of vascular disease and possible causes of hypertension. Group II tests relate to other cardiovascular risk factors or provide necessary baseline values for judging adverse biochemical effects of therapy.

Group I	Group II
Hemoglobin and hematocrit	Total and high-density lipoprotein (HDL) cholesterol
Complete urinalysis	
Serum potassium, serum creatinine	Plasma glucose (fasting if possible)
Electrocardiogram	Serum uric acid

Opinions differ regarding costs, risks, and specificity of some diagnostic procedures. An automated battery of blood chemistry tests is often used. On the basis of clinical judgment, the physician may select additional tests. Type and frequency of repeated laboratory tests should be based on the severity of target organ damage and the effects of the selected treatment program.

Secondary hypertension is rare; nevertheless, evaluation should seek to eliminate this possibility. Additional diagnostic procedures may be indicated to discover secondary hypertension (renal parenchymal disease, renovascular disease, coarctation of the aorta, primary aldosteronism, Cushing's syndrome, or pheochromocytoma) in patients: (a) in whom age, history, physical examination, severity of hypertension, or initial laboratory findings suggest secondary hypertension; (b) whose blood pressure responds poorly to drug therapy; (c) with well-controlled hypertension whose blood pressures begin to increase; or (d) with accelerated or malignant hypertension.

REFERENCES

1. Mancia G, et al.: Effects of blood pressure measurement by the doctor on patient's blood pressure and heart rate. Lancet 2:695–697, 1983.
2. Kirkendall WM, et al.: American Heart Association recommendations for human blood pressure determination by sphygmomanometers. Circulation 62:1146A–1155A, 1980.
3. Kannel WB: Some lessons in cardiovascular epidemiology from Framingham. Am J Cardiol 37:269–282, 1976.
4. Gifford RW Jr.: Isolated systolic hypertension in the elderly. J Am Med Assoc 247:781–785, 1982.
5. Rowland M, Roberts J: Blood pressure levels and hypertension in persons 6–74 years: United States, 1976–80. Advance Data from Vital and Health Statistics, No. 84. Hyattsville, U.S. Department of Health and Human Services, Public Health Service, National Center for Health Statistics, October 8, 1982, DHHS Publication No. (PHS) 82-1250.
6. Maxwell MH, et al.: Error in blood-pressure measurement due to incorrect cuff size in obese patients. Lancet 2:33–36, 1982.
7. Messerli FH, Frohlich ED: High blood pressure: A side effect of drugs, poisons, and food. Arch Intern Med 139:682–687, 1979.

---8---

VALVULAR HEART DISEASE

By MITCHELL A. KARTON, M.D.

MITRAL STENOSIS

A. **Definition.** Mitral stenosis is defined as obstruction of the mitral valve orifice. Normally the orifice size is 4 to 6 sq cm. When it is reduced to 2 sq cm or less, an increased left atrioventricular pressure gradient is required for forward blood flow.

B. **Epidemiology and General Comments.** Pure mitral stenosis is most commonly caused by rheumatic heart disease (RHD). Forty per cent of all patients with rheumatic heart disease have mitral stenosis as the primary valvular involvement. Two thirds of patients with mitral stenosis are female. After acute rheumatic fever it takes at least 2 years for mitral stenosis to occur. Symptoms usually do not appear for at least 20 years, most commonly during the patient's 30s.

C. **History.** The cardinal symptom is dyspnea on exertion. This may occur in association with fever, respiratory infection, atrial fibrillation with a rapid ventricular response, pregnancy, stress, thyrotoxicosis, or sexual intercourse. Later, patients complain of irregular beats caused by atrial fibrillation and of severe exercise limitations caused by pulmonary edema. Other complaints may include hemoptysis, symptoms of systemic emboli (20 per cent), chest pain (10 per cent), and symptoms of right heart failure (hepatomegaly, ascites, and refractory edema) caused by pulmonary hypertension.

D. **Physical Examination**

1. *General.* "Mitral facies," that is, a pinched expression with purplish cheeks, may appear. Central and peripheral cyanosis may occur if mitral stenosis is severe. The physician should look for peripheral stigmata of embolic phenomena and endocarditis.

2. *Jugular Venous Pulse.* There is a prominent a wave in the presence of pulmonary hypertension.

3. *Palpation.* Palpation indicates a small tapping left ventricle, possible right ventricular lift in the left parasternal region if there is pulmonary hypertension, and a palpable P2 in the left second intercostal space if there is pulmonary hypertension.

4. *Auscultation.* The opening snap is heard in early diastole at the base or left sternal border; the higher the left atrial pressure, the earlier is the opening snap. Opening snap may not be heard if there is significant calcification, pulmonary hypertension, or aortic regurgitation. A summary of findings of auscultation of valvular heart disease is presented in Table 8–1.

5. *Murmurs*
   a. Mid-diastolic murmur is a long low rumble heard best with the bell at the apex. If there is mild mitral stenosis, the murmur may be short and recur with presystolic accentuation.
   b. Presystolic murmur may be heard in atrial fibrillation with rapid ventricular response.
   c. Murmurs in 1 and 2 may be masked in the presence of obesity, pulmonary hypertension, or low cardiac output.
   d. The Graham-Steel murmur of pulmonary regurgitation (if there is pulmonary hypertension) is a high-pitched early diastolic blow in the left second and third intercostal spaces.

6. *Dynamic Auscultation*
   a. Diastolic murmur is made louder with tachycardia, the left lateral decubitus position, and administration of amyl nitrate. The Austin Flint murmur of aortic regurgitation fades with amyl nitrate administration.

  b. Phenylephrine or sudden standing widens the A2 opening snap interval (a split S2 narrows it).

  c. Inspiration widens the A2 opening snap interval, and frequently an "A2-P2-opening snap" sequence can be heard.

E. Laboratory Findings

  1. *Electrocardiogram (ECG).* The ECG shows P-mitrale, right ventricular hypertrophy if there is severe pulmonary hypertension, and atrial fibrillation.

  2. *Chest X-Ray.* The chest x-ray shows an enlarged left atrium associated with a straight left heart border, widening of the angle between mainstem bronchi, a prominent pulmonary artery, and a large right ventricle. If the left atrium is extremely large, mitral regurgitation should be considered.

  3. *Echocardiography.* The physician should look for calcification of the annulus. M-mode echocardiography cannot indicate severity; two-dimensional echocardiography is best for determination of mitral orifice area.

MITRAL REGURGITATION

A. Definition. Mitral regurgitation exists when the left ventricular systolic contraction sends blood backward in the left atrium.

B. Epidemiology and General Comments. Mitral valvular insufficiency may be either acute or chronic. Chronic mitral regurgitation may be caused by multiple factors that affect the valve leaflets, the mitral annulus, the chordae tendineae, or the papillary muscles, but the most common cause is rheumatic heart disease. The causes of acute mitral regurgitation are far fewer; they include ischemia or infarction involving the papillary muscles, the chordae tendineae, or the left ventricular wall; infectious endocarditis; trauma; prosthetic valve leaks; and mitral valve prolapse.

C. History

  1. Chronic mitral regurgitation is usually well tolerated for many years. Some patients complain of fatigue, exertional weakness, and dyspnea. Occasionally, symptoms of right heart failure predominate (painful hepatomegaly, ascites, and refractory edema), especially if they are associated with chronic obstructive pulmonary disease. Symptoms may increase acutely in the face of systemic hypertension.

  2. Acute mitral regurgitation is characterized by the sudden onset of severe dyspnea in the face of a febrile illness (often bacterial endocarditis) or a myocardial infarction.

D. Physical Examination

  1. *Chronic Mitral Regurgitation*

   a. Palpation. A late systolic left parasternal lift due to left atrial enlargement may combine with left ventricular retraction to produce a rocking motion of the chest.

TABLE 8-1. AUSCULTATION OF VALVULAR HEART DISEASE

Valvular Lesion	Phono-cardiogram	Murmurs Heard Best with	Point of Maximal Intensity	S1	S2	S3	S4	Other Sounds
Mitral Stenosis		Bell	Apex	Loud	Loud P2 early in disease; loud "single" S2 late in disease	Usually absent	Absent if atrial fibrillation; right-sided if pulmonary hypertension	Opening snap at lower left sternal border to apex
Mitral Regurgitation Chronic		Diaphragm	Apex radiating to axilla	Often obscured by murmur	May be widely split	Loud and low-pitched	Present if severe mitral regurgitation.	
Acute		Diaphragm	Apex, may radiate to base of spine	Normal	Loud	May be present	May be present	Graham Steell murmur; see pulmonary regurgitation
Mitral Valve Prolapse		Diaphragm	Apex, with patient in left lateral decubitus position		May be paradoxically split			Clicks may be multiple; murmurs may be absent
Aortic Stenosis		Diaphragm	2nd right inter-costal space, radiates to apex and carotids	Soft	May be paradoxically split		May be prominent	Ejection clicks heard with diaphragm at left sternal border after S1

94

	Chest Piece	Location/Murmur	S_1	S_2	S_3	S_4	Other
Aortic Regurgitation Chronic	Diaphragm—early diastolic and systolic murmurs; bell—late diastolic rumble (Austin Flint)	Left 3rd intercostal space, early diastolic murmur / Apex, Austin Flint murmur / Base, systolic ejection murmur	Normal	Normal	May be present	Rare	
Acute		Same as for chronic aortic regurgitation	Often soft	P2 may be loud	Commonly present	Commonly present	
Tricuspid Stenosis	Bell	Left SB at 4th intercostal space	Loud	Loud, late in disease	Usually absent	Right-sided if pulmonary hypertension	Opening snap at lower left sternal border just after mitral opening snap
Tricuspid Regurgitation	Diaphragm	Left SB at 4th intercostal space	May be obscured by murmur	Loud P2 if pulmonary hypertension	Often right-sided	Right-sided S4 present if severe TR	
Pulmonary Regurgitation	Diaphragm	Left SB at 2nd–4th intercostal space	Normal	Loud P2 may be obscured by murmur	Usually absent	Right-sided with pulmonary hypertension	

SB = sternal border; TR = tricuspid regurgitation.

TABLE 8–2.   USEFUL MANEUVERS FOR DIFFERENTIATING SIMILAR AUSCULTATORY FINDINGS

PROBLEM	MANEUVERS	RESULTS
Mitral stenosis vs. Austin Flint	Amyl nitrate	Murmur of mitral stenosis increases; Austin Flint murmur diminishes.
Mitral stenosis vs. tricuspid stenosis	Respiration	Murmur of tricuspid stenosis increases with inspiration; murmur of mitral stenosis does not change.
S2 and opening snap vs. widely split S2	Position, phenylephrine, respiration	A2-opening snap interval widens with phenylephrine or sudden standing; split S2 narrows; inspiration may widen A2 opening snap into A2-P2 opening snap.
Mitral regurgitation vs. tricuspid regurgitation	Respiration	Murmur of tricuspid regurgitation increases with inspiration; murmur of mitral regurgitation does not change.
Mitral regurgitation vs. aortic stenosis	Phenylephrine, amyl nitrate, cycle length	Murmur of mitral regurgitation increases with phenylephrine, diminishes with amyl nitrate; no change with cycle length; murmur of aortic stenosis diminishes with phenylephrine and increases after long cycle.
Aortic stenosis vs. mitral valve prolapse	Position, amyl nitrate	Murmur of aortic stenosis increases with sudden squatting and amyl nitrate; murmur of mitral valve prolapse is diminished and delayed with sudden squatting; it occurs earlier with amyl nitrate.
Aortic stenosis vs. hypertrophic cardiomyopathy	Valsalva maneuver, position	Murmur of aortic stenosis diminishes during the strain phase of the Valsalva maneuver and increases with sudden squatting; murmur of hypertrophic cardiomyopathy increases during strain phase of Valsalva maneuver and diminishes with sudden squatting.
Mitral valve prolapse vs. hypertrophic cardiomyopathy	Valsalva maneuver	Murmur of mitral valve prolapse begins earlier, lasts longer, and is diminished during strain phase of Valsalva maneuver; murmur of hypertrophic cardiomyopathy increases during strain phase of Valsalva maneuver.
Click of mitral valve prolapse vs. ejection click of aortic stenosis		The click of mitral valve prolapse occurs after the upstroke of the carotid pulse.

b. **Auscultation.** S1 is often obscured by murmur; otherwise it is soft or absent. S2 may be widely split. S3 is loud and low-pitched and may be associated with a low short diastolic rumble, even without mitral stenosis. S4 is heard with severe regurgitation. Opening snap, even if present, does not imply predominant mitral stenosis.

c. **Murmurs**
   1). Usually there is a holosystolic loud-blowing apical murmur radiating to axilla.
   2). The murmur may be late systolic and decrescendo.

d. **Dynamic Auscultation**
   1). The systolic murmur can be made louder with administration of phenylephrine or sudden squatting. It is made softer with administration of amyl nitrate.
   2). Murmur of mitral regurgitation increases with isometric exercise; mumur of aortic stenosis does not.
   3). Murmur of tricuspid regurgitation increases with inspiration; murmur of mitral regurgitation does not.

2. *Acute Mitral Regurgitation*
   a. **Vital Signs.** The sinus rhythm is normal.
   b. **General.** The physician should look for signs of endocarditis and right heart failure.
   c. **Pulse.** The pulse is rapid and has a small volume with brisk upstroke.
   d. **Jugular Venous Pulse.** Often there is a prominent *a* wave.
   e. **Lungs.** Rales are present.
   f. **Palpation.** There is a hyperdynamic left ventricular impulse at the apex.
   g. **Auscultation.** S1 is normal. S2 is loud; P2 is increased if there is pulmonary hypertension. S3 and S4 may be present.
   h. **Murmurs**
      1). A pansystolic apical murmur may be decrescendo, ending before A2; it is lower-pitched and softer than the murmur of chronic mitral regurgitation.
      2). The murmur may have a "seagull" quality if it is caused by rupture of chordae tendineae.
      3). The murmur may radiate to the base if rupture is of chordae to the posterior leaflet and to the spine or the top of the head if there are ruptured chordae to the anterior leaflet.

E. **Laboratory Findings**
   1. *Chronic Mitral Regurgitation*
      a. **ECG.** There is left atrial enlargement; left ventricular hypertrophy if the regurgitation is severe and long-standing (50 per cent of cases); atrial fibrillation if the regurgitation is severe and long-standing; and right ventricular hypertrophy if pulmonary hypertension is present.
      b. **Chest X-Ray.** The x-ray shows left atrial enlargement. Left ventricular hypertrophy may be present.
      c. **Echocardiography.** The left atrium and left ventricle are enlarged, with increased motion of both chambers.

2. *Acute Mitral Regurgitation*
   a. **ECG.** There may be associated acute myocardial infarction.
   b. **Chest X-Ray.** There are slight cardiomegaly, a normal left atrium, and interstitial edema with Kerley B lines.
   c. **Echocardiography.** There is hyperactivity of both left atrium and left ventricle. Ruptured chordae, flail leaflets, and vegetations may be seen.

MITRAL VALVE PROLAPSE

A. **Definition.** Mitral valve prolapse is defined as the posterior prolapse of the mitral valve leaflets into the left atrium during systole. If severe, the displacement leads to a tenting of one or both leaflets, permitting mitral regurgitation.
B. **Epidemiology and General Comments.** Primary mitral valve prolapse probably fits into a continuum of connective tissue disorders involving myxomatous degeneration of the valve; secondary mitral valve prolapse may be associated with rheumatic heart disease, ischemic heart disease, or the cardiomyopathies.

The incidence of mitral valve prolapse is thought to be approximately 10 to 20 per cent of the population, with females being more commonly affected than males. Most patients are asymptomatic, and the condition is frequently discovered incidentally during auscultation or echocardiography.

C. **History.** The most common complaint is palpitations, typically in a young female. Often patients complain of atypical chest pain that is substernal, prolonged, and not exertional. The chest pain may last for weeks at a time. Complaints of dyspnea and fatigue may indicate mitral regurgitation or bacterial endocarditis. Occasionally, patients complain of symptoms of transient ischemic attacks or amaurosis fugax.
D. **Physical Examination**
   1. *General.* General examination usually shows a thin, young female.
   2. *Musculoskeletal.* Thoracic skeletal abnormalities are sometimes seen. These include scoliosis, pectus excavatum, straight thoracic spine, and narrow anteroposterior chest diameter.
   3. *Auscultation*
      a. There is a high-frequency mid-systolic or late systolic click (possibly multiple) of short duration.
      b. The click may be followed by a late systolic high-pitched murmur that is heard best at the apex, in the left lateral decubitus position, and that peaks near S2.
   4. *Dynamic Auscultation*
      a. The click and murmur are audible earlier and with greater intensity on standing.
      b. The click comes earlier, but the murmur is longer and

softer during the straining phase of the Valsalva maneuver and with amyl nitrate administration.
c. The click and murmur are delayed and of diminished intensity with squatting.
d. The click of mitral valve prolapse may be differentiated from an ejection click because it occurs after the upstroke of the carotid pulse.
e. The murmur of mitral valve prolapse may be best differentiated from that of hypertrophic cardiomyopathy because the latter increases in intensity during the straining phase of the Valsalva maneuver and following a premature ventricular complex, whereas the murmur of mitral valve prolapse does not.

The timing, intensity, and associations of the clicks and murmurs are extremely variable. In general, it is more reliable to note the changes in timing, not intensity, during dynamic auscultation.

E. Laboratory Findings
1. *ECG.* The ECG usually has a normal appearance. Occasionally there are nonspecific ST-T wave changes in the inferior leads. Mitral valve prolapse may cause false-positive exercise ECGs. Exercise thallium-201 scans appear normal in the absence of coronary artery disease.
2. *Holter Monitor.* There is arrhythmia in 40 to 75 per cent of cases: often benign premature atrial contractions, premature ventricular contractions, supraventricular tachycardia, brady- and tachyarrhythmias, and occasionally ventricular tachycardia.
3. *Chest X-Ray.* The left atrium is large if there is chronic mitral regurgitation. Thoracic skeletal abnormalities may be present. Increased anteroposterior cardiac silhouette may be caused by pectus excavatum or straight spine.
4. *M-Mode Echocardiography.* The echocardiogram shows late systolic posterior buckling of the mitral valve leaflet (this also may be seen with mitral regurgitation). Ten to 15 per cent of M-mode echocardiograms give false-negative results.

AORTIC STENOSIS

A. Definition. Valvular aortic stenosis occurs when a narrowing of the valve orifice impedes left ventricular outflow and causes a pressure gradient between the left ventricle and the aorta during systole. A gradient of 50 mm Hg with a normal cardiac output or a valve area that is one third of normal (approximately .5 sq cm per sq m of body surface area) is usually considered to represent hemodynamically critical obstruction.
B. Epidemiology and General Comments. In patients with valvular heart disease isolated aortic stenosis is the most common finding. If there is no associated mitral valve disease, aortic stenosis is usually congenital or degenerative, not rheumatic. The vast majority of patients are male, and often they do not develop

symptoms until the fifth or sixth decade of life. The natural history involves a less than four-year survival rate once symptoms occur.

C. **History.** The cardinal symptoms, in order of appearance, are dyspnea on exertion, angina pectoris, and exertional syncope. Angina may be caused by aortic stenosis or coronary artery disease. Signs of left ventricular failure—either forward or backward—occur late in the course of the disease.

D. **Physical Examination**
1. *Vital Signs.* The pulse pressure is narrow; systemic hypertension is rare.
2. *Pulse.* The pulse has a low amplitude, slow rise, and sustained duration (pulsus parvus et tardus). An anacrotic shudder is palpable in the carotid pulse.
3. *Jugular Venous Pulse.* An *a* wave may be prominent.
4. *Palpation.* There is an active sustained left ventricular impulse with inferior lateral displacement and a double apical impulse with a systolic thrill at the base.
5. *Auscultation.* S1 is soft. S2 may be single or paradoxically split; A2 is inaudible if significant calcification exists. S4 may be prominent. The ejection click after S1 is heard with the diaphragm and at the left sternal border; the click does not vary with respiration and is rare in the elderly patient with a calcified valve.
6. *Murmur*
   a. A crescendo-decrescendo harsh mid-systolic murmur can be heard best at the second right intercostal space and is transmitted to carotids and apex; the murmur ends before A2.
   b. The higher-frequency components of the murmur may radiate to the apex and be confused with mitral regurgitation.
7. *Dynamic Auscultation*
   a. The murmur increases with squatting and administration of amyl nitrate. This finding helps to distinguish the condition from hypertrophic cardiomyopathy.
   b. The murmur decreases with the Valsalva maneuver. This finding helps to distinguish the condition from hypertrophic cardiomyopathy.
   c. The murmur changes with cycle length. This finding helps to distinguish the condition from mitral regurgitation.

E. **Laboratory Findings**
1. *ECG.* There is left ventricular hypertrophy (85 per cent of patients have severe aortic stenosis). Left atrial enlargement suggests associated mitral valve disease. The findings do not correlate with hemodynamic severity.
2. *Chest X-Ray.* The x-ray may show slight cardiac enlargement when mitral regurgitation or congestive heart failure are present; poststenotic aortic dilatation may be observable; fluoroscopy demonstrates valvular calcification.
3. *M-Mode Echocardiography.* This can be used to diagnose aortic stenosis but not to determine severity.

AORTIC REGURGITATION

A. **Definition.** Aortic regurgitation occurs when, during diastole, the left ventricle receives both a forward stroke volume from the left atrium and a retrograde regurgitant volume of blood through the aortic valve.

B. **Epidemiology and General Comments.** Aortic regurgitation may be either chronic or acute. The chronic variety has multiple causes but is usually rheumatic in origin. Other causes include syphilis, connective tissue diseases, and congenital abnormalities. If there is associated mitral valve disease, females are affected more commonly. Acute aortic regurgitation is usually caused by infective endocarditis (only rarely affecting a previously normal valve), dissection, trauma, or a prolapse or rupture of the aortic cusp.

Aortic regurgitation—both chronic and acute—may also be caused by widening of the annulus and separation of the leaflets without any valvular involvement per se. If hemodynamically significant aortic stenosis is present as well, the cause is almost always rheumatic or congenital.

In chronic aortic regurgitation, dilatation of the left ventricle provides the major hemodynamic compensation. Because the volume load develops gradually, symptoms may not appear for even up to 30 years following rheumatic fever. In acute aortic regurgitation, however, the sudden severe volume load on the left ventricle causes an acutely high filling pressure that often results in pulmonary edema, ventricular arrhythmias and interference with coronary perfusion.

C. **History**

1. *Chronic aortic regurgitation* may be associated with a childhood murmur, a family history positive for Marfan's syndrome, a history of rheumatic fever, or a history of syphilis, trauma, or endocarditis. Early in the course of the disease the patient may complain of a long-standing awareness of an uncomfortably beating heart with palpitations and head pounding, especially when in a supine position. The patient may also complain of nocturnal chest pain. Later, symptoms of left ventricular failure may predominate, including dyspnea on exertion, paroxysmal nocturnal dyspnea, and orthopnea.

2. *Acute aortic regurgitation* may be associated with a history of intravenous drug abuse, rheumatic heart disease, or trauma. The patient usually complains of severe dyspnea and weakness that is caused by sudden left ventricular failure.

D. **Physical Examination**

1. *Chronic Aortic Regurgitation*

a. **Vital Signs.** There is a widened arterial pulse pressure: systolic blood pressure may be as high as 300 mm Hg and diastolic pressure as low as 30 mm Hg. Diastolic pressure may be hard to measure because systolic sounds are audible even with the cuff deflated; however, the diastolic blood pressure correlates fairly well with blood pressure at the muffling of Korotkoff sounds.

b. **Pulse.** A rapid rise with sudden drop-off is often visible as a carotid shudder or palpable in the brachial-radial artery (Corrigan's or water-hammer pulse); other expressions of the same phenomena include head bobbing (Musset's sign), capillary pulsations seen at the base of taut fingernail beds (Quincke's pulse), auscultation of "pistol shots" over femoral arteries (Traube's sign), or Duroziez's sign (to and fro murmur over femoral arteries with light compression); pulse contour may be bisferious.

c. **Palpation.** There is a hyperdynamic left ventricular impulse that is laterally displaced. Systolic retraction may occur.

d. **Auscultation.** S1 is normal. S2 is normal or soft; P2 may be obscured by murmur. S3 may be present. S4 is rare.

e. **Murmurs.** There are three murmurs commonly heard in chronic aortic regurgitation:

   1). A high-pitched decrescendo diastolic blow is heard best with the diaphragm at the left third intercostal space, with the patient sitting forward at end-expiration. A right parasternal murmur suggests aneurysmal dilatation of the aortic root. The severity of regurgitation correlates with the duration of this murmur, not with its intensity.

   2). A harsh systolic ejection murmur occurs at the base, radiating to the carotids. The murmur peaks early and is often higher-pitched than the murmur of predominant aortic stenosis. This mumur does not imply organic obstruction.

   3). The Austin Flint murmur is an apical soft rumbling murmur in mid-diastole or with presystolic accentuation. It is probably caused by impingement on the anterior mitral leaflet by the regurgitant aortic stream.

f. **Dynamic Auscultation**

   1). The aortic regurgitation murmur (1) increases with squatting, phenylephrine administration, or isometric exercise.

   2). The aortic regurgitation murmur (1) decreases with amyl nitrate administration or the Valsalva maneuver.

   3). The Austin Flint murmur (3) fades with amyl nitrate administration. This finding helps to differentiate it from the murmur of mitral stenosis.

2. *Acute Aortic Regurgitation*

a. **Vital Signs.** These include tachypnea and tachycardia; pulse pressure is near normal, not nearly as wide as with chronic aortic regurgitation. Systolic blood pressure may be slightly increased, and diastolic blood pressure is greater than 50 to 60 mm Hg.

b. **Pulse.** Peripheral pulses are also of collapsing quality, but the dramatic physical signs seen with chronic aortic regurgitation are diminished; pulsus alternans is sometimes palpable.

    c. **Jugular Venous Pulse.** This pulse may be distended and associated with signs of pulmonary hypertension.

    d. **Palpation.** Left ventricular point of maximal intensity is nearly normal; it may be mildly displaced but without the rocking motion of chronic aortic regurgitation.

    e. **Auscultation.** S1 is often soft or absent. S2-P2 is often increased owing to pulmonary hypertension. S3 and S4 commonly are present.

    f. **Murmurs**

        1). The early diastolic murmur is lower-pitched and of shorter duration than the murmur of chronic aortic regurgitation.

        2). The mid-systolic ejection murmur is less harsh than in chronic aortic regurgitation.

        3). The Austin Flint murmur ends earlier than in chronic aortic regurgitation because left ventricular pressure exceeds left atrial pressure in diastole.

E. Laboratory Findings

  1. Chronic Aortic Regurgitation

    a. **ECG.** Left ventricular hypertrophy and lateral ST-T wave changes are present if there is severe aortic regurgitation.

    b. **Chest X-Ray.** There are left ventricular enlargement, possibly dilatation, and prominence of the ascending aorta and aortic knob.

    c. **Echocardiography.** Echocardiography shows increased left ventricular end-diastolic volume, increased septal and free wall motion, and mitral valve fluttering.

  2. Acute Aortic Regurgitation

    a. **ECG.** Often there are no signs of left ventricular hypertrophy. Nonspecific ST-T wave changes are common.

    b. **Chest X-Ray.** Mild cardiomegaly is possible. The aortic arch is normal. Interstitial edema with Kerley B lines may be seen.

    c. **Echocardiography.** Left ventricular dimensions are normal. There are premature mitral valve closure and delayed mitral valve opening, decreased E to F slope, and mitral valve fluttering. Vegetations are possible on atrioventricular cusps.

TRICUSPID STENOSIS

A. Definition. Tricuspid stenosis occurs as obstruction to right atrial outflow. When the diastolic transvalvular gradient is at least 5 mm Hg, systemic venous hypertension ensues.

B. Epidemiology and General Comments. Tricuspid stenosis generally is the result of rheumatic fever and is most commonly found in patients with concomitant mitral stenosis. The inability of the right atrium to handle a large pressure load causes symptoms and signs of right heart failure with systemic venous congestion. Low right-sided cardiac output accounts for the paucity of pulmonary signs even in the presence of mitral stenosis.

C. **History.** The complaints are predominantly those of the patient with mitral stenosis. Indeed, improvement of pulmonary congestion in a patient with mitral stenosis should suggest tricuspid stenosis. Right-sided symptoms of painful hepatomegaly, ascites, and refractory edema seem out of proportion to minimal complaints of dyspnea in the patient who is comfortable while lying flat.

D. **Physical Examination**
   1. *General.* There is evidence of right heart failure with hepatomegaly, ascites, and peripheral edema.
   2. *Jugular Venous Pulse.* There are giant *a* waves with a diminished *y* descent.
   3. *Lungs.* The lungs are relatively clear compared with those in right heart failure. There is no evidence of pulmonary hypertension.
   4. *Palpation.* There is no right ventricular lift (occasionally right atrial enlargement causes a right-sided parasternal lift). An inspiratory diastolic thrill is present at the lower left sternal border.
   5. *Auscultation.* Findings of mitral stenosis predominate. An opening snap may be heard at the lower left sternal border just after the mitral opening snap.
   6. *Murmurs*
      a. A soft diastolic high-pitched murmur with a scratchy crescendo-decrescendo presystolic component occurs at the left sternal border in the fourth intercostal space.
      b. The murmur and opening snap increase with inspiration, exercise, the right lateral decubitus position, and amyl nitrate administration. They decrease with expiration and the strain phase of the Valsalva maneuver.
      c. These changes with respiration help to distinguish the murmur from mitral stenosis.

E. **Laboratory Findings**
   1. *ECG.* There are right atrial enlargement, sometimes biatrial enlargement caused by mitral stenosis, and no right ventricular hypertrophy.
   2. *Chest X-Ray.* A prominent right atrium, superior vena cava, and azygos system are seen without enlargement of the pulmonary artery. The lungs may be clear even with evidence of mitral stenosis.
   3. *Echocardiography.* Echocardiography shows a reduced E to F slope of the anterior leaflet or tricuspid valve and paradoxic motion of the septal leaflet in diastole.

TRICUSPID REGURGITATION

A. **Definition.** Tricuspid regurgitation results from incompetence of the tricuspid valve, which allows regurgitation of blood into the right atrium during right ventricular systole.

B. **Epidemiology and General Comments.** Tricuspid regurgitation occurs most commonly as a result of right ventricular dilatation secondary to right ventricular strain or pulmonary hypertension. The tricuspid annulus is stretched, which causes separation of valve leaflets. Direct involvement of the valve leaflets is usually congenital or associated with tricuspid stenosis secondary to rheumatic fever. Occasionally in carcinoid syndrome fibrous plaques cause valve leaflet adherence to the right ventricular wall.

C. **History.** Generally patients tolerate tricuspid regurgitation well unless pulmonary hypertension coexists. Then, complaints are those of right-sided heart failure with painful hepatomegaly, ascites, and refractory edema, as well as reduced forward cardiac output.

D. **Physical Examination**
   1. *General.* Hepatomegaly, ascites, and peripheral edema are present.
   2. *Jugular Venous Pulse.* There are neck vein distension, large c-v waves with a rapid "y" descent, and hepatojugular reflux. The liver is often pulsatile before cirrhosis develops.
   3. *Lungs.* There are rales and often evidence of pulmonary hypertension.
   4. *Palpation.* There is hyperdynamic right ventricular thrust along the left parasternal border. An irregularly irregular rhythm consistent with atrial fibrillation is present.
   5. *Auscultation.* S2 has a loud P2 if there is pulmonary hypertension; S3 is often right-sided.
   6. *Murmurs*
      a. A high-pitched holosystolic murmur is heard best in the fourth intercostal space at the left sternal border; right ventricular enlargement may move the murmur closer to the apex.
      b. The murmur increases with inspiration and amyl nitrate administration; it decreases with standing and during the strain phase of the Valsalva maneuver.
      c. These changes with respiration help to distinguish the murmur from mitral regurgitation.

E. **Laboratory Findings**
   1. *ECG.* The ECG may show right atrial enlargement or right ventricular hypertrophy.
   2. *Chest X-Ray.* There is cardiomegaly caused by right atrial and right ventricular enlargement.
   3. *Echocardiography.* Right ventricular end-diastolic volume is increased, and there is paradoxic septal motion.

REFERENCES

1. Braunwald E: Mitral regurgitation: Physiologic, clinical, and surgical considerations. N Engl J Med 281:425, 1969.

This reviews basic physiology as it applies to clinical aspects of mitral regurgitation. It remains one of the clearest discussions of the subject.

2. Dohan MC, Criscitiello MG: Physiological and pharmacological manipulations of heart sounds and murmurs. Mod Concepts Cardiovasc Dis 39:121, 1970.

This review provides a thorough clinical and physiologic discussion of provocative bedside maneuvers useful in assessing valvular heart disease.

3. Johnson AD, et al.: The medical and surgical management of patients with aortic valve disease. West J Med 126:460, 1977.

This is an excellent general review of aortic stenosis and aortic regurgitation.

4. Morganroth J, et al.: Acute severe aortic regurgitation. Ann Intern Med 87:223, 1977.

This study reviews the causes, clinical features, and hemodynamic sequelae to acute aortic regurgitation. It pays particular attention to the use of echocardiography in evaluation.

5. Rapaport E: Natural history of aortic and mitral valve disease. Am J Cardiol 35:221, 1975.

An excellent brief review of the relationship between the extent of hemodynamic abnormality and the natural history of valvular diseases treated medically. Surgical implications are included for each category.

6. Rothman A, Goldberger AL: Aids to cardiac auscultation. Ann Intern Med 99:346, 1983.

This article is a critical review of the sensitivity and specificity of bedside maneuvers commonly used in physical diagnosis of valvular heart disease.

7. Selzer A, Cohn KE: Natural history of mitral stenosis: A review. Circulation 45:878, 1972.

This is still one of the best reviews of mitral stenosis.

PULMONARY CONDITIONS

9

ACUTE RESPIRATORY FAILURE

By SCOTT BARNHART, M.D.

DEFINITION

Acute respiratory failure (ARF) occurs when the body acutely fails to adequately eliminate carbon dioxide or to oxygenate the blood. As defined by arterial blood gases, ARF is an acute increase in $PaCO_2$ to > 50 mm Hg; an acute increase in $PaCO_2$ that produces a pH < 7.30; an acute decrease in PaO_2 to < 50 mm Hg; or any combination of these conditions.

EPIDEMIOLOGY AND PATHOPHYSIOLOGY

A. **Prevalence.** One survey showed that the most common nonsurgical causes of ARF were (1) drug overdoses, (2) neuromuscular disease, (3) adult respiratory distress syndrome, (4) chronic obstructive pulmonary disease (COPD), (5) pneumonia, and (6) cardiac failure.

B. **Pathophysiology.** ARF results from the interrelated processes of hypercapnia or hypoxemia.

    1. *Hypercapnia* results from hypoventilation relative to the amount of carbon dioxide that must be eliminated. Acutely it is associated with a reciprocal drop in the blood pH, which leads to respiratory acidosis. The major physiologic causes of hypercapnea include hypoventilation as a result of

        a. Neuromuscular weakness.

        b. Airflow obstruction.

        c. Increased dead space.

Increased production of carbon dioxide also contributes to hypercapnea and is frequently present in diseases leading to ARF.

    2. *Hypoxemia* has five possible physiologic causes:

        a. Decreased inspired oxygen tension

        b. Hypoventilation

        c. Ventilation-perfusion mismatch

        d. Shunt

        e. Diffusion limitation (rarely clinically significant)

More than one of these processes are often present in ARF.

DISEASES THAT CAUSE ARF

ARF can be separated into hypercapnic and hypoxemic ARF. More often than not, however, these conditions are found together. Table 9–1 presents the common causes of hypercapnia, and Table 9–2 presents the common causes of hypoxia.

TABLE 9–1. COMMON CAUSES OF HYPERCAPNIA

1. Drug overdose
2. Cerebrovascular accident, tumor, head trauma
3. Central hypoventilation
4. Myxedema
5. Diseases affecting the spinal cord
   a. Trauma
   b. Poliomyelitis
   c. Guillain-Barré syndrome
   d. Amyotrophic lateral sclerosis
6. Muscular dystrophy
7. Drug-induced neuromuscular disorders such as those secondary to aminoglycosides
8. Myasthenia gravis
9. Chest wall abnormalities:
   a. Flail chest
   b. Severe kyphoscoliosis
10. Airway obstruction
    a. Central (tracheal stenosis, tumor of the vocal cords)
    b. Peripheral (asthma, emphysema)
11. Pulmonary edema

CLINICAL MANIFESTATIONS

A. **Symptoms.** Dyspnea is frequently but not always part of the history of ARF. Symptoms associated with hypercapnia include headache, mild sedation, and confusion, which may progress to coma. Symptoms associated with hypoxia include confusion, agitation, restlessness, and dizziness.

B. **Signs.** The signs associated with hypoxia include those of a sympathetic response such as tachycardia, hypertension, and peripheral vasoconstriction, as well as sympathetic decompensation such as bradycardia and hypotension. Signs of hypercapnia include vasodilatation, diaphoresis, hypertension, and tachycardia. In addition, there is a constellation of physical signs that vary depending on the etiology of the ARF. For example, in COPD the ARF is associated with labored respirations and wheezing or decreased breath sounds on auscultation. In neuromuscular disorders a decreased rate or depth of respirations may be apparent with or without depressed consciousness.

C. **Prognostic Clinical Indicators.** Recent research has identified six specific clinical signs that have a statistically significant

TABLE 9–2. COMMON CAUSES OF HYPOXIA

1. Chronic obstructive pulmonary disease/asthma
2. Hypoventilation
3. ARDS
4. Acute pulmonary embolism
5. Pneumonia or atelectasis
6. Acute right-to-left shunt
7. Interstitial fibrosis

relationship to a need for mechanical ventilation or eventual death:

1. Pulse > 120 or < 70 beats per minute
2. Respiratory rate > 30
3. Palpable scalene muscle recruitment during inspiration
4. Palpable abdominal muscle tensing during expiration
5. Inability to perform vital capacity testing on command
6. Irregular irregularity of respiratory rhythm

RECOMMENDED DIAGNOSTIC APPROACH

When the clinician encounters a 50:50 arterial blood gas (ABG) sample in which PaO_2 and $PaCO_2$ approach 50 mm Hg, the diagnosis of ARF is suspected. If this has occurred acutely and the pH has decreased to less than 7.30, the diagnosis is confirmed. The challenge is then to establish the cause.

A. **Rule Out Life-Threatening Problems.** Problems must be ruled out that produce an immediate threat to life through marked hypoxemia, hypercapnia, and acidosis. If severe hypoxia or respiratory acidosis is present immediate steps must be taken to reverse them before an arrhythmia, circulatory collapse, or respiratory arrest occurs. Patients are evaluated for sufficient reserve to compensate for further deterioration in condition. Often respiratory failure can be reversed with the rapid institution of appropriate therapy such as oxygen for hypoxemia or bronchodilators for airflow obstruction. If this is not possible and hypercapnia and hypoxia persist, prompt intubation and mechanical ventilation are indicated.

B. **Evaluate Other Disease Possibilities**
   1. The history and physical examination usually narrow etiologic possibilities to a few diseases or processes.
   2. Anemia must be ruled out. Anemia can greatly increase the severity of ARF by producing tissue hypoxia, lactic acidosis, and eventually circulatory collapse. Rarely anemia may cause high output cardiac failure.
   3. The chest x-ray helps to limit the differential diagnoses. Many processes leading to ARF are associated with "clear" chest x-rays: airflow obstruction, pulmonary embolism, and central or neuromuscular causes of hypoventilation. Infiltrates on the chest x-ray suggest pneumonia, atelectasis, pulmonary edema secondary to cardiac failure, ARDS, or pulmonary fibrosis. Pneumothoraces also are evident on chest x-ray.
   4. An electrocardiogram helps to diagnose cardiac causes of respiratory failure, in particular, acute myocardial infarction and severe arrhythmias.

REFERENCES

1. Moser KM: Acute respiratory failure with hypercapnea. *In* Moser KM (ed.): Respiratory Emergencies. St. Louis, C V Mosby, 1982.
The most recent textbook on this subject.

2. Pontoppidan H, Geffin B, Lowenstein E: Acute respiratory failure in the adult. N Engl J Med 287:690–698, 1972.

A widely quoted review article.

3. Rogers RM, Jurers JA: Physiologic considerations in the treatment of acute respiratory failure. Basics of Respiratory Diseases, American Thoracic Society, American Lung Association 3:1–6, 1975.

The approach of a respected national organization.

---------------------10---------------------

THE ADULT RESPIRATORY DISTRESS SYNDROME

By RICHARD J. MAUNDER, M.D.

DESCRIPTION AND DIAGNOSTIC CRITERIA

A. Definition. The adult respiratory distress syndrome (ARDS) is a clinical syndrome of acute respiratory failure that occurs following major trauma, aspiration of gastric contents, systemic infection, and a variety of other precipitating and clinical events. Other terms used to describe ARDS include congestive atelectasis, shock lung, capillary leak syndrome, and noncardiogenic pulmonary edema.

B. Pathophysiologic Description. The pathogenesis of ARDS involves accumulation of inflammatory cells within the lung, followed by the release of inflammatory mediators capable of tissue injury. Damage to the alveolar-capillary membrane alters lung vascular permeability, causing accumulation of protein-rich interstitial and alveolar edema fluid. Reduced lung compliance and impaired gas exchange are the physiologic hallmarks of ARDS and are produced by the same mechanisms operative in cardiogenic pulmonary edema (see Chapter 4). Unlike congestive failure, however, the initial injury in ARDS is often followed by impaired surfactant function, cellular proliferation, disruption of alveolar architecture, and eventually lung fibrosis, which further impair pulmonary function and prolong the state of respiratory failure.

C. Criteria for Diagnosis. While a diverse spectrum of clinical events may lead to ARDS, the clinical features of the syndrome are remarkably uniform. The criteria for diagnosis are summarized in Table 10–1. Although generalized pulmonary infiltrates and hypoxemia are the key features of the syndrome, the patient must have clinical respiratory failure (tachypnea and labored breathing), and the onset must be acute, usually related temporally to a catastrophic clinical event such as the predisposing

TABLE 10–1.   DIAGNOSTIC CRITERIA FOR ARDS

1. Respiratory distress
   Tachypnea >25/minute
   Labored respirations
2. Hypoxemia
   PaO_2 <75 on FIO_2 ≥50% (0.5) or
   PaO_2/FIO_2 <175 or
   PaO_2/PAO_2 <0.3
3. Multilobar pulmonary infiltrates
4. Pulmonary artery wedge pressure ≤18 mm Hg
5. No alternative explanation for the above findings

conditions outlined in Table 10–2. Alternative explanations such as cardiac failure must be excluded.

EPIDEMIOLOGY

A. An estimated 150,000 patients develop ARDS annually.
B. The syndrome affects predominantly young people who previously had good health and occurs somewhat more frequently in males.
C. Mortality is approximately 60 per cent and has not changed appreciably over the last 20 years. Surprisingly, respiratory failure is only rarely the direct cause of death, with sepsis, often due to pulmonary infection, causing most ARDS deaths.
D. Survivors of ARDS generally do well, but approximately 40 per cent have residual abnormalities of pulmonary function, including airflow obstruction (25 per cent), low diffusing capacity (23 per cent), fall in PaO_2 with exercise (11 per cent), and reduced lung volumes.

PRESENTATION OF ARDS

A. History
   1. Clinical Risk Factors
      a. The clinical events associated with the greatest risk of ARDS are summarized in Table 10–2, along with the estimated incidence from recent series in the literature.
      b. To this list may be added more infrequent causes of the

TABLE 10–2.   RISK OF ARDS AFTER PREDISPOSING
CLINICAL CONDITIONS

Sepsis syndrome	20–40%
Aspiration of gastric contents	30–35%
Multiple transfusions (>15 units/24 hours)	26%
Long bone fractures	5– 8%
Pulmonary contusion	17%
Near-drowning	40%

syndrome such as drug overdose, pancreatitis, viral pneumonia, and various inhaled toxins (including oxygen).

c. The occurrence of multiple risks further enhances the likelihood of ARDS (26 per cent incidence with one predisposing risk, 41 per cent with two, and 54 per cent with three or more).

d. Although initially thought to be an important factor, in the absence of sepsis, shock is rarely (if ever) the only cause of ARDS.

e. The clinical events outlined in Table 10–2 are useful in predicting patients at increased risk for development of ARDS, but it is not known whether these events are related causally or are simply markers of severity of injury.

2. *Other Symptoms.* If the patient is conscious and alert, he may complain of breathlessness, but there are no other distinctive clinical features associated with ARDS. Mental status is commonly impaired in high-risk patients because of trauma, metabolic derangements, or medications. These problems make historical features of little value in the diagnosis of ARDS.

B. Clinical Features

1. The earliest sign in virtually all cases is respiratory distress. Most commonly this is associated with hypoxemia and hyperventilation (low $PaCO_2$). Since hypoxemia is predominantly caused by venoarterial shunting, PaO_2 improves minimally with increases in FIO_2. Characteristically, there is dramatic improvement with the application of positive end-expiratory pressure (PEEP), but this does not occur in all patients.

2. Most frequently, there is radiographic progression from a normal chest x-ray to a finely dispersed interstitial edema pattern, and eventually to generalized bilateral infiltrates. The process may be "patchy" in 20 to 30 per cent of cases, depending on etiology and associated conditions.

3. Reduced lung compliance occurs in most cases of established ARDS, but, particularly in the early stages, compliance may be normal.

4. Elevated pulmonary artery pressure is frequently reported, particularly in ARDS caused by sepsis. In the early stages it is probably the result of vasoactive mediators released during acute lung inflammation. Later in the course, pulmonary hypertension may be caused by thromboembolic occlusion or actual destruction of pulmonary microvasculature.

C. Timing of ARDS

1. The majority of patients who develop ARDS do so within 24 hours after the inciting clinical event. In fact, development of ARDS at later than 72 hours after risk onset should suggest the interim development of a second risk event such as sepsis or aspiration.

2. The natural history of ARDS is extremely variable. Approximately a third of patients respond to appropriate therapy of the underlying illness or injury and demonstrate steady improvement in pulmonary function and roentgenographic abnormalities in the first week. Approximately one third

(usually those with ongoing illness such as systemic infection) show progression despite treatment and never recover. Another third show initial signs of stabilization and improvement but develop complications such as sepsis, which lead to clinical deterioration. Frequently, this group develops what might be termed "chronic ARDS," with extensive pulmonary fibrosis and long-term gas exchange abnormalities. Survival depends on adequate supportive respiratory care and prevention of complications.

DIFFERENTIAL DIAGNOSIS

Table 10–3 provides a general listing of alternative explanations or diagnoses to consider for patients suspected of having ARDS.

A. **Misinterpretation of the Chest Roentgenograph.** The interpretation of chest x-rays made in critically ill patients is fraught with difficulty. The use of portable x-ray equipment, the anteroposterior projection, and supine positioning inevitably reduce the quality of the image obtained. The patient is often not able to cooperate owing to pain or obtundation. Inadequate lung inflation or motion artifact may produce a picture resembling ARDS when no abnormality is present. Pleural fluid collections in a supine patient may lead to confusion by producing diffuse haziness of the lung fields. Artifacts may appear as a result of processes outside the lung parenchyma, such as massive subcutaneous emphysema or the presence of a body cast over the thorax.

B. **Chronic Lung Disease.** The clinician must distinguish whether the process is acute or chronic. Patients with interstitial fibrosis, lymphangitic carcinoma, chronic airflow obstruction, and other respiratory conditions may meet the radiographic or gas exchange criteria outlined in Table 10–1. ARDS, on the other

TABLE 10–3.   DIFFERENTIAL DIAGNOSIS IN ARDS

1. Misinterpretation of chest x-ray
   - Poor lung inflation
   - Pleural effusions (in supine patient)
   - Inadequate x-ray penetration
2. Chronic lung disease
   - Scarring disorders (sarcoidosis, idiopathic pulmonary fibrosis, asbestosis)
   - Allergic alveolitis
   - Lymphangitic carcinomatosis
   - Chronic obstructive pulmonary disease
3. Pulmonary infection
   - Viral pneumonia
   - Diffuse gram-negative pneumonia
   - Tuberculosis
   - Disseminated fungal infection
4. Hydrostatic pulmonary edema
   - Cardiac failure
   - Volume overload

hand, represents the *acute* development of these findings, usually in association with a known precipitant.

C. **Pulmonary Infection.** A variety of pathogens, most commonly viral, can produce diffuse pulmonary infiltrates and hypoxemia, particularly in immunocompromised patients. While direct parenchymal invasion and spread is the presumed mechanism of injury, blood-borne mediators may also be involved. Most workers would include viral pneumonia as a cause of ARDS. Occasionally, however, a bacterial or fungal pneumonia may become generalized with endobronchial spread to produce a clinical picture resembling ARDS. The distinction between parenchymal infection and ARDS related to other causes is in part semantic. Alterations in pulmonary physiology and even microstructural changes may be similar, as is the approach to ventilatory management. Nonetheless, recognizing lung infection is extremely important, since specific antimicrobial therapy is often available.

D. **Hydrostatic Pulmonary Edema.** Pulmonary edema as a result of cardiac failure produces a clinical picture that often is indistinguishable from ARDS. The clinical setting, associated symptoms, and prior history may be helpful, but a firm diagnosis of ARDS requires documentation of a normal pulmonary artery wedge pressure. The cut-off in Table 10–1 (≤18 mm Hg) assures that lung edema is not entirely caused by elevated hydrostatic forces, that is, vascular permeability is definitely increased. Occasionally, volume expansion during resuscitation contributes to pulmonary edema in ARDS patients. Measurement of edema fluid protein has been used to detect altered vascular permeability when ARDS is complicated by volume overload (see the discussion of laboratory tests).

RECOMMENDED DIAGNOSTIC APPROACH

A. **Arterial Blood Gases.** Measurement of arterial blood gases is required, since hypoxemia is one of the diagnostic criteria for ARDS (Table 10–1). In the early stages, respiratory alkalosis is a characteristic finding. Long-term ARDS frequently leads to increased dead space, impairing CO_2 elimination and causing hypercarbia.

B. **Chest Roentgenograph.** Documentation of bilateral multilobar infiltrates is required for the diagnosis of ARDS. Classically, the roentgenographic changes are described as diffuse, but the process is frequently patchy. The presence of pleural effusions is unusual in ARDS and should raise the suspicion of pulmonary infection, traumatic hemothorax, or superimposed cardiac failure.

C. **Hematologic Parameters.** Thrombocytopenia occurs commonly in patients with ARDS (30 to 50 per cent). Evidence of disseminated intravascular coagulation occurs in approximately 20 per cent. There are no consistent changes in hematocrit or peripheral white cell counts.

D. **Edema Fluid Protein.** If a sufficient volume of edema fluid can be obtained, measurement of an edema fluid:plasma protein ratio may be useful in distinguishing ARDS from cardiogenic edema. A ratio of greater than 0.7 indicates increased permeability, while one of less than 0.5 suggests edema caused by elevated hydrostatic pressures.

E. **Microbiology.** Cultures of sputum or endotracheal aspirate are useful to diagnose pulmonary infection. Occasionally, more invasive techniques such as bronchoscopy or open-lung biopsy are required to obtain adequate specimens for this purpose.

REFERENCES

1. Balk R, Bone RC: The adult respiratory distress syndrome. Med Clin North Am 67:685–701, 1983.
2. Hudson LD: Causes of the adult respiratory distress syndrome—clinical recognition. Clin Chest Med 2:195–212, 1982.
3. Pepe PE, Potkin RT, Reus DH, Hudson LD, Carrico CJ: Clinical predictors of the adult respiratory distress syndrome. Am J Surg 144:124–129, 1982.
4. Petty TL, Ashbaugh DG: The adult respiratory distress syndrome: Clinical features, factors influencing prognosis, and principles of management. Chest 60:233–239, 1971.
5. Ralph D, Robertson HT: Respiratory gas exchange in adult respiratory distress syndrome. Semin Respir Med 3:114–122, 1981.
6. Rinaldo JE, Rogers RM: Adult respiratory distress syndrome—changing concepts of lung injury and repair. N Engl J Med 306:900–909, 1982.

---11---

COUGH

By SCOTT BARNHART, M.D.

GENERAL COMMENTS

Cough is defined as the sudden rapid expulsion of air through the glottis to expel mucus or other materials. It is the result of the coordination of several actions, and it acts as one of the host's respiratory defense mechanisms. There are three phases to the cough mechanism: (1) deep inspiration, (2) closure of the glottis and contraction of the muscles of expiration, and (3) opening of the glottis to allow air to rapidly exit the tracheobronchial tree and carry out materials in the airways. The neural control of the cough mechanism involves vagal afferents from receptors in the larynx, bronchi, and trachea, as well as trigeminal, glossopharyngeal, and phrenic afferents from receptors in the nose, sinuses, ear canals (vagal), pleura, stomach, pericardium, and diaphragm. Cough receptors respond to chemical and mechanical stimuli. They are most common in the larger airways and are not present beyond the respiratory bronchioles.

DIFFERENTIAL DIAGNOSIS

The most likely acute cause of a cough is a viral upper respiratory tract infection. For chronic or persistent cough the most likely causes are (1) cough secondary to postnasal drip (29 per cent), (2) asthma (25 per cent), (3) asthma and postnasal drip (18 per cent), chronic bronchitis (12 per cent), (4) gastroesophageal reflux (10 per cent), and (5) miscellaneous disorders (6 per cent). The acute and chronic causes of cough are listed in Table 11–1.

CLINICAL MANIFESTATIONS

A. History

1. **Onset and Duration.** Acute dry coughs that later become productive and are associated with flu or coldlike symptoms are likely to be caused by an upper respiratory infection. A chronic productive cough in a smoker is most likely to be caused by chronic bronchitis.

2. **Color.** Clear phlegm is evidence against infection, and yellow or green phlegm, especially if it has recently changed color, suggests infection. Bloody sputum or blood-flecked phlegm supports the diagnosis of hemoptysis and should be carefully evaluated.

3. **Amount of Phlegm.** Early viral infections, cough related to postnasal drip, psychogenic cough, and cough from irritation of receptors outside the lower respiratory tract are often dry. Deep wet coughs productive of sputum suggest a source in the lower respiratory tract. Large quantities of phlegm (up to a cup per day) may signify bronchiectasis.

TABLE 11–1.   ACUTE AND CHRONIC CAUSES OF COUGH

1. Postnasal drip
2. Asthma
3. Chronic bronchitis
4. Upper respiratory tract infection
5. Pneumonia
6. Foreign body
7. Hemoptysis
8. Pulmonary embolism
9. Aspiration
10. Reflux
11. Left ventricular failure
12. Sarcoidosis
13. Neoplastic disease, including bronchogenic carcinoma or metastatic disease
14. Inhalation of allergens or irritant gases and fumes, including cigarette smoke
15. Irritation of receptors outside the lower respiratory tract, including ear canals, diaphragm, pleura, nose, and pharynx
16. Bronchiectasis
17. Psychogenic factors

4. ***Associated Symptoms.*** Dyspnea or wheezing, or both, suggest asthma, pulmonary embolism, infiltrative disease, or pneumonia, among other causes of cough. Paroxysmal nocturnal dyspnea and orthopnea may suggest a cardiac origin. Patients with a history of allergies or hay fever are at an increased risk for sinus problems or asthma. Hoarseness suggests a lesion that directly involves the vocal cords or indirectly involves them, such as a tumor affecting the recurrent laryngeal nerve. Fever and chills suggest infection. Chest pain suggests esophageal reflux or ischemic heart disease leading to left ventricular failure and pulmonary edema.

B. **Physical Examination.** Attention should be paid to (1) vital signs, including respiratory rate and temperature; (2) tenderness of sinuses, which suggests sinusitis; (3) discharge or inflammation of the nasopharynx, (4) adenopathy suggesting infection or malignancy, (5) stridor, hoarseness, or visible lesion of the larynx on laryngoscopy, (6) the lungs, for wheezes, rales, rhonchi, or decreased breath sounds, and (7) the cardiovascular system, for evidence of heart failure with elevated jugular venous pressure, gallops, or murmurs.

LABORATORY STUDIES

A cough of acute onset and short duration associated with a history and examination suggestive of an upper respiratory infection probably does not require further evaluation unless it fails to resolve. Chronic coughs usually require further evaluation with the following studies:

A. **Sputum Examination.** This should include the general appearance and quantity, Gram's stain, culture, and acid-fast bacillus smears and culture if indicated. If an allergic cause is suspected, a Wright's stain for eosinophils may be useful.

B. **Chest X-Ray**

C. **Spirometry**

D. **Sinus Films**

E. **Bronchoscopy and Laryngoscopy**

RECOMMENDED DIAGNOSTIC APPROACH

The history and physical examination usually greatly narrow the differential diagnoses and suggest the most fruitful approach to pursue. The next step is to obtain a chest x-ray. If the chest x-ray is negative the most likely cause is asthma, which can be diagnosed by spirometry or bronchial inhalation challenge, or both. Asthma is far more likely to cause cough than is an endobronchial tumor or foreign body. If these tests are negative, one of the other potential diagnoses should be pursued, with the evaluation often including an examination of the larynx and airways by bronchoscopy.

REFERENCES

1. Irwin RS, Rosen MJ, Braman MD: Cough; a comprehensive review. Arch Intern Med 137:1186, 1977.
2. Corrao WM, Braman SS, Irwin RS: Chronic cough as the sole presenting manifestation of bronchial asthma. N Engl J Med 300:633, 1979.
3. Irwin RS, Corrao WM, Pratter MR: Chronic persistent cough in the adult: The spectrum and frequency of causes and successful outcome of specific therapy. Am Rev Respir Dis 123:414–417, 1981.
4. Poe RH, Israel RH, Utell MJ, Hall WJ: Chronic cough: Bronchoscopy or pulmonary function testing? Am Rev Respir Dis 126:160–162, 1982.

12
HEMOPTYSIS

By SCOTT BARNHART, M.D.

EPIDEMIOLOGY AND GENERAL COMMENTS

Hemoptysis is defined as the coughing of blood from below the larynx. It must be carefully differentiated from the coughing of blood that has trickled down from the nasopharynx or been vomited or derived from the upper gastrointestinal tract. Massive hemoptysis is defined as hemoptysis of 200 to 600 cc over 24 to 48 hours. Massive hemoptysis is a life-threatening process that must be aggressively evaluated and treated. Hemoptysis may arise out of sources fed by systemic or pulmonary arteries. Disruption of bronchial epithelium and capillaries by tracheobronchitis, injury to pulmonary parenchyma by infarction or necrotizing process, or acute pulmonary venous hypertension, as from mitral stenosis, all may lead to hemoptysis.

DIFFERENTIAL DIAGNOSIS

The most common cause of hemoptysis is bronchitis. Other common causes of hemoptysis include (1) chronic suppurative processes, (2) tuberculosis, (3) other infections, including necrotizing pneumonias, (4) neoplasms, and (5) pulmonary embolism. Tables 12–1 and 12–2 list the causes of hemoptysis.

CLINICAL MANIFESTATIONS

A. **History.** The history should carefully attempt to differentiate between true hemoptysis and blood arising from the gastrointestinal tract or nasopharynx. Blood from the gastrointestinal tract is frequently vomited, dark, acidic, never frothy, and may contain food particles. Important elements in the history include (1) the

TABLE 12-1. CAUSES OF HEMOPTYSIS*

1. Bronchogenic carcinoma (56)
2. Lung abscess (49)
3. Pulmonary infarct (44)
4. Bronchiectasis (43)
5. Tuberculosis (36)
6. Congenital cyst (25)
7. Empyema (24)
8. Metastatic disease
9. Arteriovenous fistula
10. Bronchitis
11. Bronchoaorto fistula
12. Broncholithiasis
13. Foreign body
14. Goodpasture's syndrome
15. Idiopathic pulmonary hemosiderosis
16. Mycetoma
17. Parasitic infection
18. Left ventricular failure
19. Trauma
20. Wegener's granulomatosis

*The frequency with which hemoptysis is associated with a disease is indicated by numbers in parentheses.

patient's age; (2) onset, duration, and amount of blood; (3) the character of the hemoptysis, that is, bright red frothy blood of small flecks mixed in with purulent sputum; (4) respiratory history, including previous history of tuberculosis; (5) smoking history; and (6) history of cardiac disease.

B. **Physical Examination.** Close attention should be paid to the following: (1) gross examination of the sputum; (2) vital signs, including respiratory rate and fever; (3) examination of the nasopharynx for a source of the bleeding; (4) adenopathy; (5) the lungs, for wheezes or rhonchi suggesting chronic obstructive pulmonary disease, rales suggesting pneumonia, and (6) the heart, for evidence of left ventricular failure or mitral stenosis. If the hemoptysis is massive, immediate attention must be directed at the patient's ability to maintain a patent airway as well as oxygenation and ventilation. Pulmonary and thoracic surgery consultations should be obtained early.

TABLE 12-2. COMMON CAUSES OF MASSIVE HEMOPTYSIS*

1. Tuberculosis (49%)
2. Bronchiectasis (22%)
3. Lung abscess (12%)
4. Carcinoma (3%)

*The figures in parentheses indicate the percentage of cases of massive hemoptysis caused by the listed disease.

LABORATORY EXAMINATIONS

The choice of laboratory examinations depends on the history and physical examination results. The following should be considered in every case of hemoptysis: (1) chest x-ray; (2) sputum, studied by Gram's stain, culture, and acid-fast bacillus smear and culture; (3) skin test with purified protein derivative; (4) complete blood count; (5) prothrombin time; (6) sputum cytology; (7) arterial blood gas; and (8) bronchoscopy.

RECOMMENDED DIAGNOSTIC APPROACH

Almost all cases should be evaluated with a chest x-ray and sputum examination and should have active or inactive tuberculosis ruled out. The next step is dictated by the history, examination, and the results of the above-mentioned studies. If it is likely that the hemoptysis is caused by bronchitis, the patient should be observed and further evaluated with bronchoscopy only if the hemoptysis is persistent (for two or more weeks), the hemoptysis is recurrent, or malignancy is suspected for some other reason, such as weight loss. Other indications include undiagnosed infections such as tuberculosis. If the chest x-ray suggests bronchiectasis or pneumonia, close observation is warranted. Signs and symptoms or radiographic evidence supporting the diagnosis of malignancy should be evaluated promptly with bronchoscopy. Other suspected etiologies should be pursued as indicated. These studies may include bronchoscopy, bronchography, tomography, ventilation-perfusion scans, angiography, sputum cytology, and examination for fungal or parasitic infection. In the case of massive hemoptysis, immediate attention is directed to (1) the assessment of airway and respiratory reserve; (2) identification of the site of bleeding, usually by rigid bronchoscopy followed by bronchial or pulmonary artery angiography as indicated; and (3) candidacy for surgery or other procedures such as arterial embolization.

REFERENCES

1. Pierson DJ: Hemoptysis, weekly update. Princeton, Pulmonary Medicine Biomedica Inc., 1978.
2. Wolfe JD, Simmons DH: Hemoptysis: Diagnosis and management. West J Med 127:383–390, 1970.
3. Lyons HA: Differential diagnosis of hemoptysis and its treatment. Basics of Respiratory Disease, American Thoracic Society, 1976.
4. Garzon AA, Gourin A: Surgical management of massive hemoptysis. Ann Surg 187:267, 1974.

PLEURAL EFFUSIONS

By SCOTT BARNHART, M.D.

DEFINITION

Whenever more than 10 to 20 mL of pleural fluid accumulates in the pleural space the patient is said to have a pleural effusion.

A. **Pathophysiology.** Up to 2 to 3 L of fluid cross the pleural space each day. The passage of this fluid through the pleural space is governed by opposing hydrostatic and oncotic pressures in the parietal, visceral, and intrapleural spaces. The net effect of these pressures is the passage of fluid from the parietal pleura into the pleural space, followed by absorption by the visceral pleura and the lymphatics. The normal pleural space has a net negative pressure, which prevents the accumulation of fluid. Any process that upsets this balance leads to the development of an effusion.

B. **Recognition.** Symptoms include breathlessness and pleuritic chest pain; signs include decreased breath sounds, dullness to percussion, and evidence of fluid on chest radiographs or ultrasound. A lateral decubitus radiograph can demonstrate the presence of free-flowing fluid.

Pleural effusions are classified as either *exudates* or *transudates*. Exudates generally result from diseases that directly involve the pleura and should be fully explained. An exudate is considered present if the fluid has one or more of the following criteria.

1. Protein concentration greater than 3 g/dL
2. Pleural fluid lactic acid dehydrogenase (LDH) to serum LDH ratio greater than 0.6
3. An LDH greater than 200 IU

Transudates result from processes that do not directly involve the pleura. Further investigation of transudates is unnecessary other than efforts to establish the primary process.

DIFFERENTIAL DIAGNOSIS

A. **Transudates.** In general, two types of processes produce transudative pleural effusions: first, diseases associated with hypoproteinemia, such as cirrhosis, nephrotic syndrome, or malnutrition, and second, diseases associated with elevated venous pressure, primarily heart failure.

B. **Exudative Pleural Effusions.** These are most likely caused by (1) inflammation of the pleura secondary to infection, as with a parapneumonic effusion or an empyema, (2) malignancy, (3) autoimmune disease, (4) pulmonary thromboemboli (which are exudative two thirds of the time and transudative one third of

121

TABLE 13–1. MAJOR CAUSES OF PLEURAL
TRANSUDATES AND EXUDATES*

Transudative pleural effusions
  A. Congestive heart failure (common)
  B. Cirrhosis
  C. Nephrotic syndrome
  D. Myxedema
  E. Hypoproteinemia
  F. Meig's syndrome
  G. Sarcoidosis

Exudative pleural effusions
  A. Infectious causes
    1. Bacterial infections
       a. *Staphylococcus aureus* (50%)
       b. *S. pneumoniae* (11%)
    2. Tuberculosis (38%)
    3. Viral, mycoplasma (less than 20%)
    4. Fungal (common with *Nocardia* and *Actinomyces*)
    5. Parasites (frequent with *Entameoba histolitica,* rare with *Pneumocystis carini* and *Echinococcus granulosus*)
  B. Neoplasms
  C. Collagen vascular
    1. Rheumatoid arthritis (rare)
    2. Systemic lupus erythematosis (20–70%)
  D. Pulmonary embolus
  E. Gastrointestinal
    1. Pancreatitis (40%)
    2. Esophageal rupture (common)
    3. Subphrenic abscess
  F. Trauma
  G. Postoperative (50% after abdominal surgery)

*Figures in parentheses indicate the percentage of a given cause that has associated effusions.

the time), and (5) pancreatitis. Table 13–1 lists the common causes of pleural effusions and gives estimates of the frequency with which an effusion is associated with the process.

HISTORY AND PHYSICAL EXAMINATION

A. **History.** Dyspnea is the most common finding. Other prominent symptoms include pleuritic chest pain and cough or symptoms associated with an inflammatory or neoplastic process. Frequently small pleural effusions are clinically silent.

B. **Signs.** Pleural effusions of less than 200 to 300 cu cm are difficult to detect by physical examination or chest radiographs. If effusions of greater than 200 cu cm are present, the patient may have dullness to percussion, decreased breath sounds at the bases, and egophony just above the level of decreased breath sounds.

RECOMMENDED DIAGNOSTIC APPROACH

A. *First, the presence of a pleural effusion must be confirmed radiographically.* Approximately 200 cu cm of fluid must accumulate in the pleural space before it becomes evident on a posteroanterior chest radiograph. The absence of free-flowing fluid does not rule out a pleural effusion, but rather suggests that the fluid has become loculated or that some other pleural process is occurring.

B. *Second, a thoracentesis is performed.* This leads to a diagnostic explanation of approximately 90 per cent of pleural effusions. A thoracentesis is omitted for patients in whom the risk of a pneumothorax from the thoracentesis is greater than the benefits of a specific diagnosis.

C. *Third, the pleural fluid is analyzed.* The fluid is classified as a transudate or an exudate with measurement of protein and LDH (see Table 13–2). The following characteristics of the fluid are examined:

1. *Appearance.* The general appearance of the fluid may serve as a guide for which additional studies should be ordered. Clear straw-colored fluid can be either exudate or transudate. Turbid fluid suggests an exudate with increased leukocytes, protein, or lipids. Frank pus is obvious and a foul odor suggests an anaerobic empyema.

2. *Bloody Effusions.* Bloody effusions are difficult to interpret, since it takes little blood (1 cu cm in 500 cu cm) to produce a pink or red tinge, and the fluid often becomes contaminated with blood from the thoracentesis. Exudative pleural effusions that are genuinely bloody suggest tuberculosis, malignancy, trauma, and pulmonary emboli. Pulmonary emboli may also induce a transudative effusion.

3. *White Cell Count and Differential Count.* More than 1000 white blood cells per cu mm suggests an exudate, and over 25,000 white blood cells per cu mm suggests an empyema. A predominance of polymorphonuclear cells is consistent with an early inflammatory lesion as would be seen in an empyema, parapneumonic effusion, pulmonary embolus, or systemic lupus. Mononuclear cells are more common in chronic inflammatory processes or in transudates. Eosinophils suggest a pneumothorax, hemothorax, asbestosis, or drug, parasitic, autoimmune, sarcoid, or fungal pleural disease.

4. *Gram's Stain and Culture.* Gram's stain and culture should be done immediately on all exudates to rule out an infected pleural space that requires early drainage. Careful bacteriologic techniques should be used when an anaerobic infection is suspected, and acid-fast bacillus and cultures should be obtained whenever tuberculosis is suspected.

5. *Glucose.* Low glucose levels are associated with pleural disease caused by rheumatoid arthritis, empyema, tuberculosis, and esophageal rupture.

6. *Amylase.* Elevated pleural fluid amylase levels suggest either pancreatic disease (pancreatitis or pseudocyst) or esophageal

TABLE 13–2. SUMMARY OF LABORATORY FINDINGS IN PLEURAL EFFUSIONS

	Appearance	White Blood Cell Count (per mm³)	Predominant Cell Type	Gram's Stain	Glucose	Other
Transudate	Serous	<1000	Mononuclear	Negative	Equal to serum	
Exudate						
Parapneumonic	Serous	5000–25,000	Polymorphonuclear neutrophil (PMN)	Negative	May be low	
Empyema	Cloudy	Innumerable	PMN	May be positive		
Tuberculosis	Serosanguinous	>1000	Mononuclear	Acid-fast bacillus	White low	
Malignancy	Serosanguinous	<1000	Mononuclear	Negative	Normal	Cytology positive (40%)
Pulmonary embolism	Serous or serosanguinous	1000–100,000	Red blood cell	Negative	Normal	
Rheumatoid arthritis	Cloudy to serous	1000–2000	Mononuclear	Negative	Low	
Pancreatitis	Cloudy	5000–20,000	None	Negative	Normal	Amylase

rupture. Amylase isoenzymes may be useful in differentiating between the sources if they are not clinically apparent.

7. *Cytology.* Cytology can establish that a neoplasm is the source of a pleural effusion. With neoplastic involvement of the pleura, the yield is approximately 50 per cent. Needle biopsy has been shown to increase the diagnostic yield to 60 to 90 per cent. The most common malignancies that produce a pleural effusion are (1) lung, (2) breast, (3) ovary, and (4) stomach.

8. *pH.* A pH of less than 7.30 suggests an exudate, especially one caused by empyema, rheumatoid disease, malignancy, or esophageal rupture.

9. *Other Studies.* Sudan stains for lipids can determine whether the thoracic duct has been ruptured. Examination for immune complexes and complement can help determine whether there is an autoimmune process.

D. *Fourth, closed pleural biopsy, pleuroscopy, or open pleural biopsy is considered.* The indication for a pleural biopsy is an unexplained exudative effusion. The biopsy is most useful to diagnose tuberculosis or carcinomatous involvement of the pleura. Needle biopsy in combination with pleural fluid cytology yields a diagnosis approximately 70 per cent of the time in tuberculosis and in up to 90 per cent of the time in malignancy. In recent years pleuroscopy has been used to diagnose the etiology of pleural effusions when results of closed needle biopsy have been negative. In an undiagnosed effusion, pleuroscopy may increase the diagnostic yield approximately 20 per cent.

REFERENCES

1. Sahn SA: The differential diagnosis of pleural effusions. West J Med 137:99–108, 1982.
2. Light RW, Macgregor I, Luchsinger PC: Pleural effusions: The diagnostic separation of transudates and exudates. Ann Intern Med 77:507–513, 1972.
3. Hirsch A, Ruffie P, Nebut M, Bignon J, Chretien J: Pleural effusion: Laboratory tests in 300 cases. Thorax 34:106–112, 1979.
4. Fraser RG, Pare JAP: Diagnosis of diseases of the chest. Philadelphia, W. B. Saunders Company, 1977, pp. 314–318.
5. Hinshaw HC, Murray JF: Diseases of the chest. 4th ed. Philadelphia, W. B. Saunders Company, 1980, pp. 883–918.

These five references are an excellent source of information on differential diagnoses of pleural effusions and the utility of the various laboratory tests.

PLEURITIC CHEST PAIN

By PATRICIA SATO, M.D.

DEFINITION

Pleuritic chest pain is caused by stretching or rubbing of the inflamed parietal pleura. It is usually described as sharp, knifelike, and superficial. It is characteristically aggravated by changes in body position, coughing, or deep inspiration because these actions stretch the pleura or oppose the inflamed surface to other structures.

The pain is easily localized and is supplied by segmental nerves. Because the parietal pleura shares innervation with other somatic afferents, it is referred to more superficial regions supplied by the intercostal nerves and thoracic segments. The pain may also be referred to the shoulder if the diaphragmatic pleura (C3 to C5) is inflamed or to the abdomen if the lower intercostals are involved. The lung parenchyma and visceral pleura are innervated by visceral afferents, which cause a vague poorly localizable pain.

DIFFERENTIAL DIAGNOSIS

A. Table 14–1 provides a comprehensive list of conditions that may manifest themselves with pleuritic chest pain. Unfortunately, the frequency of these diagnoses for the whole population has not been established. The data currently available come from a retrospective study of 97 patients below 40 years of age in whom lung scanning was performed as part of the diagnostic evaluation. In this specific patient population the most common cause was viral or idiopathic pleurisy, which occurred 53 per cent of the time. Pulmonary embolism occurred in 21 per cent of patients and infectious pneumonitis in 18 per cent.

B. The key point in evaluation is diagnosing a condition that requires specific treatment as opposed to one that only requires symptomatic relief.

TABLE 14–1. DIFFERENTIAL DIAGNOSES

Viral pleurisy	Uremia
Pulmonary embolism or infarction	Osteoarthritis of the thoracic spine
Pneumonia	Ruptured cervical discs
Pericarditis	Mediastinal tumors
Neoplasm	Mediastinitis
Pneumothorax	Subdiaphragmatic abscess
Empyema	Splenic infarction
Tuberculosis	Pancreatitis
Rib fractures	Ruptured aortic aneurysm
Costochondritis	Sarcoidosis
Connective tissue disorders	

HISTORY AND PHYSICAL EXAMINATION: DISTINGUISHING FEATURES OF SEVERAL MAJOR CAUSES OF PLEURITIC CHEST PAIN

A. **Viral Pleuritis (Usually Coxsackie B, Bornholm Disease).** This condition is preceded by an upper respiratory infection or a generalized viral prodrome and usually has a several-day history of pleuritic chest pain. A low-grade fever may be present, and the chest roentgenogram usually reveals no infiltrate and, if present, only a small effusion. The virus may be harvested from the pleural fluid to confirm the diagnosis, but usually the diagnosis is made by exclusion.

B. **Pulmonary Embolism or Infarction.** Pleuritic chest pain may be caused by pulmonary embolism or infarction. There should be greater suspicion when the risk factors of venous stasis, obesity, immobilization, surgery, oral contraceptive use, and prior cardiopulmonary disease are present. The usual history is that of sudden onset of pain with dyspnea. Physical examination may show tachypnea, tachycardia, a pleural rub, and evidence of deep venous thrombosis. The chest roentgenogram may show basilar linear atelectasis, a small pleural effusion, a new peripheral infiltrate, or normal findings.

C. **Pneumonia.** Infectious pneumonitis is often associated with pleuritic chest pain. The signs and symptoms of fever and productive cough should be present as well as an infiltrate on chest roentgenogram. Bacterial pneumonias are more likely to cause pleuritic chest pain than atypical pneumonias.

D. **Pericarditis.** The visceral and parietal pericardial surfaces are ordinarily insensitive to pain except for the lower portion of the parietal pericardium. The pain associated with pericarditis is secondary to inflammation of the adjacent parietal pleura. The physician should carefully listen for a pericardial rub and look for typical electrocardiographic findings.

E. **Neoplasm.** Tumor involvement of the pleura, either primary or metastatic, may cause pleural pain. This is a common picture in patients with a history of asbestos exposure who are ultimately found to have mesothelioma. Primary lung cancer also may directly involve the pleura. Sites of primary tumors that most commonly metastasize to the pleura are the gastrointestinal tract, breast, lung, and ovaries.

F. **Connective Tissue Disorders**

   1. *Systemic Lupus Erythematosus.* Pleural involvement occurs most commonly with lupus erythematosus and rheumatoid arthritis, in that order. The pleurisy with lupus generally occurs when the disease is active. If pleural fluid is present, initially it is an inflammatory exudate with a predominance of polymorphonuclear neutrophils with a low pH and glucose. The presence of lupus erythematosus cells in the fluid confirms the diagnosis (with 100 per cent specificity and approximately 85 per cent sensitivity). A high pleural fluid antinuclear antibody titer ($\geq$ 1:160) also supports the diagnosis.

   2. *Rheumatoid Arthritis.* Although rheumatoid arthritis is more

common in women, rheumatoid pleurisy is more common in men, particularly those with rheumatoid nodules and high rheumatoid factor titers. Pleural effusions are present in 3 to 5 per cent of rheumatoid arthritis patients, but pleurisy may occur in the absence of an effusion. Rheumatoid pleurisy usually occurs in conjunction with flare-up of articular disease. Rheumatoid factor may be detected in the pleural fluid but it is not pathognomonic. Strongly supportive evidence are a glucose level less than 30 mg/100 ml, lactic acid dehydrogenase level greater than 500 IU/l, and pH around 7.00.

RECOMMENDED DIAGNOSTIC APPROACH

A. **History.** Key points to elicit are history of a preceding viral illness, symptoms of pneumonia, predisposing factors for pulmonary embolism, chest trauma, and other systemic illnesses.

B. **Physical Examination.** Patients should be examined for pulmonary consolidation, pleural effusion, a pleural friction rub, a pericardial rub, and point tenderness of the thoracic cage, which may occur with rib fractures, costochondritis, or spinal disease. A careful abdominal examination may detect subdiaphragmatic disease manifested as pleural pain.

C. **Chest Roentgenogram.** Posteroanterior and lateral chest roentgenograms are indicated in virtually all cases of pleuritic pain. These may identify specific problems such as pneumothorax, pneumonia, asbestos-related diseases, neoplasm, or rib fractures. Also, they can confirm the presence of parenchymal involvement or a pleural effusion.

D. **Laboratory Examination.** Other screening tests that may aid in diagnosis include:

1. Complete blood count
2. Electrolytes, blood urea nitrogen, and creatinine levels
3. Gram's stain and culture of sputum
4. Purified protein derivative skin test
5. Serum amylase determination
6. Electrocardiogram

If a pleural effusion is present with pleuritic chest pain, usually it is quite small, since larger effusions tend to relieve the pain. If there is a sufficient quantity, this fluid may be aspirated and analyzed for cell count, microbiology, chemistry, cytology, and immunology to confirm or exclude a diagnosis. However, the findings still may be nonspecific (see the discussion of pleural effusions). If the cause of the pain is not readily apparent, three clinical features help point to the diagnosis of pulmonary embolism as outlined in the previously mentioned study of acute pleurisy in young adults. Lung scanning was recommended if any of the following were present: (1) pleural effusion(s), (2) history of predisposing factors or of veno-occlusive disease, and (3) physical findings indicative of phlebitis. The lung scan may rule out the diagnosis, demonstrate characteristic findings of pulmonary embolism, or give indeterminate findings (see the discussion of pulmonary embolism).

If a diagnosis cannot be confirmed and all test results remain negative, it can be presumed that the patient has viral or idiopathic pleurisy. The patient can be treated symptomatically with anti-inflammatory agents and should receive close follow-up, particularly if the pain recurs.

REFERENCES

1. Branch WT, McNeil BJ: Analysis of the differential diagnosis and assessment of pleuritic chest pain in young adults. Am J Med 75:671, 1983.
2. Novelline RA, Baltarowich OH, Athanasoulis CA, et al.: The clinical course of patients with suspected pulmonary embolism and a negative pulmonary arteriogram. Radiology 126:561, 1978.
3. Legha SS, Muggia FM: Pleural mesothelioma: Clinical features and therapeutic implications. Ann Intern Med 87:613, 1977.
4. Berger HW, Mejia E: Tuberculous pleurisy. Chest 63:88, 1973.
5. Stein PD, Willis PW, DeMets DL: History and physical examination in acute pulmonary embolism in patients without preexisting cardiac or pulmonary disease. Am J Cardiol 47:218, 1981.
6. Bain HW, McLean DM, Walker SJ: Epidemic pleurodynia (Bornholm disease) due to coxsackie B-5 virus. Pediatrics 27:889, 1961.
7. Sahn SA: Pleural manifestations of pulmonary disease. Hosp Pract 16:73, March 1981.
8. McNeil BJ, Hessel SJ, Branch WT, Bjork L, Adelstein SJ: Measures of clinical efficacy. III. The value of the lung scan in the evaluation of young patients with pleuritic chest pain. J Nucl Med 17:163, 1976.
9. Good JT, King TE, Antony VB, Sahn SA: Lupus pleuritis. Chest 84:714, 1983.

_____**15**_____

SHORTNESS OF BREATH

By SCOTT BARNHART, M.D.

GENERAL COMMENTS

Shortness of breath or dyspnea is defined as a distressing sensation associated with labored breathing or breathlessness. The assessment of dyspnea by a patient is subjective and cannot be directly measured. It is probably the most common symptom associated with cardiac or respiratory disease, or both. The sensation of dyspnea is directly related to the control of ventilation. Ventilation is dependent on the integration of afferent signals from mechanical and chemical receptors located in the small airways, skeletal muscle, pulmonary vasculature, peripheral chemoreceptors, central chemoreceptors, cortical input, and a central pacemaker. Studies of these mechanisms have led to several theories concerning the genesis of dyspnea, including (1) increased work of breathing, (2) intercostal muscle fatigue, (3) increased oxygen utilization in breathing, (4) abnormal ventilatory drives, and (5) prolonged inspiratory neuronal stimulation of the respiratory centers.

DIFFERENTIAL DIAGNOSIS

Dyspnea may arise from one or more of the following pathophysiologic processes and their associated disease states:
A. Decreased Oxygen Delivery
   1. *Nonpulmonary*
      a. Decreased inspired oxygen tension
      b. Anemia, carboxyhemoglobin, hemoglobinopathy
      c. Decreased cardiac output
   2. *Pulmonary: Airways or Pulmonary Parenchyma*
      a. Airflow obstruction
      b. Neoplasm
      c. Pneumonia
      d. Interstitial pneumonitis
      e. Emphysema
      f. Pleural effusion
   3. *Pulmonary: Vascular*
      a. Pulmonary thromboembolism
      b. Left ventricular failure
B. Increased Oxygen Demands
   1. *Exercise, Infection, Thyrotoxicosis*
C. Increased Work of Breathing
   1. *Airflow Obstruction*
   2. *Decreased Lung Compliance.* This occurs in diffuse infiltrative diseases.
   3. *Increased Carbon Dioxide Production.* This occurs with infection and increased metabolism.
D. Miscellaneous
   1. *Muscle Weakness*
   2. *Central Nervous System Stimulation*
   3. *Psychogenic Factors*
   4. *Acidosis*

CLINICAL MANIFESTATIONS

A. History
   1. *Onset.* Acute onset suggests pulmonary embolism, pneumothorax, or other processes associated with a rapid decompensation, such as heart failure from a myocardial infarction, arrhythmia, or valve failure. Chronic dyspnea is much more likely to be the result of chronic left ventricular failure, chronic obstructive pulmonary disease, or interstitial fibrosis.
   2. *Associated Symptoms.* These provide valuable clues to the diagnosis. Pleuritic chest pain may suggest pulmonary embolism, and substernal chest pain may suggest a myocardial infarction. Wheezing is often associated with asthma or

chronic obstructive pulmonary disease. Cough, fever, and chills suggest an inflammatory process.

3. *Past Conditions.* A history of pulmonary or cardiovascular disease often provides an indication of where to look for the cause of a patient's dyspnea.

B. **Physical Examination**

1. *General Appearance.* The examination should include the degree of respiratory distress and use of accessory muscles.

2. *Vital Signs.* Special attention should be given to the respiratory rate.

3. *Chest*

a. **Appearance.** Rate and depth of respirations and use of accessory muscles, splinting, paradoxic motion of the chest wall, and abdominal muscles and flail chest are noted.

b. **Percussion.** Dullness may suggest an effusion, and hyperresonance may support airtrapping from airflow obstruction or pneumothorax.

c. **Auscultation.** Wheezing, rales, and decreased or absent breath sounds may all point to the diagnosis.

d. **Cardiovascular Examination.** Elevated jugular venous pressure, cardiac enlargement, gallops, or murmurs may suggest a cardiac cause.

LABORATORY EXAMINATION

The choice of laboratory examinations generally stems from the findings of the history and physical examination. Preliminary studies usually include the folowing:

A. **Chest X-Ray:** The chest x-ray gives an indication of many abnormal processes, including abnormalities of the chest wall, pulmonary vasculature, pulmonary parenchyma, and heart size.

B. **Complete Blood Count.** Anemia representing a decreased ability to deliver oxygen must be ruled out.

C. **Arterial Blood Gas.** This is particularly valuable. The pH and $PaCO_2$ give an indication of the acid-base status, the acuteness of the derangement (acute respiratory acidosis), and the patient's ability to maintain adequate ventilation and to compensate for metabolic acidosis. The PO_2 indicates whether hypoxemia is present and whether there is a widened A-a O_2 gradient. Repeat arterial blood gas determinations following institution of oxygen therapy may give an indication of whether the problem is caused by a shunt or ventilation/perfusion $(\dot{V}/\dot{Q})$ mismatch.

D. **Electrocardiogram.** This may suggest new or old ischemic disease, left ventricular hypertrophy, or an arrythmia that could be contributing to the dyspnea.

E. **Spirometry.** Screening spirometry is useful to indicate a low vital capacity or evidence of airflow obstruction. Further pulmonary function testing, including lung volumes and diffusing capacity, may be of benefit.

Additional studies may be needed to investigate cardiac or pulmonary reserve or to evaluate extrathoracic causes, ranging from hyperthyroidism to metabolic acidosis and psychogenic causes of dyspnea. Additional studies may include exercise testing, ventilation-perfusion scans, or right or left heart catheterization.

RECOMMENDED DIAGNOSTIC APPROACH

A. Initial Evaluation
   1. *Assessment of Degree of Distress*
      a. **Acute Distress.** Emergency evaluation and support are considered.
      b. **Moderate Distress or Chronic Problem.** A full history and physical examination are indicated followed by the indicated laboratory studies.
B. Laboratory Studies
   1. *Pulmonary Studies*
      a. Chest x-ray
      b. Arterial blood gas
      c. Complete blood count
      d. Pulmonary function testing
      e. Exercise testing
   2. *Cardiac Studies*
      a. Right heart catheterization
      b. Electrocardiogram
      c. Ejection fraction
      d. Echocardiogram
      e. Left heart catheterization
      f. Exercise test

REFERENCES

1. Burki NK: Dyspnea. Clin Chest Med 1:47, 1980.
2. Moser KM: Evaluation of patients with acute or chronic dyspnea. *In* Moser KM (ed.): Respiratory Emergencies. 2nd ed. St. Louis, C.V. Mosby, 1982, pp. 214–230.
3. Hinshaw HC, Murray JF: Diseases of the Chest. Philadelphia, W. B. Saunders Company, 1980, pp. 11–14.

THE SOLITARY PULMONARY NODULE

By STEPHEN HOLLAND, M.D.,
and JAMES TALCOTT, M.D.

GENERAL COMMENTS, DEFINITION, AND DIFFERENTIAL DIAGNOSIS

A. General Comments. The asymptomatic solitary nodule proves to be malignant almost 40 per cent of the time. Early detection and diagnosis of a pulmonary nodule can lead to a five-year survival rate of 40 to 60 per cent of cases, depending on the patient's sex, the nodule's size, and the cell type. Even if the malignant nodule has metastasized to the lung, a 30 per cent or more five-year survival rate can be expected. Since the five-year survival rate is only 5 per cent for patients who have symptomatic bronchogenic carcinoma, a rational and efficient approach to the asymptomatic solitary pulmonary nodule is necessary.

B. Definition. A solitary pulmonary nodule is an asymptomatic circumscribed homogeneous density found in the periphery of the lung on chest x-ray. What is often called a "coin" lesion is actually spherical in shape with margins that may be either distinct or ill-defined. Although generally homogeneous in density, it may contain calcium or have central cavitation. The lesion should be less than 6 cm in diameter; a larger lesion is defined as a lung mass.

C. Differential Diagnosis. Many pulmonary diseases are manifested as solitary pulmonary nodules; over 50 causes have been identified. Determination of a specific cause is never as important as distinguishing a malignant nodule from a benign one (Table 16–1). This is because a malignant nodule requires resection, whereas a benign nodule can be observed and followed over time. The clinician should progress quickly and efficiently to the decision point of immediate thoracotomy or vigilant observation.

EPIDEMIOLOGY

A. Age. Carcinoma of the lung appearing as a solitary nodule in a person under the age of 35 is rare (approximately 0.3 per cent in 500 patients subject to surgery). After the age of 35 there is a steady increase in the percentage of nodules that are malignant (70 to 100 per cent of all nodules found in the eighth decade of life are malignant).

B. Sex. There is a male-to-female ratio of about 3:1 for malignant nodules.

C. Exposures. Exposure to asbestos, uranium, nickle, or plutonium increases the probability of lung carcinoma, while occupational exposure to inorganic dust increases the probability of benign pneumoconioses. Coccidioidomycosis and histoplasmosis often

TABLE 16–1. CAUSES OF SOLITARY PULMONARY NODULES*

Malignant (40%)	*Benign neoplasia* (5%)
Bronchogenic carcinoma	Hamartoma
Alveolar cell tumors	Chondroma
Solitary metastasis	Fibroma
Bronchial adenoma	Myxoma
Primary sarcoma	Xanthoma
Lymphoma	Neurogenic tumors
	Lipoma
Inflammatory (50%)	Leiomyoma
Tuberculoma	Plasmacytoma
Histoplasmoma	Histiocytoma
Coccidioidoma	Thymoma
Cryptococcus	Endometriosis
Blastomycosis	
Actinomycosis	*Other* (<5%)
Moniliasis	Hydatid cyst
Nocardiosis	Ascaris
Nonspecific granuloma	*Dirofilaria immitis*
Chronic lung abscess	Mycetoma
Lipoid pneumonia	Atrioventricular malformation
Massive fibrosis	Vascular endothelioma
Rheumatoid granuloma	Sequestered segment
Gumma	Diaphragmatic hernias
Brucella suis	Pericardial cyst
	Bronchogenic cyst
	Dermoid
	Teratoma
	Pulmonary infarct
	Mucoid impaction
	Amyloidosis
	Hematoma secondary to trauma

*Modified by the author from information in Poe RH: The solitary pulmonary nodule. *In* Poe RH, Israel RH (eds.): Problems in Pulmonary Medicine for the Primary Physician. Philadelphia, Lea & Febiger, 1982.

resolve into solitary pulmonary nodules. The frequency of malignancy in areas endemic for these organisms has been estimated at 5 to 25 per cent of discovered nodules.

D. **Smoking.** Smoking is a major risk factor for bronchial carcinoma in both men and women. Regardless of age, a greater than 40 pack-year smoking history strongly suggests a malignant lesion. Adenocarcinoma can occur in nonsmokers as well as smokers, with some predilection toward women.

E. **Nonpulmonary Malignancy.** A history of nonpulmonary malignancy raises the suspicion that a nodule is a metastatic lesion, but occasionally the nodule may prove to be a second primary or even benign. If the primary carcinoma is of the colon, rectum, or genitourinary tract, the odds favor metastasis.

HISTORY AND PHYSICAL EXAMINATION

A. **Medical History.** The history may be helpful but is rarely diagnostic (see Table 16–2). Bacterial pneumonia can resolve to

TABLE 16–2. BENIGN VERSUS MALIGNANT NODULES*

CLINICAL FEATURE	BENIGN	PRIMARY MALIGNANCY	SOLITARY METASTASIS
Age	Under 35	Over 35	Any
Size (at discovery)	Tendency to be smaller; average size 1.8 cm	Tendency to be larger; average size 3.1 cm	Either
Margin	Sharp	Ill-defined	Sharp
Calcification	Frequent; ring-shaped or popcorn pattern important	Rare	Rare
Smoking history	Not related	Usually >40 pack years	Not related
Symptoms	Rare	1 in 4	Rare
Extrapulmonary malignancy	Not usually	Not usually	Usually
Doubling time	<30 days, >500 days	30–500 days	30–500 days

*Modified by the author from information in Poe RH: The solitary pulmonary nodule. *In* Poe RH, Israel RH (eds.): Problems in Pulmonary Medicine for the Primary Physician. Philadelphia, Lea & Febiger, 1982.

leave a residual pulmonary pseudotumor. Trauma can leave occult pulmonary hematomas that have the appearance of discrete nodules. Rheumatoid lung disease can occasionally appear as a single pulmonary nodule, as can mucoid impaction or an aspergilloma in the patient with asthma. Use of oil-based nose drops or intranasal glycerine can lead to oil-droplet pulmonary granulomata.

B. Physical Examination

1. A careful breast, pelvic, genital, and rectal examination and a stool guaiac test help exclude potential extrathoracic causes.
2. Lymphadenopathy and hepatosplenomegaly point to lymphoma, leukemia, or metastatic disease as possible causes of a newly discovered solitary nodule.
3. Supraclavicular or cervical nodes and occasionally infraclavicular and axillary nodes suggest direct lymphatic extension of a primary lung neoplasm.
4. Clubbing and weight loss suggest malignancy. Combined with a history of steatorrhea, clubbing and weight loss suggest subclinical cystic fibrosis with mucoid impaction as the cause of a newly detected nodule.
5. Skin lesions of erythema nodosa suggest an active granulomatous process in the lungs.
6. Fine telangiectasia of the skin or mucous membranes suggest the small pulmonary atriovenous aneurysms or pulmonary venous lakes that are seen in hereditary hemorrhagic telangiectasia.

RECOMMENDED DIAGNOSTIC APPROACH

It is important not to forget that a shadow appearing in the midclavicular line is most often a nipple shadow, which is one of the most frequent causes of benign pulmonary nodules. Skin tags and extraneous foreign bodies are often diagnosed by a careful examination of the patient's skin or clothing or by the use of radiopaque markers or oblique films (Fig. 16–1).

A. **Step One.** Every effort should be made to obtain and review old films, since this can often prevent a potentially expensive and invasive hospitalization. A report of a negative chest x-ray is of little value, since pulmonary nodules are often missed or neglected.

1. *Growth Rates.* The rates of growth (doubling time) for various bronchogenic carcinomas and benign diseases are different. Previous x-rays can establish a doubling time and help to differentiate malignant from benign disease. When a tumor's diameter has increased by a factor of 1.26, the tumor has doubled in volume. For example, when a 1.0-cm nodule has increased to 1.26 cm in diameter it has doubled in size (a 2.0-cm nodule has doubled at a diameter of 2.52 cm, and so forth).

   a. Mean doubling times for various untreated carcinomas are 29 days for small cell, 86 days for poorly differentiated, 88 days for squamous cell, and 161 days for adenocarcinoma (range 1 to 15 months).

   b. Single pulmonary nodules that double in less than one month are almost always inflammatory. Exceptions are metastatic lesions from rapidly growing extrapulmonary primaries such as testicular cancer, osteogenic sarcomas, renal cell carcinoma, and chorionic carcinoma.

   c. If previous radiographs reveal that no increase in diameter has occurred in two or more years, it is generally safe to conclude that the nodule is benign. Close observation then becomes a prudent approach.

2. *Size.* At examination malignant nodules are larger (average diameter 3.1 cm) than benign lesions (average diameter 1.8 cm).

3. *Calcification.* The presence of calcification is fairly specific for benign lesions, although approximately 4 per cent of resected malignant pulmonary nodules are calcified. Calcification should be considered in the context of risk factors and previous chest x-rays before a lesion is assigned to a benign category for observation. A "popcorn" or speckled pattern is very characteristic of hamartomas. Histoplasmosis lesions are often calcified in a ring-shaped or laminated pattern. An eccentric pattern of calcification indicates a possible malignancy growing around another diffusely calcified benign lesion. Specificity of radiographic diagnosis can be enhanced by computed tomographic scanning of noncalcified nodules, since benign nodules tend to be more dense (mean 1 to 4 Hounsfield units).

4. *Cavitation.* Cavitation is not helpful in delineating between benign and malignant nodules.

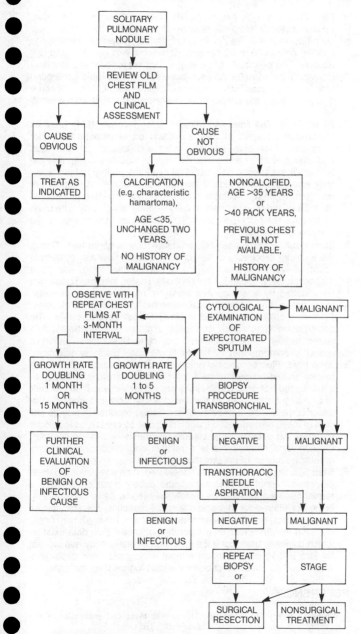

Figure 16–1. A systematic approach to work-up of a solitary nodule.

B. **Step Two.** Cytologic examination is made of expectorated sputum. Sputum cytology is highly reliable when positive (less than 2 per cent false-positive results in good hands); however, cytology is positive only in 20 to 30 per cent of patients with proven malignant disease. The sensitivity of cytology is highest for central pulmonary lesions. Because of the noninvasiveness, low cost, rapid turnaround time, and high specificity of cytology, it becomes the next procedure of choice when the suspicion of malignancy prompts further work-up.

C. **Step Three.** The risks and benefits of an invasive study must be considered. Invasive studies are designed to recover tissue for pathologic diagnosis. They all involve a degree of risk and cost, and their specificity and sensitivity vary by nodule location and the clinician's experience and technical expertise. Although their accuracy when positive is high, if they do not *disprove* malignancy (for example, when tuberculosis is present), other invasive procedures must be undertaken to unequivocally exclude malignancy. The order of invasive tests often reflects the resources and experience of the consulting physician.

D. **Step Four.** Flexible fiberoptic bronchoscopy is performed. This is the invasive procedure of first choice. It has a low risk of complication, a relatively small degree of patient discomfort, and good diagnostic yield, especially for centrally located lesions. Tissue can be obtained by washings and brushing, mucosal biopsy of suspicious areas, and fluoroscopically directed transbronchial biopsies. Positive results are obtained in up to 58 per cent of cases. The complication rate, which principally involves pneumothorax, has been reported to be less than 1 per cent. Direct visualization of bronchial anatomy may be helpful in ultimately planning resection.

E. **Step Five.** Fluoroscopically guided transthoracic aspiration needle biopsy should be performed if the diagnosis remains in doubt. In experienced hands, biopsy results are positive in about 90 per cent of all malignant nodules (in all sizes down to 1 cm in diameter). The major complication is pneumothorax. This is reported in 5 to 25 per cent of these procedures, although drainage by chest tube is seldom required. An uncorrectable bleeding diathesis is a major contraindication, and emphysema is a relative one, producing a slightly greater frequency of pneumothorax.

F. **Step Six.** Surgical resection is considered. If an unequivocal benign diagnosis cannot be established, the patient must either have a repeat needle aspiration, be closely followed by serial chest x-rays, or be considered for immediate surgical resection. Several studies using repeat needle biopsies and cytology have shown false-negative results in less than 4 per cent of cases. Few data exist on which choice is best, but if the suspicion of malignancy has led this far into a diagnostic work-up without a diagnosis, few physicians would fault curative resection as the next logical diagnostic step.

REFERENCES

1. Trunk G, Gracy DR, Byrd RB: The management and evaluation of the solitary pulmonary nodule. Chest 66:236, 1974.
  A standard approach that has not changed much in ten years.

2. Geddes DM: The natural history of lung cancer; a review based on rates of tumor growth. Br J Dis Chest 73:1, 1979.

Good information on doubling time and predicting the cause of the nodule.

3. Higgens GA, Shields TW, Keeh RJ: The solitary pulmonary nodule: Ten year follow-up of a VA-Armed Forces Cooperative Study. Arch Surg 110:570, 1975.

A study that provides helpful information on the natural history of the solitary pulmonary nodule.

4. Siegelman SS, Zerhouni EA, Leo FP, et al.: CT of the solitary pulmonary nodule. Am J Roentgenol 135:1–13, 1980.

The exact place of the CT scan in the work-up is still being determined.

5. Poe RH, Tobin RE: Sensitivity and specificity of needle biopsy in lung malignancy. Am Rev Respir Dis 122:725, 1980.

The key is a willingness to make multiple passes.

6. Poe RH: The solitary pulmonary nodule. *In* Poe RH, Israel RH (eds.): Problems in Pulmonary Medicine for the Primary Physician. Philadelphia, Lea & Febiger, 1982.

An excellent discussion and review for the primary physician.

---17---

ASTHMA

By PATRICIA SATO, M.D.

DEFINITION

The American Thoracic Society defines asthma as a "disease characterized by an increased responsiveness of the trachea and bronchi to various stimuli, manifested by airway narrowing that changes in severity either spontaneously or as a result of therapy." Asthma is episodic in nature with acute exacerbations of dyspnea, cough, and wheezing interspersed with symptom-free periods. The severity is variable and ranges from mild and infrequent symptoms to the severe airflow obstruction lasting days in so-called *status asthmaticus*.

EPIDEMIOLOGY AND GENERAL CONSIDERATIONS

A. **Incidence.** A national health survey observed that 4 per cent of the United States population has asthma. It occurs in all age groups, with 50 per cent of the cases in the pediatric age group and 75 per cent occurring before age 40. Younger patients tend to have a better prognosis, since symptomatology decreases with age. In addition, there is a group of late-onset asthmatics who have more severe disease. Most statistics show equal frequency of occurrence in both sexes. Death from asthma is uncommon, with a mortality of 0.3 per 100,000 persons.

B. **Etiology.** It is difficult to define a specific cause. All patients have a nonspecific hyperirritability of the tracheobronchial tree. However, it is clinically useful to classify patients into two groups: those with a specific allergic component—"extrinsic" asthma—and those without an allergic component—idiopathic or "intrinsic" asthma.

1. *Allergic Asthma.* This type of asthma is associated with:
   a. A personal or family history of atopy with rhinitis, eczema, or urticaria;
   b. Positive immediate hypersensitivity reactions with a wheal and flare to intradermal injections of airborne antigens;
   c. Elevated serum immunoglobulin E (IgE) levels; and
   d. A positive bronchial response to specific inhaled provocation tests. A seasonal component may be present.

The majority of cases occur in the pediatric and young adult population. Allergic asthma can be nonseasonal as well, occurring in relation to ubiquitous inhaled allergens such as dust, feathers, danders, and mold.

2. *Intrinsic (Idiopathic) Asthma.* A large segment of the asthmatic population lacks an allergic history and falls into the idiopathic category. These patients may develop asthma after an upper respiratory infection, have onset late in life, and often are more difficult to manage.

C. **Pathophysiology**

1. *Bronchospasm.* The key pathophysiologic finding in asthma is reduction in airway size as a result of bronchial smooth muscle contraction with associated edematous bronchial walls and thick tenacious secretions. These result in increased airway resistance, decreased expiratory flow rates, hyperinflation of the lungs and thorax, increased work of breathing, and a ventilation-perfusion mismatch that causes hypoxia.

2. *Neural Pathways.* The bronchospasm is mediated through neural and biochemical pathways. Provocative stimuli irritate airway nerve receptor endings and cause cough and bronchoconstriction through a vagal outflow tract. Anticholinergic drugs such as atropine act on this neural pathway. Sympathetic alpha- and beta-adrenergic receptors also help regulate bronchial smooth muscle tone, and sympathomimetic agents are a mainstay in asthma therapy.

3. *Biochemical Mediators.* Biochemical mediators are released with mast cell degranulation. These mediators are potent stimuli to airway hyperreactivity. They have recently been identified as products of oxidative metabolism of arachidonic acid. Slow-reacting substance of anaphylaxis (SRS-A) is in fact a group of leukotriene products formed by the lipooxygenase pathway of arachidonic metabolism. Prostaglandins formed by the cyclooxygenase pathway of arachidonic acid may also contribute to bronchoconstriction.

D. **Stimuli that Precipitate Bronchospasm**

1. *Airborne Allergens.* Airborne allergens are common culprits. The patient must be exposed to the allergens long enough for them to induce a state of sensitivity. Once that occurs, exposure to even very small amounts of allergens can cause bronchospasm. The antigen reacts with mucosal mast cells to cause degranulation, and irritant receptors activate the cholinergic parasympathetic system.

2. *Medications.* In a certain group of asthmatics the ingestion of aspirin or other nonsteroidal anti-inflammatory agents may cause an exacerbation. This is thought to be related to arachidonic acid metabolism and usually occurs in combination with nasal polyposis and sinusitis. In the severe form as little as 300 mg of aspirin may cause acute rhinitis, wheezing, urticaria, flushing, and hypotension.

3. *Environmental Pollutants.* Environmental pollutants may provoke attacks in individuals living in heavy industrial areas, particularly at times of temperature inversions with stagnant air masses. These attacks may be related to inhalation of sulfur dioxide or other gases or particulate matter.

4. *Occupational Asthma.* Occupational asthma may occur in one of three ways:
   a. Exposure to an antigen can cause formation of a specific IgE;
   b. Material may cause a direct release of bronchoconstrictor substance; or
   c. Inhaled work-related substances may act as general airway irritants. Treatment often requires a change in occupation.

5. *Respiratory Infections.* An upper respiratory infection is the most common event that exacerbates asthmas in both intrinsic and extrinsic types. Bacterial infections can worsen asthma, but viral infections with rhinovirus, influenza, respiratory syncytial virus, and influenza virus occur more frequently.

6. *Exercise.* Exercise can induce or worsen asthma, and exercise-induced asthma often is the presenting symptom. This phenomenon clearly is related to the environment in which the exercise is performed. Activities in cold dry air such as skiing or running are more provocative than swimming. The mechanism is not fully understood but is thought to be related to airway cooling, which occurs as the inspired air is heated and humidified. Emotional stress may precipitate asthma, and psychologic factors may increase bronchospasm in certain individuals. These objective observations have prompted the use of hypnosis and biofeedback for the treatment of some patients.

HISTORY AND PHYSICAL EXAMINATION

A. **History.** Patients classically complain of a triad of dyspnea, cough, and wheezing, which alternate with symptom-free periods. At initial evaluation, the precipitating factors should be carefully elicited, with a particular search for an allergic component. Asthma is a possible diagnosis for patients who complain of unexplained episodes of nonproductive cough or dyspnea without wheezing. A thorough medication history is required, particularly if patients are taking beta-blocker agents.

B. Physical Examination. During symptom-free periods, patients may be perfectly normal or may have wheezing only on forced expiratory maneuvers. During acute attacks patients develop a sense of constriction in the chest and soon exhibit tachypnea and cough. Respirations become labored and harsh, and the inspiratory and expiratory wheezing may be audible without a stethoscope. Air is trapped as a result of early airway closure and increases the anteroposterior diameter of the chest. As obstruction worsens, patients use the accessory muscles of breathing and develop pulsus paradoxus from the large swings in pleural pressure. These two signs signify severe compromise and should alert the physician that hospitalization may be necessary. In critical situations wheezing may lessen or disappear as a result of the marked decrease in airflow. These findings herald impending respiratory failure and the possible need for intubation and mechanical ventilation.

C. Objective Clinical Measures for Grading the Severity of Asthma. A number of recent studies have confirmed that objective physical measurements provide reasonably accurate estimates of ventilation compromise in an asthmatic patient. These measurements can predict patients who respond to therapy, have rapid relapse, or require hospitalization.

   1. Grading Scale. The following grading scale is widely used. It includes subjective symptoms, physical signs, and objective measurements. A score of four or more is considered a severe asthma attack that will probably require corticosteroids and admission to the hospital.

MEASURE		SCORE
Peak expiratory flow rate	<120 L/minute (PEFR)	1
Forced expiratory volume, one second (FEV_1)	<40 per cent of predicted value	1
Pulse rate	>120/minute	1
Respiratory rate	>30/minute	1
Pulsus paradoxus	>18 mm Hg	1
Relapse in <24 hours		1
Use of accessory respiratory muscles		1
Audible wheezing		1
Severe subjective dyspnea		1

   2. Pulmonary Function Measures. Even this scale puts a high value on physical signs and subjective symptoms, and several experts would argue that the pulmonary function measures alone should be used to guide therapy.

a. FEV_1 and PEFR correlate highly, and either is better than a combination of heart rate, respiratory rate, and pulsus paradoxus at predicting poor response to therapy.
b. Arterial blood gases provide little clinical information until the PEFR is less than 25 per cent of the predicted value, at which point they should be determined.
c. PEFR less than 16 per cent (or less than 60 L per minute) or FEV_1 less than 0.6 L should be considered severe asthma.

LABORATORY FINDINGS

A. **Laboratory Blood Work.** No single test is diagnostic of asthma. Blood and sputum eosinophilia occurs often but is not universal or specific for asthma. During an acute exacerbation, complete blood counts and blood chemistry can provide evidence of infection, dehydration, or other related problems.
B. **Arterial Blood Gases**
   1. *Arterial Blood Gases.* The arterial blood gases appear to have little use in evaluating the severity of asthma until the PEFR is less than 25 per cent of the predicted value. Arterial blood gases should always be obtained to follow the progress of patients who have severe bronchospasm at examination or who respond slowly to initial therapy.
   2. *Hypoxia.* During an acute exacerbation the usual findings are hypoxia with a widened alveolar-arterial oxygen difference $[P(A-a)O_2]$ and concomitant hypocapnia and respiratory alkalosis.
      a. The alveolar-arterial gradient should be calculated from blood gases drawn while the patient is breathing room air:
      $$P(A-a)O_2 = 150 - PaO_2 - (1.2 \times PaCO_2)$$
      b. $P(A-a)O_2$ in normal young adults is 5 to 15 mm Hg.
      c. $P(A-a)O_2$ in older adults and patients with pulmonary disease is 25 to 30 mm Hg.
   3. *Obstruction and Respiratory Failure.* A patient in whom $PaCO_2$ increases toward normal is experiencing worsening obstruction and impending respiratory failure.
C. **Skin Testing.** Patients with asthma may exhibit positive wheal and flare reactions to skin tests, but these results may not correlate with events in the chest.
D. **Chest Radiographs.** Radiographs most often appear normal in symptom-free periods but during an exacerbation typically show hyperinflation. A chest radiograph obtained during an acute attack is useful primarily to rule out other processes, such as cardiac disease, pneumonia, or pneumothorax.
E. **Pulmonary Function Tests.** The degree of airflow obstruction can be measured and its reversible nature demonstrated by studying the patient before and after inhalation of bronchodilators or during symptom-free "normal" periods. During acute exacerbations, bedside spirometry is the best method to evaluate the severity of the attack and to monitor the patient's progress.

F. Bronchial Provocation Tests. These tests are useful to detect airway hyperresponsiveness. They are performed by administering increasing concentrations of aerosolized antigen or a bronchoconstrictor agent and measuring spirometry after each dose. A dose response curve is generated that indicates airway responsiveness. Patients who have a greater response get bronchoconstriction with a lower dose. Inhalation of antigen extracts or industrial dusts may indicate specific reagin-mediated bronchospasm. A positive response to histamine or methacholine indicates nonspecific hyperresponsiveness. The histamine or methacholine tests are useful to evaluate patients with an equivocal history of asthma or those who have a chronic episodic cough but normal pulmonary function test results.

DIFFERENTIAL DIAGNOSIS

There are other causes of wheezing besides asthma. The following illnesses should be kept in mind when the patient's clinical picture is atypical for asthma:

A. Upper Airway Obstruction. When first assessing a patient with possible asthma, upper airway obstruction from a tumor, goiter, or foreign body should be considered. Laryngeal edema may appear with stridor and harsh breath sounds.

B. Localized Wheezing. This suggests endobronchial problems such as foreign body aspiration, neoplasm, or bronchial stenosis.

C. "Cardiac Wheezing." Patients in left ventricular failure may have "cardiac asthma" with wheezing.

D. Recurrent Wheezing. Recurrent episodes of wheezing can also be seen with carcinoid tumors, recurrent pulmonary embolism, and chronic bronchitis. Eosinophilic pneumonia and polyarteritis also occasionally involve asthma-like symptoms.

REFERENCES

1. Boushey HA, Holtzman MJ, Sheller JR, Nadel JA: Bronchial hyperreactivity. Am Rev Respir Dis 121:389, 1980.

   Reviews many of the causes and the physiology of bronchospasm.

2. Fischl MA, Pitchenik A, Gardner LR: An index predicting relapse and need for hospitalization in patients with acute bronchial asthma. N Engl J Med 305:783–789, 1981.

   An important study that recommends the use of objective measurements to detect patients with severe asthma who are likely to require hospitalization. Subsequent studies have not fully confirmed the original findings.

3. Nowak RM, Tomlanovich MC, Sarkar DD, et al.: Arterial blood gases and pulmonary function testing in acute bronchial asthma: Predicting patient outcomes. JAMA 249:2043–2046, 1983.

   A valuable study that showed that analysis of arterial blood gases failed to distinguish patients needing admission from those who could be safely discharged, whereas FEV_1 and PEFR could.

4. Shim CS, Williams MH Jr: Evaluation of the severity of asthma: Patients versus physicians. Am J Med 68:11–13, 1980.

Patients were more accurate than physicians in estimating the PEFR.

5. Kelsen SG, Kelsen DP, Fleegler BF, et al.: Emergency room assessment and treatment of patients with acute asthma. Am J Med 64:622–628, 1978.

This study confirmed that FEV$_1$ was a better index of degree of obstruction than physical examination or arterial blood gases.

18

CHRONIC OBSTRUCTIVE PULMONARY DISEASE

By THOMAS R. MARTIN, M.D.

DEFINITION

The term "chronic obstructive pulmonary disease" (COPD) refers to a group of disorders characterized by chronic obstruction to expiratory airflow. The common denominator is obstruction of the airways during expiration because of intraluminal secretions, thickening of airway walls, or collapse of airway walls from loss of surrounding supporting structures. Most patients with COPD have some combination of chronic bronchitis and emphysema. Chronic asthma, cystic fibrosis, and even chronic interstitial diseases can all be associated with varying degrees of chronic airflow obstruction.

A. **Chronic Bronchitis**
  1. Chronic bronchitis is defined *clinically*. The definition requires a productive cough that occurs in the absence of airway infections on most days, for at least three months of the year, for two consecutive years.
  2. Chronic bronchitis is caused by chronic exposure to inhaled agents, the most common of which is cigarette smoke. Chronic bronchitis is always associated with mucus hypersecretion and mucus gland hyperplasia in the airways. The gas exchange parenchyma of the lung is not disturbed. Most patients have subtle airflow obstruction, but only a minority of cases progress to disabling airflow obstruction. Chronic bronchitis often is reversible when the inhalation exposure ceases (such as after discontinuaton of cigarette smoking).

B. **Emphysema.** Emphysema is defined *pathologically*. Simply put, it is holes in the lung.
  1. The progressive destruction of terminal bronchioles and alveolar walls destroys the gas exchange parenchyma. Thus there is a loss of the normal support structures that tether larger airways open during exhalation. Patients with pure

emphysema complain of progressive dyspnea. In contrast with chronic bronchitis, in emphysema cough is not a prominent symptom.

2. Emphysema is thought to result from a disturbance in the balance between proteases and antiproteases in the lung parenchyma. When this balance is upset, unchecked proteolytic activity occurs over a long perod of time. For example, patients with alpha-1 antitrypsin deficiency lack the major antiprotease in serum and develop severe emphysema where blood flow is greatest. Cigarette smoke has been shown to inactivate alpha-1 antitrypsin by oxidation.

EPIDEMIOLOGY: INCIDENCE AND PREVALENCE

COPD is common in smokers and rare in nonsmokers. Although the incidence of new cases is difficult to estimate, several prevalence studies indicate that up to 27 per cent of men and 13 per cent of women in the general population have symptoms or spirometric abnormalities, or both, that suggest COPD.

CLINICAL PRESENTATION

A. Chronic Bronchitis

1. Patients with chronic bronchitis complain of chronic cough and phlegm production. Many patients have only cough and phlegm but some also develop progressive airflow obstruction that can be disabling. These patients usually have a combination of chronic bronchitis *and* emphysema. The degree of coexisting emphysema is difficult to measure clinically. It is evident only on pathologic examination of the lungs.

2. Patients with significant chronic bronchitis become hypoxemic early in the course of the disease because of ventilation-perfusion mismatching in the lung. This may lead to erythrocytosis and cor pulmonale, manifested clinically by plethora, cyanosis, dependent edema, elevation of venous pressure, right ventricular heave, accentuated pulmonic component of S_2, S_4 gallop, and hepatic congestion.

B. Emphysema

1. Patients with pure emphysema (that is, those with alpha-1 antitrypsin deficiency) complain of exertional dyspnea, but chronic cough and sputum production are rare if the patients do not smoke.

2. The patients usually appear thin and pink. They have signs of hyperinflation of the lungs, including flattened diaphragms, increased percussion note, and diminished breath sounds. The heart is usually small and in a midline position, with a subxiphoid point of maximal impulse.

3. Hypoxemia and clinical evidence of cor pulmonale are late features in emphysema because ventilation-perfusion imbalances are not as severe as in patients with predominantly chronic bronchitis.

PATHOPHYSIOLOGY

A. **Airflow Obstruction**
   1. Chronic airflow obstruction in COPD is caused by three factors:
      a. Accumulation in the airway lumen of excess secretions
      b. Thickening of the airway walls by glandular and muscular hyperplasia
      c. Loss of the elastic recoil pressure of the lung parenchyma because of destruction of terminal bronchioles and alveolar walls
   2. Excess airway secretions and bronchial wall thickening are characteristic of chronic bronchitis.
   3. Loss of lung elastic recoil is the dominant feature in emphysema.
   4. Most patients with COPD have combinations of all three pathologic features.

B. **Gas Exchange**
   1. *Hypoxemia.* Hypoxemia in COPD occurs because of abnormalities in ventilation-perfusion ($\dot{V}_A/\dot{Q}$) relationships caused by airflow obstruction. In chronic bronchitis, airway obstruction causes maldistribution of inspired gas, but perfusion of the lung parenchyma is relatively unaffected. This causes ventilation-perfusion mismatching and hypoxemia, as blood from poorly ventilated hypoxemic alveoli mixes with oxygenated blood emerging from better ventilated alveoli.
      a. Because the shape of the hemoglobin-oxygen dissociation curve is not linear, oxygenated blood from well-ventilated alveoli cannot be supersaturated to make up for desaturated blood from underventilated alveoli. Therefore, the oxygen content (mL of oxygen per 100 mL of blood) of pulmonary venous blood falls.
      b. In emphysema, destruction of respiratory bronchioles and alveolar walls results in destruction of alveolar capillaries and enlargement of air spaces. This impairs both ventilation and perfusion to the involved areas, so that the relationship between ventilation and perfusion in the whole lung may be relatively unchanged until late in the course of the disease. Consequently, hypoxemia and hypercapnia occur late in emphysema, and indicate severe loss of lung parenchyma.
   2. *Hypercapnia.* Hypercapnia in COPD is caused by severe disturbances in ventilation-perfusion relationships or by abnormalities in ventilatory drive, or by both. To evaluate

patients with hypercapnia, the clinician must distinguish between patients who "can't breathe" and those who "won't breathe."

   a. Studies of COPD patients with acute respiratory failure and progressive hypercapnia have shown that neural output from the respiratory center is usually maximal. Thus it is incorrect to attribute progressive hypercapnia to the "tiring out" of the respiratory center in such patients. Rather, these patients can't breathe, and the hypercapnia that occurs is the result of dysfunction of the respiratory bellows. Fatigue of the ventilatory muscles from the increased work of breathing may play an important role.

   b. Evidence now indicates that some patients with COPD have blunted ventilatory drives. They have less than the expected rise in ventilation in response to rises in $PaCO_2$ or falls in PaO_2. These patients won't breathe, in the sense that they do not increase ventilation in the face of hypercapnia. Whether these patients are born with "blunted" ventilatory drives, or whether the chronically increased airway resistance in COPD leads to "blunting" of existing ventilatory drives remains uncertain.

C. Lung Defense Mechanisms. COPD, particularly chronic bronchitis, is associated with delayed mucociliary clearance of particles in the conducting airways. Slowed clearance of inhaled or aspirated particles may favor the persistence of organisms in the airway and the development of pneumonia. Additionally, viral lower respiratory infections destroy the ciliated cells of the airways. This leads to severe abnormalities in mucus and particle clearance and sets the stage for bacterial superinfection in areas distal to plugged airways. As yet there is no evidence of phagocyte dysfunction in the pathogenesis of respiratory infections in these patients.

COMPLICATIONS

A. Respiratory Failure. Respiratory failure in COPD occurs when ventilation-perfusion relationships worsen in the lung or when the bellows function of the thorax fails. Often a combination of both processes occurs. Suppression of the central ventilatory drive as a result of administration of sedatives or tranquilizers can also cause respiratory failure. $\dot{V}_A/\dot{Q}$ relationships change if airflow obstruction worsens because of acute bronchitis or if pneumonia occurs in the gas exchange parenchyma. The increased work of breathing associated with worsening airflow obstruction leads directly to respiratory muscle fatigue and failure of the thoracic bellows. Neural output from the brain stem respiratory centers is increased rather than decreased in patients with COPD and respiratory failure. Consequently, ventilatory stimulants are of no use in this setting.

B. Cor Pulmonale. Cor pulmonale is heart disease caused by lung disease. In COPD, cor pulmonale occurs as a consequence of sustained pulmonary hypertension. The pulmonary hypertension is caused by the destruction of large portions of the pulmonary vascular bed, as in emphysema, or by the pulmonary vasospasm of chronic hypoxemia. The chronic hypoxemia can be reversed with oxygen therapy that maintains the oxygen saturation at greater than 85 per cent.

C. **Lung Cancer.** The incidence of lung cancer is high in patients with COPD because smoking is a common risk factor for both COPD and bronchogenic carcinoma. The risk of lung cancer is increased fivefold in smokers compared with nonsmokers. The risk of cancer decreases after cessation of smoking, even in patients without COPD, so that between five and ten years after cigarette smoking has been discontinued the cancer risk approaches that for patients who have never smoked.

COURSE AND PROGNOSIS

A. **Clues to Prognosis.** The single best prognostic indicator is the postbronchodilator forced expiratory volume of the first second (FEV_1). Patients in whom airflow rates improve after use of inhaled bronchodilators appear to have a somewhat better prognosis. FEV_1 is also a strong predictor of cardiovascular mortality, which reflects the fact that cigarette use is a risk factor not only for COPD but also for heart disease. The most common causes of death in patients with COPD include sudden death (at home), myocardial infarction, respiratory failure, pulmonary embolism, and cancer of the lung, oropharynx, and gastrointestinal tract.

B. **Course.** A single exacerbation of COPD does not have a major effect on long-term survival. However, an episode of severe respiratory failure that requires mechanical ventilation markedly worsens prognosis. Some studies have reported a one-year mortality of 50 per cent after an episode in which mechanical ventilation is required.

C. **Effects of Therapy.** The most important component of therapy for patients wth COPD is cessation of cigarette use. Chronic bronchitis often improves markedly over several months, and the accelerated annual rate of loss of airflow (FEV_1) often returns to the rate of loss seen in nonsmokers. With time (in five to ten years), the risk of lung cancer after cessation of smoking also declines to that seen in nonsmokers. Unfortunately, there is little evidence that aggressive therapy with bronchodilators prolongs life for patients with COPD. Patients who have regular medical care do better than those without regular care, but this could reflect earlier recognition and treatment of complications, rather than the benefit of medication regimens. Oxygen therapy prolongs life in hypoxemic patients, but the beneficial effect is only seen in patients who use oxygen at least 18 hours daily for more than two years.

REFERENCES

1. Petty TL (ed.): Chronic Obstructive Pulmonary Disease. New York, Marcel Dekker, 1978.

A comprehensive review of COPD with chapters by a variety of contributing authors.

2. West JB: Pulmonary Pathophysiology: The Essentials. Baltimore, Williams & Wilkins, 1982.

An excellent summary of the physiology of respiratory diseases, including pulmonary function tests, gas exchange, common lung diseases, and respiratory failure.

3. Albert RK, Martin TR, Lewis SL: Controlled clinical trial of methylpred-nisolone in patients with chronic bronchitis and acute respiratory insuf-ficiency. Ann Intern Med 92:753–758, 1980.

This study shows that methylprednisolone treatment improved FEV_1 more than placebo treatment in patients with exacerbations of COPD.

4. Traver GA, Cline MG, Burrows B: Predictors of mortality in chronic obstructive pulmonary disease: A 15-year follow-up study. Am Rev Respir Dis 119:895–902, 1979.

This study reports 200 cases of COPD followed for 15 years. After controlling for age, per cent predicted postbronchodilator FEV_1 was the best predictor of prognosis. Cor pulmonale reduced survival by half.

5. Martin TR, Lewis SL, Albert RK: The prognosis of patients with chronic obstructive pulmonary disease after hospitalization for acute respiratory failure. Chest 82:310–314, 1982.

This study shows that exacerbations of COPD do not alter the two-year prognosis in patients with COPD.

6. Nocturnal Oxygen Therapy Trial Group: Continuous or nocturnal oxygen therapy in hypoxemic chronic obstructive lung disease. Ann Intern Med 93:391–398, 1980.

A nocturnal trial of 12 hours vs. 18 hours of oxygen therapy in hypoxemic patients (P_aO_2 <55 mm Hg). Survival was improved for patients who used oxygen for at least 18 hours daily.

19

INTERSTITIAL LUNG DISEASE

By ROBERT DREISIN, M.D.

INTRODUCTION

The task confronting the clinician evaluating the patient with diffuse chronic interstitial infiltrates on the chest radiograph is formidable.

Of all patients with diffuse infiltrates on the chest radiograph, most have an acute illness (left ventricular failure, mitral valve disease, the adult respiratory distress syndrome, and atypical pneumonias). These conditions are considered elsewhere in this book. Chronic interstitial infiltration lasting for more than two months without dramatic clinical and radiographic change may be seen following occupational exposure to dusts (asbestosis, silicosis, pneumoconiosis of coal workers), or following chemical or thermal (drug-induced or radiation-induced) lung injury.

The remaining and quantitatively most important chronic infiltrative diseases of the lung are of immunologic or unknown origin. These are considered individually in this chapter (Table 19–1).

IMMUNOLOGIC AND HYPERSENSITIVITY REACTIONS

This group comprises those chronic interstitial lung reactions in which a specific endogenous or exogenous causative agent has been identified or suspected and a corresponding (inappropriate) humoral and/or cellular immune response delineated.

A. Goodpasture's Syndrome
  1. *Definition*
    a. The term "Goodpasture's syndrome" as it is generally applied is a distinct entity characterized by recurrent episodes of acute pulmonary hemorrhage, rapidly progressive glomerulonephritis, and anemia.
  2. *Etiology*
    a. Goodpasture's syndrome is defined by the presence of antibody directed at alveolar and glomerular basement

TABLE 19–1. CHRONIC PULMONARY INFILTRATES OF IMMUNOLOGIC OR UNKNOWN ORIGIN

Immunologic and hypersensitivity reactions
Goodpasture's syndrome
Hypersensitivity pneumonitis
Connective tissue disease
Rheumatoid arthritis
Systemic lupus erythematosus
Progressive systemic sclerosis
Polymyositis-dermatomyositis
Sjögren's syndrome
Ankylosing spondylitis
Idiopathic
Idiopathic pulmonary fibrosis
Sarcoidosis
Pulmonary alveolar proteinosis
Wegener's granulomatosis

*From Dreisin RB: Hypersensitivity pneumonitis (extrinsic allergic alveolitis). *In* Mitchell RS, Petty TL (eds.): Synopsis of Clinical Pulmonary Disease. 3rd ed. St. Louis, CV Mosby Company, 1982.

membranes. In the absence of demonstrable circulating or tissue-bound antiglomerular basement membrane antibody, even in the patient with the classic clinical triad, the diagnosis of Goodpasture's syndrome cannot be made.

3. *Epidemiology*
   a. Goodpasture's syndrome is overwhelmingly a disease of young and middle-aged Caucasian men.
   b. In one series the median age was 21 with a range of 16 to 61 years. The male to female ratio was 9:1, and 51 of 52 patients were Caucasian.

4. *Clinical Presentation and Course*
   a. Patients with Goodpasture's syndrome usually have recurrent *hemoptysis*. Hemoptysis is accompanied by radiographic evidence of *diffuse pulmonary infiltration,* which pathologically represents intra-alveolar blood and mild alveolar septal thickening. Initial episodes may be unimpressive, with mild blood streaking of sputum, or they may be massive.
   b. Consequently, *iron deficiency anemia* is almost always present.
   c. Hematuria, proteinuria, and azotemia characteristic of a *rapidly progressive glomerulonephritis* become apparent in several weeks, although manifestations of glomerulonephritis may occasionally antedate the pulmonary hemorrhage.
   d. **Course**
      1). The course of a typical patient with Goodpasture's syndrome is one of inexorable progression. The usual survival is less than six months, although long-term cures have been reported.
         a). Death occurs from respiratory failure associated with acute pulmonary hemorrhage.
         b). Other significant sources of morbidity and mortality are barotrauma from artificial respiration in the very stiff lungs, infection by opportunistic invaders, and renal insufficiency.

5. *Chest Radiograph*
   a. There are diffuse alveolar infiltrations in a perihilar distribution (as a result of blood in air spaces).
   b. Infiltrates initially may be localized to a single lobe or segment.
   c. Infiltrates may wax and wane.
   d. As each individual episode of bleeding ceases, the chest radiograph clears. The interstitium, however, eventually becomes accentuated with the development of pulmonary hemosiderosis.

6. *Laboratory Tests*
   a. Iron deficiency anemia is almost always present at some point in the illness.
   b. Elevated blood urea nitrogen and creatinine with proteinuria, hematuria, pyuria, and cylindruria characteristically develop after identification of the pulmonary component of the syndrome.

    c. Macrophages containing large amounts of hemosiderin are seen by iron staining of sputum.

    d. The definitive diagnosis is established by demonstration of circulating antiglomerular basement membrane antibodies.

7. **Histopathology**

    a. Alveoli are filled with blood and hemosiderin-laden macrophages. In patients with established disease, the interstitium may be thickened as well by an infiltrate of mononuclear phagocytes, edema, and foci of interstitial fibrosis.

    b. Glomeruli show typical changes of rapidly progressive glomerulonephritis with epithelial cell crescents. There is marked proliferative change within the glomerulus itself.

8. **Clues to Diagnosis.** Goodpasture's syndrome should be considered in any patient with acute pulmonary hemorrhage. The presence of diffuse pulmonary infiltrates, anemia, azotemia, or urinary sediment abnormalities singly and in combination should strengthen the suspicion.

B. Hypersensitivity Pneumonitis (Extrinsic Allergic Alveolitis)

1. **Definition**

    a. Hypersensitivity pneumonitis is the lung's reaction to antigenic organic dusts.

    b. In most patients the antigenic material is a fungal spore, although avium serum proteins and bacterial enzymes have also been implicated (Table 19–2).

2. **Etiology.** The condition is mediated by Type 3 and 4 hypersensitivity reactions.

    a. **Type 3 Reactions**

        1). These are mediated by immune complexes.

        2). Complement-fixation antibodies in sensitive individuals react with inhaled organic antigens to produce a reaction in four to six hours.

        3). These reactions are responsible for the acute manifestations of illness.

    b. **Type 4 Reactions**

        1). These are mediated by sensitized T lymphocytes present in peripheral blood and in bronchoalveolar lavage fluids of affected patients.

        2). These reactions are responsible for the development of the chronic manifestations of hypersensitivity pneumonitis.

3. **Epidemiology**

    a. Patients are exposed to antigenic material in specific occupations or hobbies.

        1). *Farmer's lung disease* occurs in farmers working in silos containing fungally contaminated hay.

        2). *Pigeon fancier's disease* affects bird shop owners or bird raisers exposed to droppings and dander.

    b. In some instances the source of exposure is less obvious, and an otherwise innocuous environmental source such as a contaminated air conditioner may be responsible for delivering the responsible agent.

TABLE 19–2. ANTIGENS, THEIR SOURCE, AND THE DISEASE ENTITIES THAT CAN PRODUCE HYPERSENSITIVITY PNEUMONITIS*

DISEASE	SOURCE OF ANTIGEN	PRECIPITINS
Air conditioner and humidifier lung	Fungi in air-conditioner and humidifiers	Thermophilic actinomycetes
Aspergillosis	Ubiquitous	*Aspergillus fumigatus, A. flavis, A. niger, A. nidulans*
Bagassosis (sugarcane workers)	Moldy bagasse	*Thermoactinomyces vulgaris*
Bird fancier's lung	Pigeon, parrot, or hen droppings	Serum protein and droppings
Byssinosis	Cotton, flax, hemp workers	Unknown
Farmer's lung	Moldy hay	*Micropolyspora faeni, T. vulgaris*
Malt worker's lung	Moldy barley, malt dust	*A. clavatus, A. fumigatus*
Maple-bark pneumonitis	Moldy maple bark	*Cryptostroma corticale*
Mushroom worker's lung	Mushroom compost	*M. faeni, T. vulgaris*
"New Guinea" lung	Moldy thatch dust	Thatch of huts
Pituitary snufftaker's lung	Heterologous pituitary powder	Heterologous antigen of pituitary snuff
Sequoiosus	Moldy redwood sawdust	*Graphium aurea basidium pullalans*
Sisal worker's lung	Unknown	Unknown
Smallpox handler's lung	Not yet demonstrated	Not yet demonstrated
Suberosis	Moldy oak bark, cork dust	Unknown
Wheat weevil disease	Infested wheat flour	*Sitophilus granarius*

*From Dreisin RB: Hypersensitivity pneumonitis (extrinsic allergic alveolitis). *In* Mitchell RS, Petty TL (eds.): Synopsis of Clinical Pulmonary Disease. 3rd ed. St. Louis, CV Mosby Company, 1982.

4. *Clinical Presentation and Course.* The specific manifestations in any patient depend more on the intensity and duration of antigenic exposure than on the identity of the eliciting antigen.
   a. **Acute Form**
      1). The classic picture of acute hypersensitivity pneumonitis is seen, for example, in the case of a sensitive farmer who enters a silo with high concentrations of fungal spores. Symptoms develop within 4 to 6 hours and consist of fever, chills, cough, dyspnea, and anorexia. Chest pain and hemoptysis are unusual. Generally these symptoms subside over the ensuing 24 to 48 hours.
      2). Physical examination shows fever and cyanosis.
         a). Rales are unusual, and wheezing is not heard unless the patient is atopic.

b. **Chronic Form**
   1). Chronic hypersensitivity pneumonitis may be extremely difficult to diagnose. Patients with this form of the disease have been exposed to low concentrations of antigen over a prolonged period of time and may have experienced an acute reaction so mild as to go unrecognized. Cough and dyspnea develop insidiously.
   2). Findings on physical examination in these patients are usually those of patients with chronic obstructive pulmonary disease, that is, hyperexpansion with diminished breath sounds. Rales are less frequently heard.
   3). The course may be progressive and irreversible unless antigen is avoided.

5. *Chest Radiographs*
   a. **Acute Form**
      1). Scattered patches of soft alveolar infiltrates are seen.
      2). With massive antigenic exposure diffuse pulmonary edema is apparent ("ARDS pattern").
   b. **Chronic Form**
      1). Hyperexpansion is present.
      2). There are increased interstitial markings. In the hyperexpanded chest this increase may be difficult to appreciate.
         a). This condition may be mistaken for the picture of chronic bronchitis and emphysema.

6. *Laboratory Data*
   a. In the acute response leukocytosis parallels the fever curve, and white blood cell counts as high as 25,000 are common.
   b. In chronic disease no leukocytosis is seen.
   c. Precipitating antibodies to the offending antigen are demonstrable in from 60 to 90 per cent of affected patients, but in hypersensitivity pneumonitis populations these antibodies may be present in unaffected exposed workers as well.
   d. Pulmonary function abnormalities are observed.
      1). In acute hypersensitivity pneumonitis the abnormalities of lung function depend on the stage at which the patient is tested. The delayed fall in vital capacity and forced expiratory volume of the first second (FEV_1) seen in a nonatopic person is depicted in Figure 19–1A, and the changes in the atopic individual are depicted in Figure 19–1B. The delayed (intermediate) response is restrictive, while the immediate response that is seen in atopic patients is obstructive.
      2). In chronic hypersensitivity pneumonitis, results are variable. In general, lung volumes are diminished, although the ratio of volume to total lung capacity may be elevated, suggesting air trapping. The diffusive capacity for carbon monoxide is impaired.

7. *Histopathology*
   a. In acute hypersensitivity pneumonitis, lung biopsy dem-

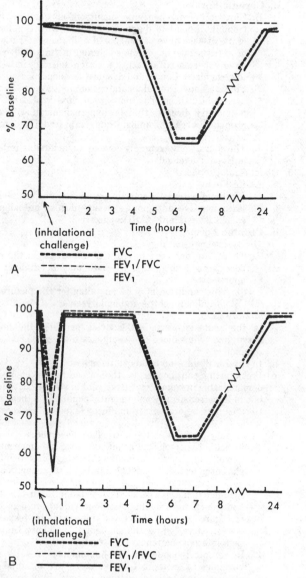

Figure 19–1. Serial spirometry following inhalational challenge in patients with hypersensitivity pneumonitis. *A,* Classic response. *B,* "Dual response" in an atopic patient. (From Dreisin RB: Hypersensitivity pneumonitis (extrinsic allergic alveolitis). *In* Mitchell RS, Petty TL (eds.): Synopsis of Clinical Pulmonary Disease. 3rd ed. St. Louis, CV Mosby Company, 1982, pp. 126–135.)

onstrates interstitial infiltration of plasma cells, lymphocytes, and occasionally neutrophils. Foamy macrophages are seen within alveolar spaces and terminal airways, and an obliterative bronchiolitis may be present. In fulminant cases hyaline membranes and intra-alveolar hemorrhage are present as well.

b. In chronic hypersensitivity pneumonitis, bronchial fibrosis and centrilobular emphysema are found. Scattered granulomata are characteristic.

8. *Clues to Diagnosis*
   a. Acute hypersensitivity pneumonitis should be considered as a possible diagnosis in any patient with an atypical pneumonia. Suspicion should be strengthened by the presence of repeated episodes in a patient in whom a source of potential antigenic contact can be historically implicated.
   b. The presence of chronic combined obstructive and restrictive lung disease in a patient with an appropriate occupational exposure should similarly alert the astute clinician to the possibility of chronic hypersensitivity pneumonitis.

C. **Connective Tissue Disease.** The connective tissue diseases are included here under the category of immunologic and hypersensitivity reactions because in the majority of cases specific abnormalities of the humoral and immune systems have been identified. In these illnesses a specific antigen responsible for the abnormalities has also been delineated (for example, double-stranded DNA or altered immunoglobulin). Each of the diseases described may appear with pulmonary illness other than that of a chronic diffuse interstitial pneumonitis. The following comments regarding the chronic interstitial forms of lung diseases in these patients should serve to direct differential diagnostic efforts but are not absolute by themselves.

1. *Rheumatoid Arthritis.* The most important intrathoracic manifestation of rheumatoid arthritis is that of slowly progressive diffuse interstitial infiltration with fibrosis. Radiographic evidence for interstitial pneumonitis is seen in 20 per cent of patients, physiologic evidence in 41 per cent, and pathologic evidence in 80 per cent. Other intrathoracic diseases are:
   a. *Pleural effusion or pleural thickening* in 20 per cent. This condition is not more prevalent in those with diffuse fibrotic disease. A very low pleural fluid glucose level is characteristic.
   b. *Rheumatoid pulmonary nodules* in patients with high titers of rheumatoid factor who also have subcutaneous nodular disease. The nodules are single or multiple and may cavitate. Despite the association between nodular disease and high-titer rheumatoid factor, there does not appear to be a significant association between rheumatoid nodules and interstitial pneumonitis.
   c. *Caplan's syndrome,* which is a rare Welsh form of rheumatoid lung disease in which rheumatoid nodules develop and cavitate fulminantly in coal miners with rheumatoid arthritis.

2. *Systemic Lupus Erythematosus.* Unlike the case in rheumatoid arthritis, pleural effusions are much more common than lupus pneumonitis per se. The interstitial pneumonitis in these patients may be overwhelming and acute but more frequently is chronic and mild. Although diffuse interstitial fibrosis has been described, serious impairment from chronic interstitial disease is very unusual.

3. *Progressive Systemic Sclerosis.* Interstitial fibrosis is present in 80 per cent of lung autopsy specimens from patients with progressive systemic sclerosis. In addition, pulmonary hypertension from intimal proliferation is seen in 20 per cent.

4. *Polymyositis-Dermatomyositis.* Interstitial pneumonitis with fibrosis is rare, occurring in less than 10 per cent of patients. Concomitant bronchiolitis obliterans is seen in a higher percentage of patients than in the other connective tissue disorders.

5. *Sjögren's Syndrome.* Sjögren's syndrome may coexist with any of the other connective tissue diseases. When it occurs alone it is most characteristically associated with a lymphocytic interstitial pneumonitis.

6. *Ankylosing Spondylitis.* Patients with ankylosing spondylitis rarely may develop fibrosis of one or both upper lung fields. The amount of apical infiltration is usually pronounced and out of proportion to the relatively mild or absent disease in the lower lung fields. Infiltrates characteristically may cavitate in advanced cases. In contrast to the pulmonary involvement seen in other connective tissue illnesses, the apical infiltrates of ankylosing spondylitis virtually always appear many years after the onset of the spondylitis itself.

IDIOPATHIC FORMS OF INTERSTITIAL LUNG DISEASE

In this group of diseases, in contrast to those described earlier, a specific etiologic agent has not been identified or suspected. While abnormalities of the immune system have been described, the antigen or agent evoking these abnormalities has not.

A. **Idiopathic Pulmonary Fibrosis (Idiopathic Interstitial Pneumonitis, Cryptogenic Fibrosing Alveolitis)**
1. *Definition.* "Idiopathic pulmonary fibrosis" is the term applied to diffuse interstitial inflammatory conditions that develop into fibrosis in patients in whom no specific cause of interstitial pneumonitis and fibrosis can be identified.
2. *Etiology.* The etiology is unknown.
3. *Epidemiology*
   a. Males are affected more often than females (5:4).
   b. The mean age is 50 years; all ages may be affected.
   c. There is no racial predisposition.
   d. It is rarely familial.
4. *Clinical Presentation and Course*
   a. Dyspnea with exertion is the most common initial symptom; dyspnea at rest is an end-stage symptom.
   b. Nonproductive cough occurs in 35 per cent of patients.

c. Systemic symptoms are unusual.

d. The course of the illness is variable. Mean duration of illness from diagnosis until death in one series was 4.8 years. Rare patients, those for whom the term "Hamman-Rich syndrome" is properly employed, have a fulminant course leading to death within six months. More commonly patients show some decrease in pulmonary function and exercise tolerance for a few months and then the condition stabilizes for many years, often in apparent response to corticosteroid and immunosuppressive therapy.

5. *Chest Radiograph*

a. Characteristically the chest radiograph shows a fine increase in interstitial markings in a reticular pattern at the lung bases. As the disease progresses the profusion and thickness of these irregularities increase and involve the rest of the lung.

b. In the end stage of the disease honeycombing develops.

c. A pattern of bilateral triangular haziness extending from both hila to the costophrenic angles is seen in *desquamated interstitial pneumonia (DIP)*, a variety of idiopathic pulmonary fibrosis.

d. Pulmonary hypertension and the radiographic findings of cor pulmonale are seen only in the final stages of the illness.

6. *Laboratory Data*

a. Polyclonal gammopathy appears in 70 per cent of cases.

b. There is an elevated erythrocyte sedimentation rate in 80 per cent of cases.

c. There are positive antinuclear and rheumatoid factors in 10 to 40 per cent of cases.

d. There are circulating immune complexes in patients with active infiltrative (as opposed to fibrotic) forms of disease.

e. Bronchoalveolar lavage may show an elevation of percentage of neutrophils and lymphocytes as compared with controls. Normal nonsmokers have less than 1 per cent neutrophils in the lavage fluids, whereas patients with idiopathic pulmonary fibrosis may have 5 to 40 per cent.

7. *Histopathology*

a. *Usual interstitial pneumonitis (UIP)*, the most common form, is characterized by a pleomorphic infiltrate of lymphocytes, plasma cells, eosinophils, and fibroblasts.

b. *Desquamative interstitial pneumonia (DIP)* is characterized by engorgement of alveolar spaces by large alveolar macrophages with varying degrees of interstitial inflammation and fibrosis. DIP may represent an early stage of the illness and therefore carry a better prognosis.

c. *Lymphocytic interstitial pneumonitis (LIP)* frequently is associated with Sjögren's syndrome and macroglobulinemia. There is a monotonous infiltrate of normal-appearing lymphocytes in the interstitium.

d. *Immunofluorescence* shows granular deposits of IgM, IgG, and complement along alveolar walls in inflamed sections of lung.

8. *Clues to Diagnosis.* Idiopathic pulmonary fibrosis involves a diagnosis of exclusion and is suspected in a case in which extensive questioning, serologic testing, and lung biopsy fail to establish an alternative cause of progressive interstitial infiltration with fibrosis.

B. **Sarcoidosis.** (Sarcoidosis is discussed in Chapter 76.)

C. **Pulmonary Alveolar Proteinosis**

1. *Definition.* Pulmonary alveolar proteinosis is a disease of unknown origin that is diagnosed histologically by the presence of proteinaceous material diffusely filling alveolar spaces.

2. *Pathogenesis.* The pathogenesis involves material collecting within alveolar spaces that contains large amounts of protein as well as lipids and glycoprotein chemically resembling normal surfactant. The disease is thought to represent a process of excessive secretion or inadequate clearance from the alveolar space.

3. *Clinical Presentation and Course*

   a. Patients may be asymptomatic at examination but generally are seen with exertional dyspnea.

   b. The majority of patients have a spontaneous remission. In the remainder, a downhill course to respiratory failure ensues. There are no extrapulmonary manifestations.

4. *Chest Radiograph.* Classically diffuse bilateral symmetrical alveolar infiltrates are seen. Unilateral disease and an interstitial radiographic appearance are less frequently seen.

5. *Laboratory Data.* More than 80 per cent of patients with pulmonary alveolar proteinosis demonstrate an isolated elevation of lactic dehydrogenase (LDH). All five isoenzymes may be responsible.

6. *Histopathology.* There is deposition of a surfactantlike material that stains pink with eosin and is strongly positive in response to the periodic acid-Schiff (PAS) reaction. Mild interstitial inflammation and fibrosis may be seen as well but are less impressive than the alveolar-filling process.

7. *Clues to Diagnosis.* Pulmonary alveolar proteinosis should be strongly considered in the differential diagnosis of any patient with chronic alveolar infiltrate. An isolated elevation of LDH should reinforce suspicion.

D. **Wegener's Granulomatosis**

1. *Definition.* Wegener's granulomatosis is a necrotizing granulomatizing vasculitis involving the upper respiratory tract, lungs, and glomeruli. Other organs may be involved as well.

2. *Etiology and Pathogenesis*

   a. The etiology is unknown.

   b. The pathogenesis is unknown.

3. *Epidemiology*

   a. Twice as many men as women are affected.

   b. The disease occurs at any age, primarily in the third to fifth decades.

   c. There is no racial or geographic disposition.

4. *Clinical Presentation and Course*

   a. Upper airway involvement includes ulcers, erosions, pseu-

dotumors, saddle nose deformity, sinusitis, and bony erosion.
  b. Lung involvement consists of nodules and cavities, unilateral or bilateral.
  c. Kidney involvement consists of focal glomerulitis, glomerulonephritis, and parenchymal masses.
  d. Less commonly involved sites:
      1). Joints: arthralgias.
      2). Skin: palpable purpura, ulcerating infarct.
      3). Eyes: granulomatous uveitis, orbital pseudotumor.
      4). Ears: serous otitis media.
      5). Heart: coronary vasculitis and pericarditis.
      6). Nervous system: mononeuritis complex, cranial neuritis.
  e. The course is fatal. Pulmonary hemorrhage, respiratory failure, and rapidly progressive glomerulonephritis appear in the untreated patient.
5. *Chest Radiograph.* There are nodules or cavities, or both. True diffuse interstitial infiltration, except by multiple discrete nodules, is not seen.
6. *Laboratory Data*
  a. Anemia, leukocytosis, and eosinophilia are present.
  b. The antinuclear factor or rheumatoid factor is positive in fewer than 10 per cent of patients.
7. *Histopathology.* There is a diffuse granulomatous vasculitis involving the medium-sized vessels, with an associated disseminated small vessel leukocytoclastic vasculitis.
  a. The necrotizing granulomas in the lung of patients with Wegener's granulomatosis are surrounded by a zone of what appears to be a usual interstitial pneumonitis. Transbronchial lung biopsy may therefore incorrectly indicate the latter diagnosis rather than the true nature of the illness.
  b. The renal lesion is that of a necrotizing focal glomerulitis with necrosis of glomerular tufts.
  c. *"Limited" Wegener's granulomatosis* has a histopathology identical to that of classic Wegener's granulomatosis. In the limited form the kidney is spared.
8. *Clues to Diagnosis.* Wegener's granulomatosis should be suspected in the middle-aged man with lung nodules, fever, night sweats, and sputum examinations that are negative for bacteria, mycobacteria, and fungi. Suspicion is strengthened by the presence of an abnormal urinalysis, symptoms of sinus drainage, and vasculitic skin lesions. The diagnosis usually is confirmed histopathologically by lung biopsy.

REFERENCE

1. Dreisin RB: Hypersensitivity pneumonitis. *In* Mitchell RS, Petty TL (eds.): Synopsis of Clinical Pulmonary Disease. 3rd ed. St. Louis, CV Mosby Company, 1982, pp. 126–135.

PULMONARY EMBOLISM

By PATRICIA SATO, M.D.

DEFINITION

Pulmonary embolism (PE) is the obstruction of the pulmonary arterial system by a thrombus that has been dislodged from a site in the deep venous system. Although a presumptive diagnosis of PE is often made from the clinical examination, the signs and symptoms associated with PE are nonspecific. Strict clinical criteria for diagnosis do not exist; rather, definitive diagnosis rests with two radiologic studies: pulmonary angiography and ventilation-perfusion scintiphotography.

EPIDEMIOLOGY AND GENERAL COMMENTS

Estimates for the incidence of PE in the United States range from 500,000 to 630,000 cases per year. Evidence of recent or old embolism is present in 25 to 60 per cent of autopsy specimens, which suggests that the true incidence is underestimated and that an antemortem diagnosis is made in less than one third of all cases. Improvement in antemortem diagnosis is needed, since the mortality rate for treated PE is approximately 10 per cent and rises to 30 per cent for untreated cases.

Three factors that contribute to thrombogenesis are stasis, vessel wall abnormalities, and alterations in coagulation. A test to determine hypercoagulability is not available, but clinical experience has demonstrated that certain conditions are associated with a higher risk of thromboembolism. These are listed in Table 20–1. In the appropriate clinical setting these conditions should raise the level of suspicion of PE.

Thromboembolism results in both respiratory and hemodynamic pathophysiologic changes. Embolic obstruction produces an area of lung that is ventilated but not perfused. This "dead space" cannot participate in effective gas exchange. Loss of lung volume also occurs and may eventually result in alveolar collapse and frank atelectasis. This is thought to be a result of bronchoalveolar hypo-

TABLE 20–1.   RISK FACTORS FOR VENOUS THROMBOEMBOLISM

Stasis	Immobilization, obesity, chronic deep venous insufficiency, congestive heart failure, chronic pulmonary disease
Estrogens	Oral contraceptives
Malignancy	Adenocarcinoma of the lung and gastrointestinal tract
Trauma	Surgery (postoperative period), burns, fractures, postpartum period

capnia and loss of alveolar surfactant in the affected lung zone. This situation contributes to ventilation-perfusion mismatch and may result in hypoxemia.

The primary hemodynamic consequence of PE is a decrease in the available cross-sectional area for pulmonary arterial blood flow. However, the pulmonary vascular bed is a large-capacity bed and is able to recruit reserve vessels. Vascular obstruction must be extensive (greater than 50 per cent) in order to result in elevation of pulmonary arterial pressure and vascular resistance. Once this does occur, pulmonary hypertension and right ventricular hypertrophy may develop.

Another factor that determines the clinical severity of an embolic event is the underlying cardiopulmonary status of the patient. Even a small embolus may have substantial pathologic effects on an individual with limited cardiac or pulmonary reserve, such as a patient with chronic obstructive pulmonary disease or cardiac valvular disease.

Death of lung tissue, that is, pulmonary infarction, rarely accompanies pulmonary embolism. The lung has three ready sources for oxygen: the pulmonary arterial circulation, the bronchial circulation, and the airways. For infarction to occur, usually there is preexisting compromise of the bronchial arterial flow or airway flow to the area of embolism, or both. The usual diseases that cause such compromise are left ventricular failure, mitral stenosis, and chronic obstructive pulmonary disease. It is thus rare to see infarction in patients without prior cardiopulmonary disease.

HISTORY AND PHYSICAL EXAMINATION

A. **History.** The two most commonly reported symptoms in patients with PE are sudden onset of shortness of breath and chest pain. The dyspnea is related to the sudden addition of alveolar dead space. Chest pain is most often pleuritic in nature and is associated with congestive atelectasis or infarction. The chest pain may be nonpleuritic and is often described as a dull substernal discomfort that is related to increases in pulmonary arterial pressure. Table 20–2 lists the incidence of symptoms from 327 patients with angiographically proven PE from the National Heart and Lung Institute's (NHLI) study of thrombolytic agents. It can be seen that the classic triad of dyspnea, chest pain, and hemoptysis is quite rare and that no single symptom or combination of symptoms is diagnostic of PE.

B. **Physical Examination.** Findings on physical examination may be minimal and, if present, are nonspecific. The most constant finding is that of tachypnea. Other findings may include tachycardia; fever; a focal area of decreased breath sounds, rales, or wheezing; and in the case of pleural involvement or infarction, a pleural friction rub. When the embolism is extensive, there may be cardiac findings of acute cor pulmonale. A right ventricular lift may be palpated or a right ventricular gallop auscultated. The pulmonic component of S2 may be accentuated (loud

TABLE 20–2. INCIDENCE OF SYMPTOMS IN PATIENTS WITH ANGIOGRAPHICALLY PROVEN PULMONARY EMBOLI

Symptom	Incidence (%)
Chest pain	88
Pleuritic	74
Nonpleuritic	14
Dyspnea	84
Apprehension	59
Cough	53
Hemoptysis	30
Sweats	27
Syncope	13

P2), and a systolic murmur may be heard over the pulmonic area. Deep venous thrombosis is an excellent indicator of concurrent pulmonary embolism, but its absence does not rule out the diagnosis. Clinical evidence of deep venous thrombosis is present in less than half of patients with PE. Table 20–3 gives the incidence of physical examination findings from the previously mentioned NHLI study of proven cases of PE.

LABORATORY STUDIES

Routine laboratory studies of blood chemistry and cell counts contribute little to the diagnosis of PE. Arterial blood gases often indicate hypoxemia, hypocapnia, and respiratory alkalosis. Patients may hyperventilate to raise the PaO_2 to a normal level, but such patients exhibit a widening of the alveolar to arterial oxygen difference $[P(A-a)O_2]$. (See Chapter 17 for a calculation method.) Thus, normal PaO_2 does not exclude the diagnosis of PE.

A. Electrocardiograms (ECGs). Findings from the NHLI study show that (1) 23 per cent of patients with submassive PE had normal ECGs, whereas only 6 per cent of patients with massive PE did; (2) one or more of the traditional findings of acute cor pulmonale (S1Q3T3, right bundle branch block, right ventricular

TABLE 20–3. INCIDENCE OF PHYSICAL SIGNS IN PATIENTS WITH ANGIOGRAPHICALLY PROVEN PULMONARY EMBOLI

Signs	Incidence (%)
Respirations 16/minute	92
Rales	58
S2P2	53
Pulse 100 beats/minute	44
Temperature 37.8° C	43
Phlebitis	32
Gallop	34
Diaphoresis	36
Edema	24
Murmur	23
Cyanosis	19

hypertrophy, P-pulmonale, or right axis deviation) occurred only in 26 per cent of patients; (3) the most common finding was either nonspecific T wave changes (42 per cent) or nonspecific RST elevation or depression (41 per cent).

Surprisingly, none of the patients had atrial fibrillation or atrial flutter. Also notable was the short duration of the changes on ECGs, with disappearance of more than 50 per cent of the abnormalities occurring by 5 to 14 days.

B. **Chest Roentgenogram.** The most common finding, which occurs approximately 50 per cent of the time, is a normal x-ray. Findings that may appear include (1) a parenchymal infiltrate with abutment against the pleural surface in patients with infarction or congestive atelectasis; (2) evidence of pleural reaction or effusion; (3) disparity in the size of comparable vessels; (4) a rat-tail appearance of a major pulmonary artery, which suggests the presence of an intraluminal organizing clot; (5) oligemia of a lung zone with hyperlucency (Westermark's sign) suggesting obstruction with increased flow to other areas; and (6) volume loss with elevation of the hemidiaphragm on the affected side, which is consistent with pneumoconstriction. The chest x-ray may provide useful information supportive of the diagnosis and can be very helpful in excluding other possible causes of the patient's symptoms such as pneumothorax or congestive heart failure. The chest x-ray so frequently appears normal in this disease that this finding should not dissuade the physician from pursuing a diagnosis of PE.

RECOMMENDED DIAGNOSTIC APPROACH

Although the clinical picture may be compelling for the diagnosis of pulmonary embolism, the history, physical examination, ECG, and chest roentgenograph are nonspecific. Diagnosis can only be made with two studies: (1) pulmonary perfusion and ventilation scintiphotography ($\dot{V}$/Q scan) and/or (2) pulmonary angiography. The appropriate approach for how and when to use these tests has been controversial at times, mainly because of the differing opinions about the specificity of ventilation-perfusion lung scanning.

A. **The $\dot{V}$/Q Scan.** The $\dot{V}$/Q scan is a valuable tool in evaluating a patient with possible pulmonary embolism. The test is highly sensitive, and perfusion scanning should be performed as part of the initial evaluation of virtually all patients. A normal six-view perfusion scan essentially excludes the diagnosis of PE. If perfusion defects are present on the scan, this confirms the presence of abnormalities in the distribution of blood flow but does not provide anatomic information. Any parenchymal disease such as pneumonia, chronic obstructive pulmonary disease, or atelectasis with reduced ventilation may show decreased blood flow. A ventilation scan can be helpful to assess ventilation in the area of abnormal blood flow. If a $\dot{V}$/Q scan demonstrates "mismatch," that is, one or more segmental or greater perfusion defects with normal ventilation to those abnormal areas, the $\dot{V}$/Q scan is characteristic of vascular obstruction and is a "high-probability" scan. Approximately 90 per cent of these patients have emboli demonstrated on pulmonary angiography. However, the results of $\dot{V}/Q$ scanning are not always so definitive.

A recent prospective study from Canada has provided information that is useful when scans demonstrate (1) one or more segmental perfusion defects with matched ventilation defects, or (2) small perfusion defects (subsegmental or smaller) with or without ventilation abnormalities. In the first group, a $\dot{V}/Q$ match on the segmental level (both abnormal ventilation and perfusion scans in the same region) did not rule out PE. Approximately 25 per cent of these patients had PE. In the case of subsegmental perfusion defects with or without ventilation mismatch, the scans were not of sufficient sensitivity or specificity to suggest high or low probability of PE. If a definitive diagnosis is to be made, pulmonary angiography must be used.

B. Pulmonary Angiography. Pulmonary angiography is an invasive procedure, but it is the only means of obtaining anatomic information about the pulmonary vasculature. It involves placement of a cardiac catheter into the pulmonary artery and injection of radiopaque dye to visualize the pulmonary vessels. It has certain limitations in that artifacts may occur and may require repeated injections, and the ability to evaluate small vessels is limited. The examiner must also be familiar with the possible angiographic findings of (1) abrupt cutoff of a vessel with or without complete obstruction, (2) filling defects in which the clot creates a negative shadow as dye flows around it, and (3) generalized decrease in filling of a lung zone. Effective use of this test depends on experience with the techniques and interpretation.

How far the physician proceeds down the diagnostic pathway is based on the clinical situation and the weighed risks and benefits of contemplated therapy. Once a diagnosis has been made, standard therapy consists of intravenous administration of heparin that is adjusted to maintain the partial thromboplastin time (PTT) at two times the control level. Other means of therapy include thrombolytic agents, which are used in the setting of massive PE, or in rare instances surgical embolectomy with venous interruption.

REFERENCES

1. Dalen JE, Haffajee CI, Alpert JS, et al.: Pulmonary embolism, pulmonary hemorrhage and pulmonary infarction. N Engl J Med 296:1431, 1977.
2. Dalen JE, Alpert JS: Natural history of pulmonary embolism. Prog Cardiovasc Dis 17:259, 1975.
3. Moser KM: Pulmonary embolism: State of the art. Am Rev Respir Dis 115:829, 1977.
4. Bell WR, Simon TL, DeMets DL: The clinical features of submassive and massive pulmonary emboli. Am J Med 62:355, 1977.
5. Stein PD, Dalen JE, McIntyre KM, et al.: The electrocardiogram in acute pulmonary embolism. Prog Cardiovasc Dis 17:247, 1975.
6. Urokinase Pulmonary Embolism Study Group: Urokinase Pulmonary Embolism Trial. JAMA 214:2153, 1970.
7. Cheely R, McCartney WH, Perry JR, et al.: The role of noninvasive tests versus pulmonary angiography in the diagnosis of pulmonary embolism. Am J Med 70:17, 1981.
8. Hull RD, Hirsh J, Carter CJ, et al.: Pulmonary angiography, ventilation lung scanning, and venography for clinically suspected pulmonary embolism with abnormal perfusion lung scan. AIM 98:891, 1983.

NEPHROLOGY

ACID-BASE DISORDERS

By RICHARD O. CUMMINS, M.D.

DEFINITION OF THE PROCESS

Clinicians often begin to suspect acid-base disorders on review of arterial blood gas or serum electrolyte findings. The challenges they face are to recognize and classify the disturbance and to determine the underlying cause.

A. **Recognition.** This depends on knowledge of three acid-base values readily available to the clinician:

1. **pH (7.40 ± 0.05).** This is a logarithmic derivative (pH = $-\log(H^+)$). Therefore, small changes in pH represent large changes in total hydrogen concentration. A change of 0.3 reflects a twofold change in H^+.

2. **pCO_2 (40 mm Hg ± 5).** This is the partial pressure of carbon dioxide dissolved in 100 ml of plasma. Alveolar ventilation regulates pCO_2; thus pCO_2 reflects the respiratory component of acid-base status.

3. **HCO_3^- (22–28 mEq per liter).** This is a measure of the free bicarbonate ion in the blood. HCO_3^- reflects the renal component of acid-base status. Most automated laboratories report this value.

4. **Relationships.** HCO_3^- and pCO_2 represent the bicarbonate buffer system. The relationship among these components is explained by the reaction

$$H_2O + CO_2 \rightleftharpoons H_2CO_3 \rightleftharpoons HCO_3^- + H^+$$

$$\text{Lungs} \qquad \text{Carbonic} \qquad \text{Kidney}$$
$$\text{(Respiratory)} \quad \text{acid} \qquad \text{(Metabolic)}$$

and by the Henderson-Hasselbalch equation

$$pH = pK + \log\left(\frac{HCO_3^-}{H_2CO_3}\right)$$

Thus changes in respiratory function alter pCO_2 and H_2CO_3, and changes in renal function, such as increased excretion of acid and increased regeneration of bicarbonate, alter HCO_3^- and H^+.

5. *Other Buffers.* The phosphate serum protein system and especially the hemoglobin buffer system also strive to maintain pH. They account for about 40 per cent of the "buffer base," that is, all substances in the blood that are able to bind excess H^+. For most clinical problems, an understanding of the bicarbonate buffer system suffices.

6. *Anion Gap.* The clinician should also search for acid-base disturbances caused by increased production, or exogenous addition, of metabolic acids. An "anion gap" results. This is calculated from serum electrolytes, although many automated laboratories supply this value routinely:

$$\text{anion gap} = Na^+{}_{\text{serum}} - (\text{chloride} + HCO_3{}^-)$$

Interpretation of the anion gap is discussed later under metabolic acidosis.

B. Classification of Acid-Base Disorders

1. *Simple Disturbances.* These involve only one driving pathologic force, often with an expected "compensatory change." A single primary abnormality with the expected compensation does not constitute a mixed acid-base disturbance.

   a. **Metabolic Acidosis.** Either metabolic acids accumulate (acid-gaining acidosis) or bicarbonate decreases (base-losing acidosis). The key abnormality is a fall in serum bicarbonate level with an elevation of serum potassium concentration.

   b. **Metabolic Alkalosis.** This is a gain of bicarbonate or a loss of metabolic acids.

   c. **Respiratory Acidosis.** Carbonic acid accumulates as a result of mismatch between reduced alveolar ventilation and carbon dioxide production.

   d. **Respiratory Alkalosis.** Carbonic acid decreases as a result of mismatch between increased alveolar ventilation and carbon dioxide production.

2. *Mixed Disturbances.* These involve either two driving pathologic forces or one primary abnormality plus medical attempts at correction.

EPIDEMIOLOGY

The epidemiology of acid-base disorders is that of the underlying pathologic processes. Acidosis, both respiratory and metabolic, is seen most often in medical practice, frequently in association with respiratory disease, renal compromise, or diabetes. Metabolic alkalosis often follows diuretic therapy, vomiting, or nasogastric drainage.

The other metabolic causes of acid-base disorders are less common, even rare, but should be considered when they are suggested by laboratory findings.

INTERPRETATION OF ACID-BASE DISORDERS

At least three approaches to the interpretation of acid-base disorders are useful: axiomatic, graphic, and tabular. Each starts where the clinician starts, with findings of abnormal blood gases or electrolytes, or both.

A. **Axiomatic Approach.** This type of approach involves simple memorization of three axioms or "golden rules" developed by the American Heart Association for its *Textbook of Advanced Cardiac Life Support*. These axioms were derived from the Henderson-Hasselbalch equation, but they are based on assumptions that may not always hold true, such as the presence of normal hemoglobin concentration and normal buffering. Memorization avoids a complicated graph or table, which is required by the other two methods.

 1. *Golden Rule #1.* A change in pCO_2 of 10 mm Hg is associated with a reciprocal change in pH of 0.08 units. For example, if pCO_2 increases 10 mm Hg from the normal value of 40 mm Hg, pH decreases 0.08 from the normal value of 7.40 to 7.32. Use of this rule permits an estimate of respiration as a driving force for abnormal pH. If the calculated pH, using Golden Rule #1, is the same as the measured pH, changes in pH are probably respiratory. If the actual pH is lower than the calculated pH, however, there must be additional acids present, which suggests metabolic acidosis in addition to a respiratory acidosis.

 2. *Golden Rule #2.* A change in pH of 0.15 is the result of a base change of 10 mEq per L. This base change is termed *base excess* or *base deficit* (also called delta base or buffer base). Here the pH change is the difference between the actual pH and the pH calculated from Golden Rule #1. To illustrate this formulation, if the pH were measured at 7.25 and the pCO_2 at 40 mm Hg, the normal pCO_2 would suggest that there was no respiratory component. The calculated pH would be 7.40 by Golden Rule #1, but the measured pH is 7.25, giving a difference of 0.15. Application of Golden Rule #2 reveals a base deficit of 10 mEq per L, thus suggesting pure metabolic acidosis.

These two axioms can be used to detect the simultaneous presence of metabolic and respiratory changes, but they cannot indicate which abnormality is primary, which is expected compensation, or whether two primary abnormalities have occurred independently. Interpretation of arterial blood gas data must occur in light of the patient's clinical status. For example, a pCO_2 of 55 mm Hg and a pH of 7.38 may be found in a patient. An increase in pCO_2 of 15 mm Hg indicates hypoventilation. Golden Rule #1 suggests that the pH should be decreased by 0.12 to a calculated value of 7.28. The difference of 0.10 pH units between the calculated pH (7.28) and the measured pH (7.38) shows a base excess of 7 mEq per L, suggesting a base-gaining metabolic alkalosis. Therefore, both respiratory acidosis and metabolic alkalosis are present. Clinical information might reveal a patient with chronic obstructive pulmonary disease, in whom respiratory acidosis was caused by carbon dioxide retention, and the metabolic alkalosis was caused by chronic renal compensation. In contrast, these values are also consistent with a previously healthy patient in cardiac arrest treated with inadequate ventilation and excessive sodium bicarbonate.

3. **Golden Rule #3.** This is a quick axiom to calculate the total body bicarbonate excess or deficit. It is based on the rough estimate that total extracellular fluid volume in liters (the distribution space of bicarbonate) is equal to one fourth of the body weight in kilograms:

$$\text{total body bicarbonate deficit (mEq)} = \frac{\text{calculated base deficit from Golden Rule \#2}}{} \times \frac{\text{weight (kg)}}{4}$$

Figure 21–1 is a flow diagram that displays the rapid application of these Golden Rules.

B. **Graphic Approach.** Graphs have been developed to display the relationship among pH (or H^+ concentration), pCO_2, and HCO_3. The nomogram of Goldberg is perhaps the most popular and is presented in Figure 21–2. As with the axiomatic approach, other clinical information is required to deduce the exact sequence of acid-base changes.

C. **Tabular Approach.** Values of pCO_2 are classified as low, normal, or high and cross-tabulated (see Table 21–1).

DIFFERENTIAL DIAGNOSIS OF ACID-BASE DISORDERS

After an acid-base disorder has been recognized and classified, the clinician must determine the primary cause, that is, the driving pathologic force.

A. **Metabolic Acidosis.** The presence or absence of an anion gap helps in the diagnosis.

1. *Increased Anion Gap (>12) (Acid-Gaining Acidosis).* The gap results from extra noncarbonic acids produced endogenously or exogenously administered (usually self-administered).

a. **Endogenous Production**
1). Diabetic ketoacidosis
2). Alcoholic ketoacidosis
3). Starvation ketoacidosis
4). Renal failure with uremic acidosis
5). Lactic acidosis

b. **Exogenous Administration**
1). Salicylate intoxication
2). Methanol intoxication
3). Ethylene glycol consumption
4). Paraldehyde intoxication

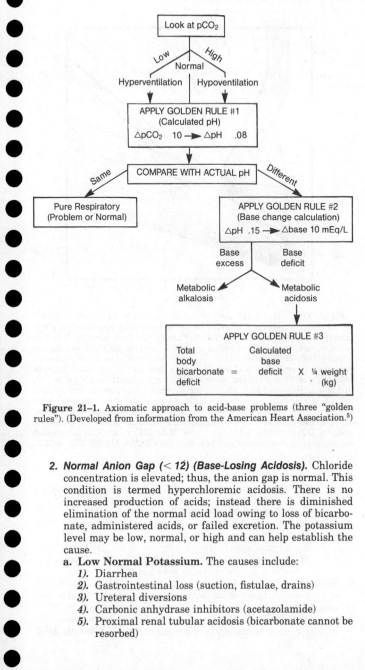

Figure 21–1. Axiomatic approach to acid-base problems (three "golden rules"). (Developed from information from the American Heart Association.[5])

2. **Normal Anion Gap (< 12) (Base-Losing Acidosis).** Chloride concentration is elevated; thus, the anion gap is normal. This condition is termed hyperchloremic acidosis. There is no increased production of acids; instead there is diminished elimination of the normal acid load owing to loss of bicarbonate, administered acids, or failed excretion. The potassium level may be low, normal, or high and can help establish the cause.

a. **Low Normal Potassium.** The causes include:
   1). Diarrhea
   2). Gastrointestinal loss (suction, fistulae, drains)
   3). Ureteral diversions
   4). Carbonic anhydrase inhibitors (acetazolamide)
   5). Proximal renal tubular acidosis (bicarbonate cannot be resorbed)

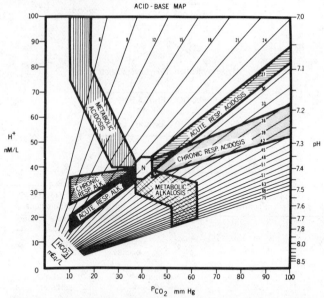

Figure 21–2. Graphic approach to acid-base disorders. The bands represent the 95 per cent confidence interval for the compensatory response to a given primary disorder. The reader should work vertically from the pCO_2 line. For example, consider a patient with a pCO_2 of 70 mm Hg, HCO_3 of 33 mEq per L, and pH of 7.30. The elevated HCO_3^- could be caused by renal compensation for a chronic respiratory acidosis. The bands show that 95 per cent of patients with pCO_2 of 70 mm Hg and chronic respiratory acidosis have a pH of 7.26 to 7.35 and HCO_3^- of 32 to 39 mEq per L, which is the case for this patient, indicating appropriate compensation. However, if the HCO_3^- were 30 mEq per L, which is outside the 95 per cent confidence band for pCO_2 of 70 mm Hg, a mixed disorder would be suggested, such as an additional metabolic acidosis. (From Goldberg M, Green SB, Moss ML, et al.: Computer-based instruction and diagnosis of acid-base disorders. JAMA 223:269–275, 1973.)

      6). Distal renal tubular acidosis (decreased acid secretion in distal tubules)

   b. High Normal Potassium. The causes include:

      1). Interstitial nephritis or chronic pyelonephritis

      2). Obstructive uropathy

      3). Adrenal insufficiency

      4). Acid administration (NH_4Cl, HCl, IV alimentation with arginine or lysine, oral $CaCl_2$)

B. Metabolic Alkalosis. The primary problem is either a loss of acid or a gain of base. With both situations serum bicarbonate concentration always rises and is the key abnormality. With sustained metabolic alkalosis an initial problem generates the alkalosis, and a secondary problem maintains the alkalosis. Most

TABLE 21-1. TABULAR APPROACH TO THE INTERPRETATION OF ACID-BASE DISORDERS*†

pCO$_2$	pH		
	Low (<7.35)	Normal (7.40 ± 0.05)	High (>7.45)
Low (<35 mm Hg)	Primary and metabolic acidosis plus either incomplete respiratory compensation or coexisting respiratory alkalosis	Primary and respiratory alkalosis plus compensatory metabolic acidosis	Primary respiratory alkalosis with or without coexisting metabolic alkalosis
Normal (40 ± 5 mm Hg)	Primary metabolic acidosis	Normal	Primary metabolic alkalosis
High (>45 mm Hg)	Primary respiratory acidosis plus either incomplete metabolic compensation or coexisting metabolic acidosis	Respiratory acidosis plus compensatory metabolic alkalosis	Metabolic alkalosis plus coexisting respiratory acidosis

*Modified from Slonim NB: Blood-gas and pH abnormalities. *In* Friedman HH (ed.): Problem-Oriented Medical Diagnosis. 2nd ed. Boston, Little, Brown & Company, 1979.

†Compensation does not remove the driving pathologic force; it returns pH toward, but never past, normal. Physiologic overcompensation does not occur.

causes of metabolic alkalosis stimulate the kidneys to reclaim more bicarbonate than they would normally, thus maintaining the alkalosis. Hypovolemia, elevated pCO_2, and chloride depletion, for example, enhance bicarbonate regeneration and are associated with most cases of metabolic alkalosis. Because chloride depletion is so often associated, urine chloride measurement is a recommended diagnostic test. Patients with low urinary chloride are called salt-responsive because administration of saline solution largely corrects the problem. High urinary chloride occurs rarely, and saline administration seldom corrects the alkalosis (salt-resistant metabolic alkalosis).

1. **Low Urinary Chloride (< 10 mEq per L), "Salt-Responsive."** This is a result of:
   a. Vomiting
   b. Gastric suction
   c. Diuretic administration (the most common cause of metabolic alkalosis)
   d. Chloride-losing diarrhea
   e. Villous adenoma of colon
   f. Carbenicillin therapy
   g. Hypercapnia

2. **High Urinary Chloride (> 10 mEq per L), "Salt-Resistant."** This occurs with the following conditions:
   a. Primary hyperaldosteronism
   b. Bartter's syndrome (secondary hyperaldosteronism)
   c. Glucocorticoid excess: (1) endogenous (Cushing's syndrome, ectopic ACTH production, hyperadrenocorticism) or (2) exogenous (glucocorticoids, ACTH, carbenoxalone, licorice ingestion, tobacco chewing)
   d. Severe potassium depletion

3. **Miscellaneous.** Miscellaneous causes of metabolic alkalosis include:
   a. Milk-alkali syndrome
   b. Rapid blood transfusion (containing sodium citrate and carbonate, which are metabolized to bicarbonate)
   c. Calcium carbonate release from bone (hypercalcemia secondary to malignancy)
   d. Decreased effective intravascular volume (leads to increased mineralocorticoid activity, for example, heart failure and hypoalbuminemia)

C. **Respiratory Acidosis.** The primary event is carbon dioxide retention from hypoventilation. Acutely (in 12 to 24 hours) tissue buffers generate HCO_3^- and the serum level rises slightly (3 to 4 mEq per L). Chronically (over 36 hours) renal excretion of H^+ and regeneration of HCO_3^- return pH toward normal. Causes include:

1. **Acute-Chronic Lung Disease.** The most common causes include:
   a. Acute mechanical obstruction of respiratory passages by foreign body, tumor, secretions, blood, or pus
   b. Severe asthma (later stages of status asthmaticus)

    c. Severe pneumonia, pulmonary edema, or bronchiolitis
    d. Chronic obstructive lung disease

2. *Central Nervous System Depression.* This may result from:
    a. Pharmacologic causes (sedatives, anesthesia, alcohol)
    b. Respiratory center lesions (ischemia, trauma, brain tumor, increased intracranial pressure)
    c. Infection (meningitis, encephalitis)

3. *Neuromuscular Disorders.* These include:
    a. Myopathies (muscular dystrophies, low potassium)
    b. Neuropathies (diphtheria, tetanus, polio, Guillain-Barré syndrome, myasthenia gravis)
    c. Intoxication (curare, succinylcholine, botulism, pesticides, nerve gas)

4. *Thoracic Cage Limitations.* These include:
    a. Kyphoscoliosis, thoracic crush injuries
    b. Scleroderma, ankylosing spondylitis
    c. Postburn contractures

5. *Lung Motion Impairment.* This results from the following conditions:
    a. Pleural effusion, pneumothorax, hemothorax, edema
    b. Hypomechanical hypoventilation
    c. Extreme abdominal distention or pain
    d. Fibrosis of pleurae or parenchymae
    e. Cardiorespiratory arrest
    f. Obesity-hyperventilation syndrome

D. **Respiratory Alkalosis.** The primary event is increased elimination of carbon dioxide as a result of hyperventilation. Acutely (within minutes) tissue buffers make H^+ available, HCO^-_3 falls by 3 to 4 mEq per L, and pCO_2 decreases to 20 to 25 mm Hg. Chronically (in three to four days) renal excretion of acid slows, endogenously produced acids accumulate, and HCO^-_3 continues to fall with normalization of pH. Causes include

1. *Pulmonary Disorders.* These consist of pneumonia, congestive heart failure, asthma, pulmonary embolism, and restrictive lung disease (early).

2. *Drugs.* Salicylates and paraldehyde intoxication, progesterones, and catecholamines are responsible.

3. *Metabolic Disorders.* Fever, exposure to high altitudes, hypoxemia, marked anemia, hyperthyroidism, liver failure, and gram-negative sepsis are responsible.

4. *Central Nervous System Problems.* Head trauma, central nervous system hemorrhage, encephalitis, and meningitis are involved.

5. *Other.* Other causes include anxiety-hyperventilation, hysteria, pregnancy, and mechanical hyperventilation.

E. **Mixed Acid-Base Disorders.** Mixed disorders are two or more simple disorders, not just a simple disorder and its compensation. The diagnostic key is knowledge of the degree of anticipated compensation for the simple disorders. The axiomatic and graphic approaches supply an estimate of expected compensation for simple disorders.

Table 21–2 presents the more common mixed disorders.

TABLE 21–2. FREQUENTLY OCCURRING MIXED ACID-BASE DISORDERS

Metabolic acidosis
1. Hyperchloremic acidosis plus high anion gap
   a. Bicarbonate loss plus lactic acidosis
   b. Early chronic renal failure (esp. interstitial nephritis)
   c. RTA with nephrocalcinosis and azotemia
   d. Resolving diabetic ketoacidosis
   e. Diarrhea with high anion gap
2. Lactic acidosis plus either ketoacidosis or methanol intoxication or ethylene glycol intoxication
3. Two or more hyperchloremic disorders
   a. RTA with diarrhea
   b. Hyperalimentation with diarrhea
   c. Gastrointestinal or renal disease plus drugs (acetazolamide, sulfamylon, oral calcium chloride)

Metabolic alkalosis plus a metabolic acidosis
Any combination of a metabolic alkalosis and either vomiting or alkali therapy
1. Diarrhea and vomiting
2. Lactic acidosis and vomiting
3. Metabolic acidosis and too much bicarbonate treatment

Combined metabolic-respiratory acidosis (pCO_2 is elevated and bicarbonate is decreased)
1. Cardiopulmonary arrest
2. Combination of renal and pulmonary disease
3. Any metabolic acidosis plus acute or chronic lung disease
4. Diabetic ketoacidosis and phosphate depletion

Metabolic alkalosis plus a respiratory acidosis
Chronic obstructive pulmonary disease patients on diuretic therapy

Metabolic acidosis plus a respiratory alkalosis
1. Pulmonary edema
2. Salicylate toxicity
3. Hepatorenal syndrome

Combined metabolic-respiratory alkalosis
1. Cirrhotic condition plus vomiting, excessive diuresis, nasogastric suction
2. Stroke patient on diuretics
3. Many intensive care unit patients
   a. Respiratory alkalosis from pain, sepsis, respirations
   b. Metabolic alkalosis from nasogastric suction, blood transfusion, lactated Ringer's solution

HISTORY, SIGNS, AND SYMPTOMS

A. In general, the history, signs, and symptoms are those of the disorders listed in the differential diagnosis.

B. However, there are some signs and symptoms that are associated with simple acid-base disorders. Although often nonspecific, they can be helpful diagnostically.

　　1. Metabolic Acidosis. Signs and symptoms include Kussmaul's breathing, ketone breath, arrhythmias, hypotension or shock, nausea and vomiting, lethargy, coma, weight loss, alcohol ingestion, "home brew" ingestion, papillitis, odor of paraldehyde on the breath, and oxalate crystals in urine (from antifreeze ingestion).

　　2. Metabolic Alkalosis. Signs and symptoms include nausea and vomiting, diarrhea, sensorium changes, tremors, convulsions, arrhythmias, hypovolemic signs, and licorice or tobacco chewing.

　　3. Respiratory Acidosis. Signs and symptoms include dyspnea, tachypnea, throbbing headache, confusion, drowsiness, coma, tremor, arrhythmias, flushed face, and tunnel vision.

　　4. Respiratory Alkalosis. Signs and symptoms include numbness and tingling of hands and feet, signs of tetany, carpopedal spasm, dizziness, psychomotor impairment, and arrhythmias.

RECOMMENDED LABORATORY STUDIES

A. An acid-base disorder must first be recognized and classified. This requires studies of the following:

　　1. Arterial pH, pCO_2, and pO_2

　　2. Serum bicarbonate and other electrolytes

　　3. Urine chloride (if metabolic alkalosis is suspected)

B. The next step is to determine the underlying pathologic process. The clinician should consider the most likely diagnosis from the differential diagnoses.

　　1. Rule-Out Tests. These tests are frequently ordered routinely and serve to rule out many diagnoses that should not be missed. Blood sugar, ketones, urine sugar, blood urea nitrogen, creatinine, calcium, hemoglobin, hematocrit, and liver function tests are examples of such routine tests.

　　2. Confirmatory Tests. These are more specific tests, and if results are positive they frequently confirm the diagnosis. These tests are only ordered if there is a good probability of disease. Salicylate level determination, urine crystal examination, intravenous pyelography, cortisol level determination, and pulmonary function tests are examples.

Confirmatory and rule-out tests for many causes of acid-base disorders are discussed in other sections of this book.

REFERENCES

1. Kassirer JP: Serious acid-base disorders. N Engl J Med 291:773–776, 1974.
2. Ravel R: Clinical Laboratory Medicine: Clinical Application of Laboratory Data. 3rd ed. Chicago, Year Book Medical Publishers, 1978.

3. Bear RA, Dyck RF: Clinical approach to the diagnosis of acid-base disorders. Can Med Assoc J 20:173–182, 1979.
4. Slonim NB: Blood-gas and pH abnormalities. In Friedman HH (ed.): Problem-Oriented Medical Diagnosis. 2nd ed. Boston, Little, Brown & Company, 1979.
5. Sladen A: Acid-base balance. In McIntyre KM, Lewis AF (eds.): American Heart Association: Textbook of Advanced Cardiac Life Support. Dallas, Texas, American Heart Association, 1981.
6. Vanatta JC, Fogelman MJ: Moyer's Fluid Balance: A Clinical Manual. 3rd ed. Chicago, Year Book Medical Publishers, 1982.
7. Goldberg M, Green SB, Moss ML, et al.: Computer-based instruction and diagnosis of acid-base disorders. JAMA 223:269–275, 1973.

22

ELECTROLYTE DISORDERS: HYPONATREMIA, HYPERNATREMIA, HYPOKALEMIA, AND HYPERKALEMIA

By STUART BURSTEN, M.D.

HYPONATREMIA

Hyponatremia indicates a problem with water, rather than a problem with sodium. In hyponatremia water has diluted the serum sodium concentration. If there is no change in tonicity, it is called *isotonic hyponatremia*; if there is a reduction in serum tonicity it is called *hypotonic hyponatremia*; and if an increase in serum tonicity has occurred, it is called hypertonic hyponatremia. If total body water has changed significantly as well, the terms "hypervolemic" and "hypovolemic" are added.

ISOTONIC HYPONATREMIA

Measured serum osmolality is normal at 280 to 295 mOsm per L. This is actually a state of "pseudohyponatremia" in which a true reduction in total body sodium has not taken place.
A. **Clinical Occurrence.** This condition occurs in states in which the solid component of serum (the ash) is increased, such as in the dysproteinemic states of Waldenström's macroglobulinemia, multiple myeloma, and hyperlipidemias.
B. **Physiologic Mechanism.** The normal solid component of serum is 7 per cent (70 mL per L). This component is not sampled when serum is analyzed for sodium. Out of a serum volume of 1 L, only 930 mL is available for analysis. This explains why if normal serum sodium is 140 mEq per L (138 to 145 mEq per L) normal saline solution (0.9 per cent NaCl) has the unusual sodium concentration of 154 mEq per L ($140/930 = 154/1000$).

1. For example, if the ash content of the serum is increased by doubling it to 14 per cent, as occurs in multiple myeloma, 140 cu cm of each liter is not available. The sodium concentration is thus determined in 860 mL (1000 − 140) and is falsely low at 129 (129/860 = 154/1000).
2. This also means that during infusions of isotonic solutions such as mannitol or glucose there is a transient dilutional hyponatremia.

RECOMMENDED DIAGNOSTIC APPROACH

When serum sodium determinations are consistently low and the serum osmolality is normal, (1) the serum should be observed for lactescence; (2) the total protein should be determined (this may be a clue to the diagnosis of multiple myeloma); and (3) the lipid fractions should be determined.

HYPERTONIC HYPONATREMIA

This rather common finding is associated with hyperglycemia, hyperosmolar hyperglycemic coma, and infusions of hypertonic mannitol (for neurosurgical patients) or glucose (hyperalimentation). The increase in glucose hypertonicity obligates water to cross into the extracellular space to dilute the serum sodium and cause hyponatremia.

A. Correction Factor

$$\text{sodium}_{(\text{corrected})} = \text{sodium}_{(\text{determined})} + \left(\frac{\text{glucose} - 100}{(100)} \times 1.8 \right)$$

B. For example, if serum sodium is 130, and the serum glucose is 750,

$$\text{sodium}_{\text{corrected}} = 130 + \left(\frac{750\text{-}100}{100} \times 1.8 \right) = 141.7.$$

HYPOTONIC HYPONATREMIA: HYPOVOLEMIC TYPE

In general, these states exist when salt is lost in greater amounts than water or when water is replaced in greater quantities than salt. Patients are placed in this category when signs of hypovolemia are present.

A. Clinical Occurrence
1. *Gastrointestinal Problems.* These include secretory diarrheas in which sodium and potassium are lost.
2. *Lung.* There is bronchorrhea, such as occurs with alveolar cell carcinoma.

3. *Skin.* There may be sweating if the person is not acclimated and still has a high-sodium–content sweat.
4. *Adrenal Insufficiency.* Renal salt-wasting occurs.
5. *Renal Problems.* Renal problems involve use of potent diuretics, chronic renal failure with salt-wasting, and postobstruction diuresis.

RECOMMENDED DIAGNOSTIC APPROACH

Virtually all patients demonstrate changes in blood pressure and pulse in relation to posture (if pulse is measured while standing, for longer than two minutes), a resting tachycardia, and diminished skin turgor.

A. **Serum Blood-Urea Nitrogen–Creatine (BUN/CREAT) Ratio.** This ratio is usually greater than 20 in this form of hyponatremia, although with renal failure it can be lower, about 10.

B. **Urine Sodium**
   1. With gastrointestinal, lung, and skin losses, urine sodium is less than 20 mEq/L.
   2. With adrenal insufficiency and renal problems the urine sodium content is greater than 20 mEq/L.

C. **Urine Osmolality.** Osmolality is usually greater than 400 mOsm per L except with renal failure when the urine is isosthenuric (280 to 300 mOsm per L).

HYPOTONIC HYPONATREMIA: ISOVOLEMIC TYPE

In this condition the volume status is normal, and there is no third spacing of fluid.

A. **Clinical Occurrence**
   1. *Water Intoxication.* This is generally found in psychotic states, particularly schizophrenia, and in some manic states.
   2. *Potassium Depletion.* As potassium shifts out of cells in hypokalemic states, sodium shifts in, producing a dilutional hyponatremia. Potassium depletion also stimulates antidiuretic hormone (ADH) secretion.
   3. *Hypothyroidism and Hypoadrenalism.* These endocrinopathies decrease the ability to excrete a water load.
   4. *Syndrome of Inappropriate Antidiuretic Hormone (SIADH) Secretion.* This can be caused by the following conditions:
      a. Ectopic ADH elaboration by tumors, particularly oat cell cancer of the lung, prostatic and pancreatic cancer, and lymphoma
      b. Inappropriate stimulation from pulmonary pathology (bacterial pneumonia, tuberculosis, lung abscesses, asthma), or drugs (vincristine, cyclophosphamide, morphine, barbiturates, nicotine, hypoglycemic agents)
      c. Uncontrolled secretion from virtually any central nervous system problem (infections, trauma, vascular disease, neoplasms), or after stress such as trauma and surgery

RECOMMENDED DIAGNOSTIC APPROACH

To suggest the diagnosis of isovolemic hyponatremia, the patient must have no signs of cardiac disease, hypovolemia, volume overload, or third spacing.

A. The physician should consider the possible causes listed above and pursue them with the appropriate diagnostic tests (see related chapters in this book).

B. SIADH has the following laboratory findings:
   1. A urine sodium concentration that is initially elevated (greater than 60 mEq per L) and that subsequently falls to a level that reflects the daily sodium intake;
   2. Urine osmolality, which should be maximally dilute, is inappropriately high;
   3. BUN and creatinine are decreased, as is the BUN/CREAT ratio;
   4. Uric acid is low, owing to an elevated glomerular filtration rate and increased tubular secretion;
   5. Serum antidiuretic hormone levels are not suppressed and are normal to high.

HYPERVOLEMIC HYPONATREMIA

This condition is associated with end-stage volume overload processes and with protein-losing states.

A. Clinical Occurrence
   1. Hypervolemic hyponatremia is frequently seen with end-stage congestive heart failure, cirrhosis, nephrotic syndrome, and severe protein-losing enteropathies with edema.
   2. *Pathophysiologic Mechanisms Include:*
      a. Excessive stimulation of antidiuretic hormone by central hypoperfusion, poor right atrial return, and increased intrathoracic pressure
      b. Reduced renal blood flow and glomerular filtration rates
      c. Loss of diluting capacity as a result of diminished delivery of solutes to the renal tubules
      d. Increased activity of the renin-angiotensin-aldosterone system

RECOMMENDED DIAGNOSTIC APPROACH

A. **Signs of Volume Overload.** The physician should examine for these signs, including peripheral edema, pulmonary edema, ascites, and hypertension.

B. **BUN/CREAT Ratio.** This ratio is greater than 20.

C. **Urine Sodium.** Urine sodium is less than 20 mEq per L.

HYPERNATREMIA

Hypernatremia is caused by either loss of water in excess of loss of salt or by a gain of salt in excess of gain in water. Like hyponatremia, hypernatremia is approached logically by consideration of the volume status. The estimated total body water deficit can be calculated as follows (desired sodium content is taken as 140 mEq per L):

$$(1\text{-sodium}_{\text{measured}}/\text{sodium}_{\text{desired}}) \times \text{total body water } (0.6 \times \text{weight in kg}).$$

For example, if the serum sodium in a 70-kg person is 160, the total water deficit is

$$(1 - 160/140) \times (0.6 \times 70) = (-20/140) \times 42 = (-1/7) \times 42 = -6 \text{ L}.$$

HYPOVOLEMIC HYPERNATREMIA

This occurs when both salt and water are lost, but with water lost in greater proportions than salt. The fluid lost is salt-poor. Hypovolemic hypernatremia may also be caused iatrogenically when the lost hypotonic fluid is replaced with hypertonic or isotonic fluid.
A. Clinical Occurrence. Hypovolemic hypernatremia occurs in the following conditions:
  1. Gastrointestinal illness, including osmotic diarrheas and vomiting.
  2. Sweating after acclimation to hot climates (low-sodium sweat).
  3. Diuretic ingestion combined with increased salt intake and poor water intake.
  4. Partial urinary tract obstruction combined with administration of hypertonic fluids.
  5. Acute or chronic renal failure with loss of concentrating ability.
  6. Urea diuresis, particularly in catabolic patients.
  7. Glycosuria: Glucose causes a urine that is 0.45 per cent sodium chloride. This is why hypernatremia is common with hyperosmolar coma and why the sodium correction for hyperglycemia must always be done. This correction permits more accurate calculation of water deficits.

RECOMMENDED DIAGNOSTIC APPROACH

A. BUN, creatinine, urine sodium, and urine osmolality should be measured.
  1. Nonrenal causes of hypernatremia produce a BUN/CREAT ratio

that is greater than or equal to 20, a urine sodium content less than 20 mEq per L, and a urine osmolality greater than 400 mOsm per L.
2. Renal causes of hypernatremia produce a BUN/CREAT ratio that is usually 10/1 because both BUN and CREAT levels are elevated, a urine sodium content greater than 20 mEq per L but less than the serum sodium content, and isosthenuric urinary osmolarity.

EUVOLEMIC HYPERNATREMIA

This condition is characterized by selective loss of water and is caused almost exclusively by one form or another of diabetes insipidus.
A. **Clinical Occurrence.** Diabetes insipidus is classified as either central diabetes insipidus or nephrogenic diabetes insipidus.
  1. Central diabetes insipidus is characterized by diminished or absent production of ADH.
    a. Primary central diabetes insipidus accounts for 50 per cent of cases.
    b. Secondary central diabetes insipidus is most often caused by cranial trauma or metastatic tumor, usually of lung or breast, and by granulomatous disease such as tuberculosis, sarcoidosis, and eosinophilic granuloma.
  2. Nephrogenic diabetes insipidus is characterized by diminished or absent renal response to ADH.
    a. Primary nephrogenic diabetes insipidus is rare, causing less than 1 per cent of cases.
    b. Secondary nephrogenic diabetes insipidus is caused by electrolyte disorders such as hypokalemia and hypercalcemia and by renal disease such as acute tubular necrosis, obstruction, or myeloma and amyloid kidney. Up to 25 per cent of nephrogenic diabetes insipidus is related to medications such as lithium carbonate (more than 50 per cent of patients taking lithium develop concentrating disorders), demeclocycline, and methoxyflurane.

RECOMMENDED DIAGNOSTIC APPROACH

A. **Twenty-Four–Hour Urine Output.** The 24-hour urine output should be measured.
  1. Central diabetes insipidus is characterized by large volumes of hypotonic urine (greater than 3 L per 24 hours); if there is complete absence of ADH the volume may be greater than 20 L per 24 hours.
  2. In nephrogenic diabetes insipidus there is diminished output of a urine that is generally isosthenuric.
B. **Water Deprivation Test.** In normal persons water deprivation causes a fall in urine volume and an increased urine osmolality proportionate to the increasing serum osmolality.

1. In central diabetes insipidus, patients have constant urine output, a rising serum osmolality, but no (or a slight) rise in urine osmolality. This is correctable with intramuscular administration of ADH.
2. Nephrogenic diabetes insipidus responds in the same manner to water deprivation, but there is no response to ADH administration.

HYPERVOLEMIC HYPERNATREMIA

A. **Clinical Occurrence.** Hypervolemic hypernatremia is almost always caused by iatrogenic administration of excess salt via hypertonic solutions. Other causes include primary hyperaldosteronism, Cushing's syndrome, and exogenous administration of steroids.
B. **Prevention.** Iatrogenic hypernatremia may be avoided by administration of properly hypotonic or isotonic solutions. Clinicians can randomly sample any body fluid loss for electrolytes throughout the day and replace exactly what is lost and no more. For urine, the free water clearance can be calculated so that the exact replacement for urine can be estimated:

$$\text{free water clearance} = \text{urine volume} - \left[\frac{(\text{urine osmoles} \times \text{urine volume})}{\text{plasma osmoles}}\right]$$

For example, 24-hour urine volume is 2 L, urine osmoles are 750, and plasma osmoles are 300:

$$\text{free water} = 2\text{ L} - \frac{(750 \times 2)}{300} = -3\text{ L}$$

(This example illustrates that free water clearance is always negative when urine osmoles are greater than plasma osmoles.)

HYPOKALEMIA

Chronic hypokalemia is associated with a variety of serious problems, including renal tubular dysfunction, chronic renal failure with interstitial degeneration, as well as cardiac arrhythmias. It can be classified into one of three types, according to whether it is caused by redistribution of potassium, by renal losses, or by losses other than renal.

REDISTRIBUTIONAL HYPOKALEMIA

In these states the total body potassium content is normal. (However, if renal wasting occurs, total body depletion may result.)

A. **Clinical Occurrence**
1. *Alkalosis.* The depletion of protons with alkalosis causes an intracellular increase of negative charges. This obligates a potassium shift into cells and leads to hypokalemia (0.6 mEq of potassium decrease per 0.1 pH increase).
2. *Insulin Administration.* Insulin acts to shift potassium into cells acutely.
3. *B_{12} Therapy.* As B_{12} stimulates myelopoiesis and rapid cell proliferation, there is a rapid sequestration of potassium in multiplying cells.
4. *Periodic Paralysis.* This is associated with thyrotoxicosis in Japanese persons and is an autosomal dominant genetic defect in whites.
5. *Epinephrine or Beta-2 Agonist Administration.* Stimulation of beta-2 receptors is associated with intracellular shifts of potassium. Renal potassium wasting can occur with long-term use of these agents.

HYPOKALEMIA FROM RENAL LOSSES

By definition the 24-hour urine potassium content is greater than 20 mEq. This occurs in two clinical states, hypertensive and normotensive.

A. **Hypertensive States.** Hypertensive states include:
1. Conditions of elevated renin, such as renovascular and malignant hypertension
2. Conditions of low renin and elevated aldosterone, such as primary aldosteronism with bilateral adrenal hyperplasia
3. Conditions of low renin and low aldosterone, such as Cushing's syndrome and after intake of exogenous mineralocorticoids, licorice (glycirrhizinic acid), chewing tobacco, and carbenoxolone

B. **Normotensive States.** Normotensive states include:
1. Renal tubular acidosis, with serum bicarbonate concentration less than 23 mEq per L
2. Alkalosis caused by vomiting, with urine chloride concentration less than 10 mEq per day
3. Alkalosis caused by diuretics, severe potassium depletion, or Bartter's syndrome
4. Drug-induced, such as by carbenicillin and its derivatives, gentamicin, amphotericin B, *cis*-platinum

HYPOKALEMIA FROM LOSSES OTHER THAN RENAL

A. These are uncommon, with the cause generally obvious from the history. The 24-hour urine potassium content is less than 20 mEq.

B. **Clinical Occurrence.** This type of hypokalemia occurs from:
1. Skin losses, without acclimation.

2. Biliary loss.
3. Secretory diarrhea (villous adenomata should be considered). This is associated with bicarbonate loss and a corresponding acidosis.

HYPERKALEMIA

Hyperkalemia always represents a potential medical emergency. The electrocardiogram (ECG) should be examined for characteristic changes immediately, since death from hyperkalemia is totally preventable. Early ECG changes are T wave peaking, with progression to QRS widening. Imminent danger of ventricular fibrillation is signaled by merging of QRS-T complexes and formation of a poorly defined sine wave pattern.

PSEUDOHYPERKALEMIA (Laboratory error)

Even if this is suspected, the ECG should be monitored while awaiting repeat laboratory test results. Serum potassium always exceeds plasma potassium by 0.1 to 0.3 mEq per L owing to release of potassium from white blood cells and platelets. To confirm this as the cause of the hyperkalemia, the plasma potassium should be compared with the serum potassium.

A. **Serum-Plasma Difference.** This difference will be 0.5 to 2.0 mEq per L with:
1. Leukocytosis greater than 50,000 per cu mm
2. Thrombocytosis greater than 750,000
3. Extensive hemolysis in the test tube

HYPERKALEMIA FROM REDISTRIBUTION

When sudden, this presents a particularly grave danger from fatal arrhythmias and must be treated.

A. **Clinical Occurrence.** This form of hyperkalemia occurs in the following conditions:
1. *Tissue Necrosis.* Crush injuries, burns, rhabdomyolysis, tumor lysis syndrome.
2. *Acidosis.* The inverse of alkalosis occurs, with extracellular shifts.
3. *Insulin Deficiency.* This is exacerbated in diabetics with simultaneous hypoaldosteronism.
4. *Medications.* Nonselective beta-blockers with blockade of beta-2 receptors can cause extracellular leak of potassium. This is characteristic of severe digitalis toxicity with inhibition of sodium-potassium ATPase.

HYPERKALEMIA FROM EXCESSIVE INTAKE AND REDUCED EXCRETION

Some degree of reduced excretion relative to the intake is present. Potassium problems are not encountered in chronic renal failure until end-stage renal disease is approached (glomerular filtration rate less than 8 to 10 mL per minute).

A. **Clinical Occurrence.** Conditions of excessive intake include:
   1. Potassium-penicillin administration
   2. Low-sodium diets
   3. Salt substitutes
   4. Transfusions

B. **Clinical Occurrence.** Conditions of reduced potassium secretion in the distal tubules and collecting ducts include:
   1. Decreased extracellular fluid volume, which is most commonly seen in elderly persons
   2. Interstitial nephritis and amyloid renal disease
   3. Use of potassium-retaining drugs, including triamterene, spironolactone, and amiloride
   4. Urinary tract obstruction

HYPERKALEMIA FROM DEFICITS IN THE RENIN-ANGIOTENSIN-ALDOSTERONE SYSTEM

These problems may be associated with renal insufficiency or may exist alone, causing hyperkalemia independent of renal function.

A. **Clinical Occurrence.** This form of hyperkalemia occurs in association with:
   1. *Decreased Renin.* Renin is decreased by:
      a. Drugs, such as beta-blockers, alpha-methyldopa, and prostaglandin inhibitors
      b. Aging
      c. Interstitial nephritis (in addition to the secretory defects mentioned above)
      d. Diabetes mellitus
   2. *Decreased Angiotensin.* Angiotensin is decreased by:
      a. Diminished glucocorticoids (Addison's disease)
      b. Hepatic failure
      c. Converting enzyme inhibitors
   3. *Decreased Aldosterone.* Aldosterone is decreased by:
      a. Addison's disease
      b. Selective adrenal hemorrhage as with heparin administration
      c. Spironolactone
      d. Hydroxylase deficiencies

RECOMMENDED DIAGNOSTIC APPROACH

The decision to obtain serum renin, aldosterone, or angiotensin values may be guided by administration of 1.0 mg per day of fludro-cortisone. If there is a response after three to five days, with kaliuresis and transition to normokalemia, the deficit is not renal, and measurements of renin, aldosterone, and angiotensin are appropriate.

REFERENCES

1. Narins RG, Jones E, Stom MC, Rudnick MR, Bastl CP: Diagnostic strategies in disorders of fluid, electrolytes and acid-base homeostasis. Am J Med 72:496–520, 1982.
2. Beck LH (ed.): Body fluid and electrolyte disorders. Med Clin North Am 65:251–448, 1981.

These are two recent and excellent summaries of the diagnostic approach to fluid and electrolyte disorders.

23
PROTEINURIA

By STEVE HOLLAND, M.D.

GENERAL COMMENTS AND DEFINITION

A. **General Comments.** The finding of protein on routine urinalysis may be either the first sign of serious renal disease or a transient and insignificant finding. In an apparently healthy individual it may reflect occult renal disease with the potential to progress to uremia or it may be transient with little, if any, prognostic significance. Persistent proteinuria may lead to denial of health insurance, rejection from some types of employment, or increased life insurance premiums. Treatable conditions must be identified and separated from conditions for which treatment does not exist or for which prognosis is benign and treatment unnecessary. The clinical picture combined with the pattern and amount of proteinuria may lead to expectant watchfulness or invasive and potentially morbid procedures.
B. **Incidence of Proteinuria.** Isolated asymptomatic proteinuria is often detected during a routine physical examination. Neither the incidence nor prevalence of proteinuria as an isolated finding among various age or population groups is certain. Estimates of the incidence of qualitative proteinuria during casual or routine urinalysis in military inductees and other adult populations have varied from 0.6 to 8.8 per cent.

C. **Definition.** Proteinuria is defined in terms of urinary protein excretion per 24 hours. Most adults excrete between 30 and 130 mg per day with upper limits of normal set at 150 mg for adults, and 140 mg per sq m of body surface area for small children.

D. **Screening for Significant Proteinuria**

1. *Dipstick.* Because of its convenience and low cost, dipstick urinalysis remains the first choice for screening for proteinuria. The indicator dye is sensitive to 30 mg of albumin per deciliter and may therefore show 1+ protein in a highly concentrated (specific gravity > 1.030) morning urine sample. This method does not detect light-chain proteins or other low molecular weight proteins, which may be present in myeloma, certain leukemias, or renal tubular disease.

2. *Sulfosalicylic Acid Test.* This protein precipitation test is more sensitive but less specific than the dipstick method and is a useful confirmatory test, especially when light-chain disease is suspected or the urine specimen is dilute. Eight drops of 20 per cent sulfosalicylic acid are added to 2 mL of urine. A white cloud of precipitate indicates a positive test.

3. *Twenty-Four–Hour Urinary Quantitative Protein Collection.* If several tests in a series of qualitative tests for protein are positive, a 24-hour urine collection for quantitative protein should be undertaken. Greater than 150 mg per day of protein is significant; greater than 3 g per day is to be considered in the nephrotic range.

4. *Urinary Creatinine Excretion.* Urinary creatinine excretion is measured to determine the adequacy of the collection. If the specimen is properly collected, it will contain an amount of creatinine appropriate to the patient's muscle mass:

   a. For young to middle-aged men this is 16 to 26 mg per kg of body weight per day (1100 to 2000 mg per day).

   b. For women this is 12 to 24 mg per kg of body weight per day (750 to 1400 mg per day).

Creatinine excretion declines with age in both sexes, reaching a rate of 8 to 15 mg per kg per day by the end of the eighth decade.

5. *Random Spot Urinary Protein-Creatinine Ratio.* In the presence of stable renal function, a random spot urinary protein-creatinine ratio of more than 3.5 represents "nephrotic range" proteinuria, and a ratio of less than 0.2 is within normal limits.

Causes of false-positive and false-negative results of tests for proteinuria are outlined in Table 23–1.

CLASSIFICATION AND DIFFERENTIAL DIAGNOSIS

Proteinuria can be classified as benign (functional), overflow, or as caused by glomerular, tubular, or interstitial dysfunction.

A. **Benign (Functional) Proteinurias.** These proteinurias are the most common cause of a positive qualitative test for urinary protein. Their pathophysiology is poorly understood, they carry no associated morbidity or mortality, and they show no evidence

**TABLE 23–1. CAUSES OF FALSE-POSITIVE (+) AND
FALSE-NEGATIVE (−) RESULTS FOR PROTEINURIA***

CLINICAL SETTING	DIPSTICK	SULFOSALICYLIC ACID
X-ray contrast media	−	(+)
Highly concentrated urine (normal)	(+)	(+)
Dilute urine (proteinuria)	(−)	+
Alkaline urine (pH > 8)	(+)	±
Gross hematuria	(+)	(+)
Metabolites of		
tolbutamide	−	(+)
sulfonamide	−	(+)
P-aminosalicylic acid	−	(+)
Penicillin analogs or cephalosporins	−	(+)
Phenazopyridine	(+)	−
Low molecular weight proteins and light chains	(−)	+
Contamination with antiseptic (chlorhexidene or benzalkonium)	(+)	−

*Modified from Abuelo JG[1] and deTorrente AM.[2]
Signs not in parentheses indicate true-positive or true-negative tests.

of systemic or renal disease. Three general categories have been described:

1. *Functional Proteinurias.* These proteinurias are transient. Occasionally they are seen with fever, strenuous exercise, exposure to cold, emotional stress, or essential hypertension. Urine protein excretion falls to normal levels with recovery from the precipitating event, and there is no loss of renal function.

2. *Idiopathic Transient Proteinuria.* This condition is common in children and young adults. Many healthy young men occasionally have dipstick tests that are positive for urinary protein if they are tested often enough. Subsequent urine specimens show no proteinuria, although these patients may have transient proteinuria at a later date. Again, there is no loss of renal function.

3. *Orthostatic or Postural Proteinuria.* This proteinuria appears only while the person is upright and may be found in some or all specimens collected in the upright position. This transient form of proteinuria causes proteinuria in 20 per cent of young men observed to be proteinuric on routine screening. The proteinuria resolves in 15 per cent of patients after 5 years and in 50 per cent after 10 years. Patients with persistent orthostatic proteinuria followed for over 20 years have shown no progression to renal failure.

B. **Overflow Proteinuria.** This can be seen with hemoglobinuria, myoglobinuria, and Bence Jones proteinuria in which increased production or concentration of low molecular weight proteins or cationic proteins overwhelms or overloads the tubule's reabsorptive capacity.

C. **Glomerular Proteinuria.** This results from increased capillary permeability to all proteins (especially albumin) and can be caused by either primary glomerulopathies such as lipoid nephrosis and membranous glomerulonephritis or secondary glomerulopathies such as amyloidosis, diabetes, or systemic lupus erythematosus. Glomerular disease is the most common cause of proteinuria associated with the serious manifestations of renal disease (hypertension, nephrotic syndrome, and renal failure).

D. **Interstitial or Tubular Proteinuria.** Interstitial or tubular dysfunction sometimes permits low molecular weight plasma proteins to escape tubular reabsorption and to appear in the urine, usually in low quantities (<2 g per day). This is seen in such disorders as chronic pyelonephritis, Fanconi's syndrome, and chronic interstitial nephritis. Albumin is usually underrepresented, and little, if any, urinary protein is detected by the dipstick method.

The causes, clinical cues, and laboratory findings in low-grade proteinuria are outlined in Table 23–2.

HISTORY AND PHYSICAL EXAMINATION

The history and physical examination may point to a familial, systemic, or primary renal cause for the proteinuria.

A. **History**
  1. *Family History.* This may reveal familial nephritis, early renal failure, and hypertension, as seen in polycystic kidney disease or other genetic protein-losing nephropathies. Proteinuria can be seen with sickle cell disease, but the finding of proteinuria rarely precedes diagnosis of the disease itself. Familial Alport's syndrome and Berger's disease (IgA nephropathy) usually appear with accompanying hematuria.
  2. *Drug History.* Drug-induced renal lesions are an important and easily corrected cause of proteinuria. Examples of associated drugs include:
     a. Gold, penicillamine, captopril (membranous nephritis)
     b. Amphotericin B, aminoglycosides (acute tubular necrosis)
     c. Probenecid, fenoprofen (lipoid nephrosis)
     d. Penicillin analogs (allergic interstitial nephritis)
  3. *Recent Infections.* Streptococcal pharyngitis or impetigo, syphilis, leprosy, or viral syndromes suggestive of hepatitis B, cytomegalovirus infection, mononucleosis, or varicella can lead to mild to moderate proteinuria. Review of travel history may uncover less common infections such as malaria, schistosomiasis, filariasis, or toxoplasmosis, all of which have been implicated in nephrotic-range proteinuria.

B. **Physical Examination.** Skin rash, heart murmur, arthralgias, and other manifestations of systemic disease should be sought during a thorough physical examination. Occasionally a primary neoplasm or evidence of spread of such tumors as lymphomas, Wilm's tumor, pheochromocytoma, or carcinoma of the colon, lung, breast, stomach, or kidney can be detected. Various man-

TABLE 23-2. LOW-GRADE PROTEINURIA*

ETIOLOGY OF PROTEINURIA	CLINICAL CUES	LABORATORY FINDING
Functional	Fever, stress, congenital hepatic fibrosis, hypertensive nephropathy, strenuous exercise	Normal renal function, normal urinary sediment except occasional white blood cells and increased hyaline casts
Idiopathic	Usually young patient, normal history and examination	Normal renal fixation, normal sediment
Orthostatic	Normal history and examination, some recovering from pyelonephritis or glomerulonephritis	No proteinuria on recumbent specimen
Chronic interstitial nephritis	Analgesic abuse, lead exposure, urinary tract infections	Pyuria
Congenital disease Polycystic kidney disease	Family history of renal failure, palpable kidneys, intermittent flank pain, and hematuria	Enlarged kidneys on intravenous pyelogram, renal cysts on ultrasound examination
Medullary cystic kidney	Family history, short stature, early renal failure	Disproportionately severe anemia, salt wasting, renal tubular acidosis
Glomerulonephritides	Streptococcal infection (skin or pharynx), symptoms of connective tissue disease (arthritis, skin rash)	Hematuria and red blood cell casts, appropriate positive serologic tests
Obstruction, stone	Flank pain with or without gross hematuria	Hematuria, prerenal renal function index
Neoplasm	Older, may be asymptomatic with normal examination or may show widespread disease	Hematuria with or without microcytic anemia
Systemic causes	Confirmatory examination and history	Appropriate laboratory tests

*Low-grade proteinuria is the excretion of less than 1 g per day of protein. Moderate proteinuria (less than 3.5 g per day) can be seen with any of these disorders in a severe advanced stage. The most common cause of moderate proteinuria is glomerular disease, although interstitial disease has also been implicated. Heavy proteinuria (greater than 3.5 g per day) is discussed in Chapter 28, Nephrotic Syndrome.

ifestations of renal disease should be considered, such as urinary symptoms, edema, hypertension, and hematuria.

RECOMMENDED DIAGNOSTIC APPROACH

A. **Repeat Qualitative Tests.** The urine should be tested qualitatively several times, over a one- to two-week period, because of the frequency of transient and benign proteinuria.

B. **Twenty-Four–Hour Quantitative Urinary Protein Collection.** This confirms and establishes the degree of proteinuria and determines the patient's diagnostic and prognostic category. Creatinine assay from the same specimen establishes the adequacy of the 24-hour collection and allows calculation of the creatinine clearance.

C. **Fasting Glucose and Protein Electrophoresis of Urine and Serum.** This procedure should be performed in older patients or when warranted by clinical suspicion.

D. **Complete Urinalysis.** A search of the urinary sediment for red blood cells, white blood cells, crystals, and cellular casts can separate proteinuric patients into two different groups: those with isolated proteinuria with (1) a normal urinary sediment or (2) with an active urinary sediment or evidence of systemic disease.

1. *Isolated Proteinuria with a Normal Urinary Sediment.* The prognosis and management of these patients depends on whether a pattern of transient, intermittent, or constant proteinuria is found.

   a. *Transient proteinuria* carries no risk of harmful sequelae and requires no further evaluation or specific follow-up.

   b. Patients with *intermittent proteinuria* show urinary protein in 50 per cent of random specimens. Histologically they make up a diverse but minimally diseased group. Most become protein-free after several years, and under the age of 30 there is no excess morbidity or mortality. Older individuals with this pattern of protein excretion carry an increased risk for death, which increases with age. All patients with a greater than normal protein loss in a 24-hour urine sample should have yearly follow-up with blood pressure measurement and urinalysis. If the pattern of excretion becomes constant, periodic assessment of renal function (blood urea nitrogen and creatinine) becomes necessary.

   c. If only random daytime urine testing is done, *orthostatic proteinuria* can easily mimic a constant pattern of protein loss. Collection should include (1) an evening sample just before retiring, (2) a sample collected while the patient is still supine the next morning, and (3) a sample collected at the next urination after ambulation. If the supine sample shows either trace or negative protein and samples 1 and 3 are positive, the patient has orthostatic proteinuria. Almost 75 per cent of young men with constant daytime proteinuria are shown to have transient orthostatic proteinuria according to this method. With less than 1 g of daily proteinuria and normal urine sediment, serious renal disease is unlikely. Follow-up every several years for blood pressure measurement and urinary protein testing should be performed. Periodic blood urea nitrogen and creatinine levels need be checked only in the small percentage of patients who later develop constant proteinuria.

d. Patients with *constant proteinuria* represent a heterogenous group with higher mortality rates and a greater risk of subsequent renal disease than those with intermittent proteinuria. Eighty per cent of patients with constant proteinuria continue to have the problem after six years, and up to 50 per cent develop hypertension over the same period. Renal insufficiency has been seen in up to 20 per cent of patients during a ten-year follow-up after diagnosis. Yearly urinalysis, blood pressure measurement, and blood urea nitrogen and creatinine determinations are recommended. An intravenous pyelogram should be obtained initially because of the occasional finding of a hydronephrotic lesion or reflux nephropathy.

2. Proteinuria with an Active Urinary Sediment or Evidence of Systemic Disease

a. The combination of proteinuria and hematuria signals glomerular inflammation. Red blood cells, red blood cell casts, and urinary protein form a nephritic urinary sediment that possesses little diagnostic specificity.

1). Serologic tests should include antistreptococcal enzyme titer, antinuclear antibody, total serum hemolytic complement, hepatitis B antigen, and venereal disease research laboratory (VDRL).

2). If the diagnosis of glomerulonephritis is not obvious from the examination, an intravenous pyelogram is obtained. This helps to exclude cystic disease, obstructive or reflux uropathy, papillary necrosis, renal tuberculosis, and renal tumors.

3). If a diagnosis does not result from a thorough clinical evaluation, percutaneous renal biopsy may be necessary. This procedure carries a minor complication rate of 5 to 10 per cent and a 0.5 to 1.0 per cent rate of serious morbidity. Death is rare. Renal biopsy may yield evidence of potentially treatable glomerular disease and also provides prognostic information.

REFERENCES

1. Abuelo JG: Proteinuria: Diagnostic principles and procedures. Ann Intern Med 98:186, 1983.

The most recent and up-to-date review.

2. deTorrente AM: The patient with proteinuria or an abnormal urinary sediment. *In* Schrier RW (ed.): Manual of Nephrology. Boston, Little, Brown & Company, 1981.

Outlines a useful and practical approach.

3. Ginsberg JM, Chang BS, Matarese RA, Garella S: Use of single void urine samples to estimate quantitative proteinuria. N Engl J Med 309:1543, 1983.
This article describes a quick and simple method that may become widely used.

_____24_____

ACUTE RENAL FAILURE

By STUART L. BURSTEN, M.D.

DEFINITION

Acute renal failure is defined as a sudden fall in renal function characterized by *azotemia.* An acute decrease in the glomerular filtration rate has usually occurred. The urine output may be normal, increased, or decreased. Acute renal failure is the final common pathway of many diverse processes and diseases that occur both extra- and intrarenally.

A. **Criteria for Diagnosis.** The initial criteria in all acute renal failure are a rising blood-urea nitrogen (BUN) and creatinine concentration, with the ratio between the two varying according to the type of renal failure (see Recommended Diagnostic Approach). Specific criteria for the classification of each type of acute renal failure are given in Table 24–1. Three important general points are:

   1. *Overlap in Laboratory Studies.* There is extensive overlap between all forms of acute renal failure. This makes absolute exclusion criteria impossible. Clinical judgment utilizing history, physical examination, and hemodynamic monitoring when indicated must be employed to define why azotemia has occurred.

   2. *Transition Between Forms.* This is common and can confuse diagnostic criteria. For example, prerenal azotemia commonly may progress to acute tubular necrosis (ATN). Late ATN may mimic chronic obstruction or chronic glomerulonephritis (in that the patient is polyuric with salt-losing nephropathy).

   3. *Hypovolemia.* Hypovolemia must always be considered and ruled out, and the possibility of obstruction must not be forgotten when there is persistent oliguria and no response to volume challenges.

CAUSES

Acute renal failure can be usefully divided into one of four larger categories:

A. **Prerenal.** This is the most common cause of acute renal failure,

TABLE 24–1. CRITERIA FOR DIAGNOSIS OF THE FOUR TYPES OF ACUTE RENAL FAILURE

Postrenal
- A. Laboratory indices similar to those in prerenal azotemia (see Table 24–3)
- B. Ultrasonographic evidence of bilateral hydronephrosis, or unilateral hydronephrosis if a single kidney is present, or evidence of intra-abdominal, retroperitoneal, or pelvic obstructing masses
- C. Evidence of bilateral obstructed flow on radiohippurate scans
- D. Evidence of obstructed flow on retrograde pyelography

Prerenal
- A. Signs on physical examination of volume depletion or effective or absolute third-spacing of fluid
- B. Volume depletion by hemodynamic criteria such as pulmonary capillary wedge pressure
- C. Urine osmoles, creatinine, sodium, and sediment consistent with pre-renal azotemia
- D. Response to volume repletion with reversal of azotemia plus, if oliguric, increase in urine output with normalization of urinary indices
- E. No evidence of obstruction on ultrasound if oliguria persists

Intrarenal: Primary Parenchymal Disease
- A. Urinalyses in accordance with Table 24–2 (urinalysis is more pathognomonic in this category than in others)
- B. Severe hypertension most commonly present as opposed to hypotension or orthostatic hypotension
- C. No evidence of obstruction on ultrasound if persistently oliguric

Intrarenal: Acute Tubular Necrosis
- A. No signs, symptoms, or hemodynamic indications of ongoing hypovolemia or following correction of hypovolemia
- B. Urinalyses in accordance with Table 24–2
- C. Urine osmoles, sodium, creatinine consistent with ATN
- D. No response to volume repletion or challenge with either resolution of azotemia or increased urine output
- E. No evidence of obstruction

representing 40 to 60 per cent of cases. Prerenal azotemia is caused by diminution in the renal blood flow (approximately 1.0 to 1.7 L per minute). Some of the major causes of prerenal acute renal failure are:

1. **Cardiac.** These include congestive heart failure, cardiogenic shock, and acute and chronic pericardial tamponade.
2. **Hepatic.** Alcoholic hepatitis or cirrhosis produce a relative decrease in intravascular volume through accumulation of ascites or a relative decrease from arteriovenous fistulae. End-stage cirrhosis may be associated with the hepatorenal syndrome.
3. **Hemorrhage.** Upper gastrointestinal bleeding or bleeding from other locations can produce acute hypovolemia that leads to acute renal failure. The increased BUN in upper gastrointestinal bleeding reflects this decreased volume more than it reflects the protein load from the breakdown of blood within the gut.
4. **Gastrointestinal Losses.** These include voluminous, frequent,

or prolonged diarrhea; persistent vomiting; intraluminal fluid in bowel obstruction; and intraluminal gut fluid and bowel wall edema in inflammatory bowel disease.

5. *Sequestration of Intravascular Volume.* This is common in burn patients and less frequent in pancreatitis.

6. *Administration of Diuretics.* Particularly potent loop-diuretics such as furosemide, bumetamide, or ethacrynic acid cause prerenal acute renal failure, but thiazide diuretics such as chlorothiazide, chlorthalidone, or metolazone may also be implicated, particularly in older people. Because of washout of the interstitial osmolar gradient, the prolonged use of diuretics results in loss of concentrating function. This is the setting in which *nonoliguric* prerenal azotemia is most often encountered. Nonoliguric prerenal acute renal failure may also be caused by inhibition of the effect of antidiuretic hormone (ADH, vasopressin) on the collecting duct by lithium or demeclocycline.

B. **Postrenal.** This category is the cause of acute renal failure in 2 to 15 per cent of patients, depending on type of hospital and patients surveyed. Postrenal acute renal failure is best described as *obstructive uropathy.* Generally, the patient is oliguric and often anuric. There may be wide fluctuations in urine output, due to changes in the obstructing lesions with the patient's position.

1. *Intraureteric Obstruction.* Causes here include (in order of frequency) stones, clots, pus, or tissue. The tissue can come from papillary necrosis of diabetes mellitus, analgesic drug excess, and the fungus balls of aspergillosis.

2. *Extraureteric Obstruction.* This is most commonly caused by tumors, which start in or extend into the retroperitoneal nodes. Examples include lymphomas and testicular carcinomas. In women, 70 per cent of the cases of obstructive acute renal failure are caused by pelvic tumors. In about 5 per cent of all patients with postrenal acute renal failure, the cause is retroperitoneal fibrosis from ergot alkaloids and radiation fibrosis.

3. *Lower Tract Obstruction.* Prostatic hypertrophy is the most common cause of obstructive acute renal failure in men (>80 per cent of the cases). Bladder lesions including adenocarcinoma and transitional cell carcinoma may uncommonly cause bilateral obstruction. Urethral obstruction, caused by stones or clots, is also a consideration.

C. **Intrarenal.** Representing 30 to 50 per cent of all acute renal failure, this category may be further subdivided into primary renal parenchymal disorders and acute tubular necrosis (ATN).

1. *Primary Renal Parenchymal Disease.* This accounts for 10 to 20 per cent of intrarenal acute renal failure in adults.

   a. **Vascular Causes.** These include glomerulonephritis, vasculitis of polyarteritis nodosa, scleroderma, malignant hypertension, thrombotic thrombocytopenic purpura, hemolytic-uremic syndrome, and embolization. Malignant hypertension once represented the most common cause of this category of acute renal failure but has now virtually disappeared as a cause, owing to aggressive treatment of hypertension.

b. **Tubulointerstitial Diseases.** The incidence of tubulointerstitial diseases, particularly *interstitial nephritis,* is increasing rapidly. They can be induced by antibiotics, particularly semisynthetic beta-lactamase–resistant penicillins, and by nonsteroidal anti-inflammatory drugs such as indomethacin and ibuprofen. Hypercalcemia and severe hypokalemia may also cause interstitial nephritis that results in acute renal failure.

c. **Crystallization Within the Tubular Lumen.** Crystallization of various compounds may result in acute renal failure: oxalate crystals, particularly in ethylene glycol ingestion, urate crystals in severe hyperuricemia (when levels of uric acid are greater than 18 to 20 mg per dL), or derivatives of methotrexate.

d. **Tumor Lysis.** Tumor lysis is an increasingly common syndrome following chemotherapy administered for large tumor masses. This syndrome is caused by urate deposition and severe hyperphosphatemia with possible calcium phosphate deposition and crystallization of oxypurinol.

e. **Deposition of Myeloma Protein.** This may result in severe acute renal failure. Diffuse interstitial nephritis is also associated with myeloma.

2. *Acute Tubular Necrosis (ATN).* The term "acute tubular necrosis" is largely a misnomer, since tubular necrosis is almost never found. Rather, vasomotor changes produce tubular ischemia, tubular dysfunction, and tubuloglomerular feedback that in turn causes decreased glomerular filtration rates.

a. **Ischemic ATN.** This is found in severe trauma, hemorrhage, hypotension, sepsis, aorta cross-clamping, or uncorrected prerenal azotemia.

b. **Toxic ATN.** Toxic ATN involves direct toxic injury to the tubular cells. Once commonly caused by exposure to heavy metals or halogenated alkanes such as carbon tetrachloride, toxic ATN now frequently results from administration of aminoglycoside antibiotics or contrast material given during radiologic procedures to dehydrated, elderly, or diabetic persons, or those with multiple myeloma.

c. **Pigment-Associated ATN.** Finally, ATN may be pigment-associated, induced by myoglobin during rhabdomyolysis or by hemoglobin during extensive hemolysis.

D. **Oliguric Versus Nonoliguric Acute Renal Failure.** Nonoliguric renal failure may be the initial presenting form, or oliguric acute renal failure may convert to nonoliguric renal failure with volume, diuretics, or spontaneously. Nonoliguric renal failure represents 30 to 40 per cent of intrarenal acute renal failure and is of interest, since the prognosis is better. Nonoliguric renal failure has a mortality of 30 to 35 per cent, whereas oliguric acute renal failure has a mortality of 55 to 65 per cent.

CLINICAL SETTING

A. Postrenal. Because bilateral obstruction is uncommon, the finding of a unilateral kidney, as with a history of congenitally absent kidney or nephrectomy, increases suspicion.

   1. History. History of nephrolithiasis, bleeding disorders, repeated pyelonephritis, or immune deficiency with fungal disease may be suggestive. Any history of a pelvic tumor in a woman or a history of lymphoma in either sex should arouse suspicion. Any tumor inferior to the diaphragm may have received radiation treatment that resulted in fibrosis, so no history of local malignancy should be ignored. A careful history of drug ingestion may be helpful (such as a history of treatment for migraine headaches with ergot alkaloids). A history in men of hesitancy, dribbling, incontinence, frequency or dysuria may suggest prostatic problems. Any history of hematuria, particularly gross hematuria, may be suggestive, since obstruction by clots may be involved.

   2. Physical Examination. Physical examination may not be helpful: flank pain and tenderness bilaterally is present in approximately 70 to 80 per cent of obstruction, but its absence cannot exclude obstruction. Bladder distention is important when present; costovertebral angle tenderness bilaterally may suggest ascending infection. Signs of inferior vena cava or lymph node obstruction (such as brawny edema or lymphedema in the lower extremities or painful swollen calves with erythema suggesting thrombophlebitis) may indicate tumor. These can occur with or without abdominal masses. Ascites in young to middle-aged women may suggest pelvic tumor.

B. Prerenal. Any history suggestive of change in volume status, such as dizziness, tiredness, syncope, edema, or ascites is important.

   1. History. A history of congestive heart failure, hepatic disease with ascites, chronic renal insufficiency, use of diuretics for any reason, or persistence of vomiting or diarrhea is helpful. Hospitalized patients with pancreatitis, burns, or postoperative status should have charts carefully surveyed for weight change, fluid input and output, and manner of nutrition, as well as diuretic use and institution of other drugs.

   2. Physical Examination. Physical examination may reveal volume depletion with postural changes in pulse and blood pressure. Signs may be more subtle in chronically hospitalized patients who may have a slowly falling blood pressure over several days and decreased pulmonary secretions. A most important sign is the daily weight. Documentation of a large decrement is an obvious indication of volume depletion, whereas long-term weight gains with falling blood pressures or edema may signal extensive shift of fluid from the intravascular space. Signs of volume overload may be present, including ascites, lower extremity or sacral edema, chronic stasis dermatitis, or ulcers in the lower extremities. Cardiac examination may reveal biventricular gallops, hepatojugular reflux, distended neck veins, or abnormal venous pulsations. Volume overload and intravascular volume depletion often coexist.

3. **Hemodynamics.** Hemodynamics help to determine prerenal acute renal failure, particularly when it is kept in mind that trends must be followed to reach valid conclusions. A persistently low pulmonary capillary wedge pressure (PCWP) suggests hypovolemia, whereas a rising or high PCWP suggests cardiac failure and renal underperfusion that is responsive to diuretics. These findings are particularly helpful in patients with cardiac or pulmonary disease, in whom physical signs may be confusing or absent or when more than one disease process is present (such as renal failure and congestive cardiomyopathy). Cardiac failure may be so delicately balanced that addition of small amounts of saline to intravascular volume may cause BUN to rise in response to falling cardiac output, whereas a fall in intravascular volume of an equally small amount may cause increasing BUN owing to renal underperfusion.

C. **Intrarenal Primary Parenchymal Disease**

1. **History.** A history of upper respiratory infection suggests postinfectious glomerulonephritis. Fever, rash, or pleuritic pain may point to vasculitis. Patients on antithrombotic agents with embolic events in other organ systems may have sustained renal emboli. Histories of drug use are important, including use of nonsteroidal anti-inflammatory drugs, lithium, antibiotics, diuretics, anticoagulants, and cimetidine. Ingestions of toxic substances, particularly ethylene glycol, or recent treatment with chemotherapeutic agents, especially cyclophosphamide or methotrexate, may also be helpful in assessment. Bone pain may suggest myeloma.

2. **Physical Examination.** Physical examination is of little help, unless evidence of specific vasculitis is found. Hypertension commonly is present (greater than 85 per cent of cases) but is nonspecific. Rashes are often present but may point to vasculitis, glomerulonephritis, or allergic nephritis (such as an allergy to antibiotics with concurrent Shwartzman reaction). Sclerodactyly suggests scleroderma.

D. **Intrarenal: Acute Tubular Necrosis.** Any hospitalized patient with azotemia, whether rapidly developing or insidious, particularly postsurgical patients, should be suspected of having ATN. A history of pre-existing prerenal azotemia may point to progression to ATN. Any trauma or hypotension, no matter how transient, is suggestive. Hypotension does not need to be documented in postsurgical patients, particularly those older than 60, in order for the physician to suspect ATN.

1. **Sepsis.** Sepsis, with or without hypotension, is a formidable risk factor. When ATN is present without a well-defined etiology, it is worthwhile to look for sepsis.

2. **Use of Aminoglycosides.** Aminoglycoside use or recent radiologic procedures using contrast material are noteworthy.

3. **Exposure to Halogenated Alkanes.** Exposure to dry cleaning

fluid or heavy metals is an often neglected historical item. A careful drug history in all cases of acute renal failure is essential.

4. **Unconsciousness.** Persons found unconscious, with or without significant bruising or pressure lesions, or alcoholics, whether or not unconscious, may have rhabdomyolysis.

5. **Seizure.** Patients with seizures, whether or not they are status epilepticus, may also sustain rhabdomyolysis, particularly with hyperthermia.

6. **Electrolyte Abnormalities.** Electrolyte abnormalities, such as hypokalemia and hypophosphatemia, may induce rhabdomyolysis in hospitalized patients.

7. **Hemolysis.** Cases with evidence of hemolysis for any reason, including tranfusion reactions, and microangiopathic hemolysis, may progress to ATN.

RECOMMENDED DIAGNOSTIC APPROACH

A. **Urinalysis.** (See Table 24–2.)

1. If red blood cell casts are present, rheumatologic studies of possible autoimmune causes or vasculitis may be indicated (see Chapter 26, Acute Glomerulonephritis). These studies include complement (total serum hemolytic complement [CH_{50}], C_3, C_4), Raji cell assay, and antinuclear antibodies.

B. **Urine Tonicity.** Urine tonicity and osmolality should be measured. Specific gravity is of little use in assessing ATN, since its accuracy may be affected by dissolved substances such as glucose and protein that are nonspecific but may cause the results to vary widely. Urine osmolality is more reliable as an indicator of changing renal function.

1. **In Prerenal Azotemia.** Eighty-five to 95 per cent of patients have urine osmolalities greater than or equal to 500 mOsm per L.

2. **In ATN.** Eighty-five to 95 per cent of patients have urine osmolality less than or equal to 350 mOsm per L (owing to loss of concentrating ability with tubular dysfunction).

3. **In Postrenal States.** The initial urine osmolality tends to resemble that of prerenal azotemia, but transition to lower osmolalities with persistent obstruction and tubular damage is almost always seen, which suggests that following urine osmolalities serially may be helpful). The large overlap in the 350- to 500-mOsm per L range makes this area useless for diagnosis, except in the context of other tests, as described later.

4. **Urine Osmolality.** Urine osmolality may also be affected by the increase in osmolality in acute renal failure caused by urea, thus giving artificially high values in the overlap range. The ratio of urine to plasma osmoles (U_{osm}/P_{osm}) has been found to be more useful and eliminates the error induced by azotemia. More than 95 per cent of ATN has U_{osm}/P_{osm} ratios of less than or equal to 1.07, whereas greater than or equal to 95 per cent of prerenal azotemia has ratios of greater than or equal to 1.25.

TABLE 24–2. URINALYSIS IN DIAGNOSIS OF ACUTE RENAL FAILURE*

	RBC	WBC (POLYS)	WBC	EPITHELIAL CELLS	PIGMENTED GRANULAR CASTS	RBC CASTS	WBC CASTS	CRYSTALS
Proliferative glomerulonephritis	++	+	0	0	0	++	+	0
Small vessel vasculitis	++	+	0	0	0	++	+	0
Obstructive uropathy	++	(esp. with infection)	0	++‡	+	0	+	+ (urate crystals if stones)
Tubulointerstitial nephritis	+	+	+++†	+	+	+	+	+
Acute tubular necrosis	++	+	0	++	++	0	+	+
Pyelonephritis	+	++	0	+	0	0	+	+
Preglomerular vasculitis	0	0	0	0	0	0	0	0
Scleroderma	0	0	0	0	0	0	0	0
Hemolytic-uremic syndrome	+	+	0	0	0	+	+	0
Tumor lysis syndrome	+	+	0	++	++	+	+	++

*All findings are transient; one must perform serial urinalyses.
†Eosinophiluria occurs in 65 to 85 per cent of patients with tubulointerstitial nephritis but is easily missed, owing to transience.
‡Inflammatory cells are common in obstruction; the physician should also look for tumor cells (i.e., lymphocytes in lymphoma or transitional cells in carcinoma).

C. Plasma Urea (BUN) and Creatinine

1. ***Creatinine.*** Creatinine is freely filtered and not readsorbed. Its production is directly proportionate to muscle mass and reasonably constant within the individual. With complete cessation of glomerular filtration, creatinine increases about 1 mg per dL per day, less with decreased muscle mass (as in an older person), and variably more up to a limit of 2.5 mg per dL per day in young muscular males.

2. ***Urea.*** Urea is freely filtered and variably reabsorbed (by 40 to 70 per cent). Reabsorption is proportionate to the flow of water in tubules, the presence of ADH, the local tubular pressure, and the peritubular blood flow. Production of urea is affected by the liver and varies widely from individual to individual. Certain clinical conditions, such as starvation, low-protein diet, and hepatic failure cause decreased production of BUN, whereas hypercatabolic states such as burns, sepsis, infection, trauma, and postsurgical condition (as well as exogenous administration of glucocorticoids) increase the rate of rise of BUN in renal failure. Thus, the rate at which BUN rises with complete cessation of glomerular filtration may be as low as 24 mg per dL per day or as high as 60 mg per dL per day, although a rate this high is unusual.

D. Plasma BUN/Creatinine Ratio. (See Table 24–3.)

1. Reabsorption of urea is increased greatly in prerenal and post-

TABLE 24–3. LABORATORY FINDINGS IN ACUTE RENAL FAILURE

	PRERENAL AZOTEMIA	ACUTE TUBULAR NECROSIS	POSTRENAL*
Osmolality	> 500 mOsm/L in 85–95%	< 350 mOsm/L in 85–95%	Initially > 500 mOsm/L but decreases
U_{osm}/P_{osm} ratios	> 1.25 in > 95%	< 1.07 in >95%	Variable
BUN/creatinine ratio (Plasma)	> 20/1 80% of the time	10/1	> 20/1 more than 80% of the time
U_{creat}/P_{creat}	≥ 20 in 80–90%	≤ 10 in 80–90%	Variable
Urine$_{Na}$	≤ 20 in 90–95%	≥ 40 in 90–95%	> 100 in postobstructive diuretic phase
Fractional excretion of sodium (FE_{Na})†	< 1% in > 90%	> 2% in > 90%	Variable

*Most of the laboratory test results are variable in postrenal acute renal failure depending on whether obstruction is complete, variable, or superimposed on an interstitial process.

$$†FE_{Na} = \frac{U_{Na}}{P_{Na}} \times \frac{P_{creat}}{U_{creat}}$$

renal azotemia, owing to low urine flow rates, high ADH levels, and low peritubular blood flow (as well as increased tubular back pressure in obstruction). With glomerular filtration rate falling in tandem, urea therefore rises out of proportion to creatinine in these forms of acute renal failure.

2. For this reason a BUN/creatinine ratio greater than or equal to 20/1 is present in prerenal and postrenal azotemia 80 per cent or more of the time. It should be noted that, owing to rapidly falling or absent glomerular filtration rate, creatinine may indeed rise at a strictly proportional rate (such as 10/1) in some instances of prerenal acute renal failure, and other diagnostic criteria must always be applied. Generally, intrarenal acute renal failure and ATN are characterized by proportionate BUN/creatinine increments (10/1) because of a direct drop-off in filtration. This is qualified by those factors, mentioned previously, that may cause a disproportionate urea rise.

E. **Urine Creatinine.** Urine creatinine is a marker of ability to concentrate urine, since creatinine is filtered without reabsorption and with only slight secretion. In prerenal states urine creatinine is usually elevated, owing to concentration of urine, and is lowered in ATN, owing to loss of diluting and concentrating ability. U_{creat}/P_{creat} less than or equal to 10 is found in 80 to 90 per cent of ATN, whereas U_{creat}/P_{creat} greater than or equal to 20 is found in 80 to 90 per cent of prerenal acute renal failure. (See Table 24–3.)

F. **Urine Sodium.** The ability to conserve sodium in proportion to the amount filtered is a marker of intact tubular function. Extreme conservation of sodium is a marker of renal underperfusion or of hypovolemia characteristic of prerenal states, or of both. Urine sodium of less than or equal to 20 mEq per L is found in 90 to 95 per cent of prerenal azotemia, whereas a value of greater than or equal to 40 mEq per L is found in 90 to 95 per cent of ATN.

G. **Fractional Excretion of Sodium (FE_{Na}).** (See Table 24–3.) A more sensitive test is the calculated fractional excretion of sodium (FE_{Na}), based on simultaneously drawn serum creatinine, serum sodium, urine creatinine, and urine sodium samples. The FE_{Na} is $U_{Na}/P_{Na} \times P_{creat}/U_{creat}$. At least 90 per cent of patients with prerenal azotemia have values under 1 per cent, whereas at least 90 per cent of patients with ATN have values greater than 2 per cent. FE_{Na} of less than 1 per cent is common in renal parenchymal disease, particularly glomerulonephritis, since the tubules retain function and attempt to compensate in response to diseased glomeruli and falling glomerular filtration rate.

H. **Other Laboratory Tests.** A clue to the presence of tubuloischemic necrosis may be hyperchloremic acidosis of rapid onset. Calcium, magnesium, phosphate, and potassium levels may give clues to causes of tubuloischemic necrosis or acute tubular necrosis, as may urate levels. Myoglobin levels in urine may confirm rhabdomyolysis. A severe anion gap metabolic acidosis with oxalate crystals in urine may indicate ethylene glycol toxicity. In addition, a postobstructive hyperchloremic tubular acidosis with hyperkalemia may be present in 75 to 85 per cent of patients with postobstructive diuresis.

I. Ultrasound. Ultrasonographic examination of the renal pelvis and ureters, the pelvic area, and the proximate abdomen may reveal the presence of obstruction and the cause in 85 per cent of cases. It must be remembered that 10 to 15 per cent of cases of obstruction are missed with ultrasound examination, and if the index of suspicion is high (as with pre-existing tumor, abdominal mass, transplantation, or a single kidney), a retrograde pyelogram may be indicated. Ultrasonography is also limited in that (1) it does not provide functional assessment or assessment of blood flow or clearance; (2) small lesions in the calyces may be missed; (3) inflammatory lesions cannot be diagnosed; and (4) the technique is extremely operator-dependent.

J. Nuclear Studies. Flow studies (pertechnetate, glucoheptonate) are indicative of renal perfusion and reliably exclude renal vascular problems. Hippurate functional studies can measure continuing renal function, suggest or confirm the presence of acute tubular necrosis, diagnose obstruction, or suggest renal transplant rejection.

K. Intravenous Urography. Intravenous urography is limited by the difficulty of giving dye to patients with marginal fluid status and by fear of exacerbating renal failure. This technique is probably less utilized than in the past, and now, owing to ultrasound, less useful.

L. Renal Biopsy. This procedure is rarely indicated in acute renal failure. It is limited in scope by the patient's total condition and the details of particular problems such as clotting status, hematocrit, functional reserve, and platelet count. Currently biopsy is reserved for oligoanuria that is extremely persistent (usually three weeks or longer) or for occasions in which clinical suspicion of a treatable disease is present (antiglomerular basement membrane Goodpasture's syndrome, lupus, and other vasculitides).

REFERENCES

1. Anderson RJ, Linas JL, Berns AS, Henrich WL, et al.: Nonoliguric acute renal failure. N Engl J Med 296:1134, 1977.
2. Brenner BM, Stein JH (eds.): Acute renal failure. *In* Contemporary Issues in Nephrology. Vol. 5. New York, Churchill Livingstone, 1980.
3. Levinsky NG, Alexander EA: Acute renal failure. *In* Brenner BM, Rector FC Jr (eds.): The Kidney. Vol. 2. Philadelphia, W. B. Saunders Company, 1976.
4. Rudnick MR, Bastl CP, Elfinbein IB, Narins RG: The differential diagnosis of acute renal failure. *In* Brenner BM, Lazarus JM (eds.): Acute Renal Failure. Philadelphia, W. B. Saunders Company, 1983.

25

CHRONIC RENAL FAILURE

By STUART L. BURSTEN, M.D.

DEFINITION, CRITERIA FOR DIAGNOSIS, AND APPROACH TO THE PATIENT

A. **Definition.** Chronic renal failure is defined as a long-term decline in kidney function. It is the final common outcome of numerous renal and systemic diseases that affect the kidney.
   1. It is the sum of glomerular, tubular, and renal endocrine failure that leads to an accumulation of toxins and products that are normally metabolized or excreted by the kidneys.
   2. These products in turn lead to multiple organ dysfunctions and accelerated disease processes, such as a volume-induced hypertension that accelerates atherosclerosis.
   3. In addition, regulatory dysfunction, such as hypocalcemia and osteodystrophy, may result from accumulation of metabolically ineffective products.
B. **Criteria for Diagnosis.** The major criterion is a slow inexorable rise in the serum blood-urea nitrogen (BUN) and creatinine levels.
   1. Most diseases that cause chronic renal failure usually appear as acute renal failure. It is now rare for patients to appear for examination unexpectedly in end-stage renal failure.
   2. A biopsy may be performed at the time that the patient is examined initially in acute renal failure. When a chronic process is suspected, or the creatinine level is already greater than 5.0, a biopsy is seldom helpful and reveals nonspecific chronic glomerulonephritis.
   3. Ultrasound can be used to examine renal size and to estimate functional reserve (small, scarred, or contracted kidneys have little functional component remaining).
C. **Approach to the Patient**
   1. *Phases of Renal Failure.* In general, three phases of chronic renal failure may be identified:
      a. **Renal Insufficiency.** There is malaise, nocturia, and mild anemia.
      b. **Frank Renal Failure.** There is progressive acidosis, hypocalcemia, hyperphosphatemia, and worsening anemia.
      c. **Uremia or End-Stage Renal Disease.** The glomerular filtration rate is less than 5 cc per minute, and there are severe symptoms and metabolic-endocrine disturbances that require dialysis.
   2. *Approach to the Patient.* This chapter emphasizes a twofold approach to patients with chronic renal failure: (1) recognition and prevention of exacerbating factors that accelerate progression to end-stage disease and (2) diagnosis and recognition of end-organ involvement and complications.

MAJOR CAUSES OF CHRONIC RENAL FAILURE

A. **Glomerular Disease.** Sixty per cent of patients with end-stage renal disease have glomerular disease as the cause of the failure.
  1. *Nephrotic Causes.* These include membranous glomerulonephritis, focal glomerulosclerosis, membranoproliferative glomerulonephritis, and chronic nonspecific glomerulonephritis.
  2. *Nephritic Causes.* These include postinfectious glomerulonephritis, IgA nephropathy, Goodpasture's syndrome, idiopathic crescentic glomerulonephritis, and non-Goodpasture's antiglomerular basement membrane disease.
B. **Vascular Disease.** Causes include diabetic nephropathy, malignant hypertension, bilateral renal artery stenosis, fibromuscular hyperplasia, polyarteritis nodosa, and Wegener's granulomatosis.
C. **Tubular Disease.** Causes include heavy metal poisoning from lead or cadmium, analgesic nephropathy, chronic hypercalcemia, chronic hypokalemia, Fanconi's syndrome, radiation nephritis, uric acid nephropathy, amyloidosis, and multiple myeloma.
D. **Intrinsic Urinary Tract Disease.** Causes include chronic pyelonephritis, chronic upper tract obstruction (stones, pus, clots, or tumors), and lower tract obstruction, most commonly prostatic.
E. **Collagen-Vascular Disease.** Causes include systemic lupus erythematosus, scleroderma, and mixed cryoglobulinemia.
F. **Congenital Processes.** These include polycystic kidneys, medullary cystic disease, and hypoplastic kidneys.
G. **Causes of Acute Renal Failure.** In general, any process that causes acute renal failure may also advance to chronic renal failure if renal damage is sufficiently severe. (Although most acute renal failure is reversible, an estimated 10 to 15 per cent of cases advance to chronic renal failure and end-stage disease.)

RECOGNITION AND PREVENTION OF FACTORS THAT ACCELERATE END-STAGE RENAL DISEASE

These factors should be suspected in any patient with a rapidly rising BUN and creatinine level when previously the patient had a slow defined rate of increase.

URINARY TRACT OBSTRUCTION

A. **Clinical Occurrence.** This is seen most often when obstruction was the original cause of the chronic renal failure. Other causes include multiple stones, urinary tract bleeding, recurrent infections, fungus balls, tumor, and retroperitoneal fibrosis. Uremic patients may also have bladder neck dysfunction and obstructive urethral edema after instrumentation.

RECOMMENDED DIAGNOSTIC APPROACH

Signs and symptoms are frequently absent. Ultrasound examination of the kidneys, pelvis, and retroperitoneal area is probably always indicated in circumstances in which the BUN and creatinine level have suddenly increased.

URINARY TRACT INFECTION

Virtually 100 per cent of patients with chronic renal failure will be infected at some time and almost universally after instrumentation.

RECOMMENDED DIAGNOSTIC APPROACH

Microscopic examination of repeated random clean-catch urine specimens for white cells, red cells, and bacteria is imperative, although urinalysis becomes increasingly unhelpful as renal failure progresses.

VOLUME DEPLETION

This is a relatively common problem in early renal insufficiency, when the ability to conserve sodium may be lost. A serious problem is created when reduced circulating volume rapidly compromises the remaining renal reserve.
A. **Clinical Occurrence.** The combination of diuretic use and acute fluid loss from vomiting, diarrhea, fever, or exercise can be particularly troublesome.

RECOMMENDED DIAGNOSTIC APPROACH

Postural changes in blood pressure and pulse may reveal volume depletion, although the autonomic neuropathy of diabetes often renders this a nonspecific finding. Careful administration of intravenous fluids may be indicated to prevent permanent loss of remaining renal function.

HYPOKALEMIA

This is also more common than is generally suspected in chronic renal failure. Potassium-excreting ability is preserved until quite late in the course of chronic renal failure, with hyperkalemia generally a sign of far advanced uremia. Preservation of volume may dictate sacrifice of potassium homeostasis.

A. Clinical Occurrence. Diuretic administration plus gastrointestinal losses can produce hypokalemia as well as the anorexia of chronic renal failure, which lead to a drastically decreased intake.

DIAGNOSIS AND RECOGNITION OF COMPLICATIONS AND END-ORGAN INVOLVEMENT

These complications should be diagnosed as they arise because they are increasingly treatable. A systematic approach prevents missed diagnoses of other separate complications of uremia. For example, the appearance of anemia in chronic renal failure may be the result of anemia of renal failure, but it may also be caused by severe gastrointestinal bleeding from platelet dysfunction.

ANEMIA

The anemia of renal failure, which is usually normochromic and normocytic, is secondary to decreased erythropoietin production primarily, but diminished maturation and faster turnover of red blood cells play a role.

A. Clinical Occurrence. Anemia usually begins early in the course of renal insufficiency with hematocrits of 25 to 32 per cent. With frank renal failure, the level drops to 19 to 25 per cent. The clinician should be particularly alarmed when there has been a rapid decline in hematocrit or when the hematocrit remains below 19 per cent for a sustained period of time.

   1. Occult bleeding with iron-deficiency anemia is always a possibility, given the platelet dysfunction of uremia and the occasional development of bone marrow toxicity.

RECOMMENDED DIAGNOSTIC APPROACH

A. The hematocrit should be followed closely for trends and changes.

B. Iron and total iron-binding capacity only reveal changes consistent with peripheral block to iron utilization.

C. Ferritin, which usually accumulates in chronic renal failure, can point to probable iron deficiency if it is in the low range of normal (less than 20 to 30).

D. Microcytosis may be a clue to bleeding or iron deficiency, although on occasion microcytosis accompanies a normal iron state in the anemia of chronic renal failure.

PLATELET AND CLOTTING DISORDERS

Chronic renal failure is often accompanied by an acquired von Willebrand's disorder, with factor VIII dysfunction and an associated platelet disorder.

A. **Clinical Occurrence.** This problem is generally observed in advanced uremia, in which the BUN is 100 to 150 mEq per L and creatinine is below 10. These problems are exacerbated by aspirin and by infection with or without sepsis. Heparin and coumarin are administered with extreme care, if at all. Antibiotics that affect vitamin K–dependent factors (cefamandole, moxalactam, and cefoperazone) should not be administered.

RECOMMENDED DIAGNOSTIC APPROACH

The key to early detection of these problems is to regularly follow the platelet count, the bleeding, and prothrombin and partial thromboplastin times.

NEUROLOGIC DISORDERS

PERIPHERAL NEUROPATHY

Peripheral neuropathy, which appears similar to the peripheral neuropathy of diabetes, exists in advanced uremic renal failure. It is probably toxin-related and is partially reversible with dialysis. It may be diagnosed by careful neurologic evaluation of vibration sense, soft touch, and position sense. An electromyelogram that shows conduction changes is confirmatory.

ALUMINUM OR TOXICITY DEMENTIA

There is also a serious central nervous system disorder, formerly referred to as *dialysis dementia* and now referred to as *aluminum* or *toxicity dementia*. This degenerative disorder is secondary to deposition of aluminum in the central nervous system.

A. **Clinical Occurrence.** Aluminum dementia is now observed prior to dialysis in advanced uremia if there have been months to years of consumption of aluminum-containing antacids for phosphate binding.

RECOMMENDED DIAGNOSTIC APPROACH

Aluminum dementia is thus far diagnosed on a clinical basis. It is manifested by a stuttering dysphasia that progresses to aphasia, seizures, and disorientation. Hemodialysis exacerbates these findings.

Serum aluminum levels are difficult to obtain, and their meaning is not fully understood.

RENAL OSTEODYSTROPHY

A. **Pathophysiologic Mechanisms.** In chronic renal failure, hypocalcemia occurs as a result of renal calcium wasting and decreased production and responsiveness to the active metabolite of vitamin D. The hypocalcemia stimulates parathyroid hormone production, and the parathormone stimulates breakdown of bone matrix by osteoclasts. With a lack of vitamin D and calcium, inefficient remodeling and fibrotic replacement of bone matrix occurs, which is a condition called *osteitis fibrosa cystica*. Aluminum deposition in bone matrix and direct toxicity to osteoblasts cause a relative vitamin D insensitivity. This leads to the *osteomalacia* of renal failure. These forms of bone disease often coexist.

B. **Clinical Occurrence.** Uremic osteodystrophy varies widely from person to person, both in onset and in patient response to vitamin D metabolites, calcium supplements, and aluminum.
   1. In young persons with uremia who have not yet had closure of the growth plates, the onset of osteodystrophy produces severe bone pain and growth retardation.
   2. In older patients osteodystrophy is usually asymptomatic until it is far advanced and pathologic fractures develop.

RECOMMENDED DIAGNOSTIC APPROACH

A. In patients with persistent hypocalcemia and hyperphosphatemia, hand radiographs should be obtained to screen for the onset of osteodystrophy.

B. Radioimmunoassay for the N-terminal parathyroid hormone may be obtained to demonstrate hyperparathyroidism.

C. Definition of the degree and type of disease requires a bone biopsy with special stains for matrix and aluminum.

METABOLIC COMPLICATIONS

In uremia a peripheral insensitivity to insulin develops with resulting hyperinsulinism and glucose intolerance. Inhibition of lipoprotein lipase by uremic toxins, plus hyperinsulinism, give rise to the hyperlipidemic state (increased very low density lipoprotein) that is characteristic of uremia. Diabetics whose condition progresses to chronic renal failure require less insulin because of reduced renal clearance.

VASCULAR COMPLICATIONS

A. **Hypertension.** The hypertension in chronic renal failure is secondary to chronic volume overload and increased peripheral resistance from altered vascular tone. The blood pressure is difficult to control, even with multiple antihypertensive agents, until dialysis is initiated.

B. **Pericardial Disease.** Because of hemodialysis, with its intermittent anticoagulation and associated hemorrhage, pericardial disease has become common, causing a marked increase in cardiac tamponade and chronic constrictive pericarditis. The echocardiogram may assist in the diagnosis of all pericardial conditions.

   1. *Acute Pericarditis.* This is a common complication of uremia that usually responds to dialysis. Symptoms include fever and typical pleuritic chest pain. A two- or three-component friction rub is present (even if intermittent) in 100 per cent of patients.

   2. *Cardiac Tamponade.* This produces a significant fall in blood pressure during dialysis, with increasing hemodynamic instability. Neck veins are monophasically elevated, with distant heart sounds. A pulsus paradoxus (greater than 15 to 20 mm Hg) is present in 75 to 80 per cent of patients. Right heart catheterization reveals equalization of diastolic pressures in all chambers.

   3. *Chronic Constrictive Pericarditis.* In this condition the neck veins are phasically elevated, demonstrating Kussmaul's elevation (a paradoxic rise during inspiration), which is not seen in cardiac tamponade. A pericardial knock caused by ventricular constriction at the end of diastole is heard. Pulsus paradoxus is rarely, if ever, present.

C. **Atherosclerosis.** This is attributed to a combination of factors found in end-stage disease: glucose intolerance, poorly controlled hypertension, hyperlipidemia, and the high prevalence of cigarette smoking (60 to 80 per cent of cases) in patients with chronic renal failure. Clinicians should remain alert for evidence of cardiac disease despite a short duration of renal failure.

INFECTION

Uremia predisposes to bacterial and viral infections through inhibition of phagocytic ability and T cell deficiency. Because fever is often suppressed in uremia, vigilance, particularly for septicemia, should be maintained with any change in the clinical status. The most frequent serious infections are: staphylococcal septicemia; staphylococcal abscesses in the urinary tract, especially perinephric abscesses; osteomyelitis; infectious endocarditis; hepatitis B; and herpes zoster.

A. Blood cultures should be obtained readily.

B. There should be a low threshold for beginning antibiotic therapy empirically, with emphasis on staphylococcal and enterobacterial coverage.

C. Renal-transplant patients on glucocorticoids or cyclosporine A are at higher risk for infections from *Candida, Aspergillus,* and atypical fungal infection, particularly pneumonias.

REFERENCES

1. Brenner BM, Stein JH (ed.): Chronic renal failure. *In* The Contemporary Issues in Nephrology Series, No. 7. New York, Churchill-Livingstone, 1981.
2. Eknoyan G (ed.): Chronic renal failure. *In* Kurtzman NA (ed.): Seminars in Nephrology. Vol. 1, No. 2. New York, Grune & Stratton, 1981.

These are two of the most thorough and complete recent reviews of this topic.

26

ACUTE GLOMERULONEPHRITIS AND THE NEPHRITIC SYNDROME

By JEFFREY B. KOPP, M.D.

INTRODUCTION TO GLOMERULOPATHY

The term "glomerulopathy" refers to a group of disorders with various causes and clinical manifestations. The common thread among the glomerulopathies is a pathologically and functionally abnormal glomerulus. Damage to the glomerulus usually results in proteinuria, which is often the only marker of glomerular disease. With further damage, cells may appear in the urine: erythrocytes, leukocytes, tubular cells, and casts. Finally, diminished renal function occurs, which is manifested as azotemia and sodium retention.

A limited variety of syndromes is seen in glomerular disease. These include: nephritic syndrome, proteinurias (see Chapter 23), nephrotic syndrome (see Chapter 28), hematuria, rapidly progressive nephritis with azotemia, and chronic renal failure (see Chapter 25).

The term "glomerulonephritis" is derived from pathology and refers to inflammatory cells within the glomerulus. Hence the diagnosis of glomerulonephritis in a strict sense can only be made from a renal biopsy. Patients with the histologic diagnosis of glomerulonephritis may have any of the syndromes of glomerular disease listed above. This chapter deals with the evaluation of the nephritic syndrome.

NEPHRITIC SYNDROME

The nephritic syndrome consists of the following features:
A. Hematuria. Hematuria is nearly always present in patients with

the nephritic syndrome. Since normal urine contains at most one to two red blood cells per high-power field of spun sediment, hematuria is defined as more than two red blood cells per high-power field. Gross hematuria occurs in about one third of cases, and the remainder have microscopic hematuria. Hematuria most commonly has other sources than glomerular pathology; in a particular patient with hematuria the key evidence that incriminates the glomerulus is the presence of red blood cell casts or proteinuria.

B. **Red Blood Cell Casts.** Although they can occur rarely in other forms of urinary system disease, such as interstitial renal disease, red blood cell casts are considered nearly pathognomonic for the nephritic syndrome. When red cells enter the tubular lumen proximal to the ascending limb of Henle's loop (the site of Tamm-Horsfall protein secretion), they may be incorporated into a protein matrix to form red cell casts. Because casts in urine may disintegrate if the specimen is agitated or allowed to sit for too long and therefore may be missed on routine urinalysis, clinicians must examine the urine themselves. First-void urine may be the most productive, since it often has the highest osmolarity and the lowest pH, which are conditions that favor the formation of casts. The best place to look for casts is at the periphery of the cover slip, since that is where the casts are carried by capillary action. If the first urine sample fails to show casts and the hematuria persists, several repeat microscopic examinations of the urine should be carried out.

C. **Proteinuria.** (See Chapter 23.) Normal 24-hour protein excretion is less than 150 mg. Patients with the nephritic syndrome usually excrete 500 mg to 3.5 g daily, but some excrete less and others exhibit nephrotic-range proteinuria, defined as excretion of greater than 3.5 g per day. In the nephritic syndrome serum albumin may be normal or reduced but rarely to the low levels that are seen in the nephrotic syndrome (see Chapter 28).

D. **Renal Insufficiency.** Depending on the extent of glomerular involvement, renal function may range from normal to markedly impaired. Perhaps half of patients have some elevation of the blood urea nitrogen or creatinine levels above the baseline values. One quarter of patients are oliguric, producing less than 500 cc of urine per day.

E. **Sodium Retention.** Positive sodium balance is typical of many patients with the nephritic syndrome. This is a result of active tubular reabsorption of sodium, which is the result of a fall in glomerular filtration. The sodium retention that results may be manifested in several ways.

1. *Edema.* This represents total body sodium excess and is seen in 90 per cent of patients. Facial edema is common, in contrast to the dependent edema that results from congestive heart failure.

2. *Congestive Heart Failure.* This condition is not seen in patients with the nephritic syndrome unless they have an underlying cardiomyopathy or are severely oliguric.

3. *Mild Hypertension.* Mild hypertension is common, but mod-

erate or severe hypertension occurs in only 10 per cent of patients.

F. Diagnostic Criteria. The diagnosis of acute nephritic syndrome can be made in the patient who has hematuria with either red blood cell casts or proteinuria in excess of 1 g per day. This description identifies some but not all of the patients for whom the eventual histologic diagnosis is glomerulonephritis. Furthermore, the conditions of some patients fit both nephritic and nephrotic syndromes. Despite these limitations, the concept of the nephritic syndrome is useful in pointing the way for further evaluation.

CLINICAL PRESENTATION

A. History. Patients with the nephritic syndrome may complain of dark urine (more often described as smoky or tea-colored than bloody), flank or loin pain, headaches, or edema. Many patients, however, are asymptomatic. Patients with nephritis as a result of systemic illness may have nonrenal symptoms, including rash in systemic lupus erythematosus, abdominal pain in Henoch-Schönlein purpura, or fever in subacute bacterial endocarditis.

B. Physical Examination. The most useful clinical signs are those of volume overload, that is, hypertension and edema. In mild cases there may be only periorbital edema, and in severe cases there may be anasarca.

RECOMMENDED DIAGNOSTIC APPROACH

A. Initial Laboratory Evaluation

   1. *Initial Tests.* These include measurement of blood urea nitrogen and creatinine, urinalysis, and a 24-hour urine collection for creatinine clearance and protein. Measuring the creatinine in the specimen allows the clinician to gauge the completeness of the collection: women should excrete 10 to 15 mg of creatinine per kg of body weight per day and men should excrete 15 to 20 mg of creatinine per kg of body weight per day.

   2. *Complement Levels.* To further elucidate the cause of the nephritic syndrome in a given patient, the level of complement is measured. The initial screen should include at least serum complement (C_3) and total serum hemolytic complement (CH_{50}); the fourth component of complement (C_4) is useful in some cases, as outlined below. The major causes of the nephritic syndrome can then be categorized according to complement levels to provide direction for further work-up. (See Table 26–1.)

B. Subsequent Evaluation. Subsequent evaluation is guided by the results of complement testing.

   1. *Low Serum Complement*

      a. **Systemic Diseases.** These disorders are usually apparent from the history and physical examination by the time the

TABLE 26–1. DISEASES ASSOCIATED WITH THE
NEPHRITIC SYNDROME

DISEASES ASSOCIATED WITH A NEPHRITIC SYNDROME THAT HAS LOW SERUM COMPLEMENT

A. Systemic diseases
    1. Systemic lupus erythematosus
    2. Focal proliferative glomerulonephritis (75%)
    3. Diffuse proliferative glomerulonephritis (90%)
    4. Subacute bacterial endocarditis (90%)
    5. Shunt nephritis (infected ventriculoatrial shunts) (90%)
    6. Cryoglobulinemia (85%)
B. Renal diseases
    1. Acute poststreptococcal glomerulonephritis (80–90%)
    2. Membranoproliferative glomerulonephritis
        Type I (50–80%)
        Type II (80–90%)

DISEASES ASSOCIATED WITH A NEPHRITIC SYNDROME THAT HAS NORMAL SERUM COMPLEMENT

A. Systemic diseases
    1. Polyarteritis nodosa
    2. Allergic granulomatosis
    3. Hypersensitivity vasculitis
    4. Wegener's granulomatosis
    5. Henoch-Schönlein purpura
    6. Goodpasture's syndrome
    7. Visceral abscess
B. Renal diseases
    1. IgG-IgA nephropathy
    2. Rapidly progressive glomerulonephritis
        RPGN associated with granular deposits
        Anti-GBM antibody-mediated RPGN
        RPGN without glomerular deposits

---

*Percentages are the approximate frequencies of depressed complement in the given disease.

nephritic syndrome is manifest. Specific signs and tests include:

    1). Systemic Lupus Erythematosus. Fever, rash, arthritis, cytopenias, antinuclear antibody, and DNA binding.

    2). Subacute Bacterial Endocarditis. Fever, heart murmurs, and positive blood cultures.

    3). Shunt Nephritis. Fever and the presence of a ventriculoatrial shunt.

    4). Cryoglobulinemia. Arthritis, purpura, and circulating cryoglobulins.

  b. Renal Diseases. Clinical distinction between the diseases in this category may be difficult.

    1). Poststreptococcal Glomerulonephritis. This condition occurs one to four weeks after pharyngitis or skin infection with Group A beta-hemolytic *Streptococcus*. Nephritis tends to be transient, lasting three to eight weeks. Features may include oliguria, gross hematuria, edema, hypertension, and encephalopathy. Although the disease is usually self-limited, perhaps 5 per cent of adult patients have intermittent or persistent abnormalities in urine samples or renal function. An even smaller number have rapidly progressive glomerulonephritis (see later discussion).

Throat and skin cultures frequently yield *Streptococcus.* The antibody response to extracellular products of streptococci is a marker for recent infection. Thus the antistreptolysin 0 titer rises above 200 in most patients with pharyngeal infection. Limitations of the ASO titer in clinical practice are that the rise following infection takes three to five weeks, the rise may be blunted by prior antibiotic therapy, and titers change little with skin infection. The complement activation in poststreptococcal glomerulonephritis occurs by the alternative pathway, resulting in a low C_3 (generally less than 50 per cent of normal values), a low CH_{50}, and a normal C_4. These low complement levels almost always return to normal by eight weeks, even when some urinary abnormalities remain. A variety of abnormal immunoproteins can be found in these patients, including immune complexes, cryoglobulins, and C_3 nephritic factor (an immunoglobulin capable of activating the alternate pathway).

> 2). ***Membranoproliferative Glomerulonephritis.*** This is a heterogeneous group of disorders. About half the patients have the nephrotic syndrome and half have the nephritic syndrome. Hypertension is less common than in poststreptococcal glomerulonephritis. Decreased renal function as evidenced by azotemia is present in about half the cases and indicates a worse prognosis. The clinical course tends to be relentless and slowly progressive. The rate of progression is variable. After ten years only 50 per cent of patients have functioning kidneys.

Whereas in poststreptococcal glomerulonephritis complement levels return to normal when the acute attack has passed, in membranoproliferative glomerulonephritis complement levels are consistently depressed. In Type I glomerulonephritis activation of complement occurs by the classic pathway, with low C_4. C_3 nephritic factor is present in only 33 per cent of cases. In Type II activation occurs by the alternative pathway, with normal C_4. C_3 nephritic factor is present in 75 per cent of cases. An elevated ASO titer is seen in 20 per cent of patients with membranoproliferative glomerulonephritis. (See Table 26–2.)

TABLE 26–2. KEY LABORATORY RESULTS IN POSTSTREPTOCOCCAL GLOMERULONEPHRITIS, MEMBRANOPROLIFERATIVE GLOMERULONEPHRITIS, TYPE I, AND MEMBRANOPROLIFERATIVE GLOMERULONEPHRITIS, TYPE II

	Post-streptococcal	Type I	Type II
C_3, CH_{50} low in:	80–90%	50–80%	80–90%
C_4	Normal	Low	Normal
C_3 nephritic factor	Some	33%	75%
Antistreptolysin titer elevated in:	70%	20%	20%
Course	3–8 weeks	Chronic	Chronic

2. Normal Serum Complement

a. **Systemic Diseases.** Involvement of other organ systems helps guide the clinician in evaluating this group of patients. Associated systemic diseases and their signs and symptoms include:

1). **Polyarteritis Nodosa.** Hypertension, arthralgias, eosinophilia, and gastrointestinal and neurologic symptoms.

2). **Allergic Granulomatosis.** Asthma and pulmonary infiltrates.

3). **Wegener's Granulomatosis.** Sinusitis and pulmonary infiltrates.

4). **Henoch-Schönlein Purpura.** Arthritis, purpura, abdominal pain, and gastrointestinal bleeding.

5). **Goodpasture's Syndrome.** Pulmonary hemorrhage.

b. **Renal Diseases.** In renal diseases the time course of the illness is a useful discriminant.

1). **Idiopathic IgG-IgA Nephropathy (Berger's Disease, Benign Recurrent Hematuria).** These patients have hematuria that is frequently gross but sometimes microscopic. Malaise, low-grade fever, and flank pain may be present. Blood pressure is usually normal and edema is absent. The hematuria follows minor viral infection, either respiratory or gastrointestinal, and resolves in two to six days. It is recurrent in 50 per cent of cases and is associated with a slow progression to renal failure in perhaps 20 per cent.

2). **Rapidly Progressive Glomerulonephritis (RPGN).** This represents a heterogeneous group of disorders manifested as the nephritic syndrome with rapid loss of renal function. In most patients with this disorder the serum creatinine level doubles in a three-month period, and some develop renal failure within weeks to months if they are untreated. Oliguria and azotemia are common at examination. Renal biopsy commonly demonstrates cellular crescents within Bowman's space, and hence the pathologic term "crescentic glomerulonephritis" is sometimes used as a synonym for the clinical term "rapidly progressive glomerulonephritis." The diagnostic approach to the patient with this syndrome must include prompt renal biopsy, since therapy that is initiated early has a better chance of success.

C. **Final Evaluation: Renal Biopsy.** The approach outlined above uses the complement levels to guide the clinician toward the diagnosis of glomerular disease. By relying on clinical history, physical examination, and serology, the clinician can in many cases make the diagnosis with a fair degree of confidence. A renal biopsy may only be needed if several diagnostic possibilities remain that involve different therapies or prognoses.

However, it is important to recognize that the results of determination of complement levels may take many days to become available and that in some cases the rapid tempo of the disease makes such a delay unacceptable. Indications for hospitalization include oliguria, elevated creatinine level, accelerated progression of hypertension, or symptomatic fluid overload. Patients with the nephritic syndrome in whom renal function is deteriorating rapidly should be evaluated for other causes of renal dysfunction such as hypovolemia, nephrotoxins, and urinary obstruction. If these causes have been ruled out, such patients generally require a renal biopsy to identify rapidly progressive glomerulonephritis.

REFERENCES

1. Couser WG: Idiopathic rapidly progressive glomerulonephritis. Am J Nephrol 2:57–69, 1982.

A recent review that includes a classification scheme and therapeutic options.

2. Glassock RJ, et al.: Primary glomerular diseases. *In* Brenner BM, Rector FC (eds).: The Kidney. Philadelphia, W. B. Saunders Company, 1981, pp. 1351–1492.

A comprehensive and detailed review, with excellent references, in the standard nephrology text.

3. Lewis EJ: Patterns of circulating complement in renal diseases. Ann Rev Med 30:445–455, 1979.

Contains a brief discussion of complement levels.

4. Madaio MP, Harrington JT: The diagnosis of acute glomerulonephritis. N Engl J Med 309:1299–1302, 1983.

Organizes the diagnostic approach to acute nephritis by complement levels.

27

NEPHROLITHIASIS

By MICHAEL KIMMEY, M.D.

DEFINITION

A. **Stone Formation.** Nephrolithiasis is defined as the presence of stones or calculi within the kidney and urinary tract. Urinary saturation with crystals of certain compounds leads to stone formation within the renal pelvis. Stones may remain within the kidney or break off and pass down the ureter. They may be asymptomatic or cause hematuria and abdominal pain. Clinicians must first recognize nephrolithiasis as the cause of the patient's symptoms, then determine the underlying reason for stone formation. Specific treatment of the metabolic problem causing stone formation can prevent the growth of more stones.

B. **Diagnostic Criteria.** Urinary stones are demonstrated by plain abdominal x-rays or intravenous pyelography. Stones may also be collected after passage in the urine. Laboratory criteria for the various causes of stone formation are listed in Table 27–1.

TABLE 27-1. ETIOLOGY OF NEPHROLITHIASIS

Stone Type	Percentage of All Stones	Metabolic Defect*	Diagnosis†
Calcium (oxalate or phosphate)	75–85	Idiopathic hypercalciuria (50)	a. Normal serum calcium b. Increased urine calcium c. Absence of processes associated with hypercalcemia (listed below)
		Hypercalcemic states 1. Hyperparathyroidism 2. Immobilization 3. Milk alkali syndrome 4. Sarcoidosis 5. Hypervitaminosis D 6. Cushing's syndrome 7. Hyperthyroidism 8. Neoplastic disorders	a. Increased serum calcium b. Other specific laboratory tests or clinical setting
		Distal renal tubular acidosis (rare)	a. Hyperchloremic acidosis b. Unable to acidify urine pH <5.5 after NH_4Cl load

		Hyperoxaluria
		1. Congenital (rare)
		    Type I (glyoolic aciduria)
		    Type II (L-glyceric aciduria)
		2. Acquired
		    Dietary (rare)
		    Gastrointestinal disease (1–2)
			a. Increased urine oxalate

Stone type†	Percentage	Cause	Diagnostic findings
		Hyperuricosuria (20)	a. Increased urine uric acid b. Gout not present
		Idiopathic (20)	a. Results of all studies in Table 27–2 normal b. Calcium stones on analysis
Uric acid	5–8	Gout (50)	a. Clinical diagnosis (75% with increased urine uric acid; 25% with increased serum uric acid)
		Idiopathic (50)	a. Clinical gout not present b. Same metabolic studies as for gout; often positive family history of gout
		Myeloproliferative disorder (uncommon)	
		Low urine output (uncommon)	
		Lesch-Nyhan syndrome (rare)	
Struvite (triple-phosphate)	10–15	Urinary tract infection	a. Bacteriuria
Cystine	1–3	Congenital defect in amino acid transport (1/7,000 births)	a. Cystine crystals on urinalysis b. Increased urine cystine

*Parentheses indicate percentage of patients with a given stone type who have the metabolic defect listed.
†Stone type may be inferred from x-ray appearance or chemical analysis. Diagnosis here refers to underlying metabolic defect.

EPIDEMIOLOGY

One out of ten males in Western countries develops a kidney stone by age 60. Women develop urinary stones one third as often as men. Two thirds of patients who have one episode of nephrolithiasis have a recurrence. Within the United States, urinary stones are most prevalent in the southeastern states and least prevalent in the northwestern states.

CLINICAL MANIFESTATIONS

A. History
1. *Signs and Symptoms.* Precise figures for the incidence of the various manifestations of nephrolithiasis are not available. Most patients have abdominal pain caused by a stone obstructing some portion of the urinary tract. Beginning as a mild ache, the pain increases in severity to reach incapacitating levels within 30 to 60 minutes. The pain generally lasts 3 to 18 hours and remains constant without a true cramping or colicky nature. As the stone passes to the distal third of the ureter, the pain may migrate to the groin, testicle, or vulva. Symptoms of dysuria and urinary frequency may be present. Nausea and vomiting are frequently associated. Fever is absent without coexistent infection. Gross hematuria is noted by the patient in about one third of cases.
2. *Clues to the Presence of an Underlying Metabolic Defect.* Highlights of the major causes of stone formation are listed below. The relative incidences of the various causes are listed in Table 27–1.
   a. **Idiopathic Calcium Nephrolithiasis.** Most commonly this is the result of hypercalciuria, which is caused by increased intestinal absorption or a renal tubular "leak" leading to secondary hyperparathyroidism. Calcium stones can also be associated with hyperuricosuria and hyperoxaluria. Urate may act as a nidus for calcium oxalate crystal growth. Hyperuricosuria in this setting is the result of excessive dietary purines (meat, fish, or poultry) in 70 per cent of patients and metabolic overproduction of uric acid in 30 per cent. Twenty per cent of patients with calcium stones have no detectable metabolic abnormality. Low fluid intake or excessive fluid losses may be involved in some of these cases.
   b. **Hypercalcemic States.** Primary hyperparathyroidism is the most common cause of hypercalcemia associated with calcium nephrolithiasis. Any hypercalcemic disorder may be the cause, although neoplasia is an unusual cause of stone formation, probably because of the short duration of hypercalcemia.
   c. **Renal Tubular Acidosis (RTA).** Type I, or distal RTA, is associated with hyperchloremic metabolic acidosis, hy-

pokalemia, hypocalcemia, hypophosphatemia, and the inability to acidify the urine. Distal RTA shows autosomal dominant inheritance and is associated with osteomalacia, rickets, and growth retardation in children.

d. **Hyperoxaluria.** Most commonly this is caused by gastrointestinal disorders associated with fatty acid and bile malabsorption (Crohn's disease, sprue, blind loop syndrome, chronic pancreatitis, small bowel resection or bypass, or biliary tract disease). Bile acids increase colonic absorption of oxalate that has not formed complexes with luminal calcium because the latter has been bound to fatty acids. Excessive dietary intake occurs in persons consuming large quantities of vegetables (especially rhubarb, spinach, or turnip greens) and small amounts of calcium. Excessive vitamin C consumption (> 4 g per day) and ethylene glycol ingestion also increase urinary oxalate concentrations. Congenital enzymatic defects leading to hyperoxaluria are rare and usually are manifested with malignant stone formation in childhood.

e. **Uric Acid Lithiasis.** Twenty-five per cent of patients have an abnormality in purine metabolism. Other causes of uric acid lithiasis include overexcretion of uric acid, excessive dietary purines, low urine volumes, persistently acid urine, and treatment with uricosuric drugs (probenecid, sulfinpyrazone, or salicylates). About 25 per cent of patients with primary gout and 40 per cent of those with gout secondary to myeloproliferative disorders develop uric acid calculi.

f. **Struvite Stones.** These stones are seen in patients with chronic or recurrent urinary tract infections caused by urease-producing bacteria. When urea is metabolized, the production of stones composed of calcium, magnesium, ammonium phosphate, and carbonate-apatite is favored. Recurrence rates of 40 per cent, calculi filling the renal pelvis (staghorn stones), chronic renal failure, and episodes of pyelonephritis are characteristic.

g. **Cystine Stones.** Cystinuria is an inherited defect in amino acid transport that leads to high urinary levels of the highly insoluble amino acid cystine. Cystine stones form early in life and cause renal colic in the second and third decades.

B. **Physical Findings.** Most patients have tenderness to percussion in the costovertebral angle. Some have tenderness anteriorly, which may mimic acute cholecystitis if tenderness is on the right side.

LABORATORY STUDIES

A. **Acute Episode**
   1. The majority of patients with abdominal pain as a result of nephrolithiasis have gross or microscopic hematuria.
   2. Elevations in blood urea nitrogen and creatinine are not

present unless there is dehydration or parenchymal renal disease.

3. The plain abdominal radiograph visualizes calcium-containing stones, which represent 80 per cent of all stones.

4. If nephrolithiasis is suspected and the plain radiograph does not show a stone, an intravenous pyelogram should be done. Additional information obtained from this study includes whether complete obstruction is present and the presence of additional unsuspected stones.

RECOMMENDED DIAGNOSTIC APPROACH

A. **Underlying Cause.** The underlying cause of stone formation is best determined after the acute episode when the patient is on a normal (outpatient) diet. Laboratory findings in the various types of stone disease are listed in Table 27–1.

B. **Acute Episode.** Patients with suggestive abdominal pain or hematuria, or both, should have a urinalysis and plain abdominal x-ray performed. If a stone is not identified on the plain x-ray, an intravenous pyelogram should be done to confirm the diagnosis.

C. **Ambulatory Protocol (for underlying metabolic defect)**
  1. *Recommended Serum and Urine Diagnostic Tests.* Table 27–2 lists the serum and urine diagnostic tests recommended for ambulatory patients who have nephrolithiasis. Whether all patients who have passed a single stone should be thoroughly evaluated is debatable. Patients with recurrent stone formation should have all of the tests listed in Table 27–2 performed.
  2. *Drug Effects.* Whenever possible, administration of drugs that may affect renal function should be stopped prior to diagnostic evaluation. These include vitamins C and D, aspirin, and diuretics. A recent intravenous pyelogram is useful as a baseline for assessment of further stone formation.

TABLE 27–2. LABORATORY EVALUATION OF ETIOLOGY OF NEPHROLITHIASIS

Serum testing	Urine testing (random)	
Calcium	Urinalysis	
Electrolytes	Urine culture	
	Cystine screen	

	Upper limits of normal (mg/24 hr)	
	Men	Women
24-hour urine collection		
Calcium	300	250
Uric acid	800	750
Oxalate	50	50
Creatinine*	20–25	16–22

*mg of creatinine per kg of lean body mass.

3. **Urinalysis.** The presence of greater than 10 white blood cells per cu mm of unspun urine indicates the presence of infection and mandates a urine culture. Infection may be a cause of the stone formation (struvite stones) or may occur secondary to the presence of stones. Crystals seen on urinalysis have a variable significance. The presence of cystine (hexagonal plates) and struvite crystals ("coffin lids") is a clue to the underlying defect. Calcium oxalate, uric acid, and calcium phosphate crystals can be seen in normal persons and thus are not useful when seen on urinalysis. The presence of cystine in the urine can be confirmed with a screening test using cyanide-nitroprusside or by chromatography.

4. **Twenty-Four–Hour Urine Collections.** These should be repeated in most cases to verify abnormal results before treatment is started. All urine collections should be checked for completeness by measuring creatinine content.

5. **Chemical Analysis of Stones.** Chemical analysis of any stones that have passed is useful but not sufficient to determine the treatment of the underlying defect. Stones may be heterogeneous, and several different metabolic defects can produce the same stone type.

REFERENCES

1. Bretland PM: Acute Ureteric Obstruction, a Clinical and Radiological Study. New York, Appleton-Century-Crofts, 1972, pp. 1–209.

A pioneering work describing clinical and radiographic features of patients with urolithiasis.

2. Coe FL: Nephrolithiasis. Contemp Issues Nephrol 5:1–275, 1980.

An excellent synopsis of all aspects and causes of nephrolithiasis.

3. Coe FL, Favus MJ: Nephrolithiasis. *In* Petersdorf RG, Adams RD, et al. (eds.): Harrison's Principles of Internal Medicine. 10th ed. New York, McGraw-Hill, 1983, pp. 1672–1676.

4. Pak CYC, Britton F, Peterson R, et al.: Ambulatory evaluation of nephrolithiasis. Am J Med 69:18–30, 1980.

28

NEPHROTIC SYNDROME

By ALAN WATSON, M.D.

DEFINITION AND DIAGNOSTIC CRITERIA

The term "nephrotic syndrome" refers to a constellation of clinical and laboratory abnormalities that are the consequences of proteinuria in excess of 3.5 g per 24 hours per 1.73 sq m. The major component of the urinary protein loss is albumin, and in the majority of cases this degree of proteinuria is sufficient to induce hypoalbuminemia.

The nephrotic syndrome per se is not an etiologic diagnosis but merely indicates abnormal glomerular permeability. This may be the consequence of a primary glomerular disease (primary or idiopathic nephrotic syndrome) or may represent a renal manifestation of a wide variety of disease processes (secondary nephrotic syndrome).

The four criteria generally regarded as necessary for the diagnosis of the nephrotic syndrome include:

1. Proteinuria: >3.5 g per 24 hours per 1.73 sq m
2. Hypoalbuminemia: <2.5 g per dL
3. Edema
4. Hyperlipidemia

However, whether the latter three features actually develop in the setting of nephrotic-range proteinuria depends not only on the urinary protein loss itself but on other factors, such as the compensatory reserve of the liver to synthesize albumin, the degree of increase in albumin catabolism, and the avidity of salt retention.

Thus, from the practical point of view, a diagnosis of nephrotic syndrome may be made in the presence of proteinuria that is greater than 3.5 g per 24 hours per 1.73 sq m of body surface area and, according to urine electrophoresis, composed predominantly of albumin.

EPIDEMIOLOGY

The incidence and causes of the nephrotic syndrome in any given population vary considerably and depend on many factors, including age, criteria for diagnosis, socioeconomic status, geographic location, and current indications for renal biopsy.

In the United States and European pediatric population (under age 16 years), the incidence of nephrotic syndrome is approximately two to five cases per 100,000 persons per year, with a male to female predominance of 2–2.5:1. Minimal-change disease accounts for over 70 per cent of these cases and for over 90 per cent of nephrotic syndrome as a result of primary glomerular disease in children between the ages of two and six years.

In adults, minimal-change disease is less common, the sex incidence is closer to unity, and secondary nephrotic syndrome is more frequently encountered. The increasing prevalence of diabetes mellitus in the adult population is largely responsible for the latter feature.

DIFFERENTIAL DIAGNOSIS

The advent of percutaneous renal biopsy as a diagnostic procedure has made it possible to classify idiopathic nephrotic syndrome into

TABLE 28–1. PREVALENCE OF PRIMARY GLOMERULAR DISEASE IN THE NEPHROTIC SYNDROME

	CHILDREN (PER CENT)	ADULTS (PER CENT)
Minimal-change disease	60	20
Membranous glomerulonephritis	6	30
Proliferative glomerulonephritis	10	30
Focal glomerular sclerosis	8	8
Membranoproliferative glomerulonephritis	10	5
Mesangial proliferative glomerulonephritis	5	6
Miscellaneous	1	1

reasonably well-defined clinicopathologic entities. The primary disorders and their relative frequencies in pediatric and adult populations are shown in Table 28–1.

The wide variety of disease states, chemical toxins, and medications that are manifested clinically as the nephrotic syndrome are outlined in Table 28–2. The most frequent causes of secondary nephrotic syndrome are diabetes mellitus, multiple myeloma, neoplastic disease, and connective tissue diseases, particularly systemic lupus erythematosus.

TABLE 28–2. MAJOR CAUSES OF SECONDARY NEPHROTIC SYNDROME

1. **METABOLIC DISEASE**
   Diabetes mellitus
   Amyloidosis
   Sickle cell disease

2. **CONNECTIVE TISSUE DISEASE**
   Systemic lupus erythematosis
   Polyarteritis
   Cryoglobulinemia

3. **INFECTION**
   Bacterial: subacute bacterial endocarditis, leprosy, syphilis
   Viral: hepatitis B, cytomegalovirus, Epstein-Barr virus
   Protozoal: malaria, toxoplasmosis
   Helminthic: filariasis, schistosomiasis

4. **NEOPLASIA**
   Lymphoma, leukemia
   Lung, colon, stomach, breast

5. **MEDICATION/TOXIN**
   Penicillamine, gold, captopril, heroin, nonsteroidal anti-inflammatory drugs
   Silver, bismuth, mercury

6. **HEREDOFAMILIAL**
   Familial nephrotic syndrome
   Alpha-1-antitrypsin deficiency
   Fabry's disease
   Nail patella syndrome

7. **VASCULAR**
   Renal artery stenosis (rare)
   Congestive heart failure
   Tricuspid incompetence
   Constrictive pericarditis
   Renal vein thrombosis

8. **MISCELLANEOUS**
   Pregnancy
   Massive obesity
   Vesicoureteric reflux

CLINICAL FEATURES

Clinical features of the nephrotic syndrome arise as a direct result of abnormal glomerular permeability and the resultant massive proteinuria.

A. Edema. The clinical hallmark symptom and sign of the nephrotic syndrome is edema, which reflects an increase in the interstitial component of the extracellular fluid compartment. Edema is usually localized to gravity-dependent areas, although in more severe instances it may become generalized (anasarca). Edema of internal organ systems may also give rise to symptoms, most notably the anorexia, nausea, and vomiting that result from edema and dysfunction of the gastrointestinal mucosa.

B. Malnutrition. Loss of lean body mass results from a persistently negative nitrogen balance (decreased intake plus increased loss and increased catabolism of albumin), which in children may be of sufficient severity to induce marasmus. The concomitant presence of edema may mask weight loss resulting from malnutrition.

C. Susceptibility to Infection. A diminution of humoral defense mechanisms (IgG, factor B, decreased opsonization) is regarded as responsible for the well-recognized susceptibility of patients with nephrotic syndrome to severe infections, notably caused by *Pneumococcus, Klebsiella,* and coliform species.

D. Thromboembolic Tendency
   1. *Renal Vein Thrombosis.* This occurs in 5 to 20 per cent of cases. Patients are commonly asymptomatic and the prognosis is poor.

Whereas in the past it was assumed that renal vein thrombosis was the causative factor in nephrotic syndrome, recent observations suggest that the syndrome precedes and predisposes to the development of renal vein thrombosis.

   2. *Other Thromboembolic Complications.* These complications occur in 20 per cent of cases. Venous complications affect the pulmonary veins and extremities. Arterial complications affect the coronary, cerebral, and peripheral veins.

E. Metabolic Complications
   1. *Accelerated Atherosclerosis.* This is related to lipid abnormalities.
   2. *Osteomalacia.* This is related to altered vitamin D metabolism.

F. Symptoms and Signs of the Underlying Disease State. These include retinopathy and neuropathy in diabetes mellitus; bone pain in multiple myeloma; arthritis and rash in connective tissue disease; and periodic chills or fevers and a history of travel in malaria.

LABORATORY FEATURES

A. Proteinuria. The proteinuria is in excess of 3.5 g per 24 hours per 1.73 sq m of body surface area and is predominantly albumin.

The diagnosis of nephrotic syndrome relies heavily on the quantification of urinary protein in a 24-hour urine collection, although it is well recognized that the amount of protein excreted can vary substantially from day to day and that errors in timing the 24-hour urinary samples are common. Moreover, such collections are cumbersome and time-consuming.

Several recent studies have demonstrated that a determination of the protein:creatinine ratio in single urine samples correlates well with the quantity of protein in timed urine collections and that a protein:creatinine ratio of greater than 3.5 (mg per mg) represents nephrotic-range proteinuria. It is thus likely that the protein:creatinine ratio of single urine samples will prove to be a satisfactory substitute for the determination of protein excretion in 24-hour urine collections.

B. **Hypoalbuminemia.** Hypoalbuminemia is less than 3.5 mg per dL (95 per cent of cases).

C. **Hyperlipidemia.** Very low-density lipoprotein and low-density lipoprotein increase; high-density lipoprotein decreases.

D. **Hypocalcemia.** The traditional concept that the observed reduction in serum calcium is solely a result of a decrease in the protein-bound fraction has been questioned recently. Losses of vitamin D–binding protein in the urine result in a decrease in serum concentrations of $25(OH)D_3$ and $1,25(OH)_2D_3$ with a resultant decrease in calcium absorption and the serum-ionized calcium fraction. For reasons that remain unclear, however, these changes are not observed in all patients with the nephrotic syndrome.

E. **Thyroid Function Studies.** Total free thyroxin and thyroxine-binding globulin increase; the level of free thyroxin is normal.

F. **Coagulation Factors.** Factors V and VII increase; antithrombin III decreases; and fibrinogen increases. This latter increase is the most consistent and important abnormality.

G. **Immunoglobulin.** Immunoglobulin G is present.

H. **Urinalysis.** Glycosuria is present (secondary to proximal tubule dysfunction). Glycosuria alone does not necessarily indicate an impaired glucose tolerance in the setting of nephrotic syndrome.

Oval fat bodies represent cholesterol esters, which appear as "Maltese crosses" on polarizing microscopy.

I. **Miscellaneous Findings.** Miscellaneous findings include hypokalemia; hypomagnesemia secondary to aldosteronism; and renal tubular acidosis.

RECOMMENDED DIAGNOSTIC APPROACH

The high incidence of minimal-change lesions as the cause of nephrotic syndrome in children allows presumptive diagnosis of this entity in the pediatric setting. The predictive value of this diagnosis is approximately 70 per cent, and a minimal-change lesion is even more likely if steroid therapy induces remission of proteinuria. In the occasional case in which steroid/cytotoxic drug therapy fails to improve the nephrotic syndrome, a renal biopsy is indicated.

In adult cases, in which a presumed cause is detected—such as diabetes mellitus or amyloidosis—biopsy is generally unnecessary unless the subsequent clinical course proves incompatible with the clinical diagnosis. In such circumstances, a renal biopsy should be performed. When no obvious cause is apparent, renal biopsy generally provides an accurate diagnosis and prognostic assessment and aids in the formulation of a rational therapeutic plan.

REFERENCES

1. Glassock RJ, et al.: Primary glomerular disease. *In* Brenner B, Rector F (eds.): The Kidney. 2nd ed. Philadelphia, WB Saunders Company, 1981, p. 1351.
2. Hutt M, Glassock RJ: Proteinuria and the nephrotic syndrome. *In* Shrier R (ed.): Fluid and Electrolyte Disorders and Renal Diseases. 2nd ed. Boston, Little, Brown & Company, 1980.
3. Glassock RJ: The nephrotic syndrome. Hosp Pract 14:105, 1979.
4. Habib R, Levy M, Gubler MC: Clinicopathologic correlations in the nephrotic syndrome. Paediatrician 8:325, 1979.
5. A Report of the International Study of Kidney Disease in Children: Nephrotic syndrome in children. Prediction of histopathology from clinical and laboratory characteristics at time of diagnosis. Kidney Int 13:159, 1978.
6. Brenner BM, Stein JH (eds.): Nephrotic syndrome. Contemporary Issues in Nephrology. Vol. 9. New York, Churchill-Livingstone, 1982.

This book provides an excellent and succinct review of the causes of primary nephrotic syndrome and of the metabolic and thromboembolic complications.

INFECTIOUS DISEASE

ACQUIRED IMMUNODEFICIENCY SYNDROME (AIDS)

By BARBARA D. KIRBY, M.D.

DEFINITION

A. The Centers for Disease Control have defined a case of AIDS as "a reliably diagnosed disease that is at least moderately indicative of an underlying cellular immunodeficiency in a person who has had no known underlying cause of cellular immunodeficiency and no other cause of reduced resistance reported to be associated with that disease." History of an underlying immunosuppressive disorder (such as Hodgkin's disease), however remote, precludes the diagnosis of AIDS. The etiologic agent of AIDS is a retrovirus, either human T cell lymphotrophic virus (HTLV-III) or the closely related lymphadenopathy-associated virus (LAV).

B. *Pneumocystis carinii* pneumonia is the most common life-threatening opportunistic infection, accounting for about one half of the primary diagnoses. Other opportunistic infections include *Mycobacterium avium-intracellulare, Toxoplasma gondii, Cryptococcus neoformans, Cryptosporidia* species, *Isospora belli,* and *Candida albicans.* Life-threatening viral infections with herpes viruses, cytomegalovirus, and hepatitis viruses also occur in AIDS patients.

C. Patients may have neoplasms, such as Kaposi's sarcoma, and lymphomas, with or without associated opportunistic infections.

D. *AIDS-related complex (ARC)* is a symptom complex consisting of malaise, fever, weight loss, diarrhea, hepatosplenomegaly, and lymphadenopathy. Patients with ARC are probably at risk to develop classic AIDS.

EPIDEMIOLOGY

A. High-risk groups for development of AIDS have been identified:
1. Homosexually active males account for 71 per cent of cases.
2. Intravenous drug users represent 17 per cent of cases overall and 51 per cent of female cases.
3. Haitians make up 5 per cent of patients.
4. Hemophiliacs make up 1 per cent of patients.
5. Sexual partners and children of high-risk groups are involved in less than 1 per cent of cases.

      6. Blood transfusion recipients are involved in less than 1 per cent of cases.

B. The incubation period may be as long as four years.

C. Transmission of AIDS appears to be similar to that of hepatitis B, occurring by intimate sexual contact, blood and blood products, and transplacentally.

D. Cases have been reported throughout the United States (with epidemic foci in New York City, Los Angeles, San Francisco, and Miami) and in Haiti, Africa, and Europe.

CLINICAL FEATURES

A. History. Social and sexual habits of patients suspected of having AIDS must be determined. Intravenous drug use and homosexuality or sexual or percutaneous contact with intravenous drug users and homosexual males are key historical points. Since the incubation period of AIDS may be quite long (years), a *remote* history of these activities should not be ignored. A history of blood transfusion during the preceding four years is potentially important.

B. Patients with AIDS may have an AIDS-related complex prior to the development of an opportunistic infection or neoplasm, or they may have only symptoms caused by opportunistic infection or tumor.

    1. *Pneumocystis carinii* pneumonia produces fever, cough, dyspnea, and pulmonary infiltrates. The pneumonia may be rapidly progressive or insidious.

    2. Kaposi's sarcoma produces a new skin lesion that is often dark blue or purple. Visceral dissemination of the tumor in association with relatively minor cutaneous involvement is not uncommon.

    3. Altered mental status and focal neurologic signs or symptoms should suggest central nervous system processes such as toxoplasmosis, cryptococcosis, herpetic encephalitis, tuberculosis, or nocardiosis.

LABORATORY FINDINGS

Impaired cellular immunity is uniformly noted. Defects include cutaneous anergy, reversal of helper to suppressor T cell ratios, and lymphopenia (less than 1500 blood lymphocytes per cu mm). The reversal of the helper to suppressor T cell ratio is caused by a decrease in absolute numbers of helper T cells. Blastogenic responses of blood lymphocytes to mitogens and antigens are abnormally low. Polyclonal hypergammaglobulinemia is frequently noted; however, humoral response to new antigens appears to be markedly impaired. Natural interferon production is reduced in some patients.

S **9964**

‖‖‖‖‖‖‖‖‖‖‖‖‖‖‖‖‖‖‖‖‖‖‖‖‖‖‖

00047489964

Inspected By: Javier_Guarin

**Sell your books at
sellbackyourBook.com!
Go to sellbackyourBook.com
and get an instant price
quote. We even pay the
shipping - see what your old
books are worth today!**

RECOMMENDED DIAGNOSTIC APPROACH

A. A white blood cell count with a differential count should be done.
B. Tests for cutaneous anergy should be performed.
C. The helper to suppressor T cell ratio (if available) should be studied.
D. Lymph node biopsy and skin biopsy are necessary if abnormalities are noted.
E. A work-up is used for specific opportunistic infection or neoplasm as indicated by the clinical presentation.

REFERENCES

1. Centers for Disease Control. AIDS: Acquired immunodeficiency syndrome. Morbid Mortal Weekly Rep 32:465–467, 1983.

Demographic data and case fatality statistics.

2. Small CB, Klein RS, Friedland GH, et al.: Community-acquired opportunistic infections and defective cellular immunity in heterosexual drug abusers and homosexual men. Am J Med 74:433–441, 1983.

Clinical features of cases of AIDS.

3. Gallo RC, Salahuddin SZ, Popovic M, et al: Frequent detection and isolation of cytopathic retroviruses (HTLV-III) from patients with AIDS and at risk for AIDS. Science 224:500–3, 1984.

Four articles from Gallo's group appeared in this issue of Science *announcing isolation of the agent of AIDS.*

4. Quinn TC: Perspectives on the future of AIDS (editorial). JAMA 253:247–248, 1985.

30

FEVER IN THE IMMUNOCOMPROMISED HOST

By OLIVER W. PRESS, M.D., Ph.D.

DEFINITIONS

A. Fever. Fever is routinely defined as an oral temperature of $\geq 100.2°$ F ($37.8°$ C) or a rectal temperature of $\geq 101.2°$ F ($38.4°$ C).
B. Immunocompromised Hosts. These are patients with any of the following types of defects in their immune defenses:
    1. Neutropenia. Neutropenia is a neutrophil count of < 500 cells per cu mm. It correlates with risk of infection more convincingly than any other risk factor.

2. *Defective Neutrophil Function.* This defect consists of abnormal chemotaxis, phagocytosis, or microbial killing and results in an increased incidence of infections, but it is less ominous than absolute neutropenia.

3. *Cellular Immune Dysfunction.* This occurs primarily in patients with abnormal T lymphocyte function.

4. *Humoral Immune Dysfunction.* This type of dysfunction results from defective production of immunoglobulins (as in disorders of B lymphocytes).

5. *Obstruction of Body Luminal Structures.* Obstruction of body luminal structures such as bowel, ureters, or bronchi promotes stasis of body fluids and overgrowth of microorganisms.

6. *Disruption of Mucocutaneous Barriers.* Such disruption, involving skin, gastrointestinal mucosa, or bronchial mucosa, results in direct microbial access to the blood stream and to other body tissues.

Table 30–1 shows common disorders in which each of these defense defects exists and typical organisms causing infection under each circumstance. In many clinical situations (bone marrow transplantation, chemotherapy), several defense systems are simultaneously impaired.

EPIDEMIOLOGY

Although exact statistics concerning the incidence of fever in immunocompromised hosts are unavailable, there is a general consensus that this entity is a common and growing problem. Cancer alone caused 20.6 per cent of all deaths (396,992 fatalities) in the United States in 1978, and of these deaths 50 to 60 per cent are attributable to opportunistic infections. With the increasing popularity of aggressive combination chemotherapy regimens and organ transplantation, the magnitude of this problem is anticipated to burgeon in coming years.

DIFFERENTIAL DIAGNOSIS OF FEVER IN THE IMMUNOCOMPROMISED HOST

A. **Infection.** Infection with bacterial, viral, fungal, or parasitic organisms can be demonstrated by culture or serology in approximately 65 per cent of febrile immunocompromised patients. (See Table 30–2 for the relative frequencies of the different types of infections.)

B. **Underlying Disease.** The underlying disease may be responsible for fever in cases of malignancy ("tumor fever") or collagen-vascular disease. This diagnosis is always one of exclusion, however, and should only be entertained after all other possibilities have been ruled out. The neoplasms most commonly associated with intrinsic fever include lymphomas, leukemias, renal cell carcinomas, adrenal carcinomas, hepatomas, and tumors metastatic to liver.

TABLE 30–1. INFECTIONS IN IMMUNOCOMPROMISED HOSTS

DEFECTIVE DEFENSE MECHANISM	TYPICAL DISEASE SETTING	TYPICAL INFECTING ORGANISMS	TYPES OF INFECTION
1. Neutropenia	Leukemia, bone marrow transplantation	*Staphylococcus epidermidis* and *S. aureus*, gram-negative rods (*Escherichia coli, Klebsiella, Enterobacter, Pseudomonas), Candida, Aspergillus*	Septicemia, pneumonia, meningitis
2. Defective neutrophil function	Uremia, alcoholism, diabetes mellitus, chronic granulomatous disease	*S. aureus, Candida*	Recurrent abscesses, septicemia
3. Cellular immune dysfunction	Hodgkin's disease, renal transplantation, acquired immunodeficiency syndrome	*Listeria, Salmonella, Nocardia, Candida, Cryptococcus,* cytomegalovirus, herpes simplex and zoster, *Pneumocystis, Toxoplasma, Strongyloides*	Septicemia, pneumonia, meningitis, cutaneous lesions
4. Humoral immune dysfunction	Multiple myeloma, chronic lymphocytic leukemia	*Streptococcus pneumoniae, Hemophilus influenzae,* gram-negative rods	Septicemia, pneumonia, meningitis
5. Obstruction of body lumens	Cancer	Gram-negative rods, *Bacteroides,* enterococcus	Septicemia
6. Disruption of mucocutaneous barriers	Burns, cancer, chemotherapy	*S. epidermidis* and *aureus,* gram-negative rods (esp. *Pseudomonas*)	Local infections, septicemia

TABLE 30-2. FREQUENCY OF VARIOUS TYPES OF INFECTIONS IN IMMUNOCOMPROMISED PATIENTS*

PATHOGEN	MULTIPLE MYELOMA PATIENTS (N = 50)	RENAL TRANSPLANT PATIENTS (N = 518)	BONE MARROW TRANSPLANT PATIENTS (SEVERAL STUDIES)
I. Bacteria (overall)	78%	16%	65%
A. Gram-negative rods			
1. *Escherichia coli*	26	1	21
2. *Klebsiella*	8	<1	21
3. *Enterobacter*	0	<1	10
4. *Pseudomonas*	12	3	48
5. Other	—	0	13
B. *Staphylococcus epidermidis*	20	1	8
C. *S. aureus*	52	<1	11
D. *Streptococcus pneumoniae*	0	<1	5–10
E. Enterococcus	0	<1	—
F. *Bacteroides*	10	<1	21
G. *Hemophilus*	4	<1	<1
H. *Mycobacterium*	0	4	47
I. Other			

II. Viruses (overall)	2%	24%	40–70%
A. Cytomegalovirus	0	21	16
B. Herpes zoster	2	2	40–50
C. Herpes simplex	0	?	40–50
D. Other	0	1	—
III. Fungi (overall)	0	4%	20–30%
A. *Aspergillus*	0	2	14
B. *Candida*	0	2	22
C. Other (*Cryptococcus, Coccidioides, Histoplasma*)	0	<1	1
IV. Protozoa (overall)	0	<1%	6%
A. *Pneumocystis*	0	<1	6
B. *Toxoplasma*	0	<1	<1
C. *Strongyloides*	0	<1	<1
D. Other	0	<1	<1

*Percentage of patients acquiring infection with the stated pathogen. Many patients had more than one infection, hence totals do not equal the sum of the individual infection incidences. (The table was compiled from Meyers, Peterson et al., Winston et al., and Twomey.)

C. **Drugs.** In immunocompromised patients drugs frequently cause fever, which may be manifested with or without pruritic maculopapular rashes and eosinophilia. Some medications predictably produce fever (bleomycin, antithymocyte globulin, and amphotericin); however, the majority of drugs cause fever idiosyncratically (trimethoprim-sulfamethoxazole, penicillin, and thiazides, for example).

D. **Transfusions.** Transfusions commonly cause febrile reactions as a result of alloimmunization to leukocyte antigens.

E. **Hematomas.** Hematomas can produce prolonged fever even if they are uninfected. Concealed hematomas are most commonly located in the retroperitoneum.

F. **Pulmonary Emboli.** Pulmonary emboli are associated with fever in 50 per cent of cases.

G. **Splenic Infarcts.** These should be suspected in patients with left-sided abdominal pain and fever.

H. **Graft Versus Host Disease.** This occurs in patients after allogeneic bone marrow transplantation (in approximately 60 per cent of cases) or rarely after transfusion with unirradiated leukocytes. The disease generally appears with fever, rash, diarrhea, and liver dysfunction.

I. **Miscellaneous Causes.** Miscellaneous causes of cryptic fever that are often overlooked include adrenal insufficiency, catheter infections, mycobacterial disease (the patient may be anergic), abdominal abscesses, and systemic viral infections, including cytomegalovirus, Epstein-Barr virus, and anicteric hepatitis (A, B, or non-A non-B).

CLINICAL APPROACH TO FEVER IN THE COMPROMISED HOST: HISTORY AND PHYSICAL EXAMINATION

A. A careful review of the patient's medical history is mandatory. Note is made of dates of initial diagnosis, dates of transplantation and invasive procedures, transfusions, drug records, and previous infection history.

B. A history of recent travel, pets, and infection exposure should be carefully elicited.

C. Localizing symptoms are of paramount importance. Particular attention should be paid to complaints of skin lesions, headache, stiff neck, visual changes, mucositis, dysphagia, abdominal pain, diarrhea, cough, dyspnea, and perirectal discomfort.

D. Careful and repeated physical examination should be performed in a search for signs of local inflammation, catheter infection, mental status changes, nuchal rigidity, lesions in the fundi and on the skin, pharyngeal abnormalities, lymphadenopathy, pulmonary rales or consolidation, hepatosplenomegaly, abdominal tenderness, or perirectal cellulitis.

E. It is important to recognize that the cardinal symptoms and signs of infection may be absent in immunocompromised patients. Neutropenic patients may not generate pus, sputum, or signs of local inflammation. Meningitis with opportunistic pathogens usually is present without meningismus (63 per cent of cases).

F. Factors that favor a microbial origin rather than an underlying disease as the cause of fever include appearance of skin lesions, mental deterioration, hypotension, hyperventilation, disseminated intravascular coagulation, hemolysis, metabolic acidosis, localized pain, and oliguria.

CLINICAL APPROACH TO FEVER IN THE IMMUNOCOMPROMISED HOST: LABORATORY EVALUATION

A. Initial Studies

1. Smears and cultures of the pharynx, perirectal area, stool, urine, sputum, blood, and other body fluids (pleural effusions and ascites) should be obtained for routine microbiologic studies for bacteria, fungi, viruses, and mycobacteria (when appropriate). Anaerobic cultures should be performed on blood and other body fluids, and blood cultures should be incubated for prolonged periods (four weeks) to allow growth of fastidious organisms. Antibiotic removal devices may be useful when patients are receiving antibiotics.
2. A chest x-ray should be done for all patients.
3. Biopsy of skin lesions should be performed for pathology and culture (bacterial, fungal, and viral).
4. The medication list should be scrutinized and unnecessary drugs discontinued.
5. Localizing sites should be investigated with appropriate studies, for example, abdominal x-ray and ultrasound in a patient with abdominal pain.
6. Empiric antibiotic administration with at least two synergistic bactericidal antibiotics (for example, ticarcillin and tobramycin) *must* be begun in all febrile neutropenic patients while awaiting culture test results.

B. Further Diagnostic Studies.
Further diagnostic studies should be considered in patients with fever that is undiagnosed by initial evaluation, as outlined below:

1. Liver function tests should be obtained to screen for hepatitis and liver metastases.
2. Serologic testing should be performed for *Legionella pneumophila,* hepatitis A and B, cytomegalovirus, Epstein-Barr virus, and toxoplasmosis.
3. Serial chest x-rays should be done to detect evolving pneumonias (such as in cytomegalovirus infection or pneumocystis). Sinus films may reveal occult sinusitis.
4. Arterial blood gases should be studied in patients with pulmonary symptoms.
5. Abdominal ultrasound or computed tomography may reveal occult abscesses, hematomas, or metastases.

6. Radionuclide scans of bone, lung, and liver and spleen are useful in cases of suspected osteomyelitis, pulmonary embolism, and splenic infarction respectively.
7. The usefulness of gallium- and indium-labeled white cell scans is controversial. Although many cases of occult infection have been diagnosed with the aid of these techniques, the frequency of false-positive and false-negative results (14 and 4 per cent, respectively for gallium) limits their utility. In addition, these methods are technically difficult and unreliable for neutropenic patients.
8. Bone marrow or lymph node biopsy may reveal histologic or microbiologic evidence of tuberculous, fungal, or *Salmonella* infection.
9. Microscopic evaluation of fresh stool specimens may demonstrate *Strongyloides stercoralis* larvae.
10. Liver biopsy should be considered for patients with hepatic dysfunction.
11. Peripheral venous and routine subclavian catheters should be removed, culture samples should be taken, and new catheters should be inserted. Right atrial Hickman and Broviac catheters need not be removed unless there is evidence of persistent catheter infection after administration of appropriate antibiotics.

C. **Diagnostic Tests for Patients with Pulmonary Infiltrates.** Further diagnostic tests that should be considered for patients with pulmonary infiltrates include the following:
1. Gram's stain and culture of sputum should be routinely ordered but frequently are difficult to obtain in neutropenic patients with mucositis. Furthermore, interpretation is difficult because of contamination with oropharyngeal flora.
2. Transtracheal aspiration may be helpful for patients who are not critically ill or severely thrombocytopenic.
3. Bronchoscopy with washings, brushings, and biopsy is frequently useful but has been associated with unacceptable rates of false-negative results and may produce massive bleeding in patients with low platelet counts.
4. Open lung biopsy is the procedure of choice for patients with acute diffuse pneumonia, since it has the highest diagnostic yield and allows better control of bleeding sites than bronchoscopic biopsy.

Typical results obtained using the aforementioned procedures are tabulated below:

PROCEDURE	DIAGNOSTIC YIELD (PER CENT)	MORBIDITY (PER CENT)
Transtracheal aspirate	5–10	2–5
Bronchoscopy		
Biopsy alone	30–75	5–20
Washings and brushings	40–84	5–20
Transthoracic needle aspirate	40–60	10–30
Open lung biopsy	80–100	5–12

D. Diagnostic Procedures for Patients with Headache, Stiff Neck, or Mental Status Changes. The procedures that should be used in these cases are outlined below:

1. Computed tomography of the head can rule out a brain abscess or hemorrhage.

2. Lumbar puncture should be performed even with minimal central nervous system symptoms so long as there is no evidence of increased intracranial pressure or severe thrombocytopenia ($< 50,000$ mm), since the common pathogens producing meningitis in compromised patients do not cause prominent meningeal symptoms. (See Chapter 35.) Cerebrospinal fluid should be analyzed for cell count, protein, glucose, acid-fast stain, India ink examination, cryptococcal antigen determination, and bacterial, mycobacterial, and fungal cultures.

REFERENCES

1. Young S: Fever and septicemia. *In* Rubin RH, Young LS (eds.): Clinical Approach to Infection in the Compromised Host. New York, Plenum Publishing Corporation, 1981, pp. 75–122.

An excellent and extensive review. Every chapter in this book is outstanding.

2. Silverberg E: Cancer statistics, 1982. CA: A Journal for Clinicians 32:15–31, 1982.

A good source of recent cancer statistics.

3. Ketchel S, Rodriguez R: Acute infections in cancer patients. Semin Oncol 5:167–179, 1978.

An excellent review, but it is a few years out of date.

4. Ebright JF, Jagmeet SS, Manoli RS: The gallium scan: Problems and misuse in examination of patients with suspected infections. Arch Intern Med 142:246–254, 1982.

A critical analysis of the utility of gallium scans.

5. Wade JS, Newman KA, Schimpf SS, et al.: Two methods for improved venous access in acute leukemia patients. JAMA 246:140–144, 1981.

A good description of the advantages and complications of Hickman catheters.

6. Springmeyer SC, Silvestri RC, Sale GE, et al.: The role of transbronchial biopsy for the diagnosis of diffuse pneumonias in immunocompromised marrow transplant recipients. Am Rev Respir Dis 126:763–765, 1982.

A good comparison of the relative yields of transbronchial and open lung biopsy for diagnosis of diffuse pneumonias occurring in patients receiving bone marrow transplants.

7. Meyers JD, Thomas ED: Infection complicating bone marrow transplantation. *In* Rubin RH, Young LS (eds.): Clinical Approach to Infection in the Compromised Host. New York, Plenum Publishing Corporation, 1981, pp. 507–551.

This chapter outlines the infectious complications seen in the largest bone marrow transplantation unit in the world.

8. Winston DJ, Gale RP, et al.: Infectious complications of bone marrow transplantation. Medicine 58:1–31, 1979.

Another good review.

9. Peterson PK, Ferguson R, et al.: Infectious diseases in hospitalized renal transplant recipients. Medicine 61:360–372, 1982.

A good review of opportunistic infections in renal transplant patients.

10. Twomey JJ: Infections complicating multiple myeloma and chronic lymphocytic leukemia. Arch Intern Med 132:562–565, 1973.

Chronicles the infections seen in 50 patients with myeloma.

---31---

FEVER OF UNKNOWN ORIGIN

By OLIVER W. PRESS, M.D., Ph.D.

DEFINITION

Petersdorf and Beeson in their classic paper of 1961 defined fever of unknown origin (FUO) as a febrile illness with a temperature of $\geq 101°F$ (38.3°C), lasting at least three weeks, that remains undiagnosed after one week of in-hospital evaluation. Strict adherence to these guidelines eliminates most transient self-limited pyrexias such as viral illness and postoperative fevers.

EPIDEMIOLOGY

Although the exact incidence of FUO is unknown, the rarity of this condition is illustrated by the fact that only 105 cases were prospectively encountered in a decade of evaluation at a large university referral center (the University of Washington) between 1970 and 1980.

DIFFERENTIAL DIAGNOSIS

Although the differential diagnosis of FUO is broad and includes many exotic conditions, Petersdorf and co-workers have repeatedly stressed that the vast majority of cases are caused by infections, neoplasms, and collagen vascular diseases. Furthermore, most elusive cases are common diseases that are manifested atypically, rather than bizarre entities. The relative frequencies of the various causes of FUOs in the United States are depicted by the following table:*

	1952–1957 (PER CENT)	1970–1980 (PER CENT)
Infections	36	30.5
1. Abdominal abscesses	11	10.4
2. Mycobacteria	11	4.7
3. Cytomegalovirus	0	3.8
4. Urinary tract infection	3	2.8
5. Sinusitis	0	1.9
6. Osteomyelitis	0	1.9
7. Endocarditis	5	0
8. Other	6	4.7
Neoplasms	19	31.1
1. Lymphoma	6	16.0
2. Leukemia	2	4.7
3. Solid tumors	9	10.4
4. Other	2	0
Collagen vascular disease	15	8.5
1. Still's disease	2	3.8
2. Systemic lupus erythematosus	5	0
3. Polyarteritis nodosa	0	1.9
4. Giant cell arteritis	2	.9
5. Rheumatic fever	6	.9
6. Other	0	.9
Granulomatous diseases (sarcoidosis, Crohn's disease, granulomatous hepatitis)	4	7.5
Miscellaneous (hematomas, pulmonary emboli, familial Mediterranean fever, myxoma)	16	6.6
Factitious fever	3	2.9
Undiagnosed	7	12.3

*Modified from Larson, et al.: Fever of undetermined origin: Diagnosis and follow-up of 105 cases, 1970–1980. Medicine 61:269, 1982.

The increase in neoplastic cases of FUO in the more recent series of cases should be noted. Among solid tumors, hypernephromas, hepatomas, and tumors metastatic to the liver are particularly likely to cause fever.

HISTORY AND SYMPTOMS

In evaluating cases of FUO, it is essential to elicit the following historical information:

A. Specific sites of organ dysfunction (abdominal pain or cough)
B. Travel history (malaria after incomplete prophylaxis during a trip to Africa; liver abscess after a visit to Mexico; babesiosis after a vacation in Cape Cod)
C. Familial illnesses (familial Mediterranean fever)

D. Medications ("drug fever")
E. Medical history (subphrenic abscess in a patient with previous abdominal surgery)
F. Extensive review of systems (transient rash, arthralgias, and lymphadenopathy in a patient with lupus)
G. Animal contact (psittacosis, brucellosis, leptospirosis, or trichinosis)

PHYSICAL EXAMINATION AND SIGNS

A. Documentation of Fever. Such documentation by the medical staff using careful precautions to avoid manipulation of the thermometer is essential in ruling out factitious fever. In a few cases scrutiny of fever curves suggests the diagnosis (Pel-Ebstein Fever in Hodgkin's disease).
B. Detection of Lymphadenopathy, Hepatosplenomegaly, and Pathologic Masses. This is of utmost utility in securing diagnoses of neoplastic, infectious, and collagen vascular origin.
C. Cutaneous Manifestations. Cutaneous manifestations occasionally suggest the diagnosis of lupus, dermatomyositis, Still's disease, chronic meningococcemia, endocarditis, or malignancy (acanthosis nigricans or tumor nodules).
D. Cardiac Murmurs. These may suggest endocarditis or atrial myxoma.
E. Bony Tenderness. This may be present in osteomyelitis or metastatic malignancy.
F. Arthritis. Arthritis is a common feature of collagen vascular disease.
G. Tender Warm Indurated Temporal Arteries. These may be present in temporal arteritis.
H. Ocular Examination. This may reveal stigmata of endocarditis, toxoplasmosis, candidiasis, lupus, or other conditions.
I. Rectal Examination. This may reveal intraluminal masses or guaiac-positive stools that indicate gastrointestinal neoplasms.
J. Serial Physical Examinations. Such examinations are important in detecting clinical clues as they evolve.

LABORATORY STUDIES AND DIAGNOSTIC TESTS

Investigation of cases of FUO commonly entails extensive diagnostic evaluation. Tests of particular utility include the following:
A. Cultures of Blood, Urine, Sputum, and Other Body Fluids. These should be routinely obtained for bacterial, fungal, viral, and mycobacterial pathogens.
B. Urinalysis. Urinalysis may demonstrate sterile pyuria (tuberculosis) or hematuria (tuberculosis or hypernephroma).
C. Liver Function Tests. These test results are commonly elevated in conditions such as liver abscesses, granulomatous hepatitis, and neoplastic disorders.

D. **Serologic Studies.** These studies may provide evidence for infections (cytomegalovirus, amebic abscesses, mononucleosis) or collagen vascular disease (antinuclear antibodies, rheumatoid factor, serum protein electrophoresis, sedimentation rate). Febrile agglutinins are rarely useful.

E. **Complete Blood Counts and Blood Film Examination.** These may indicate unusual infections such as malaria, babesiosis, or *Borrelia recurrentis*, or myelophthisis in disseminated carcinomatosis.

F. **Tuberculin Skin Tests.** Tuberculin skin tests with controls in 72 FUO patients yielded 15 positive test results. Three of these patients had active tuberculosis.

G. **Radiographic Studies.** These should be obtained for symptomatic sites. (For example, lumbosacral films in patients with low-back pain may demonstrate osteomyelitis.)

   1. Chest radiographs should be made of all patients.
   2. Barium enema and upper gastrointestinal series should be done in patients with symptoms or signs of gastrointestinal dysfunction.
   3. Intravenous pyelography or renal ultrasound should be used for patients with urinary tract abnormalities.
   4. Bone films may document osteomyelitis or metastases in patients with bony tenderness.
   5. Abdominal computed tomography may show cryptic intra-abdominal abscesses or pancreatic tumors in asymptomatic patients.

H. **Radionuclide Scans.** These are useful to study symptomatic regions or laboratory abnormalities (liver spleen scan for right-upper-quadrant pain or elevated liver function tests). Blind scanning (gallium scanning in patients with no clinical cues) often leads to diagnostic confusion owing to false-positive results. The utility of various types of radionuclide scans is shown below:

	NUMBER DONE	NUMBER HELPFUL TO DIAGNOSIS	FALSE-POSITIVE RESULTS	FALSE-NEGATIVE RESULTS
Liver and spleen scan	91	13	1	4
Gallium scan	40	7	9	3
Bone scan	23	1	0	0
Lung scan	18	1	3	0
Brain scan	11	0	0	0
Abdominal computed tomographic scan	8	0	1	3

I. **Tissue Biopsy or Laparotomy.** This procedure is most likely to yield a definitive diagnosis in cases in which abnormalities are detected on physical examination or by ancillary studies. The diagnostic yields of various types of directed biopsies are given below:

1. Bone marrow biopsy   14 per cent diagnostic
2. Liver biopsy   6 per cent diagnostic
3. Lymph node biopsy   35 per cent diagnostic
4. Other biopsy   38 per cent diagnostic
5. All tissue biopsies   22 per cent diagnostic
6. Laparotomy   48 per cent diagnostic

Although the diagnostic yield of bone marrow biopsy is relatively low, 11 of 78 biopsies indicated diagnoses that were not associated with signs or symptoms suggesting disease of the marrow. Consequently, this is the one tissue for which blind biopsy is justified. Blind laparotomy is rarely useful if symptoms and signs of intra-abdominal disease are lacking.

J. Specific Therapeutic Trials. These include antituberculous agents for suspected tuberculosis, aspirin for Still's disease or rheumatic fever, antibiotics for suspected subacute bacterial endocarditis, or corticosteroids for collagen vascular disease. Specific therapeutic trials can be employed as a last resort in difficult cases. Random administration of multiple agents cannot be condoned.

FREQUENCY AND BASES OF DIAGNOSES

The relative frequency with which the final diagnosis was achieved by employing the aforementioned diagnostic cues in 91 patients with FUO is depicted below:

1. Nonlaparotomy tissue biopsy   33 cases (36 per cent)
2. Laparotomy   19 cases (21 per cent)
3. Clinical course   12 cases (13 per cent)
4. Radiographic studies or scans   10 cases (11 per cent)
5. Autopsy   9 cases (10 per cent)
6. Nontissue culture   5 cases (5 per cent)
7. Serology   5 cases (5 per cent)
8. Other   1 case (1 per cent)

In three cases two separate sources of information were critical in adducing the correct diagnosis.

PROGNOSIS

Of 105 patients with FUO evaluated at the University of Washington between 1970 and 1980, only 9 per cent with malignancy were long-term survivors (> 12 months), whereas 78 per cent with infections and 88 per cent in other categories were alive at last follow-up.

A. Of 14 patients with FUO who remained undiagnosed after extensive evaluation, 10 were alive and well at follow-up 1 year after examination, 3 were alive but still symptomatic, and 1 had died of unrelated causes.

B. Younger patients fared significantly better than older patients, as shown below:

AGE	NUMBER OF PATIENTS	PER CENT LONG-TERM SURVIVAL
< 35 yr	28	96
35–54 yr	22	82
≥ 55 yr	22	68

C. Two thirds of patients benefited from therapeutic interventions.

REFERENCES

1. Petersdorf RG, Beeson PB: Fever of unexplained origin: Report of 100 cases. Medicine 40:1, 1961.

A superlative critical evaluation of a large series of patients with FUO. This paper established the currently accepted definition of FUO and remains the most widely quoted article in the field.

2. Larson EB, Featherstone HJ, Petersdorf RG: Fever of undetermined origin: Diagnosis and follow-up of 105 cases, 1970–1980. Medicine 61:269, 1982.

The best single recent reference that extensively reviews a large series of cases seen between 1970 and 1980. Many of the tables in this chapter are modified from this article.

3. Petersdorf RG: Fever of unknown origin (editorial). Ann Intern Med 70:864, 1969.

A brief editorial review of the advances in the understanding of FUO that occurred between 1961 and 1969.

4. Jacoby GA, Swartz MN: Fever of undetermined origin. N Engl J Med 289:1407, 1973.

An excellent review of the topic, emphasizing the importance of infections, neoplasms, and collagen vascular diseases in causing FUO.

5. John JF, Holley HJ: Fever of unknown origin. Hosp Med 27–31, 61–68, 1980.

An eminently readable well-illustrated two-part review.

6. Cunha BA: Fever of unknown origin in the elderly. Geriatrics 37:30, 1982.

A good review of geriatric FUO.

INTESTINAL INFECTIONS

By PAUL G. RAMSEY, M.D.

DEFINITION

A variety of bacteria, viruses, and parasites may cause infection of the upper or lower gastrointestinal tract. Nausea, vomiting, midepigastric bloating, and cramping characterize upper gastrointestinal tract infections. Diarrhea is the hallmark of infection of the lower gastrointestinal tract. Many clinicians find it helpful to characterize such infections by the mechanism of pathogenesis:

A. **Mucosal Ulceration.** Some microorganisms invade the intestinal wall and cause mucosal ulceration. These infections occur in the large intestine and are defined clinically by the finding of blood or polymorphonuclear leukocytes in the stool.

B. **Enterotoxin.** Other organisms cause gastrointestinal symptoms via an enterotoxin. The enterotoxin elaborated by several organisms including *Vibrio cholera* and *Escherichia coli* has been shown to stimulate intracellular cyclic adenosine monophosphate (AMP), thus leading to active secretion of electrolytes into the bowel lumen. In some cases disease is acquired by ingestion of preformed toxin (as with *Staphylococcus aureus* and *Clostridium botulinum*), while in other cases the toxin is formed after ingestion of the organism. Blood and polymorphonuclear leukocytes are absent from the stool of these patients.

EPIDEMIOLOGY

A careful history concerning epidemiologic factors is essential in the initial differential diagnosis of infectious diarrhea. Important factors include:

A. **Travel History.** This is important because of differences in geographic distribution of the organisms causing gastrointestinal infections. For example, amebiasis should be considered in an individual who has traveled to an endemic area such as Mexico.

B. **Foodborne Infections.** Such infections remain an important cause of infectious diarrhea in this country. Large outbreaks of *Salmonella* infection may be traced to restaurants or picnics. Certain foods may suggest specific infections. Travelers should avoid uncooked food such as vegetables, salad, shellfish, and partially cooked meat. A summary of bacterial, viral, and parasitic foodborne disease outbreaks reported to the Centers for Disease Control is presented in Table 32–1.

C. **Water.** Water is an important source for infection with *Giardia* and a variety of bacteria.

D. **Animal Contact.** Chickens, cats, or dogs may be a source of *Campylobacter fetus*.

E. **Host Factors.** Host factors such as decreased gastric acidity

TABLE 32–1. FOODBORNE DISEASE REPORTED TO THE CENTERS FOR DISEASE CONTROL FROM 1972 TO 1978

ETIOLOGY	NUMBER OF OUTBREAKS	NUMBER OF CASES
Bacterial		
Bacillus cereus	13	369
Clostridium botulinum	104	279
C. perfringens	70	4,573
Salmonella	261	16,172
Shigella	31	2,602
Staphylococcus	219	10,388
Streptococcus groups A & D	8	806
Vibrio parahaemolyticus	12	1,125
Yersinia enterocolitica	1	286
Other	6	55
Total	787	36,655
Parasitic		
Trichinella spiralis	80	456
Other	5	11
Total	85	467
Viral		
Hepatitis A	29	1,346
Echovirus Type 4	1	80
Total	30	1,426

(after gastric operations or in association with pernicious anemia) predispose patients to infection with *E. coli, Shigella* species, and other bacteria.

F. **Prior Antibiotic Therapy.** This raises the possibility of *Clostridium difficile* infection.

G. **Person-to-Person Contact.** This is a major source of transmission of viral infections. In child day care centers a number of infectious agents, including bacteria and parasites, may be passed.

H. **A History of Male Homosexual Activity.** Such a background introduces a large differential diagnosis *(Campylobacter,* amebiasis, herpes simplex virus, gonorrhea, *Chlamydia)* for proctitis.

I. **Immunosuppressed Patients.** Such patients may develop severe upper gastrointestinal (esophageal, gastric, and small intestinal) infections with herpes simplex virus, *Candida* species, and cytomegalovirus.

CLINICAL MANIFESTATIONS

A. **History.** Important points in the history include: (1) upper gastrointestinal symptoms (nausea and vomiting) versus lower gastrointestinal symptoms (diarrhea); (2) duration of symptoms and incubation period; (3) character of the diarrhea (volume, watery consistency, blood, or mucus); (4) presence of associated findings (fever, flatulence, epigastric bloating, severe abdominal pain); (5) health of family and close associates; (6) other epidemiologic factors (see Epidemiology).

For correlation with etiologic agents see Tables 32–2 and 32–3.

B. **Initial Differential Diagnosis Based on Stool Examination.** The absence of blood or polymorphonuclear leukocytes in the stool suggests the differential diagnosis listed in Table 32–2. The finding of blood or polymorphonuclear leukocytes (see Table 32–3) implicates a number of infectious agents, which should be treated with antimicrobial therapy (except for *Salmonella* gastroenteritis). However, the absence of blood and pus does not rule out the possibility of these organisms. For example, many patients with *Salmonella* gastroenteritis do not have blood or pus in the stool at initial examination.

RECOMMENDED DIAGNOSTIC APPROACH

The selection of diagnostic tests depends on the clinical features of a patient's illness.

A. **Examination of Stool for Polymorphonuclear Leukocytes.** Such examination can be done using a Gram's stain or methylene blue technique. In addition, Gram's stain may be useful for diagnosing *Campylobacter fetus* infection in approximately 50 per cent of patients and can be useful also for diagnosing *S. aureus* enterocolitis. However, it is important to remember that not all patients with *Campylobacter*, *Shigella*, and *Salmonella* infections have pus cells in the stool. In addition, noninfectious diseases such as ulcerative colitis and Crohn's disease can be associated with pus.

B. **Stool Culture.** Stool culture should be performed when there are signs of invasive disease (blood or pus in the stool) or systemic toxicity or if symptoms persist for more than 24 hours. Stool cultures are not necessary in all patients, especially if clinical features suggest a benign noninvasive disease. Culture techniques include:

1. Standard culture for "enteric pathogens" *(Salmonella* and *Shigella).*

2. Special culture media and temperature conditions for *Campylobacter fetus* are now included in many laboratories as part of the standard culture.

3. Special enrichment techniques are necessary to culture for *Yersinia enterocolytica* and *Vibrio* species.

4. Some laboratories can now rapidly identify *Clostridium difficile* by gas liquid chromatography.

C. **Blood Cultures.** Blood cultures should be performed if a patient has fever or systemic toxicity in association with diarrhea. Bone marrow cultures may be especially useful in the diagnosis of typhoid fever.

D. **Toxin Assay for *Clostridium difficile*.** This should be performed in addition to stool culture when this infection is suspected.

E. **Sigmoidoscopy.** Sigmoidoscopy may be useful for identifying the

TABLE 32–2. INFECTIOUS AGENTS NOT ASSOCIATED WITH BLOOD OR PUS IN THE STOOL

Organism	Incubation Period	Upper Gastrointestinal Symptoms*			Lower Gastrointestinal Symptoms*	Associated Findings
		Nausea	Vomiting	Cramps	Diarrhea	
Viral (in adults)	<7 days	+	+	++	+++	Exposure to children or family members; mild fever and myalgia are often present.
Staphylococcus aureus	1–6 hours	++++	++++	++++	++	None.
Clostridium perfringens	9–18 hours	+	+	+	+++	None.
Cholera	1–4 days	+	+	0	++++	Lower abdominal cramps and voluminous watery diarrhea.
Bacillus cereus	3–12 hours	++	++	++	++	May appear like staphylococcal or C. perfringens food poisoning.
Escherichia coli (enterotoxic)	1–2 days	+	+	+	+++	Fever and myalgia.
Giardia	7–21 days	++	0	+++	++	Midepigastric bloating, flatulence, and diarrhea may be chronic.

*Symptoms are rated on a scale of 0 to ++++, ranging from absent to most prominent.

TABLE 32–3. INFECTIOUS AGENTS ASSOCIATED WITH BLOOD OR PUS IN THE STOOL

| ORGANISM | INCUBATION PERIOD | UPPER GASTROINTESTINAL SYMPTOMS* | | | LOWER GASTROINTESTINAL SYMPTOMS* | ASSOCIATED FINDINGS |
		Nausea	Vomiting	Cramps	Diarrhea	
Campylobacter fetus	1–5 days	+	+	+ +	+ + + +	"Sheets" of polymorphonuclear neutrophils found in stool
Salmonella species	12–48 hours	+	+	+	+ + +	Fever, myalgia often present
Shigella species	1–5 days	+	+	+ +	+ + + +	Fever, myalgia, many polymorphonuclear neutrophils in stool
Escherichia coli (enteroinvasive)	>24 hours	+	+	+	+ + +	Fever, myalgia
Amebiasis	1–3 weeks	+	+	+	+ + +	Mild fever
Yersinia enterocolytica	?	0	0	+	+ +	Mesenteric lymphadenitis, reactive polyarthritis
Clostridium difficile	?	+	+		+ + +	History of recent antibiotic use

*Symptoms are rated on a scale of 0 to + + + +, ranging from absent to most prominent.

findings of *C. difficile* infection associated with pseudomembranous enterocolitis. Intestinal ulcerations found by sigmoidoscopy may suggest *Entamoeba histolytica* infection.

F. Serologic Techniques. Serologic techniques are available for infection with *E. histolytica* or *Salmonella.*

    1. Indirect hemagglutination serology to identify *E. histolytica* infection is positive in 95 per cent of patients with extraintestinal amebiasis and 80 per cent of patients with intestinal infection.

    2. Salmonella titers rise after one week of infection in 50 per cent of patients and peak by four to six weeks in 90 to 95 per cent of patients. *Salmonella* titers are most useful in patients with typhoid or paratyphoid fever.

G. Stool for Ova and Parasite Examination. Such examination should be performed if travel or sexual history suggests amebiasis or if symptoms and epidemiologic findings suggest giardiasis.

REFERENCES

1. Black RE, et al.: Epidemic *Yersinia enterocolitica* infection due to contaminated chocolate milk. N Engl J Med 298:76, 1978.
2. Blaser MJ, Reller LB: Campylobacter enteritis. N Engl J Med 305:1444, 1981.

Excellent review of all aspects of Campylobacter *infections.*

3. Blaser MJ, et al.: *Campylobacter* enteritis: Clinical and epidemiologic features. Ann Intern Med 91:179, 1979.
4. Bolen JL, Zamiska SA, Greenough WB: Clinical features in enteritis due to *Vibrio parahaemolyticus.* Am J Med 57:638, 1974.

Nice discussion of microbiologic findings including drug sensitivities.

5. DuPont HL, Hornick RB: Clinical approach to infectious diarrheas. Medicine 52:265, 1973.

General review of diagnostic and therapeutic approach.

6. Estes MK, Graham DY: Epidemic viral gastroenteritis. Am J Med 66:1001, 1979.

Excellent discussion of clinical features and transmission of this disease.

7. Harris JC, DuPont HL, Hornick RB: Fecal leukocytes in diarrheal illness. Ann Intern Med 76:697, 1972.
8. Ho DD, et al.: *Campylobacter* enteritis—early diagnosis with Gram's stain. Arch Intern Med 142:1858, 1982.
9. Hughes JM, Merson MH: Fish and shellfish poisoning. N Engl J Med 295:1117, 1976.
10. Terranova W, Blake PA: *Bacillus cereus* food poisoning. N Engl J Med 298:143, 1978.

Excellent concise review of clinical findings.

11. Wolfe MS: Giardiasis. N Engl J Med 298:319, 1978.

A brief review of diagnostic techniques, clinical findings, and treatment approaches.

LYMPHADENOPATHY

By OLIVER W. PRESS, M.D., Ph.D.

DEFINITION

Lymphadenopathy is defined as pathologic enlargement of lymph nodes. The enlargement is generally accepted to be to a size of ≥ 1 cm, although hard fixed lymph nodes of any size also are considered abnormal.

EPIDEMIOLOGY

Lymph node enlargement is a ubiquitous manifestation of numerous infectious, traumatic, and neoplastic conditions.
A. Palpable cervical lymph nodes can be detected in 56 per cent of asymptomatic adults.
B. The annual incidence of clinically significant lymphadenopathy in a typical midwestern family practice was found to be 0.5 per cent.
C. The incidence of lymphadenopathy peaks in late childhood and adolescence.

DIFFERENTIAL DIAGNOSIS

A. **Infections.** Infections are responsible for at least 69 per cent of cases of lymphadenopathy in a primary-care setting. (In an additional 29 per cent of cases no specific cause was found for lymphadenopathy.)
B. **Neoplasms.** Neoplasms are responsible for <1 per cent of all lymphadenopathy but are found in 39 per cent of nodes that come to biopsy. They occur in:
   1. Hodgkin's disease
   2. Non-Hodgkin's Lymphomas
   3. Leukemias (especially chronic lymphocytic leukemia)
   4. Carcinomas
   5. Sarcomas
   6. Histiocytic medullary reticulosis
C. **Angioimmunoblastic Lymphadenopathy**
D. **Acquired Immunodeficiency Syndrome**
E. **Storage Diseases (Gaucher's Disease, Niemann-Pick Disease)**
F. **Drug Reactions (Phenytoin, Hydralazine)**
G. **Serum Sickness**
H. **Collagen Vascular Diseases (Lupus)**
I. **Skin Diseases (Eczema) with Dermatopathic Nodes**
J. **Sarcoidosis**

INFECTIONS	PER CENT OF CERVICAL ADENITIS
1. Bacterial	
Streptococci	40
Staphylococci	10–15 (67 of nodes requiring surgical drainage)
Mycobacteria (scrofula)	0–6
Brucellosis	<1
2. Viral	
Infectious mononucleosis	0–20
Cytomegalovirus	?
Rubella	?
Varicella	?
Measles	?
Cat scratch fever	?
Herpes simplex (I and II)	?
3. Protozoal infections	
Toxoplasmosis	<1
4. Fungal infections	
Histoplasmosis	<1
Coccidioidomycosis	<1
Sporotrichosis	<1

K. Masses Confused with Lymphadenopathy
  1. *Thyroglossal Duct Cysts*
  2. *Branchial Pouch Cysts*
  3. *Dermoid Cysts*
  4. *Lipomas*
  5. *Salivary Gland (Submaxillary Gland) Enlargement*

HISTORY

A. Inflammatory nodes are usually tender, mobile, arise acutely, and resolve rapidly (in less than two weeks).

B. Lymph nodes that contain malignancy usually are nontender, may become fixed or matted, and arise insidiously with progressive enlargement.

C. Inquiry should be made with regard to associated fever, chills, sweats, pruritus, weight loss, rashes, arthralgias, jaundice, purulent node drainage, pharyngitis, cough, hemoptysis, and stool changes.

D. The medical history may divulge a history of tuberculosis, venereal disease, lupus, dental caries, scalp wounds, breast cancer, or alcohol and cigarette abuse (associated with head and neck, esophageal, and lung carcinomas).

E. Environmental exposures to measles, mumps, rubella, chickenpox, mononucleosis, cats (toxoplasmosis or cat scratch fever), or ingestion of unpasteurized milk (brucellosis or mycobacterial disease) or anticonvulsants should be considered.

F. Geographic considerations are important in assessing the likelihood of histoplasmosis (occurring in the Midwest) or coccidioidomycosis (occurring in the Southwest).

PHYSICAL EXAMINATION

A. The size, consistency, tenderness, warmth, fixation, fluctuance, and distribution of nodes should be noted.
B. Extensive otolaryngologic evaluation of the upper aerodigestive tract is mandatory in evaluating cervical nodes suspected of harboring malignancy.
C. Detection of hepatosplenomegaly, abdominal masses, jaundice, tonsillitis, pharyngitis, and rashes is important.
D. Careful search for malignancy is essential. This includes detection of breast masses, oral lesions, and guaiac-positive stool.

LABORATORY STUDIES

Laboratory studies are unnecessary in the majority of cases of lymphadenopathy, since an inflammatory origin is usually obvious. However, in instances in which the etiology of lymph node enlargement remains obscure after careful recording of the history and physical examination, the following diagnostic approach, developed by Greenfield and Jordan, is recommended.
A. **Anterior and Posterior Neck Nodes.** Enlarged cervical nodes are found in 56 per cent of cases with lymphadenopathy and are usually due to minor local infections.
   1. Facial, dental, and ear infections are sought, and antibiotics, if indicated, are administered.
   2. If there are no facial, dental, or ear infections, a throat culture should be obtained and antibiotics administered if streptococcal (or gonococcal) pharyngitis is detected.
   3. If these steps are unproductive, the blood smear should be checked for atypical lymphocytes and serologic tests for evidence of mononucleosis (monospot test and heterophile antigen performed). If atypical lymphocytosis exists but serologic tests are negative for infectious mononucleosis, repeat mononucleosis serology should be performed in seven to ten days.
   4. If the above tests are unproductive and the patient is nontoxic, further evaluation should be deferred for one to two weeks to permit minor benign inflammatory lymphadenopathy to recede before extensive and expensive testing is done.
   5. If the lymph nodes remain enlarged after one to two weeks, the mononucleosis serology should be repeated, and serologic studies for cytomegalovirus and toxoplasmosis should be performed. An intermediate-strength tuberculin skin test should be placed and a chest radiograph performed.
   6. If a diagnosis still has not been reached, excisional biopsy should be performed and examined by Gram's, fungal, and acid-fast stains; aerobic, anaerobic, fungal, and mycobacterial cultures; and frozen section and routine histology. In special

cases surface marker studies should be performed by immunofluorescence or immunoperoxidase methods (especially for lymphomas), and electron microscopy should be considered. Excisional biopsy of an entire node is far superior to needle biopsy, since node architecture is crucial in classification of lymphomas. It cannot be overemphasized that lymph node biopsy should never be undertaken in an adult unless a detailed otolaryngologic evaluation has been performed previously to exclude intraoral, laryngeal, and nasopharyngeal lesions. Explicit discussions between the internist, surgeon, and pathologist are critical prior to operation to ensure that the specimens are properly handled and processed.

B. **Submandibular Lymphadenopathy.** This condition occurs in fewer than 1 per cent of cases and usually is caused by metastatic malignancy from the thorax (breast or lung) or abdomen (stomach, colon). Early node biopsy should be performed.

C. **Axillary Lymphadenopathy.** This condition occurs in 4 per cent of cases and should prompt careful search for scratches, bites, infections, or lymphadenitis of the hands and arms as well as careful breast examination.

   1. If none of these examinations show abnormality, and the patient is nontoxic, further evaluation should be deferred, and the patient should be reexamined in one to two weeks. (Isolated axillary node enlargment is unusual for mononucleosis.)

   2. If the mass persists longer than one to two weeks, serologic tests for mononucleosis, cytomegalovirus, and toxoplasmosis should be used, a tuberculin skin test placed, a chest x-ray performed, and a node biopsy scheduled.

D. **Inguinal Lymphadenopathy.** Inguinal lymphadenopathy occurs in 16 per cent of cases. In the absence of obvious infection or tumor of the lower extremities or genitals, serologic studies for syphilis and lymphogranuloma venereum should be performed, followed by the tests described for axillary lymphadenopathy after a one- to two-week waiting period. Inguinal nodes are often difficult to assess because of the frequency with which they are enlarged in normal individuals. (Usually they are "dermatopathic nodes.")

E. **Generalized Lymphadenopathy.** This condition occurs in 24 per cent of cases. It is commonly caused by viral diseases, systemic illnesses, or drug reactions. If known viral illness is present, no work-up is indicated. Otherwise, testing should follow the sequence outlined here:

   1. Discontinuation of drugs capable of causing lymphadenopathy (phenytoin, allopurinol, hydralazine)

   2. Serology for mononucleosis, cytomegalovirus, and toxoplasmosis

   3. Other Tests
      a. Blood cultures (for endocarditis)
      b. Tuberculin skin testing
      c. Examination for antinuclear antibodies (for lupus)
      d. Chest x-ray (for sarcoidosis, tuberculosis, Hodgkin's disease)

Site	Number of Biopsies	Benign (Per Cent)	Squamous Cell Carcinoma (Per Cent)	Adeno-carcinoma (Per Cent)	Anaplastic Carcinoma (Per Cent)	Lymphoma (Per Cent)
Neck	234	63	6	8	6	18
Supraclavicular	187	37	13	18	23	9
Axillary	141	60	1	11	5	23
Groin	84	71	8	8	5	8

e. Complete blood cell count and smear
f. Liver function tests
4. Node biopsy

MALIGNANCY

Malignancy was detected in 39 per cent of 925 lymph node biopsies from patients of all ages and in 60 per cent of 226 biopsies done in patients of ages 51 to 70 years in a recent series. (ref. 4)

A. The risk of detecting malignancy in the various lymph node sites is depicted in the table opposite.

B. The fate of patients with nondiagnostic node biopsies is indicated below:

INDICATION FOR BIOPSY	LIVING AND WELL ≥1 YR AFTER BIOPSY (PER CENT)	DEVELOPED DISEASE RELATED TO INDICATION FOR BIOPSY (PER CENT)
Lymphadenopathy	82	17 (lymphomas)
Chest Disease	21	79 (mainly lung cancer)

REFERENCES

1. Linet OI, Metzler C: Incidence of palpable cervical nodes in adults. Postgrad Med 62:210–213, 1977.
2. Allhiser JN, McKnight TA, Shank JC: Lymphadenopathy in a family practice. J Fam Pract 12:27–32, 1981.

A brief analysis of 80 cases of lymphadenopathy encountered by a family practitioner, which emphasizes the benign nature of most cases of lymph node enlargement.

3. Sundaresh HP, Kumar A, Hokanson JT, Novack AH: Etiology of cervical lymphadenitis in children. Am Fam Phys 24:147–151, 1981.

A microbiologic study demonstrating the importance of group A beta-hemolytic streptococci, Staphylococcus aureus, and infectious mononucleosis as causes of cervical lymphadenitis.

4. Lee Y-T, Terry R, Lukes RJ: Lymph node biopsy for diagnosis: A statistical study. J Surg Oncol 14:53–60, 1980.

An excellent detailed analysis of 925 cases.

5. Greenfield S, Jordan MC: The clinical investigation of lymphadenopathy in primary care practice. JAMA 240:1388–1393, 1978.

A thoughtful analysis that proposes a useful algorithm for evaluation of patients with lymphadenopathy.

6. Saltzstein SL: The fate of patients with nondiagnostic lymph node biopsies. Surgery 58:659–662, 1965.

An interesting paper that addresses the prognosis of patients who have nondiagnostic lymph node biopsies.

MENINGITIS AND ENCEPHALITIS

By BARBARA D. KIRBY, M.D.

DEFINITION, ETIOLOGY, AND EPIDEMIOLOGY

A. **Meningitis.** Meningitis is defined as inflammation of the meninges. It may be caused by infections (bacterial, viral, fungal, or tubercular) or may be neoplastic or inflammatory (from sarcoidosis, vasculitis, or chemical agents). This chapter considers primarily bacterial and viral causes of meningitis.

   1. Bacterial. (See Table 34–1.)

     a. **Streptococcus pneumoniae**

       1). *S. pneumoniae* is responsible for 30 to 50 per cent of bacterial meningitis in adults, 10 to 20 per cent in children, and up to 5 per cent in infants.

       2). *S. pneumoniae* may be associated with pneumococcal pneumonia (usually bacteremic) in 25 per cent of cases or with pneumococcal endocarditis, or with both.

       3). *S. pneumoniae* may be associated with otitis media, sinusitis, or mastoiditis in 25 per cent of cases.

       4). There may be recent head injury such as skull fracture in 10 to 20 per cent of cases.

       5). Risk factors include sickle cell anemia, alcoholism, immunoglobulin deficiency, and splenectomy.

     b. **Neisseria meningitidis**

       1). *N. meningitidis* is responsible for 10 to 30 per cent of bacterial meningitis in adults and 30 to 40 per cent in children. It is rare in infants.

       2). A rash may be noted in up to 50 per cent of meningococcal infections.

       3). Peak occurrence is in winter and spring.

     c. **Hemophilus influenzae, Type B**

       1). *H. influenzae* is responsible for 1 to 3 per cent of bacterial meningitis in adults and 35 to 45 per cent in children. It is the most common cause of meningitis in children under six months of age.

       2). This form of meningitis usually occurs following upper respiratory infections (otitis media 66 per cent, pharyngitis 50 per cent) in children.

       3). There is an increased risk of development of meningitis in children who are close contacts of the patient. Therefore, prophylaxis is recommended.

     d. **Listeria monocytogenes**

       1). *L. monocytogenes* is an uncommon cause of meningitis seen in elderly debilitated patients.

       2). This form of meningitis is also seen in patients such as renal transplant recipients who are receiving immunosuppressive therapy (corticosteroids or cytotoxic agents).

TABLE 34–1. CORRELATION OF CAUSE OF ACUTE BACTERIAL MENINGITIS WITH AGE GROUP AND DIRECT INOCULATION*†

	PREMATURE AND NEONATAL (PER CENT)	2–60 MONTHS (PER CENT)	5–40 YEARS (PER CENT)	>40 YEARS (PER CENT)	EXTENSION FROM INTRACRANIAL FOCUS‡ (PER CENT)	SKULL FRACTURES§ (PER CENT)	PENETRATING INJURIES SHUNTS§ (PER CENT)	POST NEUROSURGICAL (PER CENT)
Neisseria meningitidis	—	~20 (~5)	~40 (~5)	~10 (~25)	—	—	—	—
Hemophilus influenzae	~5 (~50)	~60 (~5)	~5 (~0)	~2 (~0)	~25 (~5)	~10 (~5)	—	—
Escherichia coli	~40 (~40)	—	—⎫	~10 (~50)⎫	Occasional⎫	Occasional⎫	~5 (~60)⎫	~20 (~50)
Other Enterobacter	~20 (~60)	—	—⎭	~10 (~50)⎭	Occasional⎭	Occasional⎭	~5 (~60)⎭	~30 (~50)
Streptococcus pneumoniae	~5 (~50)	~15 (~10)	~30 (~30)	~50 (~45)	~40 (~15)	~80 (~10)		
Staphylococcus species	~2 (~60)	~2 (~25)	~10 (~50)	~13 (~40)	~10 (~25)	Occasional	~80 (~25)	~45 (~25)
Streptococcus species‖	~25 (~40)	—	~5 (~40)	~5 (~45)	Occasional	Occasional	~5	~5
Others (including Listeria monocytogenes)	~3 (~40)	~3 (~2)	~10 (~15)	~10 (~50)	~20 (~15)	~5 (~25)	~10 (~25)	~5 (~50)

*Adapted, with permission of author and publisher, from Hoeprich PD: Infectious Diseases, 3rd ed., New York, Harper & Row, 1983, p. 1036.
†The approximate fatality rate, with presently available treatment in parentheses.
‡Includes group B *Streptococcus* species.
§Antimicrobial therapy mitigates the immediate threat of acute bacterial meningitis, but appropriate surgical procedures (drainage of abscesses, excision of infected bone, repair of defects in the leptomeninges, removal of foreign bodies) are in most cases essential to cure.
‖Includes otitis media.

    3). Alcoholism is a risk factor.
   e. Staphylococcus aureus
    1). S. aureus is seen primarily in postoperative neuro-
    surgical patients and intravenous drug abusers.
   f. Staphylococcus epidermidis
    1). S. epidermidis is a major pathogen in ventricular shunt
    infection.
   g. Group B Streptococci
    1). Group B streptococci are a rare cause of meningitis in
    adults but a major pathogen in neonates.
   **h. Gram-Negative Bacilli (Escherichia coli, Klebsiella-
   Enterobacter, Proteus, Citrobacter, Pseudomonas)**
    1). These bacilli are seen in infants, postoperatively in
    neurosurgical patients, and in head injury patients,
    especially those with cerebrospinal fluid leak.
 2. *Viral Meningitis*
  a. Meningitis may be caused by a variety of viral agents.
  The most common etiologic agents are picornaviruses
  (especially enteroviruses, which are responsible for 70 per
  cent of viral meningitis, such as coxsackieviruses and
  echoviruses), paramyxoviruses (mumps), herpesviruses,
  and lymphocytic choriomeningitis (LCM).
  b. Most patients with viral meningitis are under age 40.
  c. Enteroviral infections occur predominantly in summer.
  d. Mumps meningitis is seen in winter and late spring; there
  is a predominance in males of cases of mumps meningitis.
  e. Herpes meningitis is usually associated with episodes of
  primary genital or oral herpes infection; however, it also
  may occur with recurrent herpes infections.
  f. LCM occurs throughout the year. Often there is exposure
  to animals, especially hamsters.
B. Encephalitis. Encephalitis is defined as inflammation of brain
tissue: cerebrum, cerebellum, or brain stem, or a combination
thereof.
 1. In the United States the major cause of acute nonepidemic
 viral encephalitis is herpesviruses.
 2. In the summer and early fall togaviruses, bunyaviruses, and
 picornaviruses cause encephalitis.
 3. In the winter epidemics of encephalitis are caused by vari-
 cella-zoster, Epstein-Barr virus, rubella, and paramyxovirus.
 4. California and western equine encephalitis are usually seen
 in younger patients. The vector for transmission of the disease
 is the mosquito.
 5. Other forms include eastern equine encephalitis, Japanese
 encephalitis, and St. Louis encephalitis.

CLINICAL PRESENTATION AND HISTORY

A. Bacterial Meningitis
 1. *Patterns of Onset.* There are three patterns of onset of clinical
 illness:
  a. In the first, meningitis develops over one to seven days
  and is commonly associated with respiratory symptoms.
  This pattern is noted in about 50 per cent of patients.

b. In the second, there is rapid onset of headache, confusion, lethargy, and loss of consciousness leading to hospitalization within 24 hours. These patients often do not have respiratory symptoms. This pattern is noted in about 30 per cent of patients.

c. Subacute onset occurs after one to three weeks of respiratory symptoms and is seen in 20 per cent of cases.

2. *Principal Symptoms and Signs in Adults.* These include the following:

    a. **Fever.** This is present commonly but not invariably.

    b. **Headache.** This is a very common symptom.

    c. **Seizures.** Seizures indicate a poor prognosis.

    d. **Vomiting.** This is common.

    e. **Altered Consciousness or Confusion.** Neurologic symptoms may be present in 50 per cent of patients. Fully alert patients are unusual (<5 per cent of cases).

    f. **Stiff Neck or Back.** This sign is present in 80 per cent of patients but may be a late finding. Lumbar puncture should not be withheld because of absence of Kernig's or Brudzinski's sign.

    g. **Petechiae.** Two thirds of patients with meningococcal meningitis have petechiae. However, petechiae may also be seen in viral meningitis (caused by coxsackievirus or echovirus) and other bacterial meningitis. Meningococcal meningitis may also be associated with purpura or vasculitic lesions.

3. *Signs and Symptoms in Children.* Examination may reveal fever, vomiting, and seizures. Headache may not be a chief complaint.

B. **Viral Meningitis.** Prodromal symptoms usually occur over several days. Typical symptoms include:

1. *Headache.* Headache is usually frontal or retroorbital.

2. *Malaise, Nausea, Vomiting, Listlessness, and Photophobia*

3. *Fever.* Temperature is usually elevated but need not be.

4. *Neurologic Symptoms.* Mental status is usually normal, but approximately 10 per cent of patients with viral meningitis have seizures, coma, or motor or sensory impairments.

5. *Specific Causative Agents.* Physical examination findings may suggest specific causative agents, such as:

    a. Parotitis caused by mumps.

    b. Rash caused by echovirus or coxsackievirus.

    c. Pleurodynia caused by coxsackievirus.

    d. Genital herpes caused by herpes virus.

C. **Viral Encephalitis**

1. Patients with viral encephalitis usually have signs of meningeal irritation (headache, nausea, vomiting, or nuchal rigidity) plus alterations in consciousness ranging from mild lethargy to drowsiness, stupor, or coma.

2. Focal neurologic findings and seizures are common.

3. In herpes simplex encephalitis, temporal lobe manifestations such as bizarre behavior or hallucinations may be noted.

4. Fever is usually present.

LABORATORY FEATURES

A. Cerebrospinal Fluid. Cerebrospinal fluid should be obtained from patients suspected of having meningitis or encephalitis. If brain abscess is likely, lumbar puncture should not be performed until scans (brain scan or computed tomographic scan) have excluded the diagnosis.

1. Bacterial Meningitis

   a. Cell Count. Cerebrospinal fluid leukocyte count is elevated in patients with bacterial meningitis. The number of leukocytes may be as high as 100,000 per ml but usually is in the range of 5000 to 20,000 ml. Leukocyte counts in excess of 50,000 should suggest the diagnosis of ruptured brain abscess. The leukocytes seen in patients with bacterial meningitis typically have a neutrophilic predominance. Monocytic cells may be seen in bacterial meningitis caused by *Listeria monocytogenes* as well as in partially treated or resolving meningitis.

   b. Cerebrospinal Fluid Pressure. This is typically elevated (>180 mm water).

   c. Cerebrospinal Fluid Protein. The cerebrospinal fluid protein level is usually elevated (usual range 150 to 500 mg per dL).

   d. Cerebrospinal Fluid Glucose. Cerebrospinal fluid glucose level is usually lower than 40 mg per dL (or 40 per cent of the simultaneous blood glucose concentration, provided the blood glucose concentration is less than 250 mg per dL).

   e. Gram's Stain of Cerebrospinal Fluid. This may permit rapid presumptive diagnosis. Approximately 80 per cent of untreated bacterial meningitis can be diagnosed by Gram's stain.

   f. Cerebrospinal Fluid Culture. This is positive in 70 to 80 per cent of cases of bacterial meningitis. Blood cultures should be obtained in cases of suspected bacterial meningitis. Anaerobic cultures of cerebrospinal fluid should be performed when anaerobic organisms are a possibility (as with brain abscess, middle ear infection, mastoiditis, sinus infections, malignancies, shunts, or head trauma).

   g. Counterimmunoelectrophoresis (CIE). CIE may detect the presence of capsular polysaccharide from *H. influenzae, S. pneumoniae,* and *N. meningitidis.* The false-negative rate of CIE is about 10 per cent compared with cultures; however, it may be useful in partially treated meningitis or in patients with equivocal Gram's stain results.

   h. India Ink Preparation. This should be used for immunosuppressed patients or in cases of chronic meningitis.

2. Viral Meningitis

   a. Cell Count. The cell count in cerebrospinal fluid is usually 10 to 150 cu mm but may be as high as 1000. Cells are typically lymphocytic; however, in 30 per cent of patients there may be early polymorphonuclear leukocyte predominance usually followed in 6 to 24 hours by lymphocytic predominance.

b. **Cerebrospinal Fluid Glucose.** The level of glucose is usually normal but occasionally low in patients with herpes or mumps.

c. **Cerebrospinal Fluid Protein.** The concentration of cerebrospinal fluid protein is normal or slightly elevated.

d. **Cerebrospinal Fluid Viral Cultures.** These are often negative; however, cultures of stool, urine, or throat or serologic tests may yield diagnostic information.

3. *Viral Encephalitis*

a. **Red Blood Cells and/or Xanthochromic Fluid.** These may be found in herpes simplex encephalitis.

b. **Cerebrospinal Fluid Leukocyte Count.** The usual count is 50 to 500 per cu mm.

c. **Cerebrospinal Fluid Glucose.** Cerebrospinal fluid glucose is usually normal.

d. **Cerebrospinal Fluid Protein.** Cerebrospinal fluid protein is usually elevated.

e. **Opening Pressure.** This is normal or slightly elevated.

RECOMMENDED DIAGNOSTIC APPROACH

A. **Bacterial Meningitis**
1. *Lumbar Puncture with Determination of Pressures, Cell Count, Glucose, and Protein.* Immediate Gram's stain examination should be done. Fluid should be cultured. If it is available, counterimmunoelectrophoresis should be used.
2. *Blood Cultures.* Blood cultures should be obtained.
3. *Complete Blood Count, Serum Electrolytes, and Glucose.* Bleeding parameters and platelets should be examined in patients with suspected meningococcemia.

B. **Viral Meningitis**
1. *Lumbar Puncture.* Opening pressure, cell count, glucose, and protein should be examined. When cell count shows a polymorphonuclear predominance and Gram's stain is negative, lumbar puncture should be repeated in 6 to 12 hours.
2. *Viral Culture.* This need not be done in most cases.
3. *Complete Blood Count, Serum Electrolytes, and Glucose*
4. *Culture of Cutaneous Lesions.* This may be helpful (for example, in cases of herpes infection).

C. **Encephalitis**
1. *Computed Tomography (CT).* If herpes simplex encephalitis is suspected, an emergency CT scan should be done.
2. *Brain Biopsy.* Brain biopsy of the involved area may be done for culture, fluorescent antibody, and other diagnostic studies.

REFERENCES

1. Carpenter RR, Petersdorf RG: The clinical spectrum of bacterial meningitis. Am J Med 33:262–275, 1962.

A classic report of large series of cases of bacterial meningitis.

2. Ward JI, Fraser DW, Baraff LJ, Plikaytis BD: *Hemophilus influenzae* meningitis: A study of secondary spread in household contacts. N Engl J Med 301:122–126, 1979.
3. Berk SL, McCabe WR: Meningitis caused by gram-negative bacilli. Ann Intern Med 93:253–260, 1980.

A review of 30 cases.

4. Barza M, Pauker SG: The decision to biopsy, treat or wait in suspected herpes encephalitis. Ann Intern Med 92:641, 1980.

Describes the clinical presentation of herpes encephalitis.

5. Finland M, Barnes MW: Acute bacterial meningitis at Boston City Hospital during 12 selected years, 1935–1972. J Infect Dis 136:400, 1977.

Epidemiology and bacteriology in over 500 patients.

6. Miller JR, Harter DH: Acute viral encephalitis. Med Clin North Am 56:1393, 1972.

A review of viral encephalitis.

7. Whittey R: Diagnosis and treatment of herpes simplex encephalitis. Ann Rev Med 32:335, 1981.

35

OPPORTUNISTIC INFECTIONS

By OLIVER W. PRESS, M.D., Ph.D.

DEFINITION

Opportunistic infections are microbial illnesses that develop in immunocompromised hosts. (See Chapter 30 on "Fever in the Immunocompromised Host" for discussions of the epidemiology, differential diagnosis, and clinical approach to opportunistic infections.)

OPPORTUNISTIC INFECTION SYNDROMES

A. Septicemia. This is the most common infectious syndrome observed in compromised hosts. The typical clinical picture includes sudden onset of fever, chills, sweats, malaise, pallor, and often hypotension (see chapter on Septic Shock). Subsequent complications may include renal failure, disseminated intravascular coagulation, coma, adult respiratory distress syndrome, and metastatic infection.

Listed below are the relative frequencies with which microbes were isolated from 102 septicemic patients with acute myelogenous leukemia at University Hospital in Seattle from 1979 to 1983.

Staphylococcus epidermidis	19.7%	*Bacteroides* species	4.9%
Klebsiella species	14.8%	*Candida* species	3.3%
Escherichia coli	9.8%	*Staphylococcus aureus*	3.3%
Enterobacter species	9.0%	*Serratia marcescens*	1.6%
Streptococcus viridans	9.0%	*Proteus* species	1.6%
Pseudomonas species	5.7%	*Streptococcus pneumoniae*	1.6%
Corynebacterium species	5.7%	Other	4.9%
Enterococcus species	4.9%		

Strategies that have been partially successful in decreasing the risk of bacteremia in oncology patients include:
1. Prophylactic nonabsorbable oral antibiotic administration (nystatin, gentamicin, or vancomycin) to sterilize the gut.
2. Protective reverse isolation with laminar air-flow rooms used in conjunction with prophylactic antibiotics.
3. Prophylactic administration of trimethoprim sulfisoxazole to selectively eliminate aerobic organisms from the bowel flora of neutropenic patients ("colonization resistance").
4. Prophylactic granulocyte transfusions in neutropenic bone marrow transplant recipients. This measure is controversial.

B. Pneumonia. Pneumonia is the most commonly documented localized infection in immunocompromised hosts and is responsible for 25 to 50 per cent of deaths in patients with hematologic malignancies and renal allografts. A survey of the causes of the "febrile pneumonitis" syndrome in 151 immunocompromised patients at Massachusetts General Hospital revealed the following causative agents:

	(per cent)
1. Infectious causes of febrile pneumonitis syndrome	
Conventional bacterial agents (*Pseudomonas, Escherichia, Klebsiella, Pneumococcus, Staphylococcus*)	23.8
Viral infections (cytomegalovirus, herpes simplex, adenovirus)	13.2
Fungal infections (*Aspergillus, Candida*)	10.6
Nocardia asteroides	8.6
Pneumocystis carinii	5.3
Mycobacterium tuberculosis	.7
Mixed infections	9.9
	72.2
2. Noninfectious causes of febrile pneumonitis syndrome	(per cent)
Pulmonary emboli	7.9
Recurrent tumor	5.3
Radiation pneumonitis	4.6
Pulmonary edema	4.6
Drug-induced pneumonitis	3.3
Leukoagglutinin reaction	1.3
Pulmonary hemorrhage	.7
	27.8

Clinical clues are frequently helpful in suggesting the most likely pathogens. An acute onset of pneumonitis favors conventional bacterial pneumonia, pulmonary emboli, pulmonary hemorrhage, or a leukoagglutinin reaction. A subacute onset over two to seven days suggests viral, *Mycoplasma, Pneumocystis,* or *Aspergillus* infection. A chronic course suggests fungal, nocardial, or tuberculous infection, recurrent tumor, or drug- or radiation-induced pneumonitis. Well-maintained oxygenation in the face of massive consolidation on chest x-ray is typical of pulmonary disease caused by fungi, *Nocardia,* tuberculosis, or tumor. The low response rate of infectious pneumonias (40 to 60 per cent) in the compromised host mandates aggressive diagnostic and therapeutic measures (see Chapter 31).

Allogeneic bone marrow transplant patients who develop diffuse interstitial pneumonitis represent a subset with a particularly poor prognosis. Lung biopsy studies have revealed the following statistics:

CAUSE OF DIFFUSE INTERSTITIAL PNEUMONITIS IN MARROW TRANSPLANT PATIENTS	FREQUENCY AMONG TRANSPLANT PATIENTS (PER CENT)	MORTALITY (PER CENT)
Cytomegalovirus	16	90
"Idiopathic"	13	67
Pneumocystis	8	73
Other viruses	3	80

C. **The Central Nervous System.** This is the third major site of infectious morbidity and mortality in compromised hosts and is involved in 5 to 10 per cent of patients with lymphoma or renal allografts. Appropriate management of meningitis and brain abscess in this group of patients is impeded by the low incidence of classic signs of central nervous system infections such as fever (present in only 78 per cent of patients), headache (in 58 per cent), mental status changes (in 42 per cent), focal neurologic findings (in 33 per cent), meningismus (in 27 per cent), and seizures (in 13 per cent). Furthermore, a recent analysis of 55 cases at Massachusetts General Hospital has shown that these infections are rarely caused by conventional organisms.

ETIOLOGY OF CENTRAL NERVOUS SYSTEM INFECTION	FREQUENCY (PER CENT)
Cryptococcus neoformans	27
Listeria monocytogenes	18
Aspergillus fumigatus	13
Conventional viral agents	7
JC virus (progressive multifocal leukoencephalopathy)	7
Hemophilus influenzae	5
Pseudomonas aeruginosa	4
Escherichia coli	4
Other (1 case each of *Streptococcus pneumoniae, Klebsiella,* Group D *Streptococcus, Staphylococcus epidermidis, Nocardia,* tuberculosis, *Mucor,* and *Toxoplasma)*	15
	100

Conventional bacterial meningitis *(Pneumococcus, Hemophilus)* occurred only in splenectomized bacteremic patients in this series. The patients at greatest risk of developing central nervous system infections appear to be those with Hodgkin's disease, non-Hodgkin's lymphoma, chronic lymphocytic leukemia, and those on chronic corticosteroid therapy. Mortality ranged from 47 to 77 per cent in reported series.

D. Disseminated Infections Causing Skin Lesions

1. ***Staphylococcus aureus.*** *S. aureus* classically produces hematogenously spread abscesses, infarcts, and septic embolic lesions.

2. ***Pseudomonas aeruginosa and Aeromonas hydrophila.*** These organisms can produce erythematous indurated lesions with central vesicles and areas of necrosis termed *ecthyma gangrenosum.* These lesions are particularly prone to develop in the perirectal region and the groin.

3. ***Nocardia species.*** These species commonly cause abscesses of lung, brain, and subcutaneous tissues.

4. ***Candida.*** *Candida* often produces disseminated maculopapular lesions that may coexist with endophthalmitis.

5. ***Mucormycosis.*** Mucormycosis may appear as a black necrotic nasopharyngeal or palatal eschar that rapidly invades the base of the skull to produce cranial nerve palsies, coma, hemiparesis, and death. This infection commonly develops in the setting of diabetic ketoacidosis.

6. ***Herpes Simplex and Varicella Zoster.*** Lesions from these viruses may disseminate cutaneously or to visceral organs. Diagnosis is facilitated by recognition of multinucleated giant cells on Tzank-stained preparations of vesicle scrapings and by viral culture.

E. Urinary Tract Infections. Urinary tract infections develop in 35 to 79 per cent of renal transplant patients and are responsible for 60 per cent of the observed episodes of bacteremia. The recent institution of trimethoprim sulfisoxazole prophylaxis has markedly diminished the incidence and severity of these infections. This condition is rarely the cause of serious infections or sepsis in compromised hosts other than renal transplant recipients.

DESCRIPTION OF SELECTED PATHOGENS

A. Staphylococcus epidermidis. This is a gram-positive skin commensal organism that is the most common cause of bacteremia in cancer patients. Some authors attribute the high incidence of *S. epidermidis* bacteremia to the widespread use of long-term right atrial (Hickman) catheters. Fortunately, these infections are usually easily managed using vancomycin, leading to a <1 per cent mortality.

B. Aerobic Gram-Negative Rods. Aerobic gram-negative rods, including *Pseudomonas*, remain major causes of severe bacteremia and pneumonia in compromised hosts and collectively cause approximately 50 per cent of serious infections in this patient population. Epidemiologic studies have indicated that the major portal of entry for these organisms is the gastrointestinal tract. Aspiration of gram-negative bacilli colonizing the oropharynx commonly leads to severe pneumonia, and hematogenous seeding from the gut leads to septicemia. Typical mortality for gram-negative pneumonia and bacteremia (50 and 30 per cent, respectively) is much improved over previous figures, largely as a result of empiric antibiotic administration.

C. **Mycobacterial Infections.** These infections occur in less than 1 per cent of compromised hosts. They are most commonly encountered in patients with lung cancer, lymphoproliferative disease, acute leukemia, head and neck malignancies, and stomach cancer. Most infections represent reactivation of latent disease in patients on immunosuppressive therapy. Atypical mycobacteria are responsible for up to 50 per cent of these infections in immunocompromised patients. Mortality varies from 17 to 50 per cent, with many infections being recognized only at autopsy. Isoniazid prophylaxis for compromised patients with positive tuberculin skin test prior to initiation of immunosuppressive therapy has been recommended by the Centers for Disease Control but is considered controversial by some authors.

D. **Legionella pneumophilia.** *L. pneumophilia* is a newly recognized fastidious gram-negative bacterium that causes legionnaire's disease. An increased susceptibility to this infection occurs in immunocompromised patients, particularly cancer patients, renal transplant recipients, and patients on corticosteroids. The disease generally begins with the acute onset of fever, relative bradycardia, headache, malaise, dry cough, acute pneumonia, and multiple organ dysfunction (disorientation, nausea, diarrhea, syndrome of inappropriate antidiuretic hormone, renal dysfunction, and disseminated intravascular coagulation). The diagnosis is made by:

1. Culture of the organism on Mueller Hinton media from blood, sputum, or other body fluids
2. Fourfold rise in the serum indirect immunofluorescent antibody test to ≥1:128 or a convalescent titer of >1:256
3. Direct immunofluorescent testing of respiratory secretions or lung tissue *or*
4. Dieterle staining of lung biopsy specimens

The case fatality rate nationwide is 14 per cent despite appropriate high-dose erythromycin therapy.

E. **Nocardia Infections.** These infections are acquired by the pulmonary route and may disseminate to produce pulmonary, brain, and subcutaneous abscesses. Diagnosis is difficult (sputum smears and cultures are positive in 30 per cent of cases), and biopsy is usually required. The overall survival rate is 58 per cent.

F. **Candida.** This is the most common fungal pathogen in the compromised host and commonly causes thrush, erosive esophagitis, pneumonia, and disseminated infection. Blood cultures are positive in only 25 to 50 per cent of disseminated cases, and serologic tests have poor predictive value. Consequently, documentation of invasive disease generally requires tissue biopsy (of skin lesions, lung, or esophagus). Surveillance cultures of sputum, oropharynx, stool, and urine can be used indirectly to adduce evidence for invasive *Candida* infection, since autopsy studies have shown that the risk of such infection is high if three or more of these sites grow the yeast.

G. **Invasive Aspergillosis.** This condition commonly affects the lung and occasionally the brain with rare dissemination to the gut, skin, and kidneys. *Aspergillus* is a likely pathogen when prolonged fever persists in neutropenic patients on broad-spectrum antibiotics, especially if a focal pulmonary infiltrate is present. Biopsy is required for diagnosis because sputum examination and serologic testing have many false-positive and false-negative results. These infections are usually diagnosed late in their course, and mortality has typically been 90 per cent. However, recent reports suggest that survival may be increased to 50 per cent if administration of high-dose amphotericin B is begun within 96 hours of clinical onset.

H. **Cytomegalovirus Infections.** These infections are common sequelae of bone marrow and renal transplantation and cause a variety of clinical syndromes including fever, leukopenia, mononucleosis, thrombocytopenia, hepatitis, interstitial pneumonitis, gastrointestinal ulceration, chorioretinitis, bacterial superinfection, and renal allograft dysfunction. Most episodes represent reactivation of latent virus, although primary infection acquired by transplantation of infected kidneys or marrow or transfusion of infected blood products play an important role. Diagnosis is made by culture of urine, blood, or buffy coat leukocytes, or by demonstration of a four-fold rise in complement-fixing antibody.

I. **Herpes Simplex Virus Reactivation.** This occurs in 80 per cent of renal transplant patients and in 40 to 50 per cent of marrow transplant cases. These infections are generally manifested as painful oral or genital vesicular lesions that may disseminate in a small percentage of cases to cause esophagitis, tracheobronchitis, pneumonia, eczema herpeticum, hepatitis, and meningoencephalitis. The diagnosis is generally evident on physical examination but can easily be confirmed by Tzanck preparations, culture, immunofluorescent asssays, and serologic testing.

J. **Varicella Zoster Virus.** Infection with this virus commonly causes shingles in patients with Hodgkin's disease (13 to 15 per cent), non-Hodgkin's lymphoma (7 to 9 per cent), and organ transplantation (7 to 60 per cent) and much less commonly in patients with solid tumors (1 to 3 per cent). The diagnosis can be confirmed by culture. Cutaneous or visceral dissemination is observed in 15 to 30 per cent of Hodgkin's disease cases, but mortality is low (≤1 per cent).

K. **Pneumocystis carinii.** *P. carinii* is an opportunistic protozoan that causes interstitial pneumonia that is manifested by dyspnea (91 per cent), fever (67 per cent), and nonproductive cough (50 per cent). Patients with leukemia, lymphoma, primary immunodeficiency, organ transplantation, and corticosteroid therapy are at particular risk. Rales are frequently absent despite severe tachypnea and striking radiographic abnormalities. Diagnosis usually requires lung biopsy with demonstration of organisms by methenamine silver, immunofluorescent, or toluidine blue staining. Recovery rates with appropriate therapy (trimethoprim-sulfa or pentamidine) are approximately 80 per cent.

L. **Toxoplasma gondii.** This is an obligate intracellular protozoan parasite that may cause diffuse encephalopathy, meningoencephalitis, lymphadenopathy, pneumonitis, hepatosplenomegaly, and uveitis following reactivation of latent infection, neoacquisition, or transfusion of infected blood products in compromised hosts. The cerebrospinal fluid shows nonspecific pleocytosis and protein elevation. Diagnosis is made by demonstration of trophozoites in body tissues or fluids or by specific serology (Sabin Feldman dye test or indirect immunofluorescence test). Currently the IgM-IFA test is considered the most reliable test for distinguishing acute infection. Brain computed tomography should be performed to investigate possible intracerebral mass lesions.

M. **Strongyloides stercoralis.** The intestinal threadworm is a unique nematode capable of multiplying within a host by an autoinfection cycle. Infective filariform larvae are capable of penetrating the perianal skin of the host as the larvae are passed in the stool. In this manner clinical infection may be sustained for decades after the host leaves the parasite's endemic area. Healthy subjects generally remain asymptomatic, but compromised hosts may develop severe disseminated strongyloidiasis that is manifested by pruritic erythematous skin lesions, variable eosinophilia, diffuse pneumonitis, gastrointestinal symptoms, and bacteremia associated with *Enterobacter* or *Pseudomonas* due to ulcerating enterocolitis. The diagnosis is made by observation of rhabdoid larvae in feces, duodenal aspirate, sputum, other body fluids, or tissues. Thiabendazole provides effective therapy.

References

1. Rubin RH, Greene R: Etiology and management of the compromised patient with fever and pulmonary infiltrates. *In* Rubin RH, Young LS (eds.): Clinical Approach to Infection in the Compromised Host. New York, Plenum Publishing Corporation, 1981, pp. 123–161.

A superlative chapter in an outstanding book. This textbook is the best single resource on opportunistic infections currently available.

2. Meyers J, Thomas ED: Infection complicating bone marrow transplantation. *In* Rubin RH, Young LS (eds.), Ibid., pp. 507–551.

Another superb chapter in which the infectious complications of bone marrow transplantation are delineated according to the Seattle experience.

3. Hooper DC, Pruitt AA, Rubin RH: Central nervous system infection in the chronically immunosuppressed. Medicine 61:166–188, 1982.

The best recent review available of meningitis in the compromised host.

4. Winston DJ, Dudnick DV, Chapin M, et al.: Coagulase negative staphy-

lococcal bacteremia in patients receiving immunosuppressive therapy. Arch Intern Med 143:32–36, 1983.

An excellent article documenting the emergence of Staphylococcus epidermidis *as a major cause of septicemia in immunocompromised patients.*

5. Matthay RA, Greene WH: Pulmonary infections in the immunocompromised patient. Med Clin North Am 64:529–551, 1980.

A good analysis of opportunistic infections in the lung.

6. Pennington JE: Infection in the compromised host. Semin Infect Dis 1:142–162, 1978.

A good review article.

36

OTITIS, PHARYNGITIS, AND SINUSITIS

By PAUL G. RAMSEY, M.D.

EAR INFECTIONS

A. **Definitions.** Otitis is generally divided into three categories:
  1. *Otitis Media.* Acute otitis media is a suppurative process that presumably is related to eustachian tube blockage with subsequent accumulation of fluid in the middle ear. Bacteria may gain access to the middle ear by reflux up the eustachian tube, although other pathogenic mechanisms such as hematogenous spread of bacteria occur.
  2. *Serous Otitis.* Noninfected secretory middle ear effusions are called serous otitis.
  3. *Otitis Externa.* Infection of the external ear (otitis externa) often is related to trauma.

B. **Epidemiology**
  1. *Otitis Media and Serous Otitis.* These are common problems among children less than six years of age but are uncommon in adults. The high incidence of upper respiratory tract infections in young children and the anatomy of the eustachian tube probably contribute to the incidence of ear infections in this age group.
  2. *Otitis Externa.* This is a common problem in adults and children. It is related to a number of predisposing factors, including trauma, such as in cleaning the ears with abrasive instruments; heat; humidity; excessive contact with water; and generalized skin disorders such as psoriasis or eczema.
  3. *Viral Infection.* This is an important predisposing factor for otitis media. In children, infection with respiratory syncytial virus and adenovirus and, in adults, infection with influenza virus often precede otitis media. However, viruses are isolated infrequently from middle ear effusions.

C. Etiology and Clinical Manifestations

1. *Otitis Media.* The onset is often associated with pain in the ear and fever (40 to 60 per cent of cases) and occasionally is associated with nausea, vomiting, vertigo, or hearing loss. However, the clinical features of otitis media are variable. Careful otoscopic examination of the color, contour, translucence, and mobility of the tympanic membrane is important for distinguishing otitis media from serous otitis. The organisms most commonly causing otitis media are *Streptococcus pneumoniae* and nontypable strains of *Hemophilus influenzae.* Other respiratory tract pathogens such as *Branhamella catarrhalis, Streptococcus pyogenes,* and staphylococcal species have been found in small numbers of patients. *Mycoplasma* is rarely found in middle ear isolates from patients with otitis media even when bullous myringitis is present. *S. pneumoniae* and *H. influenzae* cause the majority of cases of bullous myringitis. In the neonate and immunosuppressed adults, gram-negative bacteria and *S. aureus* may cause otitis.

2. *Otitis Externa.* Patients with otitis externa usually have pain in the affected ear but rarely have fever. Otoscopic examination reveals erythema, serosanguinous or purulent discharge, and granulation tissue in the external canal. *Pseudomonas aeruginosa* and *S. pyogenes* are common causes of otitis externa in children and adults. In addition, fungi (*Aspergillus* and *Candida* species) and viruses (herpes zoster) may cause otitis externa.

3. *Complications.* Complications of otitis include:
   a. *Mastoiditis* and temporal bone osteomyelitis.
   b. *Invasive otitis externa* secondary to infection with *P. aeruginosa* occurs in elderly diabetic patients and rarely in children and young adults. The infection spreads in the soft tissue to the base of the skull and may be associated with multiple cranial nerve palsies.

D. Diagnostic Tests.
The diagnoses of otitis media and otitis externa are usually made on the basis of clinical findings. Careful otoscopic examination of the color, contour, translucence, and mobility of the tympanic membrane is important. The otoscopic examination provides a working diagnosis in most cases. In rare situations other tests may be considered:

1. *Myringotomy.* Diagnosis of otitis media may be made most specifically by myringotomy. However, this procedure is rarely indicated. Myringotomy may be considered in the following situations:
   a. For patients with severe systemic toxicity
   b. For immunosuppressed patients
   c. For patients who have not responded to prior antibiotic therapy
   d. For patients with signs of spread of infection beyond the middle ear (mastoiditis or temporal bone osteomyelitis)

2. *Tympanometry.* This is an objective test of tympanic membrane compliance. A small probe is placed in the external auditory canal and a tone is delivered through the probe.

Accurate results can be obtained in an objective fashion. This procedure may be useful to examine individuals with chronic otitis.
3. *X-rays or Computed Axial Tomographic (CAT) Scans.* These methods may be considered if there is evidence of spread of infection beyond the ear.

PHARYNGITIS

A. **Definition.** Pharyngitis is an infection of the oropharynx that is caused by a variety of viruses and bacteria. Most infections are self-limited, but a variety of complications may occur, including:
   1. *Otitis Media and Sinusitis.* These conditions are associated with active pharyngitis.
   2. *Epiglottitis.* Epiglottitis is an infection of the epiglottis and aryepiglottic folds which may lead to airway obstruction and death.
   3. *Peritonsillar Abscess (Quinsy).* This is a complication of streptococcal pharyngitis.
   4. *Nonsuppurative Sequelae of* S. pyogenes *Infection.* Nonsuppurative sequelae include acute rheumatic fever, glomerulonephritis, and scarlet fever.
   5. *Diphtheria.* Diphtheria still occurs as a rare complication of *Corynebacterium diphtheriae* infection.
B. **Epidemiology.** Viruses cause most cases of pharyngitis, but bacteria (primarily *S. pyogenes)* may cause as many as 25 per cent of cases in epidemic situations. The distribution of etiologic agents depends on the age and clinical setting.
   1. *Age.* Pharyngitis in children is commonly caused by several different viruses, including respiratory syncytial virus, adenovirus, parainfluenza virus, rhinovirus, and enteroviruses. In adults parainfluenza virus, influenza virus, adenovirus, and enteroviruses also cause pharyngitis, but Epstein-Barr virus and herpes simplex virus should also be considered. *S. pyogenes* infections occur most frequently in school-age children, and *Mycoplasma* causes pharyngitis in individuals of ages 10 to 25.
   2. *Clinical Setting.* In crowded living conditions (in schools and military settings) adenovirus is the most important cause of pharyngitis. *S. pyogenes* infections also occur frequently in these settings, with the highest incidence in the winter.
C. **Clinical Manifestations and Microbiology**
   1. *Symptoms and Physical Findings.* Sore throat, the hallmark symptom of pharyngitis, usually develops acutely. General malaise, myalgia, fever, and upper respiratory tract symptoms including coryza, cough, and laryngitis may be present. Findings on physical examination may include tender anterior cervical lymphadenopathy and oropharyngeal erythema often in association with a patchy or confluent exudate. Although symptoms and physical findings do not allow diagnosis of a specific etiology for pharyngitis, there are suggestive findings.

2. **Tender Cervical Lymphadenopathy.** Tender cervical lymphadenopathy with an exudative pharyngitis and leukocytosis (white blood count greater than 15,000 cu mm) suggests streptococcal infection.

3. **Findings of Scarlet Fever.** A bright erythematous rash with a sandpaper feel involving the trunk and face and skin folds (Pastia's lines) also suggests streptococcal infection. The rash usually spares the palms and soles and desquamates in the resolving phase.

4. **Exudative Pharyngitis.** This is *not* a specific finding for streptococcal infection. It can be seen with Epstein-Barr virus, adenovirus, herpes simplex virus, and other viral infections. Many patients with Epstein-Barr virus infection may also have beta-hemolytic streptococci isolated from the pharynx.

5. **An Adherent Gray Black Membrane.** An adherent gray black membrane with edema of the fauces suggests diphtheria. The onset of this infection is abrupt with rapid spread of the tonsillar exudate. Symptoms and signs include severe lethargy, stridor, cranial and peripheral nerve palsies, and airway obstruction.

6. **Peritonsillar Abscess (Quinsy).** Adults in the second or third decade of life may develop peritonsillar abscesses (quinsy) secondary to infection with beta-hemolytic streptococci and rarely with *S. aureus*. The superior pole of the tonsil is the common location for abscess formation. Symptoms include sore throat, dysphagia, and impaired paletal motion. Trismus may result from irritation of the internal pterygoid muscle. Physical examination reveals a fluctuant mass, and the uvula is often displaced from the midline.

7. **N. gonorrhoeae.** These organisms may be found occasionally in the appropriate epidemiologic setting.

8. **Dysphagia.** Dysphagia with sore throat, fever, and cervical adenopathy suggests the possible diagnosis of *epiglottitis*. Dysphagia may be out of proportion to the signs of pharyngitis noted on physical examination. On physical examination patients appear anxious and tend to sit leaning forward. Breathing may be quiet or respiratory stridor may be present. Secretions can be seen in the back of the oral cavity, and epiglottitis can be confirmed by the presence of an erythematous epiglottis projecting over the tongue. However, the tongue must be depressed to see the epiglottis, and this maneuver may lead to complete airway obstruction. If epiglottitis is suspected, this procedure should be performed only if personnel and equipment are available for emergency endotracheal intubation or tracheostomy.

D. **Diagnostic Tests and Differential Diagnosis.** It is important to distinguish self-limited benign infections (viral and *Mycoplasma* infections) from infections associated with morbidity and potential mortality.

1. **Throat Cultures.** Throat cultures are necessary to diagnose group A streptococcal pharyngitis. Throat swabs should be cultured also for *N. gonorrhoeae* if the clinical setting suggests this diagnosis.

2. **Lateral Neck X-rays.** Recognition of the complications of pharyngitis depends primarily on the history and physical examination. However, lateral neck x-rays are important for diagnosing epiglottitis. These roentgenograms demonstrate an enlarged epiglottis and may also show extension of infection into the prevertebal tissues. Patients should be observed carefully while the x-rays are taken.

SINUSITIS

A. **Definition.** Bacterial, viral, and occasionally fungal infections of the paranasal sinuses may cause acute or chronic sinusitis. The bacterial causes of acute and chronic maxillary sinusitis have been established by sinus puncture technique. *H. influenzae, S. pneumoniae,* and other streptococci are the primary pathogens causing acute sinusitis, and anaerobic organisms and *S. aureus* have been implicated in cases of chronic disease. It is often difficult to distinguish infectious sinusitis from noninfectious allergic conditions. Sinusitis can be categorized according to the anatomy of the paranasal sinuses:

1. **Maxillary Sinusitis.** This form is extremely common (it has been estimated that 1 per cent of "colds" are complicated by acute maxillary sinusitis). However, complications related to maxillary sinusitis are rare.

2. **Frontal Sinusitis.** This form is unusual but may be complicated by potentially life-threatening infections (as in cranial osteomyelitis, brain abscess, frontal subperiosteal abscess, epidural abscess, or subdural abscess).

3. **Bacterial Infection of the Ethmoid Sinus.** This is a common cause of orbital cellulitis.

4. **Sphenoid Sinusitis.** Although this form is rare, the relationship of the sphenoid sinus to critical structures, including the pituitary gland, optic canals, dura mater, and the cavernous sinus leads to severe complications.

B. **Epidemiology.** A variety of conditions predispose adults and children to sinusitis:

1. **Associated Infection.** Most cases follow viral upper respiratory tract infection. Symptoms of viral infection that persist longer than seven days should raise the question of sinusitis.

2. **Mechanical Problems.** Deviated nasal septum, facial trauma, and nasal polyps disrupt the normal sinus drainage pattern, predisposing patients to sinusitis.

3. **Allergies.** Allergies are an important predisposing condition for infectious sinusitis.

4. **Extension of Odontogenic Infections.** This may lead to complicated bacterial sinusitis.

5. **Cystic Fibrosis.** Most patients with cystic fibrosis develop bacterial sinusitis.

6. **Immunosuppressed Patients.** Immunosuppressed patients may be prone to develop complications of sinusitis that occa-

sionally are related to unusual organisms (for example, fungal infections in diabetes).

7. **"Nosocomial Sinusitis."** This is an important cause of fever and morbidity in hospitalized patients. Sinusitis should be considered in all patients with fever in association with prolonged nasotracheal intubation.

C. **Clinical Features.** The clinical features of sinusitis depend on the anatomic location of infection.

1. **Maxillary Sinusitis.** This form is associated with facial pain, purulent nasal discharge, and altered facial sensation. Facial pain may be aggravated by stooping. Headache and fever occur in a minority of patients. Sinus transillumination is helpful in diagnosing cases of acute maxillary sinusitis but is less helpful in the setting of chronic disease. Transillumination findings are divided into three categories: normal, dull, and opaque. Finding of opaque sinuses correlates with active purulent infection as determined by sinus puncture.

2. **Frontal Sinusitis.** Patients with acute frontal sinusitis often have symptoms of pain and tenderness over the frontal sinus. Fever, purulent nasal discharge, and signs of involvement of the maxillary sinuses may be seen. Pitting edema over the forehead suggests a possible diagnosis of a subperiosteal abscess ("Pott's puffy tumor"). Sinus transillumination can be a valuable part of the physical examination in adults.

3. **Ethmoiditis.** Ethmoiditis may be associated with orbital complications, including:
   a. Edema or cellulitis of the eyelid
   b. "Orbital cellulitis" characterized by tenderness of the eye, ophthalmoplegia, chemosis, proptosis, and erythema and edema of the lids
   c. Severe proptosis related to subperiosteal abscess
   d. Orbital abscess
   e. Other complications such as meningitis, epidural abscess, or cavernous sinus thrombosis

4. **Headache.** Headache is the most common initial symptom in patients with **sphenoid sinusitis**. Pain is often unilateral and may involve the frontal, temporal, or occipital regions. On physical examination patients may have unexplained tenderness over the vertex of the skull or over the mastoid. Fever is present frequently in patients with acute sphenoiditis but may be absent in patients with chronic infection. Extension of infection from the sphenoid sinus may lead to cavernous sinus thrombosis, pituitary insufficiency, bitemporal hemianopsia, subdural abscess, internal carotid infection, and meningitis. Clinical features of septic cavernous sinus thrombosis include abrupt onset of photophobia, headache, ophthalmoplegia, chemosis, and proptosis. *S. aureus* has been the most frequent cause of septic cavernous sinus thrombosis, but gram-negative organisms and anaerobes have also been implicated.

D. **Diagnostic Tests.** Most cases of acute maxillary sinusitis can be diagnosed by sinus transillumination. However, radiologic examination remains the most sensitive and specific test. The

Water's view provides the best examination of the maxillary sinuses. Findings of opacity or air fluid level or mucosal thickening greater than 8 mm have been correlated with findings of purulent material and microbial pathogens by sinus puncture. X-ray examination is essential for diagnosing frontal, ethmoid, and sphenoid sinusitis. In addition, polytomographic examinations or CAT scans may be needed for diagnosis of sphenoid sinus infection. Direct sinus aspiration is the only procedure that can provide accurate information concerning etiology. Nasal swab cultures in general do not correlate with cultures of material obtained by direct sinus aspiration.

REFERENCES

1. Berg O, Bergstedt H, Carenfelt C, et al.: Discrimination of purulent from nonpurulent maxillary sinusitis: A clinical and radiographic diagnosis. Ann Otolaryngol 90:272–275, 1981.
2. Caplan ES, Hoyt NJ: Nosocomial sinusitis. JAMA 247:639–641, 1982.

A discussion of 33 cases of hospital-acquired sinusitis emphasizes the predisposing factors and microbiologic findings.

3. Dobie RA, Tobey DN: Clinical features of diphtheria in the respiratory tracts. JAMA 242:2197, 1979.

A nice review of clinical findings.

4. Doroghazi RM, Nadol JB, Hyslop NE, et al.: Invasive external otitis: Report of 21 cases and review of the literature. Am J Med 71:603–614 1981.

Excellent review of all aspects of this unusual but important infectious process.

5. Evans FO, Sydnor JB, Moore WEC, et al.: Sinusitis of the maxillary antrum. N Engl J Med 293:735–739, 1975.

Excellent clinical study of acute maxillary sinusitis.

6. Frederick J, Braude AI: Anaerobic infection of the paranasal sinuses. N Engl J Med 290:135–137, 1974.

Discussion of microbiologic findings in patients with chronic sinusitis.

7. Gorfinkel HJ, Brown R, Kabins SA: Acute infectious epiglottitis in adults. Ann Intern Med 70:289–294, 1969.
8. Hamory BH, Sande MA, Sydnor A, et al.: Etiology and antimicrobial therapy of acute maxillary sinusitis. J Infect Dis 139:197–202, 1979.

A follow-up article to the study by Evans et al.

9. Klein JO: Microbiology and antimicrobial treatment of otitis media. Ann Otol Rhinol Laryngol (Suppl 84) 90:30–35, 1981

A concise review of otitis media.

10. Levy ML, Ericsson CD, Pickering LK: Infections of the upper respiratory tract. Med Clin North Am 67:153–171, 1983.

A recent review of sinusitis, otitis, and pharyngitis.

11. Lew D, Southwick FS, Montgomery WW, et al.: Sphenoid sinusitis—a review of 30 cases. N Engl J Med 309:1149–1153, 1983.
12. McCurdy JA: Peritonsillar abscess. Arch Otolaryngol 103:414–415, 1977.

SEPTIC ARTHRITIS AND OSTEOMYELITIS

By PAUL G. RAMSEY, M.D.

DEFINITION

Septic arthritis is an infection involving the joint space. Findings of inflammation including erythema, swelling, tenderness, and limited range of motion are usually present. Although polyarticular involvement occurs, a single joint is involved in most cases. Septic arthritis may mimic noninfectious inflammatory joint diseases and should be distinguished also from *septic bursitis,* which involves the olecranon or prepatellar bursa. In patients with septic bursitis, inflammatory signs are usually limited to the bursa, and there is normal range of motion of the joint.

Osteomyelitis is an infection of the bone and marrow. Osteomyelitis is classified according to route of infection, acute versus chronic, or by clinical setting.

A. Route of Infection

1. ***Hematogenous.*** The infection is hematogenous in 19 per cent of adult cases, most commonly involving the long bones in children and the vertebrae in adults.

2. ***Contiguous Spread.*** This occurs in 47 per cent of adult cases and is common in the pelvis, skull, and mandible. Implantation (puncture wounds) and postoperative infections are classified in this category.

3. ***Vascular Insufficiency.*** This accounts for 34 per cent of cases in adults, often in diabetics. The feet are involved most commonly.

B. Acute Versus Chronic. Cases are classified as acute during the first occurrence of osteomyelitis. The duration of symptoms before examination varies depending on the route of infection. Cases of patients who have a history of prior osteomyelitis are classified as chronic.

C. Clinical Settings. Several special clinical settings of osteomyelitis are recognized: (1) vertebral osteomyelitis; (2) intravenous drug abuse; (3) sickle cell anemia; (4) artificial joints; (5) hemophiliacs; (6) osteitis pubis; and (7) puncture wounds.

EPIDEMIOLOGY

Factors to be considered in a patient with septic arthritis, septic bursitis, or osteomyelitis are outlined below.

A. Septic Arthritis

1. ***Age.*** Gonococcal infection is the most common cause of septic arthritis in the 15- to 40-year age group.

2. ***Inflammatory Joint Disease.*** Rheumatoid arthritis, trauma,

and gout are predisposing factors for infection and make the diagnosis of septic arthritis more difficult.

3. *Infection of a Prosthetic Device.* This condition is difficult to diagnose, since fever is often absent. Joint tenderness may be the only clue to an infected prosthesis.

4. *Sexual History.* Sexual history is important because of the risk of gonococcal infection.

5. *Concurrent Infections.* Concurrent infections are often found in patients with septic arthritis: bacteremia (50 per cent of cases), pneumonia (5 per cent), urinary tract infections (15 per cent), decubitus ulcers (15 per cent), and skin ulcer (10 per cent).

6. *Intravenous Drug Use*

B. **Septic Bursitis.** Most patients with septic bursitis involving the olecranon or prepatellar bursa are young to middle-aged men with a history of trauma to the site. They are often plumbers, carpet layers, carpenters, gardeners, and so forth. Some patients may have a history of other diseases involving the bursa, and a few patients have developed infection after intrabursal corticosteroid injection.

C. **Osteomyelitis**

1. *Age.* There are two age peaks: childhood (85 per cent of cases) and old age. Bone involvement depends on age: long bones are affected in children and vertebrae in adults.

2. *Predisposing Factors.* Depending on the route of infection, a number of predisposing factors may be involved.

   a. Predisposing conditions for *hematogenous infection* include antecedent trauma, genitourinary tract infections, drug addiction, and hemoglobinopathies.

   b. Precipitating factors for osteomyelitis secondary to a *contiguous focus* of infection include postoperative infections (60 per cent of cases), soft tissue infections, infected teeth, paranasal sinus infections, and radiation therapy.

   c. Most patients with osteomyelitis related to *vascular insufficiency* are diabetic and older than 50.

CLINICAL MANIFESTATIONS

A. **Septic Arthritis.** The relationship of clinical findings to microbiology is important in this condition.

1. *Neisseria gonorrhoeae.* *N. gonorrhoeae* accounts for 90 per cent of cases in patients aged 15 to 40. Seventy-five per cent of patients are female. Gonococcal arthritis is one manifestation of disseminated gonococcal infections (DGI). Patients usually have fever; pustular, papular, or petechial skin lesions (fewer than 30 in number); and joint involvement of the wrist, fingers, knees, or ankles. *Tenosynovitis* is an early finding. Septic arthritis usually follows with monoarticular involvement of the knees, ankles, or wrists. In women disseminated gonococcal infections occur in association with menstruation.

2. *Staphylococcus aureus.* *S. aureus* accounts for approximately

70 per cent of cases of bacterial but nongonococcal septic arthritis in adults. In elderly adults with rheumatoid arthritis, *S. aureus* accounts for more than 90 per cent of cases. In these patients signs of joint inflammation may be attributed to the underlying arthritis, and fever is often absent.

3. **Beta-Hemolytic Streptococci (Groups A and B).** These organisms may cause mono- or polyarticular septic arthritis, especially in association with bacteremia.

4. **Gram-Negative Bacteria.** These bacteria have accounted for increasing numbers (10 per cent) of cases of septic arthritis in recent years. Patients with host defense abnormalities, chronic diseases, intravenous drug use, and other noninfectious inflammatory joint disease are at risk of developing gram-negative infections. *Hemophilus influenzae* is a common cause of septic arthritis in children but is uncommon in adults.

5. **Fungal and Mycobacterial Septic Arthritis.** Fungal (in immunosuppressed patients and intravenous drug users) and mycobacterial (in patients with underlying inflammatory joint disease) septic arthritis occur infrequently.

B. **Septic Bursitis.** Swelling (100 per cent of cases) and pain (95 per cent) of the prepatellar or olecranon bursa suggest this diagnosis. Fever (50 per cent) and chills are less common. Although cellulitis is common (approximately 75 per cent of cases), joint motion is nearly normal. Some patients with septic bursitis (50 per cent) have a break in the skin. *S. aureus* and rarely beta-hemolytic streptococci cause septic bursitis.

C. **Osteomyelitis.** The clinical features and microbiology vary greatly with age, route of infection, and predisposing illness.

1. **S. aureus.** *S. aureus* is responsible for 80 per cent of childhood and 50 per cent of adult cases of hematogenous infection. As many as 10 per cent of patients with *S. aureus* sepsis develop osteomyelitis. Streptococci (10 per cent of cases), enteric gram-negative rods (8 per cent), *Salmonella* (2 per cent), and other miscellaneous bacteria account for smaller numbers of cases. Clinical findings depend on the organism, the patient's age, and predisposing factors. In general, patients with acute hematogenous osteomyelitis develop signs and symptoms localized to the involved bone. Fever, chills, and general malaise are found in less than half the patients. Some patients may have more prolonged symptoms that last several months before examination. Several special circumstances are described:

   a. *Vertebral osteomyelitis* accounts for 2 per cent of adult hematogenous osteomyelitis. Most patients (90 per cent) have localized continuous pain lasting longer than three months (50 per cent). In bacterial osteomyelitis, the adjacent vertebrae are frequently involved.

   b. Hematogenous osteomyelitis related to *intravenous drug abuse* often involves the vertebrae (including the cervical vertebrae), sternoclavicular joint, sacroiliac joint, or the os pubis. These infections are often gram-negative (*Pseudomonas* in 60 per cent), and only 15 per cent are caused by *S. aureus.* Patients usually have localized pain without systemic symptoms.

  c. In patients with *sickle cell anemia,* it is difficult to distinguish bone infarction associated with crisis from osteomyelitis. *Salmonella* osteomyelitis should be suspected in patients with sickle cell disease or other hemoglobinopathies.

 2. **Contiguous Focus of Infection.** Osteomyelitis secondary to a contiguous focus of infection is more common in older patients. *S. aureus* is the most common bacterial isolate (50 per cent of cases), but many patients have polymicrobial infection. *S. epidermidis* should be considered a pathogen when it is isolated from bone, especially in the setting of a prosthetic device. *Pseudomonas aeruginosa* osteomyelitis of the bones in the feet occurs secondary to puncture wounds, and anaerobic osteomyelitis may be seen in relation to decubitus ulcers, bites, trauma to the head, and intra-abdominal infections. Wounds and draining sinuses are important clues to osteomyelitis secondary to a contiguous focus of infection. Local inflammatory signs usually are present, although fever often is absent and many patients have subacute indolent courses.

 3. **Vascular Insufficiency.** Osteomyelitis related to vascular insufficiency in diabetic patients is associated with local pain and inflammatory findings, including cellulitis. An open wound, draining sinus, or crepitus of the soft tissues should raise the possibility of osteomyelitis in a diabetic patient. Most infections are polymicrobial with a mixture of staphylococci, streptococci, gram-negative organisms, and anaerobic bacteria.

 4. **Prosthetic Device Infections.** These infections are especially difficult to diagnose. Fever and inflammatory signs are often absent, and symptoms of local pain appear in an indolent fashion. *S. epidermidis* is an important pathogen in this setting.

DIAGNOSTIC TESTS

The utility of diagnostic tests may be divided into two general categories:

A. Confirmation of the Infectious Process

 1. **Joint Aspiration.** In diagnosing septic arthritis, joint aspiration is mandatory. The synovial fluid findings are useful in distinguishing septic arthritis from other inflammatory conditions (Table 37–1). Radiographic examination may be helpful for demonstrating concomitant osteomyelitis, the presence of joint effusion (especially helpful in cases of hip infections), and loosening of a prosthetic device. Technetium-99 scanning can be used to define an inflammatory process in a deep-seated joint such as the sacroiliac joint.

 2. **Aspiration of Bursal Fluid.** This procedure is necessary to make the diagnosis of septic bursitis. The findings are variable, ranging from serous material to thick pus.

TABLE 37–1. CHARACTERISTICS OF ARTHROCENTESIS FLUID*

Condition/Disease	Appearance	Viscosity	Leukocytes (per mL)	Glucose (mg/dL)	Comments
Normal	Clear, straw-colored	High	75(15% PMNs)	Nearly equal to blood	
Noninflammatory diseases					
Osteoarthritis, traumatic arthritis	Clear	High	1000 (15–25% PMNs)	Nearly equal to blood	Acute trauma, often grossly bloody with RBCs on microscopy
Inflammatory diseases					
Rheumatoid arthritis	Translucent-opaque, light yellow	Low	2000–75,000 (60–75% PMNs)	25 mg/dL lower than blood	"Rice bodies" seen
Gout, pseudogout	Translucent-opaque, white	Poor	10–75,000 (60–75% PMNs)	25 mg/dL lower than blood	*Gout:* Needlelike negative birefringent crystals *Pseudogout:* Rhomboid weakly positive birefringent crystals
Infectious diseases					
Bacterial septic arthritis	Opaque, gray, or yellow	Variable	100,000 (>75% PMNs) but lower with partial treatment, low-virulence organisms	25 mg/dL lower than blood	

*Reprinted, with permission of author and publisher, from Eisenberg M, Copass M: Emergency Medical Therapy. 2nd ed. Philadelphia, W. B. Saunders Company, 1983.

3. **X-Ray Findings.** The diagnosis of osteomyelitis can be suggested by x-ray findings. However, abnormalities apparent on x-ray examination are delayed at least ten days after initial symptoms. Early abnormalities include periosteal elevation and soft tissue swelling. After one month, sclerotic areas of bone appear. The sensitivity of x-rays in the first few weeks of osteomyelitis has been reported as 30 per cent, with a specificity of 89 per cent. Technetium-99 bone scans may suggest osteomyelitis within 48 hours of symptom onset and, with hematogenous osteomyelitis in children, the sensitivity and specificity have been approximately 90 per cent. However, specificity may be less in adults with osteomyelitis related to contiguous infections. There is little published data on indium-111 white cell scans, but these scans may prove valuable.

B. Microbiologic Diagnosis

1. **Gram's Stains.** Gram's stains of synovial fluid are positive in approximately 60 to 70 per cent of cases. Aerobic and anaerobic cultures should be performed on all joint fluid aspirates, with particular attention paid to cultures for gonococci in the appropriate age groups. In selected patients with underlying chronic joint disease and indolent symptoms, mycobacterial cultures of the synovial fluid should be performed. However, synovial biopsy cultures have a higher yield. Acid-fast smears of synovial fluid have a low yield for tuberculosis (20 per cent). Blood cultures and cultures from other sites of infection should be performed in patients with septic arthritis.

2. **Culture of Bursal Fluid.** In patients with septic bursitis, culture of the bursal fluid is necessary for microbiologic diagnosis. Gram's stain of fluid is often negative, and culture may grow only a few colonies of *S. aureus*. In some patients initial joint fluid culture may be negative. However, if clinical findings are suspicious, repeat cultures should be performed and treatment initiated. Blood cultures are rarely positive in patients with infectious bursitis.

3. **Bone Biopsies.** Bone biopsies are the "gold standard" for defining the cause of osteomyelitis. Bone biopsies should be considered in most cases unless the results of blood culture are positive. Sinus tract cultures generally do not predict the findings of bone biopsy culture. The same organism was found in the sinus tract and bone in only 44 per cent of patients in one study. However, if *S. aureus* is isolated as a single organism from a sinus tract, it can be found in 78 per cent of bone biopsy cultures.

REFERENCES

1. Canoso JJ, Sheckman PR: Septic subcutaneous bursitis. Report of sixteen cases. J Rheumatol 6:96, 1979.
2. Enarson DA, et al.: Bone and joint tuberculosis: A continuing problem. Can Med Assoc J 120:139, 1979.
A good discussion of clinical features.

3. Goldenberg DL, Cohen AS: Acute infectious arthritis. A review of patients with nongonococcal joint infections (with emphasis on therapy and prognosis). Am J Med 60:369, 1976.

Excellent review of microbiologic findings in relation to clinical setting.

4. Ho G, Jr., Tice AD, Kaplan SR: Septic bursitis in the prepatellar and olecranon bursae: An analysis of 25 cases. Ann Intern Med 89:21, 1978.

Presentation of clinical features and treatment.

5. Holzman RS, Bishko F: Osteomyelitis in heroin addicts. Ann Intern Med 75:693, 1971.

Description of anatomic involvement and microbiology.

6. Leonard A, et al.: Osteomyelitis in hemodialysis patients. Ann Intern Med 78:651, 1973.

Emphasizes clinical clues that may lead to early diagnosis.

7. Lewis RP, Sutter VL, Finegold SM: Bone infections involving anaerobic bacteria. Medicine 57:279, 1978.

A detailed review of the role of anaerobes.

8. Mackowiak PA, Jones SR, Smith JW: Diagnostic value of sinus-tract cultures in chronic osteomyelitis. JAMA 239:2772, 1978.

An excellent article that documents the need to obtain bone biopsy in patients with osteomyelitis.

9. Miller EH, Semian DW: Gram-negative osteomyelitis following puncture wounds of the foot. J Bone Joint Surg 57A:535, 1975.
10. Pichichero ME, Friesen HA: Polymicrobial osteomyelitis: Report of three cases and a review of the literature. Rev Infect Dis 4:86, 1982.
11. Raff MJ, Melo JC: Anaerobic osteomyelitis. Medicine 57:83, 1978.

Extensive review of this topic.

12. Sapico FL, Montgomerie JA: Pyogenic vertebral osteomyelitis: Report of nine cases and review of the literature. Rev Infect Dis 1:754, 1979.

An excellent review of the clinical course of this infection.

13. Waldvogel FA, Medoff G, Swartz MN: Osteomyelitis: A review of clinical features, therapeutic considerations, and unusual aspects. N Engl J Med 282:198, 260, 316, 1970.

An outstanding review of all aspects of osteomyelitis.

14. Waldvogel FA, Vasey H: Osteomyelitis: The past decade. N Engl J Med 303:360, 1980.
15. Ward JR, Atcheson SG: Infectious arthritis. Med Clin North Am 61:313, 1977.

An excellent general review.

SEPTIC SHOCK

By OLIVER W. PRESS, M.D., Ph.D.

DEFINITION

Septic shock is defined as severe generalized impairment of vital organ perfusion, which ensues as a result of hematogenous microbial infection. Typical findings include arterial hypotension (systolic blood pressure <90 mm Hg), oliguria (<25 cc of urine per hour), mental obtundation, fever, tachypnea, and metabolic acidosis.

Sepsis exposes the circulation to a variety of toxic bacterial products (endotoxin and exotoxin) that activate the complement, coagulation, fibrinolytic, and kinin pathways and that may result in vasodilation, increased vascular permeability, and disseminated intravascular coagulation. Prolonged hypotension often leads to irreversible end organ damage (acute tubular necrosis, cerebral infarction, "shock liver," rhabdomyolysis, bowel infarction, and adult respiratory distress syndrome).

EPIDEMIOLOGY

A. **Incidence.** The annual incidence of gram-negative bacteremia has risen progressively with increased use of invasive monitoring, indwelling catheters, immunosuppression, and aggressive surgery to approximately 100,000 to 300,000 cases per year.[1] Roughly 40 per cent of these patients develop septic shock.[2] Analogous figures for gram-positive bacteremia and shock are unavailable.

B. **Risk Factors.** Attributes that predispose to the development of septic shock in patients with bacteremia include advanced age, antecedent immunosuppressive therapy, pre-existing cardiac or renal disease, and bacteremia with gram-negative (as opposed to gram-positive) organisms:[3]

BACTERIAL SPECIES	NUMBER OF CASES OF BACTEREMIA	PER CENT DEVELOPING SHOCK
1. Gram-negative bacilli	780	42
2. *Staphylococcus aureus*	58	29
3. *Streptococcus pneumoniae*	123	14

DIFFERENTIAL DIAGNOSIS

A. **Cardiogenic Shock.** This occurs in myocardial infarction, arrhythmias, cardiomyopathy, and valvular heart disease.

287

B. **Obstructive Shock.** This occurs in tamponade, constrictive pericarditis, and pulmonary embolism.
C. **Hypovolemic Shock.** This occurs in hemorrhage, vomiting, diarrhea, pancreatitis, peritonitis, ascites, polyuric renal failure, diabetes insipidus, diuretics, Addison's disease, diaphoresis, and burns.
D. **Anaphylactic Shock**
E. **Neurogenic Shock.** This occurs in conditions such as spinal cord injury.
F. **Metabolic Shock.** This occurs with drug overdose, severe acidosis, or alkalosis.
G. **Microcirculatory Impairment.** This occurs with polycythemia vera and hyperviscosity.
H. **Toxic Shock Syndrome.** See also Chapter 40.

DIAGNOSIS

Diagnosis of septic shock is based on the clinical syndrome of tissue hypoperfusion (hypotension, oliguria, confusion, acidosis, and tachypnea) in the setting of documented or suspected infection with fever, chills, and positive blood cultures occurring in the absence of overt primary cardiac disease, hemorrhage, anaphylaxis, drug overdose, or neurologic injury.

SYMPTOMS AND SIGNS

Symptoms and signs in septic shock and their frequencies of occurrence are outlined below.[4]

SYMPTOMS AND SIGNS	FREQUENCY (PER CENT)
Fever	91
Pallor and cyanosis	44
Vomiting and diarrhea	35
Chills	34
Tachypnea or respiratory distress	31
Jaundice	18
Bloody stools	10
Hypothermia	6

LABORATORY FINDINGS IN SEPTIC SHOCK[4, 5]

A. Blood cultures are positive in 75 per cent of cases after a single culture and in 98 per cent after three blood cultures.[1]
B. Leukocytosis is found in most patients with an average initial count of 13,000 and a peak value of 23,000. Leukopenia may either precede leukocytosis or signal terminal sepsis.

C. Acidosis is present in 62 per cent of patients with an average pH of 7.30.

D. Uremia is common with an average initial blood urea nitrogen of 55 and a peak value of 72 mg per cent.

E. Hyperamylasemia occurs in 42 per cent of cases owing either to pancreatitis or more commonly to impaired renal clearance.

F. Hyperbilirubinemia and transaminasemia were found in 15 per cent of patients with septic shock.

G. Thrombocytopenia occurs in 46 per cent of patients with sepsis and is often associated with elevated levels of platelet-associated immunoglobulin G.[6]

H. Electrocardiographic abnormalities, particularly ST-T wave changes suggestive of ischemia, are seen in 92 per cent of cases.

BACTERIOLOGY OF SEPTIC SHOCK*

BACTERIAL SPECIES	NUMBER OF ISOLATES	PER CENT
Gram-negative bacteria		
Escherichia coli	33	20
Klebsiella species	17	10
Proteus species	16	10
Enterobacter species	10	6
Pseudomonas species	7	4
Neisseria meningitidis	6	4
Bacteroides fragilis	5	3
Salmonella species	3	2
Other gram-negative bacteria	6	4
	103	63
Gram-positive bacteria		
Streptococcus pneumoniae	23	14
Staphylococcus aureus	18	11
Streptococcus pyogenes	6	4
Other streptococci	7	4
Enterococci	3	2
Clostridium species	2	1
	59	36

Of special interest is the observation that *Staphylococcus epidermidis* is not reported to be a common cause of septic shock despite the fact that it is a common cause of bacteremia in opportunistic infections (see Chapter 35).

---

*This section was compiled from four separate published series.[6–9]

PRIMARY FOCI OF INFECTION IN CASES DEVELOPING SEPTIC SHOCK[6-9]

SITE	NUMBER OF CASES	PER CENT
Urinary tract infection	24	32
Pneumonia	23	31
Bowel diseases	7	9
Cholangitis	5	7
Endocarditis	4	5
Line sepsis	1	1
Facial cellulitis	1	1
Unknown	10	13
	75	100

RECOMMENDED DIAGNOSTIC APPROACH

A. Patients with suspected septic shock require emergent evaluation and treatment in an intensive care setting.

B. A careful history and physical examination must be performed with special emphasis on detecting the primary focus of infection (pneumonia; urinary tract infections, including pyelonephritis and prostatitis; enteritis; cholangitis; skin infections; and line sepsis). History of a recent urinary instrumentation or manipulation of an infected wound is particularly pertinent.

C. Specimens should be obtained immediately for Gram's stain and culture of blood (at least two specimens should be taken 15 minutes or more apart), urine, sputum, body fluids (pleural or joint effusions, ascites), cerebrospinal fluid (if there are symptoms or signs of meningitis), and skin lesions (ecthyma gangrenosum in *Pseudomonas* sepsis, purpura in meningococcemia, pustules in staphylococcal sepsis, and bullae in clostridial infection).

D. Examination of Gram's stain of buffy coat blood smears may demonstrate the causative organism in cases with high-level bacteremia and guide antibiotic choice. Unfortunately, cases with positive buffy coat smears usually pursue a fulminant course: mortality in this subgroup was 100 per cent in a recent series.[10]

E. New technologic advances that may assist in efficient early detection of sepsis include processing of blood culture samples with an antimicrobial removal device (in patients already receiving antibiotics), lysis-centrifugation of blood culture specimens, and use of counterimmunoelectrophoresis to detect specific microbial antigens.

F. Indwelling intravenous catheters should be removed and their tips cultured semiquantitatively.

G. Chest radiographs should be used to detect pneumonia or developing adult respiratory distress syndrome.

H. Arterial blood gas measurements are essential in monitoring respiratory alkalosis, metabolic acidosis, and impending respiratory failure.

I. Hourly urine output must be assessed (usually Foley catheterization is necessary) to guide resuscitative efforts with fluids and low-dose dopamine.

J. Fluid resuscitation should be begun immediately to prevent irreversible end organ dysfunction. In most circumstances hemodynamic monitoring with an arterial line and Swan-Ganz catheter is required to optimize fluid management.

  1. Several hemodynamic patterns have been delineated by measurement of the parameters shown below:[3]

	SVR*	CO*	SV*	CVP*	ACID-BASE STATUS*
a. Early gram-negative shock	↓↓	↑↑	↑↑	↓	Respiratory alkalosis
b. Late gram-negative shock	↑	↓	↓	↑	Metabolic acidosis
c. Gram-positive shock	variable	normal or slight increase	slight increase	variable	variable

*SVR = systemic vascular resistance; CO = cardiac output; SV = stroke volume; CVP = central venous pressure.

  2. Patients with early shock often have hyperdynamic cardiac function and low peripheral resistance, which give the skin and extremities a well-perfused appearance ("warm shock").

  3. Later, cardiac output diminishes, systemic vascular resistance increases, and the classic picture of "cold shock" with cool cyanotic clammy skin supervenes.

K. Immediate empiric broad-spectrum antibiotic administration (such as a beta-lactamase–resistant penicillin and an aminoglycoside) should be initiated without waiting for culture results.

L. The roles of massive doses of corticosteroids, naloxone, and antisera to endotoxin remain controversial.

PROGNOSIS

Despite aggressive modern management, mortality for septic shock remains at 40 to 60 per cent. Studies have shown that particularly high fatality rates are seen in patients over age 55, in cases with polymicrobial bacteremia, and in cases with oliguria or severe acidosis.

REFERENCES

1. Ellner JJ: Septic shock. Pediatr Clin North Am 30:365–371, 1983.

A compact recent review of the subject.

2. Kreger BE, Craven DE, McCabe WR: Gram negative bacteremia. IV. Re-evaluation of clinical features and treatment of 612 patients. Am J Med 68:344–355, 1980.

A detailed analysis of a large group of patients with gram-negative bacteremia, 44 per cent of whom had septic shock. Information on gram-positive infections is not included.

3. McCabe WR, Treadwell TL, De Maria A: Pathophysiology of bacteremia. Am J Med 75 (Suppl):7–18, 1983.

A superb pathophysiologic analysis of bacteremia and septic shock with a penetrating review of the literature.

4. Weil MH, Shubin H, Biddle M: Shock caused by gram negative organisms. Ann Intern Med 60:384–398, 1964.

A comprehensive but dated analysis of 169 cases of septic shock.

5. Sanford JR, Hodgin UG: Gram Negative Rod Bacteremia: An Analysis of 100 Patients. Septic Shock Workshop 1964, National Academy of Sciences and National Research Council, Washington, D.C., pp. 67–76, 1964.

An older study with a good analysis of risk factors.

6. Kelton JG, Neame PB, Gauldie J, Hirsh J: Elevated platelet-associated IgG in the thrombocytopenia of septicemia. N Engl J Med 300:760–764, 1979.

The best paper available on the thrombocytopenia of sepsis.

7. Shanson DC: Aetiological agents and laboratory diagnosis of bacteraemic shock. J Clin Pathol 33:888–889, 1980.

A succinct description of 58 cases of septic shock.

8. Winslow EJ, Loeb HS, Rahimtoola RH, et al: Hemodynamic studies and results of therapy in 50 patients with bacteremic shock. Am J Med 54:421–432, 1973.

A careful analysis of the cardiovascular parameters in a large group of patients with septic shock.

9. Leon C, Rodrigo MU, Tomasa A, et al.: Complement activation in septic shock due to gram negative and gram positive bacteria. Crit Care Med 10:308–310, 1982.

Activation of the complement system through the classic pathway is documented in 19 patients with septic shock. There were no differences between patients with gram-negative and gram-positive shock.

10. Reik H, Rubin SJ: Evaluation of the buffy coat smear for rapid detection of bacteremia. JAMA 245:357–359, 1981.

Eight patients with positive buffy coat smears were detected over a six-year period. All eight died of sepsis.

39

SKIN INFECTIONS

By PAUL G. RAMSEY, M.D.

DEFINITION

Categories of primary cutaneous infections include *cellulitis, impetigo, folliculitis, furunculosis, ulcerative lesions,* and *cutaneous mycoses.* Trauma such as surgery, puncture wounds, burns, and bites often provide the site of entry for infectious agents, although in many patients no entry site is apparent. The primary skin lesions must be distinguished from skin lesions that appear as manifestations of systemic infections. Maculopapular, vesicular, nodular, petechial, and ulcerative lesions often are associated with a variety of systemic viral, bacterial, fungal, and parasitic infections. However, the majority of primary skin infections are caused by bacteria and fungi. The classification of primary cutaneous infections is made by the appearance of the lesion as outlined here:

A. **Cellulitis.** Cellulitis is a spreading superficial erythematous lesion that is warm to the touch. Subclassifications of cellulitis including *erysipelas* and *erysipeloid* are described later.

B. **Impetigo.** Impetigo appears as a confluent group of vesicles or pustules with a characteristic superficial crust.

C. **Folliculitis.** Folliculitis represents a purulent infection of hair follicles and appears as small pustular lesions in the distribution of body hair.

D. **Furuncles.** Furuncles or common *boils* are cutaneus abscesses related to obstructed hair follicles or sebaceous glands, and *carbuncles* are large furuncles.

E. **Ulcerative Lesions.** These are deep erosions with dermal destruction. A crust of necrotic material may cover the base of an ulcer.

F. **Cutaneous Mycoses.** Cutaneous mycoses involve a variety of clinical findings as discussed later.

EPIDEMIOLOGY

Several factors may be related to the possible causes of primary skin infections:

A. **Age.** Young children are more likely than adults to develop facial cellulitis and frequently acquire and spread impetigo.

B. **Associated Conditions.** Adults with venous insufficiency, peripheral vascular disease, superficial mycoses, and primary skin diseases are likely to develop cellulitis of the extremities.

C. **Risk of Surgical Wound Infection.** Risk is related to type and length of surgery as well as to the skill of personnel.

D. **Prolonged Bed Rest.** This predisposes patients to ischemic necrosis of the skin surface, that is, to decubitus ulcers.

E. **Animal Exposure.** This is an important risk factor for unusual bacterial infections such as tularemia or anthrax.

F. **Occupation.** Acquisition of unusual bacteria may be related to occupation.

G. **Puncture Wounds.** Puncture wounds are associated with risk of developing anaerobic infections (tetanus) and are associated with acquisition of unusual organisms (*Pseudomonas aeruginosa* infection of the feet).

CLINICAL MANIFESTATIONS OF PRIMARY SKIN INFECTIONS

A. **Cellulitis: Microbiology and Types of Infection**
   1. *Erysipelas.* This is an erythematous indurated inflammatory lesion that often has a shiny appearance. The sharply demar-

cated raised border is a distinguishing feature. Bullous lesions may appear and rupture, leaving weeping erosions. Group A beta-hemolytic streptococci probably cause most cases of erysipelas. Usually, no obvious entry site is found. Erysipelas may involve the face (either one or both cheeks) or the lower extremities.

2. **Hemophilus influenzae.** *H. influenzae* is a common cause of a purplish cellulitis in children. The margins are not sharply demarcated, differentiating this cellulitis from streptococcal erysipelas. *H. influenzae* cellulitis often involves the face and may be associated with sepsis and meningitis.

3. **Staphylococcus aureus.** *S. aureus* and beta-hemolytic streptococci (usually group A but occasionally groups B, C, D, G, and F) are the most common causative agents involved in cellulitis. Typical skin findings include erythematous warm spreading lesions with indistinct borders. A primary skin lesion (secondary to trauma, superficial mycoses, or ischemic disease) is often present. Lymphangitic spread and regional adenopathy may be present. In many patients beta-hemolytic streptococci and *S. aureus* may be present together.

4. **Gram-negative Bacteria.** Gram-negative bacteria including *E. coli, Pseudomonas, Klebsiella,* and *Enterobacter* may cause cellulitis in patients with venostasis disease, ischemia, diabetes mellitus, or after surgery. Gas formation in the soft tissues may develop with these organisms.

5. **Synergistic Cellulitis.** This condition, which is caused by combinations of anaerobic bacteria and gram-negative organisms, may occur in the settings described above. Gas formation is characteristic.

B. **Impetigo.** Impetigo is caused by group A streptococci or *S. aureus*. Breaks in the skin may be obvious in patients with staphylococcal disease but absent with streptococci. The vesiculopustular lesions of impetigo are usually perioral but may involve the extremities. Spread of impetigo among children and from children to adults is enhanced by crowded living conditions and poor hygiene.

C. **Erysipeloid.** Erysipeloid is a distinctive type of purplish cellulitis with raised well-defined borders that occurs on the hands or fingers of fishermen or meat handlers. It is caused by *Erysipelothrix rhusiopathiae.*

D. **Folliculitis.** Most episodes of folliculitis are caused by *S. aureus* or *Candida* species. However, *Pseudomonas aeruginosa* acquired from bathing in hot tubs and spas causes a severe form of folliculitis, called *hot tub folliculitis,* that is associated with fever and systemic symptoms.

E. **Erythrasma.** This is an infection of intertriginous skin that is characterized by red or brownish patches and caused by *Corynebacterium* species.

F. **Furuncles.** Furuncles caused by *S. aureus* commonly occur in the axilla, the groin, and around the nose and lips. Some individuals are prone to chronic staphylococcal carriage and recurrent furunculosis. Furuncles usually are not associated with systemic findings, but carbuncles may be accompanied by fever, constitutional symptoms, and bacteremia.

G. **Ulcerative Skin Lesions.** These lesions, often associated with fever and regional lymphadenopathy, may be caused by tularemia, anthrax, swimming pool granuloma, or sporotrichosis.

1. *Tularemia.* Tularemia is associated with a history of animal (especially rabbit) or tick exposure. The primary skin lesion is a pruritic red papule. An ulcer with sharply defined edges and a depressed center appears four days after inoculation.

2. *Anthrax.* Anthrax is associated with a history of exposure to hairs, hides, animal products, fertilizer, and herbivores. A "malignant" pustule appears two to five days after inoculation. The characteristic skin lesion begins as a red papule, which vesiculates and forms a black eschar surrounded by a rim of nonpitting, nonpainful brawny edema.

3. *Swimming Pool Granuloma.* This form of granuloma is caused by *Mycobacterium marinum* and is acquired from fish tanks or swimming pools. The incubation period has not been well defined. Skin lesions consist of groups of papules on an extremity, which progress to ulceration and scab formation.

4. *Sporotrichosis.* Sporotrichosis may be acquired from exposure to plants (including decaying vegetation). After an incubation period ranging from 1 to 12 weeks, papular skin lesions appear. These lesions often ulcerate and are usually arranged in a "lymphocutaneous" distribution extending from the hand up the forearm.

H. **Trichophyton and Microsporum Species.** These species cause the majority of cases of superficial mycoses. These fungal infections of epidermal tissues occur anywhere on the body, parasitizing all keratinized tissues (skin, hair, and nails). These specialized fungi are not capable of invading deeper tissues. Invasion of the web space between the toes (tinea pedis) is a common predisposing factor for development of cellulitis of the lower extremity.

RECOMMENDED DIAGNOSTIC APPROACH

Clinical appearance of skin infections and epidemiologic factors allow the clinician to make a diagnosis in many patients without the use of other diagnostic tests. However, cultures and other tests are important in selected situations. It is particularly important to be aware of systemic sequelae of primary skin infections such as sepsis (from *S. aureus, H. influenzae,* and so forth), glomerulonephritis *(Streptococcus pyogenes),* and deep tissue invasion (myonecrosis or fasciitis).

A. **Blood Cultures.** Blood cultures should be performed if a patient has signs of systemic toxicity, especially in the setting of possible *H. influenzae* cellulitis or staphylococcal abscesses.

B. **Culture of Purulent Material.** In cases with folliculitis, cutaneous abscesses, or ulcerative lesions, this method should be considered if the patient is acutely ill or immunosuppressed.

C. **Vesiculopustular Lesions.** In patients with impetigo, cultures should be performed by swabbing the base of the vesiculopustular lesions after removing the crust.

D. **Needle Aspiration.** The yield of culture of needle aspirate of the advancing edge of cellulitis is low. A skin biopsy improves the yield but should be reserved for patients at risk for unusual organisms (diabetics) or with unusual clinical features.

E. **Serologic Tests.** Serologic tests such as streptozyme are useful in documenting sequelae of streptococcal disease but are not useful in the clinical management of primary skin infections.

F. **Wood's Lamp.** Wood lamp examination may assist in making the diagnosis of erythrasma (a red fluorescence is seen) and infections with *Microsporum* species (blue-green fluorescence is seen).

G. **Potassium Hydroxide (KOH) Preparation.** This is useful in the diagnosis of superficial mycoses.

H. **Special Cultures or Serology.** These procedures are indicated in select circumstances such as for tularemia, anthrax, sporotrichosis, or swimming pool granuloma.

I. **X-Ray Examination.** This may be indicated if gas-forming organisms or underlying osteomyelitis are suspected.

REFERENCES

1. Dellinger EP: Severe necrotizing soft-tissue infections: Multiple disease entities requiring a common approach. JAMA 246:1717, 1981.

A review of clostridial and mixed aerobic and anaerobic infections with an outline of the surgical approach.

2. Fierer J, Daniel D, Davis C: The fetid foot: Lower-extremity infections in patients with diabetes mellitus. Rev Infect Dis 1:210, 1979.

A summary of the microbiology in patients with diabetes mellitus.

3. Fisher JR, et al.: Necrotizing fasciitis: Importance of roentgenographic studies for soft-tissue gas. JAMA 241:803, 1979.

4. Fleisher G, Ludwig S, Campos J: Cellulitis: Bacterial etiology, clinical features, and laboratory findings. J Pediatr 97:591, 1980.

Microbiologic findings of cellulitis in children are documented by culture of material obtained by needle aspiration.

5. Galpin JW, et al.: Sepsis associated with decubitus ulcers. Am J Med 61:346, 1976.

A nice review of microbiology and clinical features of these infections.

6. Ginsberg MB: Cellulitis: Analysis of 101 cases and review of the literature. South Med J 74:530, 1981.

A retrospective study of clinical features.

7. Louie TJ, et al.: Aerobic and anaerobic bacteria in diabetic foot ulcers. Ann Intern Med 85:461, 1976.

8. Meislein HW, et al.: Cutaneous abscesses: Anaerobic and aerobic bacteriology and outpatient management. Ann Intern Med 87:145, 1977.

A nice discussion of clinical management and microbiologic findings.

9. Peter G, Smith A: Group A streptococcal infections of the skin and pharynx. N Engl J Med 297:311, 1977.

An excellent review of all aspects of streptococcal infections.

10. Reuler JB, Cooney TG: The pressure sore: Pathophysiology and principles of management. Ann Intern Med 94:661, 1981.
11. Swartz MN: Cellulitis and superficial infections. *In* Mandell GL, Douglas RG, Jr., Bennett JE (eds.): Principles and Practice of Infectious Disease. 1st ed. New York, Wiley, 1979, pp. 803–806.

A concise review of clinical features, microbiologic findings, and management of all types of skin infections.

12. Uman SJ, Kumin CM: Needle aspiration in the diagnosis of soft tissue infections. Arch Intern Med 135:959, 1975.

Demonstrates the potential benefit of needle aspiration cultures in patients at risk of infection from unusual organisms.

40

TOXIC SHOCK SYNDROME

By BARBARA D. KIRBY, M.D.

DEFINITION

Toxic shock syndrome is a systemic illness whose pathophysiology, although poorly understood, appears to be caused by a toxin produced by *Staphylococcus aureus*. Although the syndrome was first described in 1927, an epidemic occurring in menstruating women was recognized in the late 1970s. The Centers for Disease Control have established criteria for the diagnosis of toxic shock syndrome (TSS).

A. Major Criteria. These conditions must be present:
1. Fever (temperature greater than or equal to 38.9° C)
2. Rash (diffuse macular erythroderma)
3. Desquamation, notably on the palms and soles of the feet, which appears one to two weeks after onset of illness (assuming the patient survives to convalescence)
4. Hypotension (systolic blood pressure less than or equal to 90 mm Hg for adults or less than a fifth percentile for age in children under 16 years old, or orthostatic syncope)

B. Additional Criteria. Additional criteria consist of involvement of three or more of the following organ systems:
1. Gastrointestinal (vomiting or diarrhea at onset of illness)
2. Muscular (severe myalgia or elevation of creatine phosphokinase to at least twice normal concentration)
3. Mucous membrane (conjunctival, oropharyngeal, or vaginal hyperemia)
4. Renal (elevation of creatinine or blood urea nitrogen to at least twice normal level; greater than five white blood cells per high-power field in urine in the absence of urinary tract infection)
5. Hepatic (elevation of serum glutamic oxaloacetic transami-

nase or serum glutamic pyruvic transaminase level to at least twice normal)
  6. Hematologic (platelet count less than 100,000 per cu mm)
  7. Central nervous system (disorientation or altered consciousness without focal neurologic findings)
C. **Negative Test Results.** Negative results of the following tests, if obtained:
  1. Blood, throat, or cerebrospinal fluid cultures for other pathogens
  2. Serologic tests for Rocky Mountain spotted fever, leptospirosis, or measles

EPIDEMIOLOGY

The majority (90 per cent) of cases of TSS have been reported in menstruating women. Tampon use is a significant risk factor. Onset of illness usually begins on the fourth day of the menstrual period. However, in recurrent episodes onset often occurs earlier.

Cases occurring in nonmenstruating women, men, and children occur in the setting of established *S. aureus* infection or colonization. Examples include wound infections, nasal packs, osteomyelitis, abscesses, infected burns, cellulitis, bursitis, empyema, and septic abortion. In addition, postpartum cases have been described that occur after vaginal or cesarean delivery associated with vaginal infection or mastitis.

The causative agent of TSS is *S. aureus*. The disease appears to be toxin-mediated; however, the exact type and nature of the toxin(s) remains to be defined.

DIFFERENTIAL DIAGNOSIS

Diseases to be considered in the differential diagnosis of TSS are febrile illnesses associated with rash:
A. **Scarlet Fever**
B. **Meningococcemia**
C. **Rocky Mountain Spotted Fever**
D. **Kawasaki Disease.** Kawasaki disease, while similar to TSS, occurs in young children and does not involve hypotension.
E. **Measles and Other Viral Exanthems**
F. **Severe Drug Eruptions**

SYMPTOMS AND SIGNS (See Definition.)

A. **Symptoms.** The severity of illness may range from mild to rapidly life-threatening. Over 90 per cent of patients describe gastrointestinal symptoms (nausea, vomiting, and diarrhea), which usually begin at the onset of illness. The presence of other symptoms depends on involvement of other specific organ systems.

B. **Signs.** Evidence of vasomotor instability may range from an orthostatic fall in blood pressure to frank shock. The characteristic rash of TSS is an erythroderma (a sunburnlike rash). Conjunctival and mucous-membrane hyperemia are common. In cases associated with menstruation, vaginal discharge is sometimes present.

LABORATORY FINDINGS

Characteristic laboratory features are described in the section on Definition.

A. **Thrombocytopenia.** This is one of the most common laboratory abnormalities. The nadir in platelet count usually occurs several days into the course of illness.

B. **Staphylococcus aureus.** Isolation of *S. aureus* from vaginal cultures (in menstruation-associated cases) and from wounds or other infected sites may suggest the diagnosis of TSS but is by no means diagnostic or required for diagnosis. *S. aureus* is usually found if appropriate cultures are obtained.

RECOMMENDED DIAGNOSTIC APPROACH

A. **Blood Tests.** A complete blood count with platelets, liver function tests, urinalysis, and serum creatinine should be obtained. Arterial blood gases should be measured if pulmonary involvement is noted.

B. **Culture.** Culture should be done from the vagina (in menstruation-associated cases) or other potentially infected sites such as an abscess, wound, or blood.

C. **Tests to Rule Out Other Causes.** In certain patients tests may be indicated to rule out other possible causes such as meningococcemia, scarlet fever, Rocky Mountain spotted fever, leptospirosis, or viral exanthems.

REFERENCES

1. Centers for Disease Control: Follow up on toxic shock syndrome. Morbid Mortal Weekly Rep 29:441–445, 1980.
   The case definition.

2. Tofte RW, Williams DN: Toxic shock syndrome: Clinical and laboratory features in 15 patients. Ann Intern Med 94:149–156, 1981.
   Clinical features of toxic shock syndrome are described.

3. Fisher RF, Goodpasture HC, Peteire JD, Voth DW: Toxic shock syndrome in menstruating women. Ann Intern Med 94:156–163, 1981.
   Clinical and epidemiologic features.

4. The toxic shock syndrome (symposium). Ann Intern Med 96:831–996, 1982.
   A comprehensive symposium describing clinical, epidemiologic, and therapeutic aspects.

5. Wannamaker LW: Toxic shock: Problems in definition and diagnosis of a new syndrome. Ann Intern Med 96:775–777, 1982.
   An editorial discussing problems in diagnosis.

6. Reingold AL, Dan BB, Shands KN, et al.: Toxic-shock syndrome not associated with menstruation: A review of 54 cases. Lancet 1:1–4, 1982.

41

INFECTIVE ENDOCARDITIS

By EDWARD W. HOOK III, M.D.

DEFINITION

Infective endocarditis (IE) is an infection characterized by continuous bacteremia originating from a platelet-fibrin vegetation on the endothelial surface of the heart (primarily the cardiac valves).

EPIDEMIOLOGY AND CLASSIFICATION

A. **Acute and Subacute Forms.** Traditionally IE has been divided clinically into acute and subacute forms depending on whether untreated patients could be expected to survive for more or less than eight weeks. Other differential points are outlined opposite.

B. **Cardiac Status Classification.** Currently the acute-subacute distinction has blurred, owing to decreased incidence of rheumatic heart disease (RHD); increased survival of patients with predisposing diseases including congenital (CHD), rheumatic, and atherosclerotic heart disease; increased use of antibiotics prior to hospitalization; increased public awareness and earlier initiation of therapy; increased prevalence of intravenous drug abuse; advances in cardiac surgery; increased use of intravenous hyperalimentation and central catheters; increased general longevity; and improved microbiologic laboratory techniques.

Instead, a typology based on premorbid cardiac status provides a more useful conceptual framework. (See table on pages 302 and 303.)

C. **Prosthetic Valve IE (PVE).** This form of IE deserves additional comment. It is relatively uncommon but severe. The attack rate has gradually decreased from involving 3.2 per cent of all prosthetic valves in the 1960s to 2.1 per cent in the 1970s. Late onset (more than two months from surgery) is more common (64

FEATURE	ACUTE BACTERIAL ENDOCARDITIS	SUBACUTE BACTERIAL ENDOCARDITIS
Symptoms	Rigors, sweats, chills, back pain, arthritis, meningismus	Anorexia, weight loss, fatigue, cough, malaise
Underlying cardiac disease	Often none (60–70%)	Rheumatic heart disease; occasionally calcific aortic stenosis, idiopathic hypertrophic subaortic stenosis, click murmur; mitral stenosis
Fever	Nearly always	Most (exceptions: antibiotics, uremia, congestive heart failure, old age, central nervous system bleed)
Petechiae	15–45%	20–70%
Splenomegaly	30%	70%
Splinter hemorrhages, Roth's spots, Janeway's lesions, Osler's nodes	Rare	Rare
Murmur	Absent in ⅓ of patients with left heart lesions and ⅔ with tricuspid lesions	85%
Change in murmur	7%	17%
Pericardial rub	Rare (myocardial abscess, embolic myocardial infarction, root dissection)	10% (nonspecific pericarditis)
Erythrocyte sedimentation rate	99%	80–90%
Anemia	50–60%	80–90%
Leukocytosis	80%	40–50% (often with left shift, toxic granules, monocytes)
Thrombocytopenia	Frequent	Rare
Globulins, + rheumatoid factor	Rare	50–60%
Microorganisms	S. aureus, S. pneumoniae, N. meningitidis, S. pyogenes, H. influenzae	S. viridans, enterococci

per cent of all PVE) than early onset (less than two months, 36 per cent). The most frequent infecting organisms in PVE are staphylococci, Gram negative rods, and fungi (early onset) and S. viridans and enterococci (late onset). Blood cultures are positive in only 85 per cent of cases.

For reasons that are unclear, the aortic valve is more frequently involved than the mitral valve (the aortic valve is involved in 40 to 70 per cent of cases in different series). Mortality is high at about 55 per cent overall in most series.

	PREDISPOSING ENDOCARDIAL DISEASE	INTRAVENOUS DRUG ABUSERS	PROSTHETIC VALVE (POSTSURGICAL)
Incidence	1/1000 hospital admissions Age: 40–60 Approx. 70% all IE	Unknown Age: 20–40 Estimated 1.52 cases/1000 addicts per year	2–9% of prosthetic valves Age: 40–60 Approx. 12% all IE
Underlying disease	RHD 60% CHD 10% Other 10% None 20%	70% with no underlying heart disease Approx. 25% with RHD and CHD Approx. 5% with previous IE	Mostly RHD and CHD
Valve involved	Mitral 40% Atrial 20% Mitral + atrial 30% Tricuspid <5%	Tricuspid alone or with other valves 50% Atrial + mitral 18% Atrial 17% Mitral 14%	Mitral 20% Atrial 40–70% Atrial + mitral 30% Tricuspid 5%

Infecting organisms	Streptococci 59%	S. aureus 60%	S. aureus 20/10%*
	Streptococcus viridans 35%	Pseudomonas aeruginosa 10%	Staphylococcus Epidermidis 30/25%
	Enterococci 7%	Candida 5%	Gram-negative bacilli 20/10%
	Other 17%	S. viridans 10%	S. viridans 10/40%
	Staphylococci 21%	Enterococci 5%	Fungi 13/5
	S. aureus 18%	Other gram-negative bacilli 5%	
	Gram-negative bacilli 5%	Serratia 5%	
	Fungi <5%		
	Negative cultures 15%		
Mortality	20–25%	10–15%	50–60% (80% early onset and 40% late)
Other	Mitral valve prolapse	Presentation mostly pulmonary owing to septic pulmonary emboli (70–100%), rare systemic emboli; right atrial catheter can easily displace vegetations	Heterograft more resistant to IE; fewer ring abscess and perivalve leaks; more easily sterilized once infected

*Early or late onset.

D. Etiologic Agents

1. *Penicillin-sensitive Streptococci.* Penicillin-sensitive strep-tococci (minimal inhibitory concentration for penicillin <0.1 μg per mL) are the most common cause of IE and are isolated from more than 45 per cent of all cases of endocarditis. Species included in this category include *Streptococcus sanguis, S. bovis,* and *S. equinus.*

2. *Enterococci.* Enterococci, a subset of Group D streptococci, are less sensitive to penicillin and cause 10 to 20 per cent of all IE. Among enterococci, *S. faecalis* is the most common offender. The most common predisposing situations to this infection are in old men after a genitourinary manipulation and in young women after an obstetric-gynecologic procedure. Infection with enterococci may occur after gastrointestinal intervention or with intravenous drug abuse. Infection generally occurs in patients with pre-existing heart disease, although in some series up to half have normal valves. The condition is usually subacute at initial examination.

3. *Staphylococci.* Infection with staphylococci is relatively common, accounting for 25 to 30 per cent of IE and 60 per cent of IE related to intravenous drug abuse. The disease may follow a fulminant acute course with multiple complications (congestive heart failure from valve destruction, renal failure, metastatic infection, emboli, and splenomegaly, among others) and high mortality (overall about 40 per cent). Among intravenous drug abusers, IE is usually right-sided, and in nonaddicts, usually left-sided. Among nonaddicts approximately 50 per cent of staphylococcal IE has no identifiable portal of entry.

Staphylococcal bacteremia occurs more than five times as often as IE, so positive blood cultures do not necessarily mean IE. Factors that may help distinguish the two are outlined in the following table:

**FACTORS THAT DISTINGUISH *S. AUREUS*
ENDOCARDITIS FROM BACTEREMIA**

Diagnostic of endocarditis
1. New pathologic or changing heart murmur
2. Major embolic event(s)
3. New splenomegaly (rare)
4. Peripheral microembolic signs (rare)

Characteristic of endocarditis
1. Intravenous drug use
2. Prosthetic valve
3. Meningitis *(de novo)*
4. Severe renal failure, microscopic hematuria (especially casts)
5. Cardiac conduction defects, peri-carditis, congestive heart failure
6. Teichoic acid antibodies (sub-stantial titer)

Supportive of endocarditis
1. Rheumatic valvular heart murmur
2. Community-acquired bacter-emia, delayed treatment, no primary site of infection

Suggestive of bacteremia
1. Hospital-acquired bacteremia
2. Promptly treated bacteremia related to wounds or use of intravenous devices

4. *Gram-Negative Bacteria.* Gram-negative IE has been distinctly uncommon in the past (1 to 3 per cent). In recent years the incidence has increased (5 to 10 per cent in natural valves and 17 per cent in prosthetic valves) as a result of increasing narcotic addiction, cardiac valve replacement, immunosuppressive therapy, and widespread use of antibiotics.

5. *Culture-Negative IE.* The incidence of persistently negative blood cultures has in numerous series remained 15 to 20 per cent. In recent years the improved microbiologic techniques have been offset by the increased use of preculture outpatient antibiotics and by the increased occurrence of nonbacterial IE.

Causes of apparently culture-negative endocarditis include:

1. Prior antimicrobial treatment
2. "Fastidious" bacteria
3. Q fever
4. Fungi
5. Acid-fast bacteria
6. *Chlamydia*
7. Noninfective endocarditis
8. ? L forms of bacteria
9. ? Virus

While no consensus exists as to how far to look for a microbiologic diagnosis before declaring the case culture-negative, the Mayo Clinic recommends:

a. Review of history of previous antibiotics, intravenous drug abuse, exposure to gonococcus, brucellosis, psittacosis, nongonococcal urethritis or cervicitis, Q fever, and recent dental or dermatologic manipulation
b. Gram's stain, biopsy, and culture any cutaneous lesions
c. Obtaining blood culture results from the referring hospital if possible
d. Use of nutritional supplements in the culture and continuation of incubation for three to four weeks with blind subcultures and Gram's stains
e. Obtaining two blood cultures each for *Brucella, Neisseria,* and fungi
f. Repeating two sets of routine blood cultures
g. Obtaining serologies for the organisms listed above
h. Echocardiography
i. Bone marrow biopsy and culture

6. *Fungi.* Infection with fungi is generally uncommon as a cause (1 per cent of cases involving the native valve), but there is increasing incidence with prosthetic valves (18 per cent of early and 5 per cent of late onset disease). There is increasing incidence also with intravenous drug abuse and intravenous hyperalimentation. Among nonaddict patients, fungal species include *Candida albicans* (found in normal gastrointestinal flora, presumably unsuppressed when antibiotics destroy normal limiting bacterial flora), and *Aspergillus* species (common

airborne organisms, presumably causing contamination intra-operatively). In addicts, the chief fungi are *C. parapsilosis, C. tropicalis,* and *C. stellatoidea.* These have been occasionally recovered from drug packages and mucosal surfaces that may contaminate the skin during intravenous injection.

Fungal IE characteristically produces bulky vegetations. Major emboli occur frequently (in 18 of 24 patients in one series). Tissue invasion is also frequent. Mortality without surgery is almost 100 per cent and even with surgery is 80 per cent.

7. *Other Organisms.* Numerous case reports of uncommon organisms exist, often found retrospectively at autopsy in cases of "culture-negative" endocarditis. These include *Corynebacterium*, Q fever organisms, *Brucella, Chlamydia,* and *Legionella.*

PATHOGENESIS

A. **Pathogenesis of IE.** The pathogenesis involves several steps:
   1. *Endothelial Valve Damage.* Normally highly resistant to infection, endothelium becomes susceptible when disrupted by foreign bodies (such as catheters, prosthetic valves), abnormal hemodynamic patterns (Venturi, jet effects from incompetent valves, ventricular septal defects, or atrial septal defects) and other unknown factors (possibly metabolic, immunologic) that expose connective tissue and release tissue factors that promote thrombus formation.
   2. *Sterile Platelet-Fibrin Thrombus Formation.* This condition—so-called nonbacterial thrombotic endocarditis—provides a potential meshwork haven for microorganisms. Without infection, the thrombus tends to spontaneously regress, and the susceptibility to IE decreases.
   3. *Bacteremia Leads to Colonization.* A wide variety of events such as dental extractions, tooth brushing, barium enemas, cystoscopy, and insertion of an intrauterine device produce bacteremia that is usually transient and spontaneously resolving.
   4. *Infection of Thrombus.* The likelihood of infection varies with several parameters:
      a. Age of thrombus: experimentally, younger thrombi are more susceptible.
      b. Location of thrombus: for unknown reasons, infection is most likely in atrial or mitral valves, less likely in tricuspid or pulmonary valves, and least likely with extracardiac endothelial vegetations (vascular grafts).
      c. Different organisms have various likelihood of causing infection, presumably because of variation in adherence factors.
      d. Within the vegetation, infecting organisms exhibit geographically varying metabolic rates; superficially located organisms replicate rapidly and produce the characteristic

continuous bacteremia. However, deep organisms are in the lag phase of growth and require long-term treatment.

e. Finally, infection is enhanced by local agranulocytosis. The vegetation's meshwork is too small to allow polymorphonuclear neutrophils to enter, permitting unimpeded bacterial growth.

5. *Immunopathologic Mechanisms.* A number of mechanisms appear to be involved, but the details and clinical significance of these are not well established. Antimyocardial antibodies, antimicrobial antibodies, circulating immune complexes, and some evidence of cell-mediated immune reactions have been documented.

DIAGNOSIS

A. **Clinical Presentation.** Typical symptoms and signs from several series are pooled in the following table:

SYMPTOMS	PER CENT	PHYSICAL FINDINGS	PER CENT
Fever	80	Fever	90
Chills	40	Heart murmur	85
Weakness	40	Changing murmur	5–10
Dyspnea	40	New murmur	3–5
Sweats	25	Embolic phenomena	>50
Anorexia	25	Skin manifestations	50
Weight loss	25	Osler's nodes	10–23
Malaise	25	Splinter hemorrhages	15
Cough	25	Petechiae	20–40
Skin lesions	20	Janeway's lesions	<10
Stroke	20	Splenomegaly	20–57
Nausea and vomiting	20	Septic complications (pneumonia, meningitis, etc.)	20
Headache	15		
Myalgia and arthralgia	15	Mycotic aneurysms	20
Edema	15	Clubbing	12–52
Chest pain	15	Retinal lesion	5–10
Delirium and coma	10	Signs of renal failure	10–15
Hemoptysis	10		
Back pain	10		
Abdominal pain	10–15		

The actual constellation of manifestations varies considerably among different patient populations, and some authorities estimate that reliance on the classic diagnostic criteria would result in failure to suspect IE in up to 90 per cent of cases. Consequently, heavy reliance must be placed on the laboratory findings.

B. **Laboratory Findings**

1. *Blood Cultures (BC).* Blood cultures remain the principal diagnostic test for IE. Success of pathogen recovery depends on the number of cultures, volume of blood obtained per culture, processing techniques, type of pathogen involved, and

preculture use of antibiotics. Not significant in IE are the time of culture and the site.

a. Number of BC. The standard data come from the 1967 work of Werner et al. In 178 cases of IE, the percentages of positive cultures were:

Organism	First BC (Per Cent)	First Two BC (Per Cent)
Streptococci	96	98
Staphylococci	88	100
Other	82	100

With fastidious or nonbacterial pathogens, or when preculture antibiotics have been given, a greater number of blood cultures may be necessary. Overall, current recommendations suggest routine two to three blood cultures in the first 24 hours.

b. Volume of Blood. There is an approximately linear relationship between the bacterial yield and the blood volume cultured. Ten mL is the minimun essential volume per culture. Some institutions recommend as much as 30 cu cm per culture.

c. Preculture Antibiotics. In a study of 32 patients eventually diagnosed to have IE with positive blood cultures, 17 had received outpatient antibiotics in the two weeks before admission and 15 had not. There was a significant reduction in the positivity of initial blood culture results in the treated group, although the treatment did not halt the disease or prevent the ultimate positivity of the culture.

d. Timing of Blood Culture. Because bacteremia from IE is continuous, there is no increased yield from cultures obtained over specified intervals or with acute temperature elevations.

e. Site of BC. It has been shown that there are measurably but not significantly greater numbers of bacteria in arterial versus venous blood. Arterial blood cultures give no advantage over venous cultures.

2. *Immunologic Tests*

    a. Nonspecific laboratory indicators of immune processes have long been recognized:

	Per Cent
Anemia	70–90
Erythrocyte sedimentation rate (mean 57)	90–100
Rheumatoid factor	40–50
Hypergammaglobulinemia	20–30
Hypocomplementemia	5–15
Proteinuria	50–65
Microscopic hematuria	30–50
Red blood cell casts	12

b. Recently more sophisticated assays have been devised; however, the nature and clinical significance of these are poorly understood.

3. **Echocardiography.** Echocardiography has been extensively evaluated for its utility in the initial diagnosis of IE, the diagnosis of complications of IE, the choice and timing of therapeutic interventions (medical versus surgical) and prognostication.

   a. **Initial Diagnosis of IE.** Some bacteremic patients without clinical findings of IE in fact have vegetations that can be demonstrated by echocardiography. This group is small (less than 10 per cent). Echocardiography is not routinely useful in bacteremia but is indicated with clear clinical evidence of IE, with clear risk factors for IE, and with intravascular source or unidentified source of bacteremia.

   b. **Diagnosis of Complications of IE: Vegetations.** The overall sensitivity and specificity of two-dimensional and M-mode echocardiography have been widely estimated and range from 13 to 83 per cent and 60 to 90 per cent, respectively.

The best study of echocardiography to date is from Come et al., who prospectively evaluated with M-mode echocardiography 189 febrile patients who were then subsequently diagnosed on clinical grounds to have either IE (51 of 189) or non-IE (138 of 159). The calculated sensitivity was 37 per cent, specificity 96 per cent, predictive value of a positive test 76 per cent, and predictive value of a negative test 80 per cent.

The diagnosis of vegetations is particularly difficult with abnormal underlying valves. In one study of 85 patients with mitral valve prolapse, abnormal echoes consistent with vegetations were seen on the anterior leaflet in 11, in the posterior leaflet in 18, and in both in 5; however, only 1 patient had clinical IE. Thus, in approximately 40 per cent of mitral valve prolapse, false-positive echocardiograms can result. Two-dimensional echocardiography appears more specific in mitral valve prolapse.

In general, echocardiography provides another adjunctive test that is useful for confirming the diagnosis of IE when it is suspected on clinical grounds or by the presence of established risk factors. This method is helpful in identifying complications of IE and population groups with worse prognoses.

4. **Cardiac Catheterization.** Indications for catheterization include preoperative hemodynamic assessment in patients with congestive heart failure, persistent sepsis, or recurrent embolism. Cardiac catheterization is also useful for evaluation of concurrent coronary artery disease, left or right shunts, ruptured sinus of Valsalva aneurysms, valve ring abscesses, mycotic aneurysms, and for quantitative culture on both sides of tricuspid and pulmonary valves in right heart IE with negative echocardiographic results.

5. **Electrocardiogram (ECG).** The ECG is useful for detecting conduction disturbances resulting from myocardial abscesses

(partial or complete heart blocks, premature ventricular contractions) or emboli causing myocardial infarction.

RECOMMENDED DIAGNOSTIC APPROACH

A. **History (High Index of Suspicion Required).** Important factors include:
 1. Malaise, weight loss, low-grade fever
 2. Underlying heart disease (rheumatic, valvular, or congenital)
 3. Intravenous drug abuse
 4. Procedures (dental, urologic, or gastrointestinal manipulations)
 5. Prior antibiotic use
B. **Physical Examination.** This should cover:
 1. Vital signs
 2. Cardiac: presence or changed murmur, signs of new congestive failure
 3. Peripheral stigmata of disease: petechiae, splinter hemorrhage, and splenomegaly
C. **Laboratory Tests.** Laboratory tests should include:
 1. Blood cultures (three times)
 2. Leukocyte count
 3. Urinalysis (presence of red blood cells or red blood cell casts)

REFERENCES

1. Mayo Clinic Proceedings 57:4–175, 1982.

An extensive symposium covering a wide variety of topics, including the following articles:

a. Pruitt RS: William Osler and his Gulstonian lectures on malignant endocarditis. pp. 4–9.
b. Wright AJ, et al.: Experimental animal endocarditis. pp. 10–14.
c. Hermans PE: The clinical manifestations of IE. pp. 15–20.
d. Washington JA: The role of the microbiology lab in the diagnosis and antimicrobial treatment of IE. pp. 22–32.
e. Wilson WR, et al.: General considerations in the diagnosis and treatment of IE. pp. 81–85.
f. Johnson CM, et al.: Pediatric endocarditis. pp. 86–94.
g. Wilson WR, et al.: Treatment of penicillin-sensitive streptococcal IE. pp. 95–100.
h. Wilkowski CJ: Enterococcal endocarditis. pp. 101–105.
i. Thompson RL: Staphylococcal IE. pp. 106–114.
j. Geraci JE, et al.: Endocarditis due to gram-negative bacteria. pp. 145–148.
k. Van Scoy RE: Culture-negative endocarditis. pp. 149–154.
l. Wilson WR, et al.: Prosthetic valve endocarditis. pp. 155–161.
m. Wilson WR, et al.: Management of complications of IE. pp. 162–170.
n. Keys TF: Antimicrobial prophylaxis for patients with congenital or valvular heart disease. pp. 171–175.

2. Come PC, et al.: Diagnostic accuracy of M-mode echo in active IE and prognostic implication of ultrasound-detectable vegetations. Am Heart J 103:839, 1982.

Prospective evaluation of sensitivity, specificity, and diagnostic accuracy of M-mode diagnosis of vegetations.

3. Scheld WM: Bacterial adherence in the pathogenesis of endocarditis. J Clin Invest 61:1394, 1978.

Review of interaction of bacterially produced dextran, platelets, fibrin, and IE.

4. Werner AS, et al.: Studies on the bacteremia of bacterial endocarditis. JAMA 202:199, 1967.

The first study of rate on blood culture positivity in IE; the basis of the "2 BC" tradition.

5. Bayer AS: Staph bacteremia and endocarditis. Arch Intern Med 142:169, 1982.

Suggests an algorithm for separating staphylococcal IE from non-IE bacteremia.

42

INFECTIOUS MONONUCLEOSIS

By RICHARD O. CUMMINS, M.D.

DEFINITION

Infectious mononucleosis (IM) is a specific infection caused by the Epstein-Barr (EB) virus, a member of the herpes group. For years, however, the term "infectious mononucleosis" has been applied to nonspecific clinical syndromes that consist of generalized lymphadenopathy, absolute and relative lymphocytosis with an increased number of atypical lymphocytes, fever, sore throat, and transient heterophil antibody responses. These "mononucleosis-like" syndromes may or may not have heterophil antibody responses and may or may not be caused by the EB virus.

A. Criteria for Diagnosis

  1. Unequivocal diagnosis is established if one of several anti-Epstein-Barr virus antibodies is identified. These antibody titers have helped define the epidemiology of EB virus infection, but in practice there are few reasons to obtain them.
  2. The presence of the classic clinical, hematologic, and serologic picture noted below under Clinical Manifestations is sufficient for diagnosis. It should be noted, however, that 5 to 10 per cent of patients with documented EB mononucleosis have negative heterophil tests—so-called heterophil-negative IM.

EPIDEMIOLOGY

A. IM is worldwide in distribution. In economically underdeveloped areas a subclinical or nonspecific infection occurs in virtually all young children. In middle and upper socioeconomic groups, however, only 50 to 60 per cent of adolescents have antibodies to EBV. Moreover, infection in young adults (15 to 25 years old)

produces the familiar clinical picture only 30 to 50 per cent of the time. Most clinical cases (60 per cent) occur in 15- to 24-year-olds.
B. Transmission usually occurs by salivary exchange during close personal contact. The disease, however, is not very contagious, with an annual incidence of less than 15 per cent among susceptible college students.
C. The incubation period is 30 to 50 days in adults and 10 to 14 days in children.

CLINICAL MANIFESTATIONS

A. **History**
   1. Clinicians usually first suspect IM when patients who complain of pharyngitis are noted to have a more generalized lymphadenopathy associated with fever and malaise.
   2. In the typical case a three- to five-day prodrome of fatigue, myalgia, and malaise occurs, followed by a frankly clinical 7- to 20-day period in which the major subjective symptoms are sore throat, fever, headache, and weakness.
B. **Classic Features.** The classic features of IM, and the basis for diagnosis, include the following triad (numbers in parentheses show the expected frequency of findings in documented cases of IM):
   1. *Clinical Signs and Symptoms*
      a. Lymphadenopathy (90 per cent), splenomegaly (50 to 60 per cent)
      b. Sore throat (70 per cent), exudative pharyngitis (40 per cent), malaise (50 per cent)
      c. Fever: over 38.3° C in 70 to 80 per cent and lasting over a week in 90 per cent of the febrile cases and over two weeks in 50 per cent
   2. *Hematologic Picture*
      a. Absolute lymphocytosis: over 4000 per cu mm (>90 per cent)
      b. Relative lymphocytosis: over 50 per cent (> 90 per cent)
      c. Atypical (Downy cell) lymphocytes: over 10 per cent (>90 per cent)
   3. *Elevated Titers of Heterophil Antibody.* (See laboratory studies.) Titers are greater than (a) 1:56 in 80 per cent of cases, (b) 1:224 in 65 per cent, and (c) 1:896 in 35 per cent.
C. **Pharyngitis.** In patients with pharyngitis, four physical findings occur significantly more often in heterophil-positive patients than in heterophil-negative patients (numbers in parentheses show frequency in heterophil-positive patients):
   1. Inguinal adenopathy (53 per cent)
   2. Posterior auricular adenopathy (33 per cent)
   3. Palatine petechiae (27 per cent)
   4. Marked axillary adenopathy (20 per cent)

D. **Other Signs and Symptoms.** Vigorous pursuit of the diagnosis is really only necessary when IM is suspected as the cause of these other manifestations (numbers in parentheses show the expected frequency of the finding in documented cases of IM):

   1. Hepatomegaly (50 per cent).
   2. Jaundice (4 per cent).
   3. Rash (urticarial and morbilliform; 2 per cent).
   4. Neurologic problems occur in only 2 per cent of cases but can be quite alarming. They include aseptic meningitis, encephalitis, cranial nerve paralysis, transverse myelitis, and Guillain-Barré syndrome.
   5. Other problems that occur in less than 1 per cent of cases include pericarditis, myocarditis, arteritis, pulmonary infiltrates and effusions, hilar adenopathy, renal nephritis, hepatitis, pancreatitis, hemolytic anemia, thrombocytopenia, and splenic rupture (0.5 per cent).

DIFFERENTIAL DIAGNOSIS

Infectious mononucleosis exists as part of the differential diagnosis for two conditions:

A. **Sore Throats and Pharyngitis.** Infectious mononucleosis causes few of the sore throats and pharyngitis cases seen by most clinicians (usually less than 2 per cent). If suggestive history and physical findings are absent, the possibility that IM caused the pharyngitis is remote, and diagnostic tests—especially tests for heterophil antibodies—are not indicated. (See Chapter 36.)

B. **Prolonged Malaise, Low-grade Fever, Upper Respiratory Infections, Unexplained Viral Illnesses, and Lymphadenopathy.** This clinical picture occurs frequently in general medical practice. Infectious mononucleosis is among several diseases that occasionally cause these complaints and findings:

   1. *Febrile Pharyngotonsillitis.* This can be caused by streptococcal or viral infection, diphtheria, or Vincent's angina.
   2. *Blood Dyscrasias.* These are particularly common in leukemia.
   3. *Rubella.* The rash of IM spares the face, whereas the rash of rubella regularly affects the face.
   4. *Cytomegaloviral Infection.* Fever, splenomegaly, hepatitis, and atypical lymphocytes occur with cytomegaloviral infection. However, an older age group is usually involved, pharyngitis and cervical adenopathy are rare, and a history of multiple blood transfusions is often present.
   5. *Toxoplasmosis.* Fever, generalized lymphadenopathy, atypical lymphocytosis, splenomegaly, and malaise occur with toxoplasmosis. Pharyngitis, however, is absent or minimal.
   6. *Heterophil-negative Infectious Mononucleosis.* This term is applied to patients who have virtually all of the classic signs and symptoms of IM, especially lymphocytosis with atypical lymphocytes, but who have negative heterophil reactions.

This can occur in up to 10 per cent of "classic" cases. There are several causes of these heterophil-negative mononucleosislike illnesses:

a. **True EB Virus Infection.** This occurs in 30 to 50 per cent of cases, but other serologic tests are required to make this diagnosis, which is more common in children and the elderly. Repeat Monospot testing is often positive.

b. **True Cytomegaloviral Infection.** This occurs in 20 to 40 per cent of cases. Specific complement-fixing antibody tests are needed to confirm this diagnosis.

c. **Miscellaneous Causes.** Miscellaneous causes account for 10 per cent of cases. Causes include toxoplasmosis, rubella, listeriosis, hepatitis, mumps, adenovirus, serum sickness, and several drug reactions (with isoniazid, para-aminosalicylic acid, and phenytoin).

LABORATORY TESTS

A. **The Serology of Mononucleosis.** In 1932 Paul and Bunnell first demonstrated that the serum of patients with mononucleosis agglutinated the red blood cells of sheep and horses (*heterophil agglutination test* or the *"presumptive test"*).

1. *Other Diseases That May Produce Sheep Cell Agglutinins.* Persons with serum sickness, hepatitis, Hodgkin's disease, rubella, leukemia, sarcoidosis, rheumatoid arthritis, adenoviral infections, and even normal people may have low titers (the nonspecific Forssman's antibody).

2. *Specific Differentiation.* Additional tests are used:

a. Beef red blood cells remove IM heterophil antibodies; guinea pig kidney cells do not.

b. Beef red blood cells do not remove the heterophil antibodies in normal people; guinea pig kidney cells do.

c. Both beef red blood cells and guinea pig kidney cells remove the heterophil antibodies of serum sickness.

d. Thus the *Davidsohn exclusion test* is occasionally used. (1) The heterophil agglutinin titer is measured with horse or sheep red blood cells. If the titer is elevated, generally over 1:28, then (2) the titer is measured after serum is mixed first with beef red blood cells and then with guinea pig kidney. (3) A decrease in the original titer after beef red blood cell absorption (two to three tube dilutions) but not after guinea pig kidney absorption (titer remains at or above 1:64) is diagnostic of IM.

3. *Monospot Test.* In practice, the Monospot test* (with horse red blood cells) is generally used to detect heterophile antibodies and has virtually replaced the Paul-Bunnell and Davidsohn tests. A positive reaction is 1:80. Monospot test parameters that have emerged from population studies of United

---

*Ortho Diagnostic Systems, Inc., Raritan, New Jersey.

States college students in whom the prevalence of probable EB virus infection was 25 to 30 per cent include:
   a. Sensitivity and specificity of 95 per cent.
   b. Positive and negative predictive values of 95 per cent.
   c. The false-positive tests probably represent low titers from previous infection.
   d. The false-negative tests are usually positive when repeated.

4. *Heterophil Agglutinins.* Heterophil agglutinins are often present during the first week of illness but may be delayed. In one study of documented cases of IM, 38 per cent of patients had antibodies during the first week of clinical signs, 60 per cent during the second week, and 80 per cent during the third week.

B. **The Hematologic Picture.** It should be noted that the levels of absolute and relative lymphocytosis mentioned earlier, as well as the percentage of atypical lymphocytes, are dynamic levels. They generally occur at some stage of the disease, but not necessarily at the time that blood samples are taken from a particular patient. Specific values for the lymphocytosis may have been obtained before or after a patient's peak level. Clinical judgment therefore is required.

RECOMMENDED DIAGNOSTIC APPROACH

A. White blood cell and differential counts should be performed.
B. If the following are found, the Monospot test should be used:
   1. Elevated (>10 per cent) atypical lymphocytes, *plus*
   2. Absolute lymphocytosis (>4000 per cu mm), *or*
   3. Relative lymphocytosis (>50 per cent).
C. If the Monospot test result is greater than 1:80, diagnosis is confirmed. Only 25 to 30 per cent of patients with this peripheral blood picture have positive Monospot test results.

REFERENCES

1. Jordan MC: Nomenclature for mononucleosis syndromes. JAMA 234: 45–46, 1975.
2. Henke CE, Kurland LT, Elveback LR: Infectious mononucleosis in Rochester, Minnesota, 1950 through 1969. Am J Epidem 93:483–490, 1973.
3. English EC, Geyman JP: The efficiency and cost effectiveness of diagnostic tests for infectious mononucleosis. J Fam Pract 6:977–981, 1978.
4. Aronson MD, Komaroff AL, Pass TM, et al.: Heterophil antibody in adults with sore throat: Frequency and clinical presentation. Ann Intern Med 96:505–508, 1982.
5. Niederman JC: Epstein-Barr virus infection, including mononucleosis. Chap. 212. *In* Harrison's Principles of Internal Medicine. 10th ed. New York, McGraw-Hill, 1983, pp. 1170–1174.
6. Weinstein L, Branch WT, Jr.: The infectious mononucleosis-like syndrome and other causes of fever, pharyngitis, and lymphadenopathy. *In* Branch WT (ed.): Office Practice of Medicine. Philadelphia, W. B. Saunders Company, 1982, pp. 48–56.
7. Niederman JC: Infectious mononucleosis. *In* Wyngaarden JB, Smith LH,

Jr. (eds.): Cecil's Textbook of Medicine. 16th ed. Philadelphia, W. B. Saunders Company, 1982, pp. 1651–1654.

8. Horwitz CA, Henle W, Henle G, et al.: Heterophile-negative infectious mononucleosis and mononucleosis-like illness. Laboratory confirmation of 43 cases. Am J Med 63:947–949, 1977.

9. Gantz NM: Infectious mononucleosis: Differential diagnosis. *In* Gantz N, Gleckman RA (eds.): Manual of Clinical Problems in Infectious Disease. Boston, Little, Brown & Company, 1979.

43

PNEUMONIA

By BARBARA D. KIRBY, M.D.

DEFINITION

Pneumonia is defined as infection of the lung parenchyma.

A. Etiology. A large number and variety of bacterial, mycoplasmal, chlamydial, rickettsial, mycobacterial, fungal, viral, and parasitic pathogens may cause pneumonia.

B. Pathogenesis. Microorganisms gain entry to the lung through one of four means:

1. *Aspiration of Oropharyngeal or Nasopharyngeal Microorganisms.* This is the most common cause of bacterial pneumonia.
2. *Inhalation of Microbes.* This is a common cause.
3. *Hematogenous Spread.* Hematogenous spread is less common.
4. *Direct Spread from Contiguous Site of Infection.* This is the least common means.

CLUES TO ETIOLOGIC DIAGNOSIS

A. Demographic Data

1. *Age*
   a. **Mycoplasma pneumoniae.** *M. pneumoniae* is a major cause of pneumonia in children, the most common cause in persons of ages 18 to 40, and uncommon in patients older than 40.
   b. **Legionnaires' Disease.** This disease is rare in children and represents up to 15 per cent of community-acquired and nosocomial pneumonia in adults.
   c. **Pneumococci.** These organisms are the most common cause of pneumonia in adults over 40 years old.
2. *Sex.* There is a male to female predominance (2 to 3:1) in most bacterial pneumonias.

B. Family History

1. *Incubation Period.* The incubation period for *M. pneumoniae*

is 14 to 21 days. A history of upper respiratory infection in a family member may suggest this cause.

C. **Social Habits**

1. *Alcohol and Cigarette Use.* These are risk factors for development of pneumonia and for increased morbidity. Fifty per cent of all cases of *Klebsiella* pneumonia (generally an uncommon form of pneumonia) occur in alcoholics.

2. *Intravenous and Recreational Drug Use*

   a. **Decreased Consciousness.** Episodes of decreased conciousness increase risk for aspiration.

   b. **Pulmonary Infiltrates.** Pulmonary infiltrates in an intravenous drug user may be hematogenously spread from endocarditis (usually caused by *Staphylococcus aureus*).

3. *Sexual Preference.* Pneumonia in a homosexual male indicates the possibility of acquired immunodeficiency syndrome (AIDS) associated with *Pneumocystic carinii* or other opportunistic infections.

D. **Season**

1. *Influenza.* Influenza usually occurs in winter, although episodic cases may occur in other seasons.

2. *Pneumococcal Pneumonia.* This form has peak incidence in late winter and early spring.

3. *Legionnaires' Disease.* This form has a peak in summer and fall.

E. **Exposure to Animals**

1. *Psittacine Birds.* Exposure can cause psittacosis (*Chlamydia psittaci*).

2. *Pigeons.* Exposure can lead to cryptococcosis (*Cryptococcus neoformans*).

3. *Livestock.* Exposure to goats, sheep, or cattle can cause Q fever (*Coxiella burnetti*).

4. *Small Animals (Rabbits) and Ticks.* Exposure can cause tularemia (*Francisella tularensis*).

5. *Rodents and Fleas.* Rodents and fleas may carry plague (*Yersinia pestis*).

F. **Occupational Risk Factors.** Construction work is a risk factor for legionnaires' disease.

G. **Travel History**

1. *Overnight Travel.* During the incubation period (two to ten days) this is a risk factor for legionnaires' disease.

2. *Travel to Endemic Areas*

   a. **Southeast Asia.** Meliodosis and tuberculosis are prevalent.

   b. **Ohio and Mississippi Valley.** Histoplasmosis is endemic to this area.

   c. **Lower Sonoran Life Zone.*** Coccidioidomycosis is endemic to this area.

   d. **Southwestern United States.** Plague is endemic to this region.

---

*In the United States includes areas of California, Arizona, New Mexico, and Texas.

H. Setting. The setting in which the pneumonia is acquired may provide a clue to the origin.

1. *Community-acquired*
    a. **Pneumococcal Pneumonia (Streptococcus pneumoniae).** This is the primary community-acquired bacterial pneumonia.
    b. **Mycoplasma pneumoniae.** This organism infects children and young adults in closed environments such as military barracks, dormitories, or family settings.
    c. **Other.** Other sources of pneumonia include *Legionella pneumophila* (legionnaires' disease), *Hemophilus influenzae, Klebsiella pneumoniae, S. aureus* (especially following influenza outbreaks), anaerobic bacteria, and tuberculosis.
2. *Nosocomial (Institutional or Hospital-acquired).* In the hospital setting there is increased frequency of staphylococcal and gram-negative enteric bacilli (*Pseudomonas aeruginosa, Proteus, Escherichia coli, Serratia),* and depending on the host, opportunistic fungi and parasites.

I. Predisposing Factors
1. *Underlying Illness*
    a. **Diabetes Mellitus, Chronic Obstructive Pulmonary Disease, Congestive Heart Failure.** Patients with these conditions have increased risk for pneumonia.
    b. **Cystic Fibrosis.** This condition is associated with an increased incidence of *P. aeruginosa* and *S. aureus* pneumonia.
    c. **Specific Defects in Host Defenses.** These defects may be either disease- or drug-induced (corticosteroid, cytotoxic chemotherapy).
        1). **Leukopenia.** Leukopenia predisposes to bacterial or *Aspergillus* pneumonia.
        2). **Humoral Defects.** These defects predispose to *S. pneumoniae* or *H. influenzae* pneumonia.
        3). **T cell Defects.** T cell defects may result in bacterial *(L. pneumophila)*, fungal *(Aspergillus, Candida, Cryptococcus neoformans, Histoplasma),* parasitic (*P. carinii, Strongyloides stercoralis),* or viral (cytomegalovirus, herpes virus) pneumonia.
2. *Decreased Gag Reflex.* In the following situations this condition predisposes to aspiration: seizure disorder, endotracheal intubation, cerebrovascular accident, other neurologic disorders, or if it is drug-induced (from narcotics or alcohol).
3. *Recent Influenza Infection.* This factor predisposes to bacterial superinfection. Because of damage to normal lung host defenses, the course of the subsequent bacterial pneumonia is unusually virulent and often fatal.
4. *Excavation.* Excavation near the patient's residence is a risk factor for legionnaires' disease.

CLINICAL PRESENTATION

(See the later discussion of Specific Pathogens for classic presentations of common pneumonias.)

A. **Symptoms**
1. *Recent Upper Respiratory Tract Infection.* This finding is common in patients with bacterial pneumonia (except for legionnaires' disease).
2. *Fever.* Temperature elevation occurs in most patients with pneumonia. Major exceptions include elderly and debilitated patients with overwhelming infection.
3. *Cough.* Most patients have cough. The character of cough may be helpful in etiologic diagnosis.
   a. **Hacking, Troublesome, or Nonproductive.** This type of cough is associated with *M. pneumoniae.*
   b. **Nontroublesome and Nonproductive.** This type of cough is characteristic of legionnaires' disease.
   c. **Productive.** This type is common to most bacterial pneumonias.
4. *Chills.* Shaking chills are common in bacterial pneumonias. A single chill at onset suggests pneumococcal pneumonia.
5. *Vital Signs*
   a. **Temperature Curve.** The temperature curve may suggest a diagnosis (for example, it is continuous in legionnaires' disease).
   b. **Heart Rate.** In adults heart rate increases 10 beats per minute for each Fahrenheit degree of temperature elevation (15 beats per minute per centigrade degree). A relative bradycardia suggests legionnaires' disease, *Mycoplasma* infection, tularemia, or influenza.
   c. **Respiratory Rate and Effort**
6. *Physical Examination*
   a. **Mental Status Changes.** This may suggest hypoxemia or concomitant meningitis, or both.
   b. **Cyanosis.** Presence of cyanosis suggests hypoxemia.
   c. **Chest.** The chest should be examined to detect rales, signs of consolidation, or signs of pleural fluid.
   d. **Abdomen.** The abdomen should be examined for ileus (pneumococcal pneumonia), splenectomy scar (pneumococcal sepsis or *Hemophilus* sepsis), and hepatic tenderness (may be found in pneumococcal pneumonia).

LABORATORY FINDINGS

A. **Sputum.** Gross and microscopic examination is critical to determine the etiologic agent.
1. *Color.* The sputum may be bloody (in patients with legionnaires' disease); rusty ("classic" pneumococcal pneumonia); the color of currant jelly ("classic" *Klebsiella* pneumonia); yellow-green (typically seen in patients with bacterial pneumonia); or like anchovy paste (amebae).
2. *Amount.* The amount of sputum produced is often scant in *Mycoplasma* or pure viral pneumonias.
3. *Consistency.* The sputum may be purulent (most bacterial pneumonias), watery (*Mycoplasma,* legionnaires' disease), or mucoid (*Klebsiella,* pneumococcal).

4. *Odor.* Feculent sputum suggests anaerobic organisms.
5. *Stains.* A "good" sputum sample has less than 10 epithelial cells and more than 25 polymorphonuclear leukocytes per high-power field.
   a. **Gram's Stain.** The presence of a predominant organism with morphologic and staining characteristics of a known bacterial pathogen suggests that this is the etiologic agent. Interpretation of Gram's stain tests must be done by an experienced microbiologist, technician, or clinician. Gram's stain examination of patients with legionnaires' disease does not reveal the gram-negative *Legionella*.
   b. **Direct Fluorescent Antibody Stain.** This method is useful in diagnosis of legionnaires' disease; in a single sputum specimen the sensitivity of the stain (if appropriate conjugates are used) is 60 per cent and the specificity is 95 per cent.
   c. **Fungal Stains**
   d. **Acid-fast Stains**
   e. **Examination for Parasitic Ova**
B. **Sputum, Blood, Cerebrospinal Fluid, and Pleural Fluid Cultures.** These cultures are done as indicated. Culture of blood and sputum should be done in all hospitalized patients. Cerebrospinal fluid should be examined in patients with altered mental status, headache, or other signs of central nervous system involvement.
C. **Radiograph.** "Classic" x-ray findings may suggest a diagnosis, but the overlap in radiographic findings is sufficiently great that use of the radiograph is misleading. Examples include:
   1. *Lobar Involvement.* This suggests pneumococcal pneumonia or legionnaires' disease.
   2. *Right Upper Lobe Consolidation with Bulging Fissure.* This suggests *Klebsiella* infection.
   3. *Involvement of Superior or Basilar Segments of Lower Lobes or Posterior Segments of Upper Lobes.* This suggests aspiration pneumonia.
   4. *Pneumatoceles.* This finding indicates staphylococcal pneumonia in children.
   5. *Perihilar Infiltrates.* These suggest *Mycoplasma* infection.

SPECIFIC PATHOGENS

A. **Streptococcus pneumoniae (Pneumococcal Pneumonia).** This is the primary community-acquired bacterial pneumonia.
   1. *Clinical Presentation.* The condition has an abrupt onset characterized by a single shaking chill (80 per cent of cases), rapidly rising temperature, cough (75 per cent), pleuritic pain, and dyspnea. Sputum may be rusty, bloody, pink, or green and mucopurulent. Herpes labialis may be noted.
   2. *Laboratory Findings*
      a. **Leukocytosis.** Leukocytosis is typical. Absence of leukocytosis or leukopenia are poor prognostic signs.

B. **Legionella pneumophila (Legionnaires' Disease)**
   1. *Clinical Presentation*
      a. **Anorexia, Malaise, and Weakness.** These symptoms occur in 100 per cent of cases.
      b. **Cough.** Nontroublesome, initially nonproductive cough is present in 92 per cent of cases. Later the cough becomes productive of watery often bloody or blood-tinged sputum.
      c. **Chills.** Seventy-seven per cent of patients have chills, which are characteristically recurrent.
      d. **Diarrhea.** Diarrhea that is watery, without blood, mucus, white blood cells, or abdominal discomfort occurs in 47 per cent of cases.
      e. **Pleuritic Pain.** The symptom complex of pleuritic pain with bloody sputum (33 per cent of cases) may suggest diagnosis of pulmonary embolus with infarction.
      f. **Temperature.** Temperature is in excess of 103° F in 80 per cent of patients. The temperature curve is continuous (not spiking).
      g. **Relative Bradycardia.** This occurs in 60 per cent of cases.
      h. **Altered Mental Status.** Mental status is altered in 38 per cent of cases.
   2. *Laboratory Findings*
      a. **Leukocytosis.** Leukocytosis is typical; leukopenia is a poor sign.
      b. **Serum Glutamic Oxaloacetic Transaminase (SGOT), Serum Glutamic Pyruvic Transaminase (SGPT), and Alkaline Phosphatase.** There are mild to moderate abnormalities of SGOT, SGPT, and alkaline phosphatase.
      c. **Hyponatremia and Hypophosphatemia.** Hyponatremia and hypophosphatemia each occur in 50 per cent of cases.
      d. **Radiographic Features**
         1). Unilobar infiltrate progressing to consolidation occurs in 66 per cent of cases.
         2). Multifocal areas of bronchopneumonia are present in 33 per cent of cases.
   3. *Diagnosis*
      a. **Culture.** Charcoal yeast extract agar is used.
      b. **Stain.** Direct fluorescent antibody is used but is of retrospective value only. A diagnostic fourfold rise to 1:128 or greater occurs three to six weeks after the onset of illness.
C. **Mycoplasma pneumoniae.** This disease is common in children and young adults.
   1. *Clinical Presentation.* The disease may develop insidiously.
      a. **Fever, Headache, and Malaise.** These signs and symptoms predate cough by two to four days.
      b. **Cough.** The cough is hacking, paroxysmal, and troublesome. Sputum is scant and may be blood-tinged.
      c. **Shaking Chills.** These are rare.
      d. **Temperature.** Temperature rarely exceeds 102° F.
      e. **Bullous Myringitis.** Bullous myringitis occurs in 10 per cent of cases.

    f. Examination of the Chest. The chest may be normal despite radiographic evidence of pneumonia.

  2. Diagnosis

    a. Culture. Culture is possible but not usually done.

    b. Mycoplasma. There is a fourfold rise in *Mycoplasma* complement fixation titers, which occurs between two and four weeks after the onset of illness.

    c. Cold Agglutinins. Cold agglutinins are nonspecific; however, titers of 1:128 or greater in a patient with compatible clinical illness are suggestive. (These are detectable between the second and third weeks of illness.)

D. Influenza

  1. Influenza A, B, and C. Influenza A is most common and causes the most serious illness.

  2. Clinical Presentation

    a. Sudden Onset of Severe Headache. This is frequently associated with retroorbital pain.

    b. Diffuse Myalgia. Diffuse myalgia occurs in 50 per cent of cases.

    c. Fever. Temperature is elevated to 100 to 103° F and rarely to 106° F.

    d. Chilliness. Occasionally there are true rigors.

    e. Relative Bradycardia. Relative bradycardia may be noted.

    f. Respiratory Symptoms. Respiratory symptoms usually appear as systemic symptoms subside.

      1). Cough. Cough, present in 75 per cent of cases, is productive of mucoid sputum in one third.

      2). Substernal Chest Pain. This affects 50 per cent of patients.

    g. Radiographic Features

      1). Influenza Virus. Perihilar infiltrates can be seen.

      2). Bacterial Superinfection. This may be rapidly progressive.

  3. Diagnosis. Diagnostic tests need not be done if the clinical diagnosis is not in doubt such as in cases of typical illness in a setting of known community spread.

    a. Culture. Culture is done of throat swab or nasopharyngeal wash.

    b. Complement Fixation

    c. Hemagglutination Inhibition. Hemagglutination inhibition is most reliable. Acute and convalescent sera should be submitted.

REFERENCES

1. Cassell GH, Cole BC: Mycoplasmas as agents of human disease. N Engl J Med 304:80–89, 1983.

A comprehensive review.

2. Foy HM, Kenney GE, McMahan R: *Mycoplasma pneumoniae* in an urban area. JAMA 214:1666–1672, 1970.

Epidemiologic data in a large study.

3. Kirby BD, Snyder KM, Meyer RD, Finegold SM: Legionnaires' disease: Clinical features of twenty-four cases. Ann Intern Med 89:297–309, 1978.
4. Kirby BD, Snyder KM, Meyer RD, Finegold SM: Legionnaires' disease: Report of sixty-five nosocomially acquired cases and review of the literature. Medicine 59:188–205, 1980.
5. Murray HW, Masur H, Senterif L, et al.: The protean manifestations of *Mycoplasma pneumoniae* infection in adults. Am J Med 58:299, 1975.

A description of extrapulmonary manifestations of the illness.

6. Murray PR, Washington JA II: Microscopic and bacteriologic analysis of expectorated sputum. Mayo Clin Proc 50:339–344, 1975.
7. Tew J, Calenoff L, Berlin BS: Bacterial or nonbacterial pneumonia: Accuracy of radiographic diagnosis. Radiology 124:607, 1977.
8. Stulbarg MS: Problems in diagnosing pneumonia—Medical Staff Conference, University of California, San Francisco. West J Med 140:594–601, 1984.

A discussion of diagnostic tests.

44

SEXUALLY TRANSMITTED DISEASE*

By MICKEY S. EISENBERG, M.D., Ph.D.

GENERAL COMMENTS

A. Diagnosis of sexually transmitted diseases (STDs) is complicated by several factors.
   1. Symptoms resulting from STDs overlap considerably, thus making it difficult to clinically distinguish the pathogenic organism on the basis of symptoms alone.
   2. Laboratory tests to identify all pathogenic organisms are not readily available. Thus, it is a practical necessity to sometimes make a presumptive diagnosis without laboratory confirmation.
   3. Patients may have infections with more than one pathogen.
   4. Patients may have infections involving more than one site, and symptoms from various sites may be minimal or more intense.
B. This chapter presents information on selected STDs with emphasis placed on criteria for presumptive and definitive diagnosis. At the end of the chapter the diagnostic approach to common STD-associated symptoms is presented using algorithms.

---

*Portions of this chapter are adapted from material generously supplied by Walter Stamm, M.D., and the Seattle Sexually Transmitted Disease Training Program, Harborview Medical Center, Seattle, Washington.

DIAGNOSIS OF STD

Criteria for presumptive and definitive diagnosis are presented. A presumptive diagnosis is sufficient grounds for initiation of therapy.* A list of STDs is shown in Table 44–1. (Not all STDs are covered in this chapter.)

A. Gonorrhea

1. *Etiology.* *Neisseria gonorrhoeae*, a gram-negative diplococcus.
2. *Epidemiology.* One million cases are reported annually in the United States. Actual incidence is probably two to three times higher.
3. *Typical Clinical Presentation.* Men usually have dysuria, frequent urination, and purulent urethral discharge but may be asymptomatic. Women may have abnormal vaginal discharge, abnormal menses, dysuria, or may be asymptomatic. Anorectal and pharyngeal infections are common in homosexual men and heterosexual women. Often these are asymptomatic; proctitis generally produces mild rectal pain or discharge.
4. *Diagnosis*

PRESUMPTIVE	DEFINITIVE
Microscopic identification of typical gram-negative intracellular diplococci on smear of urethral or rectal exudate (men) or endocervical material (women)	Growth on selective medium demonstrating typical colony morphology, positive oxidases reaction, typical Gram's stain morphology, and confirmed by sugar utilization, coaggulatination or antigonococcal fluorescent antibody (FA) testing
Sensitivity of Gram's stain: male urethritis (98%), female cervix (50%), rectal (20%)	
Growth on selective medium demonstrating typical colony morphology, positive oxidase reaction, and typical Gram's stain morphology	A definitive diagnosis is required if the specimen is extragenital, from a child, or medicolegally significant.

B. Pelvic Inflammatory Diseases (PIDs)

1. *Etiology.* PID is caused by *N. gonorrhoeae, Chlamydia trachomatis, Mycoplasma hominis*, and anaerobic bacteria either alone or in combination.
2. *Epidemiology.* Between 600,000 and 1 million cases of PID are estimated to occur in the United States each year. These cases cause the most important sequelae of STDs in women, namely involuntary infertility and ectopic pregnancy.
3. *Typical Clinical Presentation.* The patient may have pain and tenderness involving the lower abdomen, cervix, uterus, and adnexae, often with fever, chills, and elevated white blood cell count and erythrocyte sedimentation rate. The diagnosis

---

*Material in this section is adapted from the Centers for Disease Control Sexually Transmitted Diseases Summary, 1982.

TABLE 44–1. CLASSIFICATION OF STDs

Bacteria	Viruses
Neisseria gonorrhoeae	Herpes simplex virus
Treponema pallidum	*Molluscum contagiosum*
Chlamydia trachomatis	Hepatitis A
Mycoplasma hominis	Hepatitis B
Ureaplasma urealyticum	Cytomegalovirus
Hemophilus ducreyi	Genital warts
Calmmatobacterium granulomatis	Protozoa
Shigella species	*Trichomonas vaginalis*
Campylobacter fetus	*Entamoeba histolytica*
*Gardnerella vaginalis**	*Giardia lamblia*
Streptococcus, group B*	*Phthirus pubis* (crab louse)
	Sarcoptes scabiei (scabies mite)

*May not be associated with sexual transmission.

is more likely if the patient has multiple sexual partners, a history of PID, uses an intrauterine device (IUD), or is in the first five to ten days of the menstrual cycle. Many women with PID lack the entire constellation of symptoms and signs outlined here; the physician should thus have a low "threshold" for findings suggesting diagnosis.

4. Diagnosis

PRESUMPTIVE	DEFINITIVE
Unilateral or bilateral adnexal tenderness on examination in association with evidence of lower genital tract infection and without associated evidence of other diagnosis (ectopic pregnancy, appendicitis).	Direct visualization of inflamed (edema, hyperemia, or tubal exudate) fallopian tube(s) at laparoscopy or laparotomy makes the diagnosis of PID definitive. A culture of tubal exudate establishes the cause.
Cervical cultures for *N. gonorrhoeae* and/or *Chlamydia trachomatis*, if positive, support the diagnosis.	

C. Syphilis

   1. Etiology. *Treponema pallidum.*

   2. Epidemiology. There are 30,000 cases annually in the United States. Most new cases occur in homosexual or bisexual men.

   3. Typical Clinical Presentation

      a. Primary. The classic chancre is single, painless, indurated, and located at the site of exposure. Many are rectal. All genital lesions of this type should be suspected to be syphilitic until proved otherwise.

      b. Secondary. Patients may have a highly variable skin rash, mucous patches, condylomata lata, diffuse lymphadenopathy, or other signs.

      c. Latent. Patients have no clinical signs.

4. Diagnosis

PRESUMPTIVE	DEFINITIVE
Primary: Patients have typical lesion(s) and either a newly positive serologic test for syphilis (STS) or an STS titer that is at least four-fold greater than the last, or there has been syphilis exposure within 90 days of lesion onset. *Secondary*: Patients have the typical clinical presentation and a strongly reactive STS. *Latent*: Patients have serologic evidence of untreated syphilis without clinical signs.	Primary and secondary syphilis are definitively diagnosed by demonstrating *T. pallidum* with darkfield microscopy or FA techniques in material from a chancre, regional lymph node, or other lesion, or by demonstrating a newly positive venereal disease reaction level and fluorescent treponemal antibody. A definitive diagnosis of latent syphilis cannot be made under usual circumstances.

D. Nongonococcal Urethritis (NGU)

1. **Etiology.** Primarily *C. trachomatis* and *Ureaplasma urealyticum* and less commonly herpes simplex virus and *Trichomonas vaginalis* are causes.
2. **Epidemiology.** This is the most common cause of urethritis in men, with an estimated three million cases annually. This condition is more common in heterosexual than in homosexual men.
3. **Clinical Presentation.** Men usually have dysuria, frequent urination, and mucoid to purulent urethral discharge. Some men have asymptomatic infections.

   Female sexual partners of men with chlamydial NGU are likely to have chlamydial endocervicitis.
4. **Diagnosis**

PRESUMPTIVE	DEFINITIVE
Men with typical clinical symptoms are presumed to have NGU when the urethral Gram's stain is negative for gonorrhea. Asymptomatic men with negative tests for gonorrhea (Gram's stain and/or culture) are also presumed to have NGU if they have at least four white blood cells per oil immersion field on an intraurethral smear.	Recovery of *C. trichomatis* from the male urethra or demonstration of *T. vaginalis*. Note: gonococcal and nongonococcal urethritis often coexist in the same patient.

E. Mucopurulent Cervicitis

1. **Etiology.** Cervicitis without vaginitis is primarily a result of chlamydial or gonococcal infection. Ulcerative cervicitis is caused by herpesvirus.
2. **Epidemiology.** This is the most common STD syndrome in women. Cases of mucopurulent cervicitis are similar to ureth-

ritis in men. Most cases are caused by *C. trachomatis*; the next most common cause is *N. gonorrhoeae*; and a small percentage are caused by herpesvirus. In one third of cases the cause is obscure.

3. **Clinical Presentation.** There is a vaginal discharge and lower abdominal pain.

4. **Diagnosis.** Mucopurulent discharge is seen at the cervical os with increased polymorphonuclear leukocytes seen on Gram's stain. The presence of five or more polymorphonuclear neutrophils per oil immersion microscopic field suggests cervicitis. Cervical ectopy is a common sign of mucopurulent cervicitis caused by *C. trachomatis*. Presumptive and definitive diagnosis of *Neisseria gonorrhoeae* is found on page 324. If gonococcal infection cannot be documented, *C. trachomatis* infection should be strongly suspected and a presumptive diagnosis made. If available, chlamydial cultures can be the basis for a definitive diagnosis of the infection.

F. **Vaginitis**

1. **Etiology.** Common organisms causing infection are *Trichomonas vaginalis, Candida albicans,* and *Gardnerella vaginalis* (with anaerobic bacteria). Other infectious, chemical, allergenic, and physical agents may cause vaginitis.

2. **Epidemiology.** This is an exceedingly common infection in young women, often from unknown causes. It is not always sexually transmitted.

3. **Typical Clinical Presentation.** (See Table 44–2.) Findings on examination vary from no signs or symptoms to erythema, edema, and pruritus of the external genitalia. Excessive or malodorous discharge is a common finding.

4. **Diagnosis.** See Table 44–2.

PRESUMPTIVE	DEFINITIVE
Trichomoniasis: Profuse grayish discharge with odor	*Trichomoniasis:* Typical motile trichomonads are identified in a saline wet mount of vaginal discharge, or a vaginal culture is positive for *T. vaginalis.*
Gardnerella vaginitis: Foul-smelling vaginal discharge (fishy odor); identification of "clue cells" in a saline wet mount; positive whiff test (a mixture of vaginal discharge and 10 per cent potassium hydroxide liberates an "amine-like" or "fishy" odor); vaginal pH ≥ 4.7	
	Candidiasis: Microscopic identification of yeast forms (budding cells or hyphae) in Gram's stain or potassium hydroxide wet mount preparations of vaginal discharge.
Candidiasis: The presumptive criteria are typical clinical symptoms of vulvovaginitis (marked itching).	

G. **Granuloma Inguinale**

1. **Etiology.** *Calymmatobacterium granulomatis.*

2. **Epidemiology.** This condition is exceedingly rare in the United States (fewer than 50 cases per year) and usually occurs in people from Asia, Africa, or the tropics.

TABLE 44-2. LABORATORY FEATURES OF VAGINITIS*

	NORMAL	TRICHOMONIASIS	*Gardnerella* VAGINITIS	CANDIDIASIS
Appearance of discharge	Clear or whitish-gray, nonhomogenous	Grayish-white, homogenous; may be frothy	Grayish-white, homogenous	White, clumped, cottage–cheese–like
Amount of discharge	None	Large	Large	Scant
pH of discharge	<4.7 (≥5 during menses)	≥4.7	≥4.7	<4.7
Amine (fishy odor) when 10% KOH is added to discharge	Negative	Positive	Positive	Negative
Microscopy saline and 10% KOH preparations	Epithelial cells	Motile trichomonad Clue cells† may be leukocytes	Clue cells	Leukocytes ± yeast and pseudomycelia

*Reprinted with permission, from Handsfield H: Hosp Pract Jan. 111–118, 1982.
†Clue cells are epithelial cells with a ragged and refractile appearance that are caused by a large number of adherent bacteria. Up to 10 per cent of Clue cells among epithelial cells may be seen normally.

3. *Typical Clinical Presentation.* Granuloma inguinale appears initially as single or multiple subcutaneous nodules at the site of inoculation. Nodules erode to form beefy, exuberant, granulomatous, heaped ulcers, which are painless, bleed on contact, and enlarge slowly. Spread by autoinoculation is common.

4. *Diagnosis*

PRESUMPTIVE	DEFINITIVE
The typical clinical presentation is sufficient to suggest the diagnosis. Resolution of the lesions, following specific antibiotic therapy, supports the diagnosis. A history of travel to the tropics (particularly India or Papua New Guinea) among patients or their partners helps to substantiate the clinical impression.	Scrapings or biopsy specimens from the ulcer margin reveal the pathognomonic Donovan bodies on microscopic examination. These appear as gram-negative bacteria in vacuolar compartments within white blood or plasma cells.

H. Lymphogranuloma Venereum (LGV)

1. *Etiology.* *C. trachomatis* (LGV serotype).
2. *Epidemiology.* LGV is rare in the United States.
3. *Typical Clinical Presentation.* The primary lesion of LGV is a 2 to 3 mm painless vesicle or nonindurated ulcer at the site of inoculation. Patients commonly fail to notice this primary lesion. Regional adenopathy follows within a week to a month later and is the most common clinical observation. Most patients have bilateral painful adenopathy. Sensation of stiffness and aching in the groin, followed by swelling of the inguinal region, may be the first indication of infection for most patients. Adenopathy may subside spontaneously or proceed to the formation of abscesses that rupture to produce draining sinuses or fistulae.
4. *Diagnosis*

PRESUMPTIVE	DEFINITIVE
The LGV complement fixation test is sensitive: 80 per cent of cases have titers of 1:16 or higher. Since the sequelae of LGV are serious and preventable, treatment should not be withheld pending laboratory confirmation.	A definitive diagnosis of *C. trachomatis* infection from an appropriate specimen (lymph node aspirate) and confirmation of the isolate as an LGV immunotype; however, such laboratory diagnostic capabilities are not widely available.

I. Molluscum Contagiosum

1. *Etiology.* Molluscum contagiosum virus.
2. *Epidemiology.* Epidemiology is poorly defined.
3. *Typical Clinical Presentation.* The lesions are 1 to 5 mm, smooth, rounded, shiny, firm, flesh-colored to pearly white papules with characteristically umbilicated centers. They are most commonly seen on the trunk and anogenital region and are generally asymptomatic.

4. Diagnosis

PRESUMPTIVE	DEFINITIVE
Usually on the basis of the typical clinical presentation	Microscopic examination of lesions or lesion material reveals the pathognomonic *Molluscum* inclusion bodies.

J. Condylomata Acuminata
1. *Etiology.* Human papilloma virus.
2. *Epidemiology.* Epidemiology is poorly defined.
3. *Typical Clinical Presentation.* Condylomata acuminata appears as single or multiple soft, fleshy, papillary or sessile painless growths around the anus, vulvovaginal area, penis, urethra, or perineum.
4. *Diagnosis*

PRESUMPTIVE	DEFINITIVE
A diagnosis may be made on the basis of the typical clinical observations. The possible diagnosis of condylomata lata is excluded by obtaining a test for syphilis.	A biopsy, although usually unnecessary, is required to make a definitive diagnosis. Biopsy should be done for very atypical lesions, for which neoplasia is a consideration, before initiation of therapy.

K. Herpes Genitalis
1. *Etiology.* Herpes simplex virus (HSV) types 1 and 2.
2. *Epidemiology.* There are an estimated four to six hundred thousand primary infections annually and two to three million recurrent episodes annually.
3. *Typical Clinical Presentation.* Multiple vesicles appear anywhere on the genitalia. Vesicles spontaneously rupture to form shallow ulcers, which may be very painful. Lesions resolve spontaneously without scarring. The first occurrence is termed *initial infection* (mean duration 12 days). Herpes genitalis is often associated with local pain, fever, dysuria, lymphadenopathy, and so forth. Subsequent, usually milder, occurrences are termed *recurrent infections* (mean duration 4 to 5 days). The interval between clinical episodes is termed *latency*. Viral shedding occurs intermittently during latency.
4. *Diagnosis*

PRESUMPTIVE	DEFINITIVE
When typical genital lesions are present or a pattern of recurrence has developed, herpes infection is likely. Presumptive diagnosis is further supported by direct identification of multinucleated giant cells with intranuclear inclusions in a clinical specimen prepared by Papanicolaou's or other histochemical stain.	An HSV virus tissue culture demonstrates the characteristic cytopathogenic effect (CPE) following inoculation of a specimen from the cervix, the urethra, or the base of a genital lesion. The isolates can be identified as type 1 or type 2 by FA, neutralization, or other serologic techniques.

L. Chancroid

1. **Etiology.** *Hemophilus ducreyi.*
2. **Epidemiology.** Chancroid is rare in the United States but has occurred in epidemics or clusters of cases in the last few years; otherwise, it appears in travelers to the tropics, Southeast Asia, and Africa.
3. **Typical Clinical Presentation.** A single or multiple superficial painful ulcer appears and is surrounded by an erythematous halo. Ulcers typically have a white necrotic base with ragged serpiginous borders. Accompanying painful adenopathy is unilateral or bilateral. A characteristic inguinal bubo that may rupture occurs in 25 to 60 per cent of cases. Ulcers usually occur on the coronal sulcus, glans, or shaft. Females are usually asymptomatic.
4. **Diagnosis**

PRESUMPTIVE	DEFINITIVE
When the only organisms seen in an aspirate from a bubo are arranged in chains or clumps along strands of mucus and are morphologically similar to *H. ducreyi*, the diagnosis is highly likely. A clinical picture consistent with chancroid involving the genitalia or a unilateral bubo, or both, is suggestive. Since many STDs cause genital ulcers, it is crucial to differentiate between them. All such ulcers should be examined by dark-field microscopy. Gram's stain of ulcer is not diagnostic.	The diagnosis is definitive when *H. ducreyi* is recovered by culture. Biopsy may be diagnostic but is not usually performed.

M. Pediculosis Pubis

1. **Etiology.** The condition is caused by an infestation with *Phthirus pubis* (pubic or crab louse), an ectoparasite 1 to 4 mm long with segmented tarsi and claws for clinging to hairs.
2. **Epidemiology.** Epidemiology is poorly defined.
3. **Typical Clinical Presentation.** Symptoms range from slight discomfort to intolerable itching. Erythematous papules, nits, or adult lice clinging to pubic, perineal, or perianal hairs are present and often are noticed by patients.
4. **Diagnosis**

PRESUMPTIVE	DEFINITIVE
A history of recent exposure to pubic lice in a patient with pruritic erythematous macules, papules, or secondary excoriations in the genital region	Finding of lice or nits attached to genital hairs

N. Scabies

1. **Etiology.** This is caused by *Sarcoptes scabiei,* the itch mite. The female mite is 0.3 to 0.4 mm long and the male is somewhat smaller. The female burrows under the skin to deposit eggs.
2. **Epidemiology.** Epidemiology is poorly defined.
3. **Typical Clinical Presentation.** Symptoms include itching, which is often worse at night, and the presence of erythematous papular eruptions. Excoriations and secondary infections are common. Reddish-brown nodules are caused by hypersensitivity and develop one or more months after infection has occurred. The primary lesion is the burrow. When not obliterated by excoriations, it is most often seen on the fingers, penis, and wrists.
4. **Diagnosis**

PRESUMPTIVE	DEFINITIVE
The diagnosis is often made on clinical grounds alone. A history of exposure to a patient with scabies within the previous two months supports the diagnosis.	Definitive diagnosis is made by microscopic identification of the mite or its eggs, larvae, or feces in scrapings from an elevated papule or burrow.

RECOMMENDED DIAGNOSTIC APPROACH

A. Urethritis in Men

1. Nongonococcal urethritis (NGU) accounts for a majority of urethritis in men. *Chlamydia* causes approximately 40 per cent of NGU, *Ureaplasma urealyticum* causes approximately 10 to 20 per cent, and a small percentage is caused by herpesvirus and *Trichomonas.* The remaining cases are caused by other pathogens that are poorly characterized.
2. The urethral Gram's stain is the most useful test to distinguish gonococcal from nongonococcal urethritis. (See Fig. 44–1.)

B. Ulcerative Genital Lesions

1. Most ulcerative genital lesions are caused by herpesvirus infection. Ten to 15 per cent of genital ulcers may be traumatic in origin. Syphilis is less common, and chancroid and other infectious causes are rarely seen. (See Fig. 44–2.)
2. Genital herpes is supported by a history of vesicular lesions becoming ulcerative over several days or by recurrences in the same area.
3. Dark-field examination should be performed on all ulcerative lesions, regardless of the presence of pain, unless genital herpes seems quite likely.
4. Lymphadenopathy is often present but is of little help in distinguishing among the various causes.

C. Nonulcerative Genital Lesions

1. Nonulcerative lesions in the genital region are caused by a

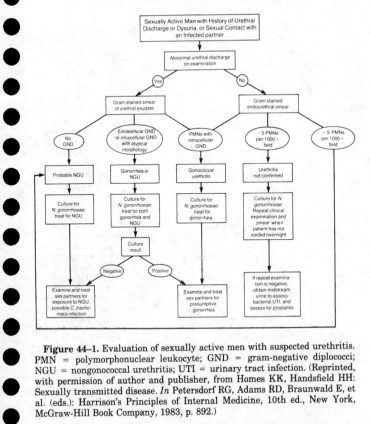

Figure 44–1. Evaluation of sexually active men with suspected urethritis. PMN = polymorphonuclear leukocyte; GND = gram-negative diplococci; NGU = nongonococcal urethritis; UTI = urinary tract infection. (Reprinted, with permission of author and publisher, from Homes KK, Handsfield HH: Sexually transmitted disease. *In* Petersdorf RG, Adams RD, Braunwald E, et al. (eds.): Harrison's Principles of Internal Medicine, 10th ed., New York, McGraw-Hill Book Company, 1983, p. 892.)

variety of sexually and nonsexually transmitted diseases. The numerous causes do not lend themselves to an algorithmic diagnostic approach. Instead, important causes of nonulcerative skin lesions are considered, as listed in Table 44–3.

D. Vaginitis

1. As outlined earlier, vaginitis is predominantly caused by *Trichomonas, G. vaginalis,* and *Candida* species. Symptoms include increased vaginal discharge, abnormal color or odor of the discharge, vulvar itching, dysuria, and often dyspareunia.

2. Findings on physical and microscopic examination of the discharge usually allow characterization of the vaginitis. (See Fig. 44–3.)

3. There is often considerable overlap of symptoms among vaginitis, urethritis, cervicitis, and salpingitis. Hence, other causes of vaginal discharge, dysuria, and other signs and symptoms should be considered if the suspected vaginitis does not respond to therapy.

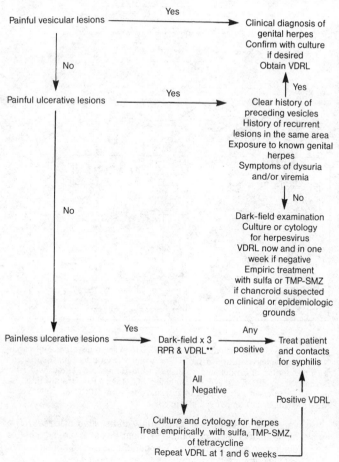

Figure 44–2. Evaluation and management of ulcerative genital lesions: *10 to 15 per cent of genital ulcers may be traumatic in origin, with no infectious cause proven; however, all ulcers should be evaluated for potential infectious cause regardless of a history of trauma. **Positive rapid plasma reagin card tests (RPRs) and venereal disease reaction levels (VDRLs) should be confirmed with a fluorescent treponemal antibody (FTA) or microhemag-glutination-*Treponema pallidum* test (MHA-TP). All patients should have a quantitative VDRL done. TMP-SMZ = trimethoprim plus sulfamethoxazole.

E. Cervicitis

1. Major causes of cervicitis are *C. trachomatis, N. gonorrhoeae,* herpesvirus, *Candida,* and *Trichomonas.*
2. Cervicitis may occur alone or in combination with vaginitis. *Candida* and *Trichomonas* are common causes of cervicitis combined with vaginitis. *Gonorrhoeae* and *Chlamydia* usually

TABLE 44–3. THE MOST COMMON NONULCERATIVE SKIN LESIONS*

DISEASE	APPEARANCE	GENITAL DISTRIBUTION	ITCHING	TIME COURSE	DIAGNOSTIC TEST	TREATMENT	OTHER
Scabies	Red, linear, excoriated areas, often with papules, pustules, and burrows	External genitalia, often on webs between fingers, thighs, lower abdomen, and buttocks	Marked, often worse at night or in a warm room	Days	Demonstration of mite in burrow on skin scraping	Common benzene lotion	Should launder sheets and clothes and treat other sex partners or household contacts simultaneously
Genital warts	Ranges from flat-topped to verrucous, to frondlike, well-elevated, well-demarcated lesions	Around glans, distal penis, intraurethral in men; introitus and vagina in women; perirectal	Mild or none	Weeks to months	None	Podophyllin, liquid nitrogen, or resection	May recur if not treated adequately
Candida infection	Flat, reddish-brown, well-demarcated, slightly scaly lesions; often satellite lesions	Glans and under foreskin in men; labia and vulva in women; occasional perirectal lesions	Moderate to marked	Days	KOH preparation	Topical nystatin, clotrimazole, or miconazole	Partner should be examined and treated also
Molluscum contagiosum	Pearly-white papular smooth-surfaced	Anywhere on genitals	Minimal	Weeks	None; may be possible to press a discharge	Curettage	Often become superinfected, particularly if

Table 44–3 continued on following page

TABLE 44-3. THE MOST COMMON NONULCERATIVE SKIN LESIONS* *Continued*

Disease	Appearance	Genital Distribution	Itching	Time Course	Diagnostic Test	Treatment	Other
	umbilicated papules				from the central core		manipulated; often multiple lesions in genital and nongenital areas
Lichen planus	Annular, polygonal, flat-topped, violaceous lesion	Singular or multiple, usually on penile shaft or glans	Mild to moderate	Days	None	None; may use topical steroids to control itching	History of similar lesions; lesion on nongenital areas
Psoriasis	Well-demarcated papulosquamous plaques with silver scale; usually bleeds if scale is removed	Penile shaft, scrotum, perirectal area	Moderate	Days to weeks, may wax and wane	None	Dependent on severity of disease; refer to dermatologist	Usually has psoriatic lesions elsewhere (elbows, knees, lower back); history of episodic lesions; may have pitted nails
Fixed drug eruption	Erythematous, well-demarcated area; may evolve from erythema to	Any part of genitalia, but glans and penile shaft most	Moderate	Days sudden onset	None	None, or topical steroids in severe cases	Often a history of previous similar reactions in

	vesicles or blebs	common in men; labia in women					same location; may have nongenital lesions; history of new drug within ten days of onset; most common with sulfa drugs, barbiturates, and tetracycline
Superficial mycoses	Brownish red; well-marginated, often scaling	Medial thighs, scrotum, in gluteal folds; usually symmetric	Moderate to marked	Weeks	KOH preparation	Topical Tinactin, miconazole, or oral griseofulvin	Often foot lesions also; worse in hot humid weather or under occlusive clothing
Deep mycoses	Sharply marginated, indurated, often raised, irregular, verrucous lesions; may ulcerate	Scrotum and penile shaft in gluteal folds; external genital lesions rare in women	Minimal	Weeks to months	KOH test, culture, biopsy	Dependent on type of fungus	May have nongenital skin lesions or visceral lesions also
Carcinoma	Sharply demarcated, variegated, firm, raised, irregular	Any part of external genitalia	Minimal	Weeks to months	Biopsy	Dependent on type of carcinoma	May have firm, hard, regional lymph nodes; may have

Table 44–3 continued on following page

TABLE 44–3.   THE MOST COMMON NONULCERATIVE SKIN LESIONS* *Continued*

Disease	Appearance	Genital Distribution	Itching	Time Course	Diagnostic Test	Treatment	Other
							systemic signs of weight loss, weakness
Reiter's syndrome	Multiple, inflamed, tender, elevated, moist papules	Lesions characteristically around the glans penis; circinate balanitis	Moderate	Days	None	None	Associated with arthritis, conjunctivitis, and after other skin lesions on the soles of the feet

*Reprinted with permission of the Seattle STD Training Program, Harborview Medical Center.

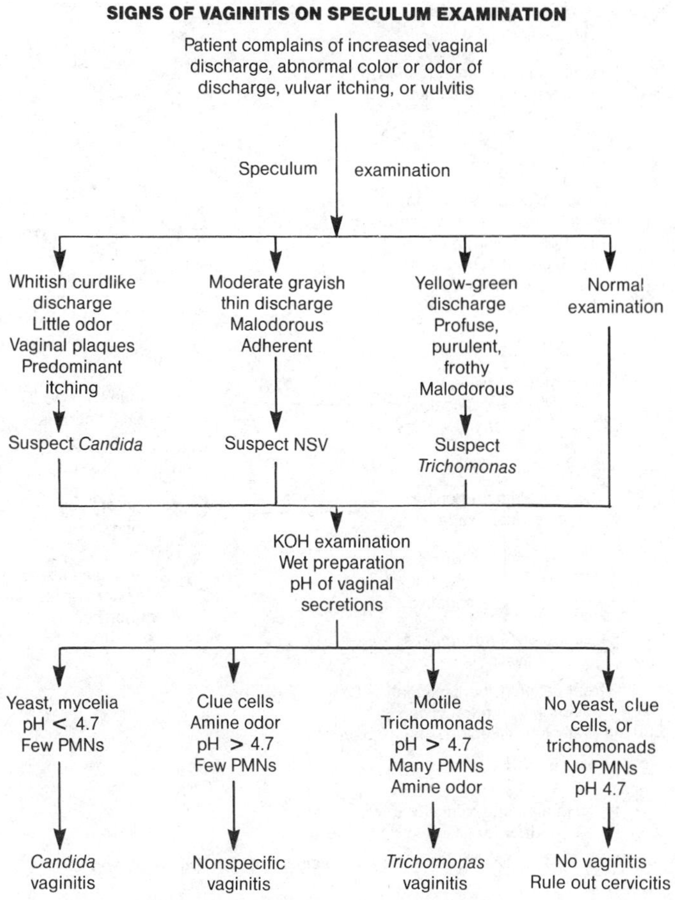

SIGNS OF VAGINITIS ON SPECULUM EXAMINATION

Patient complains of increased vaginal
discharge, abnormal color or odor of
discharge, vulvar itching, or vulvitis

Speculum   examination

Whitish curdlike discharge Little odor Vaginal plaques Predominant itching	Moderate grayish thin discharge Malodorous Adherent	Yellow-green discharge Profuse, purulent, frothy Malodorous	Normal examination
Suspect *Candida*	Suspect NSV	Suspect *Trichomonas*	

KOH examination
Wet preparation
pH of vaginal
secretions

Yeast, mycelia pH < 4.7 Few PMNs	Clue cells Amine odor pH > 4.7 Few PMNs	Motile Trichomonads pH > 4.7 Many PMNs Amine odor	No yeast, clue cells, or trichomonads No PMNs pH 4.7
Candida vaginitis	Nonspecific vaginitis	*Trichomonas* vaginitis	No vaginitis Rule out cervicitis

Figure 44–3. Evaluation of suspected vaginitis.

cause nonerosive cervicitis without vaginitis. Herpesvirus as a
cause of cervicitis produces ulcerative necrotic lesions that are
easily seen on pelvic examination.

3. Gonococcal infections, when present, can be diagnosed by
Gram's stain 60 per cent of the time and by culture 80 to 90 per
cent of the time. If gonococcal infection cannot be diagnosed,
Chlamydia infection should be considered and empiric treatment
begun (and/or culture, if available). (See Fig. 44–4.)

F. **Pelvic Inflammatory Disease (PID)**
   1. PID is conveniently categorized into gonococcal and nongonococcal forms. Nongonococcal PID is caused by *C. trachomatis*

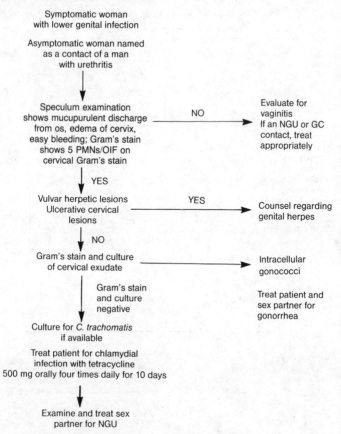

Symptomatic woman
with lower genital infection

Asymptomatic woman named
as a contact of a man
with urethritis

Speculum examination
shows mucupurulent discharge   NO   Evaluate for
from os, edema of cervix,   vaginitis
easy bleeding; Gram's stain   If an NGU or GC
shows 5 PMNs/OIF on   contact, treat
cervical Gram's stain   appropriately

YES

Vulvar herpetic lesions   YES
Ulcerative cervical   Counsel regarding
lesions   genital herpes

NO

Gram's stain and culture   Intracellular
of cervical exudate   gonococci

Gram's stain
and culture   Treat patient and
negative   sex partner for
         gonorrhea

Culture for *C. trachomatis*
if available

Treat patient for chlamydial
infection with tetracycline
500 mg orally four times daily for 10 days

Examine and treat sex
partner for NGU

Figure 44–4. Evaluation and management of mucopurulent cervicitis.

(sexually transmitted) and by *Bacteroides fragilis* and anaerobic gram-positive cocci (nonsexually transmitted).
2. PID should be considered in all women with lower abdominal pain. Pain is usually bilateral. Vaginal discharge, menometror-rhagia, dysuria, onset of pain associated with menses, and fever are common symptoms.
G. **Infectious Proctitis in Homosexual Men**
   1. Major infectious causes of infectious proctitis, primarily occurring among homosexual men, are *N. gonorrhoeae* and herpesvirus. Other sexually transmitted microorganisms include enteric path-ogen (*Shigella* and *Salmonella*) and parasites (*Giardia lamblia* and *Entamoeba histolytica*). The role of *C. trachomatis* as a cause of proctitis is unclear.

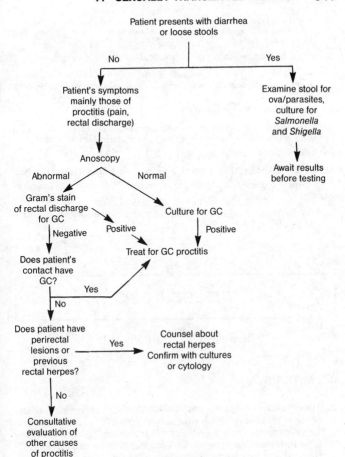

Figure 44–5. Evaluation of patients with proctitis or diarrheal illness in homosexual men.

2. Anoscopy is a key diagnostic procedure in defining the cause of proctitis. (See Fig. 44–5.)
3. Gram's stain detects only 10 to 25 per cent of patients who have positive rectal gonococcal cultures.

REFERENCES

1. Sexually transmitted diseases: Treatment guidelines. Morbid Mortal Weekly Rep 31:25, 1982.
An up-to-date review of STD guidelines.

2. Corey L, Homes KK: Genital herpes simplex virus infections: Current concepts in diagnosis, therapy and prevention. Ann Intern Med 98:973–983, 1983.

Up-to-date and comprehensive discussion from acknowledged authorities.

3. Corey L, Holmes KK: Genital herpes simplex virus infections: Clinical manifestations, course, and complications. Ann Intern Med 98:958–972, 1983.

An up-to-date and comprehensive article.

4. Jacobs NF, Kraus SJ: Gonococcal and nongonococcal urethritis in men: Clinical and laboratory differentiation. Ann Intern Med 82:7, 1975.

The value of Gram's stain is discussed.

5. Handsfield JJ: Sexually transmitted diseases. Hosp Pract 17:99–116, 1982.

A good general discussion of STD and an excellent discussion of diagnosis of vaginitis.

6. Sexually Transmitted Diseases Summary 1982. Centers for Disease Control, Atlanta, Georgia, 1982.

45
TUBERCULOSIS

By RICHARD ALBERT, M.D.

DEFINITIONS

A. Tuberculosis Infection and Tuberculosis. Tuberculosis is an acute or chronic infection caused by *Mycobacterium tuberculosis*. The American Thoracic Society distinguishes between tuberculosis infection (the tubercle bacillus has become established but there are no symptoms or evidence of active disease, and bacteriologic studies are negative) and tuberculosis (an infected person has a disease process involving one or more organs, and bacteriologic studies are positive).

B. Acquisition of Disease. Patients with pulmonary tuberculosis generate organisms in small particles (droplet nuclei), 1 to 4 μm long, whenever they cough or speak. These particles can remain suspended in the air and when inhaled by susceptible hosts can multiply without initial resistance. Subsequently, the organisms become engulfed by phagocytes but may remain viable within the intracellular environment. During the initial infection, the bacilli spread through lymphatics to regional lymph nodes and through the blood throughout the body. In a small percentage of patients (about 5 per cent), initial control is inadequate and progressive disease results. Usually the cell-mediated immunity that develops is able to limit further multiplication of the

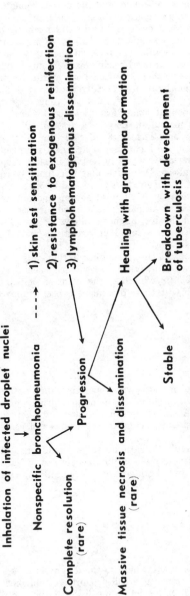

Figure 45-1. Results of infection with *M. tuberculosis*. When an infected droplet nucleus is deposited in the alveolus of a susceptible person, a nonspecific asymptomatic area of bronchopneumonia—the primary focus—develops initially. Tubercle bacilli from the primary focus drain to regional lymph nodes. Subsequently, lymphatic drainage delivers tubercle bacilli to the systemic circulation and then, potentially, to all organs of the body. In about 5 per cent of newly infected persons the pulmonary process progresses and becomes radiographically or clinically apparent. Rarely, the lymphohematogenous spread of large numbers of bacilli throughout the body may lead to miliary tuberculosis or other extrapulmonary manifestations. By far the most common outcome for the initial infection with *M. tuberculosis* is healing with granuloma formation. In most persons, the healed granulomas remain stable and with time may calcify; overt disease never occurs. In about 5 to 15 per cent of cases, one of the granulomas—in the lung or elsewhere in the body—breaks down; tubercle bacilli multiply and the person becomes ill with tuberculosis. (Reprinted, with permission of author and publisher, from Glassroth J, Robin AG, Snider DE: Tuberculosis in the 1980s. N Engl J Med 302:1441–1450, 1980.)

organisms, the infection is controlled, and the patient remains asymptomatic with the only evidence of disease being conversion of the tuberculin test result to positive. In a small percentage of patients who acquire asymptomatic disease (5 to 15 per cent), active tuberculosis develops after an interval that may vary from a few years to decades. Factors favoring reactivation include old age, immunosuppressive therapy, alcoholism, and undernutrition. The most common location for recurrent disease is the upper lung zones. However, other areas of the lung may be involved, as may other nonpulmonary foci. (See Fig. 45–1.)

C. **Definitive Diagnosis.** Tuberculosis may be a systemic disease with protean manifestations. The data collected from history, physical examination, routine laboratory tests, chest roentgenograms, and skin testing are frequently helpful in suggesting the presence of tuberculosis. Definitive diagnosis usually requires demonstration of *M. tuberculosis* in tissues by histologic examination or in secretions or body fluids by stains and culture. The need for definitive diagnosis, particularly by culture, cannot be overemphasized. A definitive diagnosis allows exclusion of other diseases having similar clinical presentations and also enables testing of drug susceptibility.

D. **Other Mycobacterial Disease.** Disease similar to that caused by *M. tuberculosis* can be caused by other mycobacteria such as *M. kansasii* and *M. avium-intracellularae*. The transmission and pathogenesis of infection with these organisms is poorly understood.

EPIDEMIOLOGY

In 1983, 23,532 cases of tuberculosis were reported to the Centers for Disease Control. With the exception of the period during which large numbers of southeast Asian refugees immigrated to the United States, there has been a steady decline in the number of cases reported.

Despite the decline, tuberculosis continues to be a public health problem. It is estimated that over ten million people are infected with *M. tuberculosis* in the United States. They have a lifelong risk of developing disease.

HISTORY

The history usually does not contribute to the diagnosis unless contact with a patient with active tuberculosis can be established. Many patients with active disease come to medical attention only through case finding activities (investigation of contacts of patients with active disease) or by further investigation of patients who have conversion of the tuberculin skin tests.

SIGNS AND SYMPTOMS

Although active disease may be found in asymptomatic individuals, symptoms of disease are usually present. Unfortunately, these symptoms may have an insidious onset and frequently may be ignored. When symptoms are present, they are usually generalized and include fatigue, anorexia, and weight loss, which may have been noted for weeks to months.

Patients may have an acute febrile illness resembling influenza or they may have a low-grade fever. Some patients have fever of undetermined origin. (See Chapter 31.) Other findings depend on the organ system involved.

A. **Pulmonary Tuberculosis.** Cough productive of mucoid or mucopurulent sputum is the most common manifestation of pulmonary tuberculosis (except in children, in whom cough is unusual). Hemoptysis is rare. When it is observed in patients with chest roentgenographic evidence of posttuberculous scarring, the possibility of an aspergilloma should be considered.

B. **Meningeal Tuberculosis.** Tuberculous meningitis usually causes fever, a change in mental status, headaches, or seizures. Cranial nerve abnormalities (especially III and VI) are common. Pulmonary or miliary disease is usually present, and the purified protein derivative (PPD) test is usually positive. In 1980 356 cases of meningeal tuberculosis were reported to the Centers for Disease Control. This represented 1.2 per cent of the total cases of tuberculosis reported that year.

C. **Peritoneal Tuberculosis.** Ascites, fever, and abdominal pain are the characteristic findings. Finding of a doughy abdomen is rare. Most patients have no evidence of pulmonary disease, but pleural effusions may be present. Only 138 cases were reported in 1980 (0.5 per cent).

D. **Genitourinary Tuberculosis.** Genitourinary tuberculosis should be considered whenever patients have dysuria, pyuria without bacteriurea, unexplained hematuria or proteinuria, a beaded vas deferans on palpation, or epididymitis. Women may have menorrhagia, oligomenorrhea, amenorrhea, pelvic inflammatory disease, or infertility. Abnormal calices, pelvis, ureters, or bladder may be seen on excretory pyelography. In 1980 610 cases were reported, which represented 2.2 per cent of total cases.

E. **Lymph Node Tuberculosis.** Any lymph node may be involved. Hilar or mediastinal adenopathy may be present during the initial pulmonary infection, particularly in children. Cervical and supraclavicular adenopathy is common and usually occurs in patients without roentgenographic evidence of pulmonary involvement. Nodes in these areas may spontaneously drain. In adults, *M. tuberculosis* is almost always the causative organism. In children, mycobacteria other than tuberculosis may be responsible. In 1980 1026 cases were reported.

F. **Bone and Joint Tuberculosis.** The skeleton (most commonly the lower spine and weight-bearing joints) is affected in approximately 1 per cent of patients with tuberculosis. About half of these have no evidence of pulmonary involvement. In 1980 333 cases were reported (1.2 per cent).

G. Pericardial Tuberculosis. Most, but not all, patients with tuberculous pericarditis are dyspneic and have extensive pulmonary involvement. Symptoms may include orthopnea and chest pain, and constriction with impaired right ventricular filling may result. Mortality is high.

H. Laryngeal Tuberculosis. Patients with laryngeal tuberculosis have hoarseness or a sore throat. Extensive pulmonary involvement is usually seen. Sputum smears are markedly positive.

I. Miliary Tuberculosis. Patients may have acute onset of fever and shortness of breath or may only describe nonspecific generalized symptoms. Miliary tuberculosis may occur at any age and may precede the development of the miliary pattern seen on chest roentgenographs. Patients may have hepatomegaly, splenomegaly, generalized lymphadenopathy, or meningitis and may be pancytopenic or have leukemoid reactions. In 1980 177 cases were reported (0.6 per cent).

J. Other Organs. Tuberculosis rarely may cause adrenal insufficiency, chronic otitis media, mastoiditis, perirectal abscesses, or fistulae. *M. bovis* has been associated with disease in the small intestine, usually in the iliocecal area.

LABORATORY AND X-RAY STUDIES

Diagnosis can only be established by culture of tuberculous bacilli or by their observation on histologic examination of tissue. In children with hilar adenopathy in the appropriate setting (contact with known disease), bacteriologic proof may not be required.

A. Chest X-Ray. Pulmonary tuberculosis is often first suspected on the basis of chest x-ray findings. In general, inactive disease often shows a hilar node with a peripheral calcification (Gohn complex), and apical scarring may be present. Active disease may show an apical lesion (often mottled in appearance), which may go on to cavitate. Laminograms may identify suspected cavitary lesions. Unfortunately, the roentgenographic classification of disease into active or inactive categories is imprecise. Virtually any roentgenographic abnormalities can be caused by tuberculosis.

B. Sputum, Gastric Fluid, and Urine. Specific instructions regarding collection of material brought up from the lung are needed. Three good-quality early morning specimens are sufficient. Sputum production can be induced by inhalation of hypertonic saline solution (3 to 10 per cent) or collected by nasotracheal suction or bronchoscopy. Brushings can be obtained for culture during this procedure. Tissue can be obtained by transbronchial biopsy for histologic examination as well as for culture. Aspiration of gastric fluid after an eight- to ten-hour fast can be cultured for tuberculosis. For urinalysis, the first specimen voided in the morning is preferred. Several collections are required. Broad-spectrum antibiotics in the urine may result in negative cultures.

C. Other Specimens. Pleural, cerebrospinal, peritoneal, and pericardial fluids should be analyzed for protein and glucose and compared with simultaneous blood glucose determinations. Also, cell and differential counts should be obtained. A high protein level (greater than 3 g), lymphocytosis, and low glucose levels are usually found in patients with tuberculous infections. However, neither the presence nor the absence of these findings is diagnostic. To increase diagnostic yield, biopsy of pleural and peritoneal tissues should be performed at the time of thoracentesis or paracentesis. Specimens should also be acquired from the lung, pericardium, lymph nodes, bones, joints, bowel, salpinges, and epididymis when noninvasive techniques fail to establish the diagnosis. In cases in which hematogenous or miliary disease is being considered, bone marrow, lung, or liver biopsy for histologic examination and culture should be considered.

D. **Tuberculin Skin Testing.** The cell-mediated immune response to infection with mycobacteria produces delayed hypersensitivity to culture extracts. Reactive patients are not all infected with *M. tuberculosis* since cross-reactivity to mycobacteria other than *M. tuberculosis* can occur. The larger the reaction, the more likely it is that it is caused by *M. tuberculosis*.

The area of induration should be determined 48 to 72 hours after injection of 0.1 mL of tween-stabilized purified protein-derivative (PPD) containing 5 tuberculin units (also known as intermediate-strength PPD), just beneath the surface of the skin. Finding of an area of induration greater than 10 mm in diameter indicates infection; it does not document the presence of active disease. The infection may have occurred as long ago as from two weeks previously to in the far distant past. In evaluation of close contacts of patients with active disease, a reaction of 5 mm is considered positive. A negative test does not exclude infection, even in the absence of anergy. First- and second-strength tuberculin tests have limited, if any, diagnostic use.

The PPD test should be used to determine the rate of tuberculosis in various populations, in periodically repeated surveillance, and in case finding.

E. **Staining Techniques and Culturing for Tuberculosis.** Water-soluble dyes are taken up through the wall of the tubercle bacillus and cannot be eliminated by an acid wash. Hence, "acid-fastness" is not a property exclusive to *M. tuberculosis*. Nontuberculous mycobacteria, nocardia, and the recently described Pittsburgh pneumonia agent can also be stained in this way. Culturing is considerably more sensitive than use of an acid-fast smear to detect the presence of mycobacteria. Culturing is essential to distinguish *M. tuberculosis* from other mycobacteria, as well as to test for drug susceptibility. Several weeks to months may be needed before the cultures can be interpreted as being positive and before the mycobacterial species and drug susceptibility can be determined. Two recently described techniques to identify tuberculosis organisms in sputum cultures after only a few days of inoculation are being evaluated. (See references by Odham and Snider[9, 10].)

RECOMMENDED DIAGNOSTIC APPROACH

The diagnostic approach must be customized to the patient's clinical findings and type of tuberculosis suspected.

A. **Low Suspicion of TB.** A chest x-ray is an adequate initial procedure. Three early morning sputum specimens for staining and culture are indicated when the chest x-ray is suggestive of TB.

B. **High Suspicion of Pulmonary TB.** Chest x-ray and collection of three early morning sputum specimens for staining and culture are initial diagnostic steps. If tuberculosis is not proved, the next diagnostic steps should be based on the availability of specimens (pleural fluid, pleural tissue, and so forth), as suggested by the signs and symptoms and seriousness of the illness. It is useful to culture for tuberculosis when urinalysis is abnormal without explanation or if intravenous pyelography suggests tuberculosis.

REFERENCES

1. Khan AM, Kovnat DM, Bachus B, Whitcomb ME, Brody JS, Snider GL: Clinical and roentgenographic spectrum of pulmonary tuberculosis in the adult. Am J Med 62:31–38, 1977.

Demonstrates the varied roentgenographic manifestations of active pulmonary tuberculosis.

2. Weg JG, Farer LS, Kaplan AI, Mathews JH, Sbarbaro JA (American Thoracic Society and Centers for Disease Control): Diagnostic standards and classification of tuberculosis and other mycobacterial diseases. Am Rev Respir Dis 123:343–358, 1981.
3. Bailey WC, Albert RK, Davidson PT, et al. (American Thoracic Society and Centers for Disease Control): Treatment of tuberculosis and other mycobacterial diseases. Am Rev Respir Dis 127:790–796, 1983.
4. Farer LS, Flynn JP, Bailey WC, Albert RK: Control of tuberculosis. Am Rev Respir Dis 128:336–342, 1983.

References 2, 3, and 4 are joint statements by the American Thoracic Society and the Centers for Disease Control providing a comprehensive review of all aspects of tuberculosis.

5. Glassroth J, Robins AG, Snyder DE: Tuberculosis in the 1980s. N Engl J Med 302:1441–1450, 1980.

Reviews recent literature on tuberculosis.

6. Centers for Disease Control: Morbid Mortal Weekly Rep 38:6–9, 1983.

Contains epidemiologic data for 1983.

7. Proudfoot AT, Akhtar AJ, Douglas AC, Horne NW: Miliary tuberculosis in adults. Br Med J 2:273–276, 1969.

A review of a large series.

8. Goren MB, Cernich M, Brokl O: Cell observations on mycobacterial acid-fastness. Am Rev Respir Dis 118:151–154, 1978.

Demonstrates lack of specificity in acid-fast staining as an indicator of tuberculosis.

9. Odham G, Larsson L, Mardh P-A: Demonstration of tuberculostearic acid

in sputum from patients with pulmonary tuberculosis by selected ion monitoring. J Clin Invest 63:813–819, 1979.

10. Snider DE, Good RC, Kilburn JD, et al.: Rapid drug-susceptibility testing of mycobacterium tuberculosis. Am Rev Respir Dis 123:402–406, 1981.

In references 9 and 10 new techniques aimed at speeding up microbiologic identification of tuberculosis are described.

11. Kwan KL, Kurt DS, Stottmeier KD, Sherman MS, McCabe WR: Mycobacterial cervical lymphadenopathy: Relation of etiologic agents to age. JAMA 251:1286–1288, 1984.

Mycobacterium tuberculosis clearly preponderates as the cause of mycobacterial cervical adenitis in adults, while other mycobacteria are the cause of most adenitis in children.

12. Powell KE, Meador MP, Farer LS: Recent trends in tuberculosis in children. JAMA 251:1289–1292, 1984.

Incidence data for children are given.

46

URINARY TRACT INFECTIONS

By BARBARA D. KIRBY, M.D.

DEFINITION

Infections of the urinary tract are very common and range in severity from asymptomatic bacteriuria to life-threatening bacteremic pyelonephritis. Complicated infections of the urinary tract result from anatomic or physiologic obstruction (renal calculi, anatomic anomalies, indwelling urinary catheters, or urologic manipulation), or both.

A. Asymptomatic Bacteriuria
1. Asymptomatic bacteriuria occurs in 1 to 2 per cent of children, 2 to 5 per cent of child-bearing women, and in 5 to 15 per cent of older women.
2. Asymptomatic bacteriuria during pregnancy is found in 2 to 10 per cent of women and poses a special problem. The onset of bacteriuria is usually during the first trimester. Twenty to 40 per cent of pregnant women who develop first-trimester asymptomatic bacteriuria develop pyelonephritis during pregnancy if the bacteriuria is not eradicated. Less than 1 per cent of women without bacteriuria during early pregnancy develop pyelonephritis.

B. Acute Uncomplicated Cystitis
1. This is an infection of the bladder, typically occurring in otherwise healthy young women.
2. The usual pathogens are *Escherichia coli* and *Staphylococcus saprophyticus*.

C. Acute Uncomplicated Pyelonephritis
1. This is an infection of renal parenchyma without anatomic or physiologic abnormality or foreign body.
2. The usual pathogen is *E. coli.* If the pyelonephritis is recurrent, potential pathogens, in addition to *E. coli,* include *Proteus* sp., *Enterobacter* sp., and enterococci.

D. Complicated Infections
1. Pathogens associated with renal calculi include *Proteus* sp., *Klebsiella* sp., enterococci, and *Staphylococcus aureus.*
2. Pathogens associated with urologic manipulation, obstruction, indwelling urinary catheter, and nosocomial infections include *Proteus* sp., *Klebsiella* sp., *Enterobacter* sp., *Serratia* sp., *Pseudomonas* sp., *Staphylococcus aureus,* enterococci, and fungi, including *Candida albicans.*

EPIDEMIOLOGY

A. Infections of the urinary tract are very common in females.
B. Pregnancy is a risk factor for asymptomatic and symptomatic infections.
C. Urinary tract infections in males under age 45 are almost always associated with urologic abnormalities.
D. Urinary tract infections are a leading cause of nosocomial infection (40 per cent of cases). Of nosocomial urinary tract infections, 75 per cent of cases are associated with indwelling urinary catheters. The remainder are attributable to urologic manipulation. Two per cent of patients with catheter-associated bacteriuria develop bacteremia. Pathogens responsible for nosocomially acquired urinary tract infections demonstrate marked resistance to antimicrobial agents.

DIFFERENTIAL DIAGNOSIS

Evaluation of patients with symptoms of dysuria should include consideration of:
A. Urethritis. This may be caused by *Neisseria gonorrhoeae* or *Chlamydia trachomatis.*
B. Vaginitis. This may be caused by *Gardnerella vaginalis* and vaginal anaerobes (nonspecific vaginitis), *Trichomonas vaginalis,* or *C. albicans.*
C. Genital Herpes Infection

CLINICAL FEATURES

Because of overlaps in signs and symptoms between patients with upper tract (pyelonephritis) and lower tract (cystitis) infection, signs and symptoms cannot be relied upon for localization of site of infection. However, typical clinical pictures exist.

A. **Acute Uncomplicated Cystitis.** Urgency, frequent urination, dysuria, suprapubic discomfort in the absence of fever, flank pain, or systemic symptoms are common.

B. **Acute Pyelonephritis.** Fever, flank (costovertebral angle) pain, shaking chills, nausea, vomiting, and myalgia are typical. Urgency, frequent urination, dysuria, and suprapubic pain are often absent in patients with pyelonephritis. Patients may have septic shock from gram-negative bacteremic pyelonephritis.

LABORATORY FEATURES

A. **Pyuria**
   1. Determination of the presence or absence of pyuria is essential to the diagnosis of urinary tract infection. Recent studies have shown that patients with pyuria almost always have infected urine. The presence or absence of pyuria is particularly important, since the criterion of greater than or equal to 100,000 colonies of bacteria per cu mm of urine for diagnosis of urinary tract infection is no longer absolute.
   2. The hemacytometer method can be used to measure pyuria.
      a. It is simple and reliable.
      b. Fresh, uncentrifuged urine is examined in a hemacytometer chamber.
         1). Fewer than eight white blood cells per cu mm usually correlates with sterile urine in asymptomatic women.
         2). More than eight white blood cells per cu mm are present in most patients with acute cystitis (most patients have more than 60 cells per cu mm according to this technique).

B. White blood cell casts are commonly seen in pyelonephritis and are not seen in patients with lower tract disease.

C. Hematuria may be present in both cystitis (50 per cent) and pyelonephritis.

D. There may be bacteriuria; the presence of one bacterium per high power field of uncentrifuged urine correlated with 100,000 bacterial colonies per cu mm when cultured.

E. **Culture**
   1. One hundred thousand bacterial colonies per cu mm is no longer an absolute requirement for the diagnosis of bacterial infection of the urinary tract.
   2. Colony counts of 100 to 10,000 bacteria in patients with pyuria and a compatible clinical picture can have diagnostic importance and must be interpreted in the clinical context.
   3. Quantitative cultures of urine specimens should be done.

RECOMMENDED DIAGNOSTIC APPROACH

A. **Cystitis**
   1. *Urinalysis.* Urinalysis shows the presence of pyuria (hemacytometer method) and bacteriuria.

    2. Gram's Stain of Urine. Morphologic and staining characteristics of bacteria that are seen direct the selection of an antimicrobial agent.

    3. Urine Culture. Urine culture may confirm the appropriateness of antibiotic therapy or suggest a need to alter therapy. If urine culture is negative, other causes of symptoms should be considered such as urethritis or chlamydial infection.

B. Pyelonephritis

    1. Urinalysis. Urinalysis shows the presence of pyuria, white blood cell casts, and bacteriuria.

    2. Gram's Stain of Urine. This has the same role as for cystitis.

    3. Urine Culture

    4. Ill Patient and/or Complicated Pyelonephritis

      a. Blood cultures should be done.

      b. White blood cell count with differential count should be determined.

C. Bladder Washout and Antibody-coated Bacteria Tests. These procedures are not routinely done but may be of value in localization of infection in selected cases.

REFERENCES

1. Brumfitt W: Urinary cell counts and their value. J Clin Pathol 18:550–553, 1965.

The Hemacytometer technique is described.

2. Latham RH, Running K, Stamm WE: Urinary tract infections in adult women caused by *Staphylococcus saprophyticus.* JAMA 250:3063–3066, 1983.

A description of infection caused by this pathogen.

3. Stamm WE, Counts GW, Running KR, et al.: Diagnosis of coliform infection in acutely dysuric women. N Engl J Med 307:463–468, 1982.

An approach to diagnosis of acute cystitis is described.

4. Farrar WE: Infections of the urinary tract. Med Clin North Am 67:187–201, 1983.

An overview of approach and management.

—————————47—————————

VIRAL HEPATITIS

By RUSSELL McMULLEN, M.D.

DEFINITION

A. Hepatitis A and Hepatitis B. A number of viral agents are now known to be responsible for acute hepatocellular infection, damage, and dysfunction. Previously, it was thought that there were two types of viral hepatitis: "infectious" and "serum." Infectious hepatitis is now referred to as hepatitis A and serum hepatitis as hepatitis B. In addition, non-A non-B hepatitis, epidemiologically similar to hepatitis B, is recognized. However, the specific viral agents that are responsible for the infection have not been serologically isolated. Also recently recognized is the delta agent, a defective virus that utilizes the hepatitis B virus in order to replicate and produce clinical infection.

B. Criteria for Diagnosis. Hyperbilirubinemia and elevated transaminase levels often lead to a presumptive diagnosis of viral hepatitis, especially with epidemiologic support, but by themselves are not definitive. Other less common infectious, toxic or drug-induced liver dysfunction, and hepatobiliary tract disease must be considered and ruled out.

1. Serologic testing is available to detect antibody to the hepatitis A virus (HAV) and can differentiate acute from past infection.

2. Screening for various antigenic components of the hepatitis B virus (HBV), and antibodies to them, can determine whether acute HBV infection is present, whether infection has occurred in the past, or whether ongoing infection persists.

3. Assays for antibody to the Epstein-Barr virus (EBV) and cytomegalovirus (CMV), which can cause a picture similar to the more common types of viral hepatitis, are available.

4. There is no definitive test for non-A non-B hepatitis (NANBH). This remains a diagnosis of exclusion.

5. Serologic testing for the delta agent is available only in selected research settings.

EPIDEMIOLOGY

A. Hepatitis A

1. Hepatitis A is caused by a 27-nm RNA virus. The usual mechanism of spread is by the fecal-oral route. Waterborne infection (including infection from contaminated shellfish) can occur.

2. The disease is present worldwide, but is most prevalent in areas with crowding and poor sanitation. Greater than 50 per cent of urban adult Americans of low socioeconomic status have antibody to hepatitis A virus (HAV). In contrast, the rate is 2 to 3 per cent in young adult Scandinavians.

3. The incubation period is two to six weeks, with peak infectivity occurring in the week prior to the onset of jaundice and during the early clinical illness. However, most infections are subclinical and undiagnosed, tending to perpetuate the spread of the disease.

4. There is no carrier state.

B. Hepatitis B

1. Hepatitis B is caused by a 42-nm DNA virus (HBV), also known as the *Dane Particle*. It is composed of a surface antigen (HBsAg), which can circulate independently, and the core

antigen (HBcAg). The core also includes a DNA polymerase molecule, as well as the "e" antigen (HBeAg).

2. Transmission of HBV is often parenteral. However, many body fluids besides blood contain the virus; saliva and semen probably transmit the disease via inoculation through inapparent mucosal lesions. The incubation period is two to six months.

3. The following identifiable groups are at risk for infection with HBV:

   a. Those receiving blood products: The risk is less than formerly, given that banked blood is screened for HBsAg.
   b. Parenteral drug abusers.
   c. Hemodialysis patients.
   d. Organ-transplant recipients.
   e. Certain groups of health care workers, especially those with contact with blood products or high-risk patients.
   f. Household contacts of infected individuals.
   g. Male homosexuals with multiple partners.
   h. Infants of infected mothers may acquire the virus by third-trimester maternal-fetal transmission.

4. There are definite patterns of infection throughout the world. Ten per cent of the adult population of the United States carries antibody to HBsAg. Some Southeast Asian populations have greater than 90 per cent evidence of past infection.

5. A carrier state exists for hepatitis B. The rate for adults in the United States is 0.2 per cent, reflecting an incidence of less than 10 per cent after initial infection. Populations with high rates of past infection, such as Southeast Asians, have a high carrier rate (10 to 15 per cent).

C. Non-A Non-B Hepatitis (NANBH)

1. Agents of non-A non-B hepatitis have not been definitely identified, but several appear to exist.

2. The type of NANBH common in the United States has an epidemiology similar to hepatitis B. It is the leading cause (90 per cent) of hepatitis associated with blood products. There is a 3 to 7 per cent risk of transmission with a single unit of volunteer donor blood. Similar groups are at risk with NANBH as with HBV infection: drug abusers, hemodialysis patients, transplant recipients, health care workers, homosexuals with multiple contacts, and close household contacts of infected individuals. Maternal-fetal transmission also occurs.

3. The rate of the carrier state is quite high. In addition to the 3 to 7 per cent incidence of infection from blood from volunteer asymptomatic carriers, there is a greater than 20 per cent incidence of infection following transfusion with blood from paid donors.

D. Delta Agent

1. Delta agent is a defective virus that uses the reproductive mechanism of the HBV to facilitate replication. Delta agent superinfection occurs in carriers of hepatitis B and during acute HBV infection.

2. Transmission of delta agent appears to occur by percutaneous methods or by inapparent skin inoculation.
3. A persistent delta infection frequently leads to chronic active hepatitis (in 60 to 90 per cent of cases). Fulminant hepatitis and death (25 per cent of cases) are much more common when delta agent infection is combined with acute HBV infection.
4. Delta agent is endemic in Italy, North Africa, and South America. Some cases have occurred in intravenous drug abusers in Europe and the United States.

CLINICAL MANIFESTATIONS

A. Prodrome

1. The common types of viral hepatitis have a similar prodrome. However, the onset is fairly abrupt in hepatitis A and more indolent with HBV and NANBV infections. Incubation periods following infection are different: HAV, 2 to 6 weeks (mean 3.7 weeks); HBV, 2 to 6 months (mean 11.8 weeks); NANBV, 6 to 12 weeks (mean 7.8 weeks).
2. Patients with HAV are infectious for two to three weeks before the onset of icterus and less so for one week afterwards. HBV-infected individuals are infectious when HBsAg can be detected in the serum, usually six weeks before symptoms develop. The onset of infectivity for NANBH is undefined.
3. Early clinical manifestations include fever (37.5 to 38.5° C), fatigue, and malaise. Desire for cigarettes may decrease. Gastrointestinal complaints include anorexia, nausea, and occasionally diarrhea. Hepatomegaly (70 per cent of cases) and right upper quadrant tenderness (90 per cent) follow, with splenomegaly (20 per cent) in severe cases.
4. Arthralgia and urticarial rash occur in hepatitis B (10 per cent of cases) caused by HBsAg-antibody immune complex formation. Similar findings are rarely seen with HAV (1 per cent of cases) and have been reported in NANBH.

B. Icteric Phase

1. This phase occurs in less than half of all types of infection (probably in 10 to 20 per cent).
2. From the time of initial transaminase elevation, patients may show a progression from dark urine (bilirubinuria) to acholic stool and then jaundice. Palatine and scleral icterus may be noted first on examination. Pruritus, caused by cutaneous bilirubin deposition, mirrors the serum concentration.
3. Systemic symptoms begin to resolve at this point in hepatitis A.

C. Convalescent Phase

1. There is a gradual return to well-being in the infections that resolve.
2. Bilirubin rapidly normalizes after HAV infection, and enzymes normalize in 80 to 90 per cent of cases by four months after onset of symptoms.

3. Hepatitis B can have a slower resolution. Serum bilirubin roughly reflects levels of HBsAg, which persists for 6 to 20 weeks in resolving symptomatic infections. Five to 10 per cent of patients become chronic carriers.
4. NANBH can resolve quickly or may show a smouldering pattern of enzyme elevation. The latter finding suggests development of a carrier state.

D. Fulminant Hepatitis

1. Fulminant hepatitis is an overwhelming infection that destroys large numbers of hepatocytes. Manifestations include deep jaundice with initial high enzyme levels, prolonged prothrombin time, persistent jaundice following enzyme normalization, and hepatic encephalopathy.
2. Fulminant hepatitis is a rare complication of hepatitis but is more common in hepatitis B (1 to 3 per cent of cases) than in hepatitis A (0.5 to 1 per cent) or NANBH (rare).
3. When it does occur, fatality rates are greater for NANBH (90 per cent) than for hepatitis A (60 per cent) or hepatitis B (70 per cent). (Superimposed delta infection can increase mortality to 90 per cent in HBV infection.)

E. Chronic Hepatitis

1. Development of a carrier state may occur after acute infection with HBV or NANBV. It does not occur after hepatitis A.
2. Five to 10 per cent of patients with acute hepatitis B go on to be chronically positive for HBsAg. The percentage may be highest in those with parenteral inoculation. Carriers are at risk of developing immune-complex–mediated disease such as membranous glomerulonephritis. HBsAg is found in 40 to 50 per cent of persons with polyarteritis nodosa. Chronic carriers, especially those who develop cirrhosis, are 300 times more likely to develop hepatocellular carcinoma.
3. The rate of chronicity appears higher in NANBH (perhaps as high as 50 per cent). Approximately 3 to 7 per cent of adults in the United States may be carriers (this is inferred from the likelihood of acquisition of NANBH after blood transfusion).
4. HBV and NANBV infection can result in chronic persistent hepatitis. This is a mild inflammation of the portal areas of the liver parenchyma. It does not progress or carry risk of cirrhosis.
5. HBV and NANBV infection can result in chronic active hepatitis. This involves more extensive cellular damage, bridging of inflammation between portal areas, and eventual development of fibrosis. Twenty per cent of cases are caused by chronic HBV infection and an unknown number by NANBH. The chronic hepatitis associated with NANBH is more likely to be chronic-active (50 per cent of cases), although histologically more benign when it does occur.

DIFFERENTIAL DIAGNOSIS

The differential diagnosis of viral hepatitis includes any cause of acute jaundice. Besides infection with HAV, HBV, and NANBV (delta agent infection is rare in this country), there are several sources of hepatic disease to be considered.

A. **Other Viruses**
   1. *Epstein-Barr Virus.* The syndrome of infectious mononucleosis, typically seen in young adults, can involve the liver. Mild enzyme abnormalities are common, but hepatomegaly (10 per cent of cases) and jaundice (4 per cent) can occur. Significant hepatic sequelae are rare.
   2. *Cytomegalovirus.* In a nonimmunosuppressed adult, parenteral transmission of CMV can result in a picture similar to that seen in EBV infection (that is, hepatomegaly and mild jaundice). There is some evidence that CMV hepatitis can progress to chronic liver disease. In immunosuppressed patients the disease can be much more striking.
   3. *Yellow Fever.* Jaundice is a common manifestation of the severe form of yellow fever. The incubation period is short (three to six days). It should be suspected only in recent travelers from endemic areas of Africa and South America.
   4. *Herpes Simplex.* Disseminated infection can include hepatic involvement with hepatic necrosis.
   5. *Coxsackievirus.* Hepatitis may be seen in severe systemic infection.

B. **Nonviral Infections**
   1. *Typhoid.* Jaundice as a result of diffuse hepatic involvement has been reported. It should be differentiated from the cholecystitis often seen in typhoid.
   2. *Syphilis.* Liver function abnormalities, most typically alkaline phosphatase, can be seen in secondary syphilis (10 per cent of cases).
   3. *Leptospirosis.* This is a biphasic illness. During the second, "immune," phase, Weil's syndrome with marked hyperbilirubinemia and modest liver enzyme elevation can be seen. Mortality increases with age, approaching 40 per cent.
   4. *Q Fever.* The disease is caused by the rickettsia *Coxiella burnetti.* It is spread to humans by exposure to aerosols at the time of parturition of infected goats, cows, and sheep. Exposure to their hides can also spread the disease. Hepatomegaly and jaundice may be prominent symptoms; the hepatic lesions are granulomatous.
   5. *Toxoplasmosis.* Hepatic involvement is usually not severe unless the patient is immunosuppressed.
   6. *Malaria.* Hepatomegaly and marked jaundice are most common in falciparum malaria.
   7. *Liver Abscess.* Both bacterial and amebic liver abscess tend to have focal hepatomegaly and tenderness. Bilirubin level may be elevated, although transaminases tend to be normal. A history of cholangitis or travel to endemic areas may suggest the diagnosis.

C. **Toxic Hepatitis**
   1. *Acute Alcoholic Hepatitis.* This type of hepatitis occurs after increased intake by someone with a regular consumption of 60 g per day of ethanol. Fever, marked hepatomegaly, and a strikingly elevated white blood cell count are typical.

2. *Medications*
    a. **Hepatocellular Injury.** This condition is similar to viral hepatitis and can be caused by a number of agents, including:
        1). *Halothane.* Halothane probably causes a hypersensitivity reaction. Likelihood of the reaction increases with increased number and frequency of exposures.
        2). *Isoniazid.* The likelihood of injury increases with age. Prophylaxis for tuberculosis is not recommended for those older than 35.
        3). *Methyldopa*
        4). *Phenytoin*
        5). *Phenylbutazone*
        6). *Sulfonamides*
    b. **Cholestatic Jaundice.** This condition can be caused by:
        1). *Erythromycin Estolate*
        2). *Chlorpromazine*
        3). *Antithyroid Agents (Propylthiouracil and Methimazole)*
        4). *Estrogenic and Androgenic Steroids*
    c. **Hepatotoxic Agents**
        1). *Acetaminophen.* Hepatocellular injury occurs as a result of suicide attempts as well as chronic overdose, owing to the drug's presence in many over-the-counter medications.
        2). *Vitamins.* The fat-soluble vitamins A and D are especially hepatotoxic.
3. *Other Hepatotoxins.* These include the industrial agent carbon tetrachloride as well as the toxin of *Amanita phalloides* from mushroom poisoning.

D. **Biliary Tract Disease.** Causes of obstructive or "surgical" jaundice should be considered.

E. **"Benign Postoperative Jaundice" or "Reactive Hepatopathy."** This condition is seen in markedly ill patients with nonhepatic disease. It is characterized by elevation of bilirubin and alkaline phosphatase levels with normal or nearly normal transaminase levels.

F. **Gilbert's Syndrome.** The syndrome is found in 7 per cent of the population and is caused by deficient hepatic uptake of bilirubin and defective glucuronyl transferase activity. It is seen after fasting or mild illness and is characterized by an elevated indirect bilirubin concentration in association with normal hepatic enzymes.

G. **Jaundice Associated with Pregnancy.** Two conditions can occur in the third trimester:
    1. *Cholestatic Jaundice of Pregnancy:* This is a relatively benign condition. Bilirubin elevation is low, as are transaminase levels.
    2. *Acute Fatty Liver.* This condition has a high mortality. Bilirubin, enzymes, and prothrombin time are usually quite abnormal. The picture is one of total hepatic collapse. The cause is unknown.

LABORATORY TESTS

A. General Tests

1. *Transaminases.* Aspartate aminotransferase (AST; serum glutamic oxaloacetic transaminase [SGOT]) and ALT (alanine aminotransferase; serum glutamic pyruvic transaminase [SGPT]) are markers for hepatocellular injury. Used as screening tests, they can detect otherwise subclinical hepatitis. Values in acute hepatitis may range from the low hundreds to several thousand international units (IU). Generally, ALT is greater than AST (SGPT>SGOT); a useful exception occurs in alcoholic hepatitis, in which levels are rarely higher than 300 IU and AST>ALT (SGOT>SGPT). With exceptions, decreasing transaminases reflect gross resolution of disease.

2. *Bilirubin.* Elevation of bilirubin can be indicative of the degree of hepatic injury and usually parallels transaminase increase. However, bilirubin rises in many hepatobiliary disorders; fractionation is of limited value, since almost all hepatobiliary diseases have significant elevation of direct bilirubin. An exception occurs with Gilbert's syndrome, in which indirect bilirubin is the predominantly elevated fraction. The same is true in hemolysis.

3. *Prothrombin Time.* The concentrations of liver-synthesized clotting factors determine the prothrombin time. It has some utility as a parameter of the severity and progression of liver dysfunction (if parenteral vitamin K is made available to eliminate potential malabsorption).

4. *Alkaline Phosphatase.* This enzyme is elevated in almost all hepatobiliary and some systemic disorders. It is of little value in diagnosis of hepatitis, although it may be markedly elevated in biliary tree disease or cholestasis. It is also found in bone; 5'-nucleotidase or γ-glutamyl transpeptidase can confirm the source as hepatic.

B. Specific Tests and Diseases

1. *Hepatitis A*

   a. In acute infection with HAV, an IgM antibody (anti-HAV) is produced, beginning at the time that jaundice appears (or approximately two weeks after fecal shedding begins). The antibody remains detectable in serum for several months.

   b. Following an acute infection, IgG antibody to HAV develops and probably lasts for life. If present, the antibody indicates remote infection with HAV. It is presumed to confer immunity from reinfection and militates against the diagnosis of hepatitis A in an acute episode of jaundice.

   c. Transaminase and bilirubin values are typically high in hepatitis A but generally resolve within weeks. The course of hepatitis A is diagrammed in Figure 47–1.

2. *Hepatitis B.* There are several serologic markers for antigenic components of the hepatitis B virus, as well as antibodies to

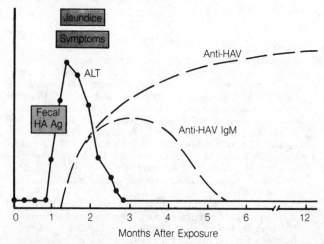

Figure 47–1. The clinical, serologic, and biochemical course of typical type A hepatitis. HA Ag = hepatitis A antigen; ALT = alanine aminotransferase; Anti-HAV = antibody to hepatitis A virus. (Reprinted, with permission of publisher, from Hoofnagle JH: Perspectives on Viral Hepatitis, Vol. 2, 1st ed. Rahway, New Jersey, Abbott Laboratories, 1981, p. 4.)

those components. Those that are generally commercially available include:

a. **HBsAg**
   1). Hepatitis B surface antigen (HBsAg) from the outer coat of the HBV can be found in the serum several weeks before onset of symptoms, perhaps as early as one week after inoculation. The HBsAg disappears with resolution of the infection. Continued presence in serum suggests the carrier state (although assay may be negative in the very low-level carrier state).

b. **Anti-HBs**
   1). Antibody to the HBsAg (anti-HBs) is indicative of recovery from HBV infection and immunity from reinfection.
   2). It is generally not seen until one to four months, or longer, after HBsAg is cleared from the serum. Occasionally the test can be positive at the time of clinical illness; arthralgia and urticaria are then more common.
   3). In subclinical infections, anti-HBs appears early and HBsAg may never be detectable.

c. **Anti-HBc**
   1). Antibody to the core of HBV (anti-HBc) appears three to four weeks after HBsAg is found in serum, generally just before clinical illness develops.
   2). During acute infection, a portion of anti-HBc is IgM; this finding may become a significant diagnostic tool.

   3). Anti-HBc decreases after resolution of symptoms, but chronic carriers of HBV frequently have high levels.

   4). After HBsAg disappears, and before anti-HBs appears, anti-HBc may be the only marker of HBV infection present (the "core window").

  d. HBeAg

   1). A portion of the core of HBV that can circulate freely.

   2). This occurs in acute infection and is indicative of a high degree of infectiousness.

   3). HBeAg disappears with resolution of symptoms. If present for longer than ten weeks after resolution, there is a strong likelihood that the patient may become a chronic carrier. Chronic carriers often remain positive for HBeAg (25 to 50 per cent of patients).

  e. Anti-HBe

   1). Antibody to HBeAg (anti-HBe) indicates probable resolution of infection.

   2). Anti-HBe generally disappears within one to two years following acute infection.

   3). If a carrier converts from HBeAg to anti-HBe, this suggests that the chronic disease is reaching an inactive phase with low infectivity.

The three common courses a hepatitis B infection may follow are diagrammed in Figures 47–2 to 47–4.

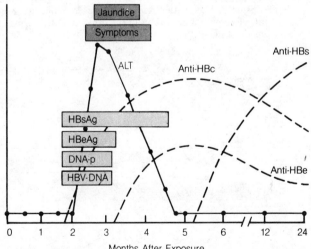

Figure 47–2. The clinical, serologic, and biochemical course of typical acute type B hepatitis. ALT = alanine aminotransferase; HBsAg = hepatitis B surface antigen; HBeAg = hepatitis B e antigen; DNA-p = serum hepatitis B virus DNA polymerase activity; HBV-DNA = serum hepatitis B virus DNA; Anti-HBs = antibody to HBsAg; Anti-HBe = antibody to HBeAg; Anti-HBc = antibody to hepatitis B core antigen. (Reprinted, with permission of publisher, from Hoofnagle JH: Perspectives on Viral Hepatitis, Vol. 2, 1st ed. Rahway, New Jersey, Abbott Laboratories, 1981, p. 6.)

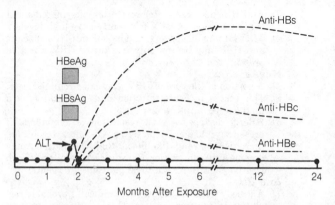

Figure 47–3. The clinical, serologic, and biochemical course of a subclinical asymptomatic hepatitis B virus infection. (Reprinted, with permission of publisher, from Hoofnagle JH: Perspectives on Viral Hepatitis, Vol. 2, 1st ed. Rahway, New Jersey, Abbott Laboratories, 1981, p. 7.)

3. Non-A non-B Hepatitis

   a. There are no specific markers for the unidentified virus. The diagnosis of this form of hepatitis remains a diagnosis of exclusion.

   b. Transaminase elevation and severity of jaundice are generally less pronounced than in the other common forms of infectious hepatitis.

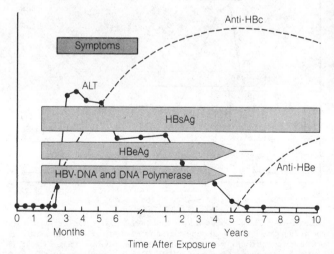

Figure 47–4. The clinical, serologic, and biochemical course of a chronic type B hepatitis infection. (Reprinted, with permission of publisher, from Hoofnagle JH: Perspectives on Viral Hepatitis, Vol. 2, 1st ed. Rahway, New Jersey, Abbott Laboratories, 1981, p. 8.)

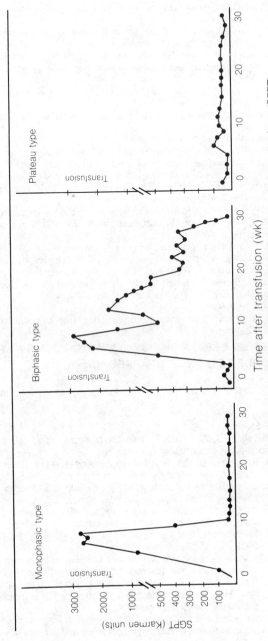

Figure 47–5. Three patterns of change in the concentration of serum glutamic pyruvic transaminase (SGPT) in patients with posttransfusion non-A non-B hepatitis. (Adapted, with permission, from Tateda A, et al.: Non-B hepatitis in Japanese recipients of blood transfusions: Clinical and serologic studies after the introduction of laboratory screening of donor blood for hepatitis B surface antigen. J Infect Dis 139:511–518, 1979.)

c. Several patterns of transaminase elevation may occur (see Fig. 47–5).

1). Monophasic, in which an acute rise is followed by permanent return to normal levels.

2). Biphasic or multiphasic, in which periodic elevations are seen between returns to near-normal enzyme levels.

3). Plateau, in which smouldering low-level elevations persist.

The latter two patterns may have greater likelihood of progression to a carrier state.

4. Mononucleosis (Epstein-Barr Virus)

a. The Monospot test for heterophile antibodies may be positive but can be negative in the first one to two weeks of clinical illness. As many as 10 per cent of cases of infectious mononucleosis caused by Epstein-Barr virus (EBV) remain heterophil-negative.

b. EBV antibodies, measured in both acute and convalescent sera, can suggest the diagnosis with less likelihood of negative results.

c. Absolute lymphocytosis, relative lymphocytosis (>50 per cent), or greater than 10 per cent atypical lymphocytes on a white blood cell differential count are frequently seen in mononucleosis. Unfortunately, these findings can be seen in other viral illnesses, including hepatitis.

5. Cytomegalovirus

a. Specific acute and convalescent antibody titers can confirm the diagnosis.

RECOMMENDED DIAGNOSTIC APPROACH

A. History. Specific questioning should be directed as outlined in Table 47–1.

B. Laboratory Studies

1. Initial Studies

a. AST (SGOT), ALT (SGPT), bilirubin, complete blood count, and alkaline phosphatase are analyzed.

1). If symptoms and physical examination suggest biliary tract disease, amylase levels should be determined and ultrasound, radionuclide imaging, or computed tomography considered. Further work-up should be done as directed. If hepatic abscess is suggested, an ultrasound study should be made for an evaluation.

2). Prothrombin time is obtained if AST (SGOT), ALT (SGPT), and bilirubin are abnormal.

3). If transaminases are normal and bilirubin is increased, Gilbert's syndrome (indirect bilirubin determination) or other disorders of bilirubin metabolism should be considered. Hemolysis or ineffective erythropoiesis can be ruled out with a complete blood count.

4). The complete blood count and differential may suggest mononucleosis, although lymphocytosis and atypical lym-

TABLE 47–1.   HISTORICAL CLUES IN DIAGNOSIS OF
HEPATITIS

Recent travel history
Ethnic background and birth place (especially Asian, Oceanic, or North
  African; or close exposure to these individuals)
Sexual orientation and patterns of contact
Known exposure to an infectious agent causing hepatitis (including health
  care workers with high risk exposure)
Past or current medical conditions
  Previous hepatitis, including type (if known); other liver disease
  History of or symptoms suggestive of biliary tract disease
  Transfusions or administration of blood products
  Hemodialysis
  History of organ transplantation
  History of recent surgery (benign postoperative jaundice?)
  History of frequent previous jaundice (Gilbert's syndrome?)
  Current pregnancy (third trimester—consider cholestatic jaundice of
    pregnancy or acute fatty liver of pregnancy)
Drug history
  Illicit drug usage (especially parenteral)
  Prescription medications (include oral contraceptives)
  Over-the-counter medications (include vitamins)
Toxin exposure
  Alcohol usage
  Occupational exposure
  Mushroom ingestion

phocytes can be seen in viral hepatitis. A strongly suggestive history coupled with a positive Monospot test result
can indicate the diagnosis.

  5). If the history suggests an uncommon infectious hepatitis,
acute serum should be obtained for appropriate studies.

  6). If other medical illness is suggested (Wilson's disease,
sarcoidosis, complications following ileojejunal bypass,
acute congestion secondary to heart failure), appropriate
evaluation should be initiated.

2. *Hepatitis Screen*

  a. If the history *strongly* suggests hepatitis A (such as jaundice
that develops after an appropriate incubation period following
exposure to a known case of hepatitis A), tests for anti-HAV
can be done. A positive IgM fraction confirms acute infection.
However, a positive IgM test does not rule out other acute or
chronic concomitant infection in a patient with acute hepatitis
A.

  b. Therefore, it is usually advisable to obtain a full battery of
hepatitis serologic studies. Besides HAV testing, this should
initially include HBsAg, anti-HBs, and anti-HBc. HBsAg alone
is insufficient: it can be positive in a chronic carrier state and
therefore not diagnostic of acute HBV infection. Also, HBsAg
can be undetectable in subclinical infections (if abnormal
chemistries are the reason for the evaluation). Complete
serologic evaluation can determine the status of present,
past, or ongoing HBV infection. (See Table 47–2.)

TABLE 47–2. INTERPRETATION OF HEPATITIS B SEROLOGIC TESTS

SEROLOGIC TEST			SUGGESTED DIAGNOSES AND FOLLOW-UP
HBsAg	**Anti-HBs**	**Anti-HBc**	
+	−	−	Early hepatitis B infection: probably preclinical or early clinical illness. HBeAg/anti-HBe testing possibly indicated: If −/− ("e window") or −/+: resolution likely If +/−: still highly infectious Needs follow-up testing until anti-HBs is positive (+), i.e., acute infection has resolved.
+	−	+	Diagnostic of either of the following: 1. Acute HBV infection: has not developed anti-HBs yet. Consider "e" antigen testing as outlined above. Needs follow-up testing for anti-HBs until positive. 2. Chronic HBV carrier Consider NANBH or HAV as diagnosis of the acute hepatitis. Consider other virus or toxin.
+	+	+	Acute hepatitis B Atypical pattern; usually HBsAg is gone by the time anti-HBs appears; should resolve, since antibody is present.
−	+	+	Remote hepatitis B infection Recovery is indicated by positive anti-HBs. Consider HAV, NANBH, other virus, or other cause of acute hepatitis.
−	−	+	One of the following: 1. Remote HBV infection: anti-HBs now at undetectable level. If HBeAg is negative, assume remote infection and consider HAV, NANBH, other virus, or other cause of acute hepatitis. 2. Immediate past HBV infection: the "core window" after HBsAg disappears but before anti-HBs appears. A positive test for HBeAg suggests this diagnosis. While the patient is still infectious (positive HBeAg), it is in the process of resolution, since HBsAg has disappeared. Follow-up is needed to be sure anti-HBs becomes positive.

Table continued on opposite page

TABLE 47–2. INTERPRETATION OF HEPATITIS B
SEROLOGIC TESTS *Continued*

| SEROLOGIC TEST | | | SUGGESTED DIAGNOSES AND FOLLOW-UP |
HBsAg	Anti-HBs	Anti-HBc	
			3. Low-level carrier state: HBsAg is too low to measure. If acute infection is present, consider HAV, NANBH, other virus, or other cause.
–	+	–	Either of the following: 1. Remote HBV infection: anti-HBc now too low to detect. 2. Past immunization with hepatitis B vaccine: the vaccine contains low levels of HBsAg only. If acute infection is present, consider HAV, NANBH, other virus, or other cause of hepatitis.
–	–	–	No evidence of HBV infection Consider HAV, NANBH, other virus, or other cause of hepatitis.

3. **Follow-up Studies**
   a. If the hepatitis screen does not suggest acute HAV or HBV infection, paired sera should be obtained for EBV and CMV. A Monospot test should be considered if one has not already been done or should be repeated in case it has converted.
   b. If tests for EBV and CMV are negative, probable diagnosis is NANBH. Toxic or other liver disease should be reconsidered.
   c. Enzymes should be followed to document resolution of infection.
   d. Liver biopsy should be reserved for cases in which significant diagnostic doubt exists. Continued evidence of liver enzyme elevation or deteriorating condition may prompt biopsy.

REFERENCES

1. Dienstag JL: Non-A, non-B hepatitis. I. Recognition, epidemiology, and clinical features; II. Experimental transmission, putative virus agents and markers, and prevention. Gastroenterology 85:439–462, 743–768, 1983.

An extremely complete review article.

2. Feinstone SM, Hoofnagle JH: Editorial: Non-A, maybe-B hepatitis. N Engl J Med 311:185–188, 1984.

Continued controversy over the etiology of NANBH.

3. Hadler SC, Monzon M, Ponzetto A, et al.: Delta virus infection and severe hepatitis: An epidemic in the Yucpa Indians of Venezuela. Ann Intern Med 100:339–344, 1984.

A discussion of an outbreak of a disease with serious implications for populations at risk of HBV infection.

4. Krugman S, Overby LR, Mushahwar IK, et al.: Viral hepatitis, type B: Studies on natural history and prevention re-examined. N Engl J Med 300:101–106, 1979.

An excellent discussion of serologic testing and relation to disease course.

5. Mosley JW, Redeker AG, Feinstone SM, et al.: Multiple hepatitis viruses in multiple attacks of acute viral hepatitis. N Engl J Med 296:75–78, 1977.

The postulated existence of NANB viruses is discussed; the pattern of hepatitis serologic evaluation described mirrors methods that are available today.

6. Seeff LB, Hoofnagle JH: Immunoprophylaxis of viral hepatitis. Gastroenterology 77:161–182, 1979.

Evaluation of efficacy and recommendations for prophylaxis of viral hepatitis.

7. Szmuness W, Dienstag JL, Purcell RH, et al.: Distribution of antibody to hepatitis A antigen in urban adult populations. N Engl J Med 295:755–759, 1976.

Demonstrates increased incidence of HAV infection in lower socioeconomic classes.

8. Szmuness W, Stevens CE, Harley EJ, et al.: Hepatitis B vaccine: Demonstration of efficacy in a controlled clinical trial in a high-risk population in the United States. N Engl J Med 303:833–841, 1980.

Demonstrates the utility of vaccine for hepatitis B as well as the risk of HBV and NANB transmission in sexual contact.

9. Zimmerman HJ: Hepatotoxicity: The adverse effects of drugs and other chemicals on the liver. New York, Appleton-Century-Crofts, 1978.

An exhaustive work covering all aspects of toxic liver disease.

48

AMENORRHEA

By MITCHELL KARTON, M.D.

DEFINITION

Amenorrhea is classified as primary or secondary.

A. Primary Amenorrhea. The patient has never menstruated. Primary amenorrhea is classified as:

1. Absence of menses by age 16, even in the presence of normal growth and normal secondary sexual characteristics, or
2. Absence of menses at age 14, associated with lack of normal growth or absence of normal secondary sexual development, or both.

B. Secondary Amenorrhea. Secondary amenorrhea is defined as:

1. Absence of menstruation for six months (or for a duration equal to three consecutive cycles) in a woman with a history of regular menses, or
2. Absence of menstruation for 12 months in a woman with previous irregular menses.
3. Physiologic causes of secondary amenorrhea include pregnancy, puerperal amenorrhea, and normal menopause. Secondary amenorrhea in women of child-bearing age should be considered the result of pregnancy until proved otherwise.

EPIDEMIOLOGY

A. Primary Amenorrhea. This is a rare disorder. Over 95 per cent of normal girls have their first period by age 15. Approximately 60 per cent of cases of primary amenorrhea are caused by errors in gonadal or genital development, which include, in order of decreasing frequency: gonadal dysgenesis, 30 per cent (including Turner's syndrome); Müllerian dysgenesis, 20 per cent; and errors in genital development such as male pseudohermaphroditism, 10 per cent. The other 40 per cent of patients have primary amenorrhea caused by hypogonadotropism (10 per cent), and other systemic causes such as endocrinopathies, gonadal resistance syndromes, and outflow tract abnormalities. Some conditions classically associated with secondary amenorrhea, such as polycystic ovarian disease, may develop early enough to prevent even the first menstrual cycle.

B. Secondary Amenorrhea. Secondary amenorrhea (excluding pregnancy and menopause) is much more common than primary amenorrhea. The list of causes of secondary amenorrhea is long, but it can be divided into anatomic abnormalities, primary ovarian failure with high gonadotropins, secondary ovarian failure with low gonadotropins (owing to either pituitary or hypothalamic disease), or chronic anovulation with increased ovarian steroid production such as from tumors or polycystic ovary disease. (Fifty to 60 per cent of patients with anovulation are amenorrheic.)

DIFFERENTIAL DIAGNOSIS

Table 48–1 lists the numerous causes of primary and secondary amenorrhea.

HISTORY AND SIGNS AND SYMPTOMS

A helpful approach for the clinician evaluating the patient with amenorrhea is to group the causes of amenorrhea according to where

TABLE 48–1.   CAUSES OF PRIMARY AND SECONDARY AMENORRHEA*

Primary amenorrhea
A. Fetal errors in genital differentiation
   1. Male pseudohermaphroditism caused by deficient testosterone synthesis
     a. 20, 22-desmolase
     b. 3β-hydroxy-steroid dehydrogenase
     c. 17α-hydroxylase
     d. 17, 20-desmolase
     e. 17-ketosteroid reductase
   2. Male pseudohermaphroditism caused by 5α-reductase deficiency
   3. Male pseudohermaphroditism caused by androgen resistance
     a. Complete testicular feminization
     b. Incomplete testicular feminization
     c. Familial incomplete male pseudohermaphroditism (type 1)
   4. Female pseudohermaphroditism with fetal and postnatal androgen excess
B. Fetal errors in gonadal development
   1. True hermaphroditism
   2. Gonadal dysgenesis with stigmata of Turner's syndrome
   3. Mixed gonadal dysgenesis
C. Fetal errors in gonaductal development
   1. Müllerian dysgenesis
D. Ovarian follicles insensitive to gonadotropins
   1. 17α-hydroxylase deficiency
   2. "Resistant ovary syndrome"
E. Hypothalamic-pituitary diseases
   1. Familial hypogonadotropic hypogonadism
   2. Pituitary tumors
   3. Idiopathic panhypopituitarism
F. Unknown
   1. Polycystic ovary disease (chronic anovulation)
   2. Delayed menarche
   3. Systemic diseases

Table continued on opposite page

TABLE 48–1. CAUSES OF PRIMARY AND SECONDARY AMENORRHEA* *Continued*

Secondary amenorrhea
A. Anatomic abnormalities
  1. Intrauterine synechiae (Asherman's syndrome): postsurgical, postinfective, postabortive, posttraumatic, or after IUD use
  2. Müllerian abnormalities or agenesis
  3. Testicular feminization
  4. Hysterectomy
B. Primary ovarian failure (with high gonadotropins)
  1. Congenital: gonadal dysgenesis, gonadotropin resistance
  2. Acquired: premature primary ovarian failure (postinfectious, postoperative, postchemotherapy, postradiation, autoimmune oophoritis, gonadotropin resistance)
C. Secondary ovarian failure (with low or normal gonadotropins)
  1. Galactorrhea-amenorrhea syndromes with high prolactin
  2. Intrinsic disease
    a. Hypothalamus: tumors, trauma, postsurgical or postradiation effects, Sheehan's syndrome, empty-sella syndrome
  3. Extrinsic disease: psychogenic; from starvation (anorexia nervosa); exercise; after oral contraceptive pill use; excessive estrogen from obesity, age, or thyroid disease; endocrinopathies; intercurrent systemic disease; drug-induced; idiopathic
D. Chronic anovulation with increased ovarian steroid production
  1. Ovarian tumors, both feminizing and masculinizing
  2. Polycystic ovary disease (continuous estrus syndrome)

*Adapted from Williams R, et al.: Textbook of Endocrinology. 6th ed. Philadelphia, W. B. Saunders Company, 1981.

the problem arises: in the outflow tract, ovary, pituitary gland, or hypothalamus.

A. Outflow Tract
  1. Asherman's Syndrome
    a. **History.** Endometritis, surgery (including cesarean section and myomectomy), rarely tuberculosis or schistosomiasis, and use of an intrauterine device are associated with this condition.
    b. **Diagnosis.** The diagnosis is made by hysteroscopy or hysterosalpingography.
  2. Müllerian Dysgenesis
    a. **History.** There is cyclic abdominal pain and distention from hematocolpos, hematometra, or hematoperitoneum; puberty, growth, and development are normal.
    b. **Physical Examination.** Careful pelvic examination is used to determine the presence or absence or abnormalities of imperforate hymen; the presence of a vagina (if present, its patency); and the presence and patency of the cervix and uterus.
    c. **Laboratory Findings.** There is a normal female karyotype, 46XX (to differentiate from male pseudohermaphroditism).
    d. **X-Ray.** Frequent urinary tract abnormalities and spinal and musculoskeletal malformations are ruled out.
    e. **Ultrasound.** This is used to rule out endometriomas.

3. Male Pseudohermaphroditism

a. History. Puberty is normal or minimally delayed. Often there is a positive family history of sexual immaturity and infertility and a possible history of inguinal hernia.

b. Physical Examination. Examination shows variable virilization due to the possibility of some androgen effect, but usually there is a normal female phenotype. The patient may be tall with a eunuchoidal tendency; if there is complete testicular feminization, the female external genitalia are immature, and if incomplete, clitoromegaly may be present. Fifty per cent of patients have inguinal hernias (cryptorchid testes).

c. Laboratory Findings. There is a normal male karyotype, 46XY. Male testosterone levels are normal or slightly elevated.

B. Ovaries

1. Gonadal Dysgenesis (Turner's Syndrome)

a. History. There is a history of delayed puberty, edema of the extremities in the neonatal period, and growth retardation that became evident by the third or fourth year of life.

b. Physical Examination. Examination shows short stature, webbed neck, shield chest, increased carrying angle, and immature female external genitalia and secondary sex characteristics. The physician should check for symmetry of peripheral pulse and blood pressures in all four extremities.

c. Laboratory Findings. There is a karyotype for 45XO. Gonadotropins are elevated.

d. X-Ray. The chest x-ray should be observed for signs of coarctation of the aorta, skeletal malformations, and urinary tract abnormalities.

e. Other. The presence of Y chromosome must be determined by karyotyping in all cases of elevated gonadotropins in women under the age of 30. The Y chromosome is associated with testicular tissue within the gonad, which indicates a predisposition to virilization and malignant tumor formation (25 per cent of cases). Thirty per cent of patients with a Y chromosome show no evidence of virilization. Therefore, even normal-appearing adult females with ovarian failure and high gonadotropin levels (if less than 30 years of age) should be karyotyped.

2. Premature Ovarian Failure

a. History. The patient should be questioned regarding signs and symptoms of other autoimmune diseases such as rheumatoid arthritis, diabetes mellitus, Addison's disease, thyroiditis, hypoparathyroidism, pernicious anemia, and myasthenia gravis.

b. Laboratory Findings. Laboratory tests should cover complete blood cell count with erythrocyte sedimentation rate; electrolytes; Ca^{++}, PO_4^{-}; thyroid function tests, including thyroid-stimulating hormone and antithyroid antibodies; A.M. cortisol; rheumatoid factor; antinuclear antibodies; and antiacetylcholine receptor antibodies.

3. *Polycystic Ovary Disease*
   a. **History.** There are normal growth, development, and puberty; reports of association with diabetes mellitus; dysfunctional uterine bleeding.
   b. **Physical Examination.** Examination shows hirsutism, with occasional evidence of virilization. There are reports of association with acanthosis nigricans.
   c. **Laboratory Findings.** There is a normal female karyotype. The luteinizing hormone/follicle-stimulating hormone (LH/FSH) ratio may be elevated.
4. *Ovarian Tumors*
   a. **History.** There are occasional symptoms as a result of thyroid or serotonin excess in benign cystic teratomas.
   b. **Physical Examination.** There are signs of virilization with arrhenoblastoma and hypertension and diabetes associated with lipoid cell tumors; many tumors are palpable on pelvic examination.

C. **Pituitary**
1. *Tumors*
   a. **History.** There is a history of headache, blurry vision, bitemporal hemianopsia (usually these symptoms occur with larger, more rare tumors such as craniopharyngiomas; also hemianopsia is a very late finding); occasionally symptoms of hypothyroidism, adrenal insufficiency, and diabetes insipidus (especially with craniopharyngiomas); and galactorrhea (prolactin-secreting micro- and macroadenomas).
   b. **Physical Examination.** Examination reveals visual field defects; occasional evidence of acromegaly; Cushing's syndrome; sexual infantilism (craniopharyngioma); and galactorrhea.
   c. **Laboratory Findings.** There may be alterations in adrenocorticotropic hormone (ACTH), cortisol, growth hormone (GH), thyroid-stimulating hormone (TSH), and antidiuretic hormone (ADH). Prolactin is elevated in 20 per cent of women with secondary amenorrhea and in 50 per cent of patients with galactorrhea-amenorrhea.
   d. **X-Ray.** Skull series show calcification (craniopharyngioma); a coned-down view of sella should be used if there is elevated prolactin. If the sella is abnormal, a computed axial tomographic (CAT) scan should be used.
2. *Idiopathic Panhypopituitarism*
   a. **History.** There is a history of previous operations, pituitary radiation, and postpartum hemorrhage (Sheehan's syndrome).
   b. **Physical Examination.** There is evidence of hypothyroidism, adrenal insufficiency, and loss of axillary and pubic hair.
   c. **Laboratory Findings.** TSH, ACTH, GH, and gonadotropin levels are low.

D. **Hypothalamus**
1. *Anorexia Nervosa*
   a. **History.** There are no other medical problems; a high-

achievement family; bulimia; self-induced vomiting; light-headedness; and constipation, usually between 10 and 30 years of age.

   b. **Physical Examination.** Anorexia is associated with a 25 per cent weight loss or weight 15 per cent below normal for age and height; hypotension; bradycardia; lanugo; and yellowish palms from hypercarotenemia. Mental status examination is notable for denial, rigidity, a distorted body image, and thought content often focused on hoarding or unusual handling of food.

   c. **Laboratory Findings.** There are low gonadotropins; elevated cortisol; normal prolactin; normal TSH and T_4, but with low T_3 and elevated reverse T_3.

2. Anorectic Reaction Associated with Exercise

   a. **History.** The patient exercises regularly and makes a conscious attempt to lower body weight and percentage of body fat. There are high stress levels.

   b. **Physical Examination.** The mental status examination is notable for insight into the problem and absence of denial.

   c. **Laboratory Findings.** Exercise is associated with elevated prolactin, ACTH, and GH levels and decreased gonadotropins.

3. Post-pill Amenorrhea. Work-up is recommended only after six months following discontinuation of use of oral contraceptive pills or 12 months after the last injection of Depo-Provera.

RECOMMENDED DIAGNOSTIC APPROACH

A. Initial Steps

1. History and Physical Examination. (See Fig. 48–1.) The physician should look specifically for a family history of genetic abnormalities, normal reproductive tracts, abnormal patterns of growth and development, unusual stress factors, malnutrition, other systemic illnesses, evidence of central nervous system disease, medications, and exercise history.

2. Possible Pregnancy. If the history and physical examination are normal, pregnancy must be ruled out.

3. TSH and Prolactin Level. If the patient is not pregnant, a TSH sample and a prolactin level must be drawn. Only a few patients have otherwise clinically inapparent hypothyroidism, but the test is inexpensive and the condition is easily reversible. Elevated prolactin levels may occur for many reasons (see Table 48–2).

4. CAT Scan. If the prolactin level is greater than 100 mg per mL, a CAT scan should be obtained to rule out a pituitary adenoma. If the prolactin level is mildly elevated and associated with galactorrhea or central nervous system abnormalities, a lateral projection of a coned-down view of the sella tursica should be used. Galactorrhea alone also requires a coned-down sellar view. If the sellar view is abnormal, a CAT scan should be obtained.

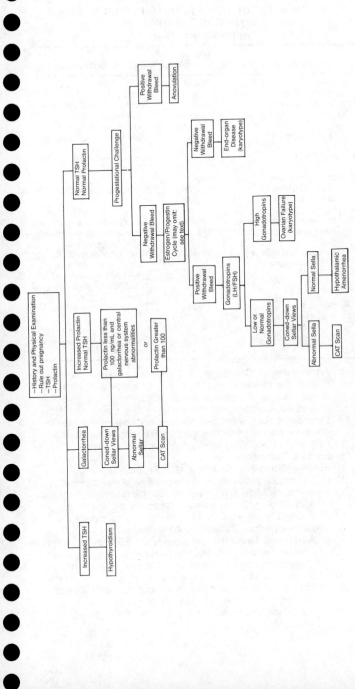

Figure 48–1. Flow diagram for evaluation of amenorrhea.

TABLE 48–2. PROLACTIN LEVELS UNDER VARIOUS ABNORMAL CONDITIONS
(Approximate Ranges)

Condition	Range (ng/mg of blood)	Comments
1. Primary hypothyroidism	30–100	Confirm with elevated TSH
2. Polycystic ovarian disease	20–50	About 30–50% of patients have elevation; others are in normal range.
3. Anorexia nervosa	10–50	Often have mild elevation of GH as well.
4. Renal failure	10–50	Probably decreased clearance.
5. Pituitary tumors		
Microadenomas	20–200	Not a firm distinction.
Macroadenomas	>200	
6. Drug use		
Phenothiazines or other neuroleptics	20–200	Usually there is a dose-related return to normal after discontinuation.
Birth control pills or other estrogens	15–50	About 1/3 of patients have mild elevations; if there is no return to normal, evaluate for pituitary tumor.
Reserpine, amphetamines, and methyldopa	15–30	Usually mild elevations.
Morphine-methadone	10–75	With chronic use, levels tend to be higher.

5. *Progestational Challenge.* If TSH and prolactin levels are normal, the patient should receive a progestational challenge (either 100 mg of progesterone in oil parenterally or medroxy-progesterone acetate, 10 mg orally for five days). Within the subsequent week, withdrawal bleeding confirms an endometrium adequately primed with endogenous estrogen, a patent outflow tract, and a functioning hypothalamic-pituitary-ovarian axis.

B. **Secondary Evaluation**

1. *Positive Withdrawal Bleeding After Progestins*

   a. **Chronic Anovulation.** In the absence of galactorrhea, and with normal TSH and prolactin levels, the diagnosis of chronic anovulation (almost always caused by polycystic ovarian disease) is made. No further evaluation is necessary.

2. *Negative Withdrawal Bleeding After Progestins*

   a. **Abnormal Genitalia or Significant History of Infection or Trauma (including curettage).** A cyclic course of estrogens and progestins should be given. If no withdrawal bleeding occurs, there is anatomic disease of the endometrium or outflow tract. This rarely occurs, but if it does, a karyotype should be obtained. (In the presence of a normal history and examination, this progestin-challenge test is unnecessary.)

b. **Gonadotropin Levels**
1). If these are elevated, the diagnosis of primary ovarian failure is made. A karyotype should be obtained.
2). If normal or low, radiologic evaluation should be done for pituitary or hypothalamic tumors. If a coned-down sellar view is abnormal, a CAT scan should be obtained; if the sellar view is normal, the diagnosis of functional hypothalamic amenorrhea can be made.

REFERENCES

1. DeGroot LJ, et al.: Endocrinology. New York, Grune & Stratton, 1979.

This is one of the classic texts on endocrinology, notable for detailed discussions of laboratory tests covering indications, methods, and causes of normal and abnormal values.

2. Speroff L, et al.: Clinical Gynecologic Endocrinology and Infertility. 3rd ed. Baltimore, Williams & Wilkins, 1983.

This text offers a good clinical discussion of the evaluation of amenorrhea, complete with recommendations and evaluations of treatments including hormone replacement.

3. Williams R, et al.: Textbook of Endocrinology. 6th ed. Philadelphia, W. B. Saunders Company, 1981.

This is one of the definitive discussions of amenorrhea, presented within the context of ovarian function and dysfunction.

4. Odell WD, Federman DD (eds.): Symposium on adolescent gynecology and endocrinology. West J Med 131:401–416, 516–532, 1979.

This symposium offers complete discussion of sexual maturation and amenorrhea, hirsutism, and DES exposure—all from a physiologic point of view.

5. Kleinberg D, et al.: Galactorrhea: A study of 235 cases, including 48 with pituitary tumors. N Engl J Med 296:589–600, 1977.

A retrospective analysis of 235 patients with galactorrhea. This study is exceptionally well organized in its discussion of several groups of patients with amenorrhea, including their responses to stimulation and suppression tests, the character of their menses, prolactin levels, and a brief consideration of the mechanisms causing galactorrhea.

49

BREAST NODULE

By STEPHEN K. HOLLAND, M.D.

GENERAL COMMENTS AND EPIDEMIOLOGY

A. **Definition of the Problem.** The discovery of a breast lump by a patient during self examination or by a physician during a routine examination requires a rapid and precise plan for diagnostic work-up and ultimate therapy. Over 90 per cent of these women, however, will not have breast cancer, and 70 per cent of all women coming to biopsy for a suspicious breast mass have benign disease. Early determination of whether a breast nodule is cancerous offers more cures, increased long-term survival, and the need for less extensive surgery and adjuvant therapy.

B. Epidemiology

1. *Incidence of Breast Cancer.* Breast cancer accounts for 27 per cent of all cancers that develop in women, with 1 out of every 11 women developing breast cancer in her lifetime. In 1985 alone, almost 120,000 new cases were anticipated in the United States. Of all breast cancers found at biopsy, the distribution in one series was Paget's disease, 1 to 4 per cent; minimal breast cancer, 5 per cent; infiltrating duct carcinoma, 78 per cent; and inflammatory carcinoma, 2 per cent.

2. *Breast Lumps.* Over 60 per cent of women have discernible lumps in their breasts. Some authors have argued that the lumpy breast is actually a normal finding. Although a vast majority of these lumps are benign, from 80 to 90 per cent of all cancerous breast biopsies came from breast lumps discovered by the patient or by her physician.

3. *Geography.* Breast cancer is truly a Western disease. The incidence and mortality rates are approximately five times higher in North America and Northern Europe than in most Asian and African countries. The rates in Southern Europe and South American countries fall in between these two extremes.

4. *Risk Factors.* See Table 49–1.

5. *Prevalence Studies of Benign Breast Disease.* One study of biopsied lumps found the following distribution:

LESION	FREQUENCY (PER CENT)	MEDIAN AGE (YEARS)
Chronic cystic mastitis	34	41
Fibroadenoma	27	27
Acute or chronic inflammation	16	34
Miscellaneous, including inter-ductal papilloma and ductal ectasia	10	early 40's

HISTORY AND PHYSICAL EXAMINATION

A. History. A thorough review of the risk factors outlined in Table 49–1 is important. The clinician should also concentrate on:

1. *Pain.* Breast cancer is not usually painful, but there are exceptions. It should not be assumed that painful lesions are always benign. A cyclic fullness or pain with menses that is bilateral and diffuse suggests fibrocystic disease. Cervical or dorsal radiculitis causes a sharp radiating pain; costochon-

TABLE 49–1. BREAST CANCER RISK FACTORS*

1. Family history
   A. Maternal family member with postmenopausal breast cancer: risk 1.5 times general population's.
   B. Maternal family member with premenopausal breast cancer: risk 3.5 times general population's.
   C. Maternal family member with bilateral disease at diagnosis: risk 5.5 times general population's.
   D. Maternal family member with premenopausal bilateral disease at diagnosis: risk 9 times general population's.
2. Age of occurrence
   A. Younger than 20: a surgical oddity (less than 0.1% of all breast cancers).
   B. Age 20 to 30 years: one of every 100 biopsies done for suspicious lumps will be malignant.
   C. Age 30 to 60 years: overall risk for these three decades is approximately 5.5 to 6 that of the general population, with the risk rising each year. Median age at diagnosis is 48 years, with delay in diagnosis calculated to average 9 months.
   D. Older than 70: suspicious lesions almost always malignant.
3. Early menarche (age 11) or late natural menopause: risk greater than 2 times general population's (oophorectomy before age 35 seems to reduce subsequent risk of breast cancer).
4. Nulliparous women: risk 4 times general population's.
5. Older than 30 years at first pregnancy: risk 5 times general population's.
6. Benign breast disease: risk 4.5 to 5 times general population's (if the benign disease has been biopsied: risk 8 times general population's).
7. Previous breast cancer: risk breast cancer in remaining breast 5 times general population's.
8. North American and Northern European women: risk 5 times that of Asian and African women and 2.5 times that of South American women and Southern European women.
9. Ionizing radiation greater than 100 rads, especially if exposure occurred before age 20: linear dose response curve with risk ratios ranging from 1.7 to 10.5.
10. Estrogen therapy for longer than 10 to 15 years in women: risk slight but inconsistent elevation (no increased risk seen with use of combination-type oral contraceptives).
11. Postmenopausal obesity: risk statistically increased.

*Adapted from Hatfield H, Guthrie H: Breast cancer concepts. Am Family Physician 30:195–200, 1984; Modan B: Epidemiology of breast cancer—preventative aspects. Isr J Med Sci M: 804–809, 1981.

dritis has a more aching quality; infection produces a throbbing sensation; and with ductal ectasia, patients often experience itching, burning, or drawing. Pain from trauma is often described as sore, bruised, or stabbing. An organizing hematoma can produce a soft tissue mass with accompanying retraction of nipple or skin that is suggestive of an invasive carcinoma.

2. **Nipple Discharge.** Over 80 per cent of premenopausal women experience some discharge when the nipple is manipulated. The discharge may vary in color, ranging from dark (often mistakenly called bloody) to more clear serous material. The color and consistency are rarely helpful diagnostically. *The key clinical question is whether the discharge is associated with a mass.* A spontaneous discharge in the presence of a

mass is a worrisome sign, especially if the woman is older than 50. A spontaneous discharge without a palpable mass is caused by an intraductal papilloma in over 90 per cent of cases. Surgery is usually indicated, but the patient can be assured that the incidence of papillary carcinoma in this situation is extremely low. In women over age 60, however, the risk increases, and 30 per cent of women with nipple discharge and no palpable mass are eventually found to have cancer.

3. **Nipple Ulceration.** Nipple ulceration may indicate Paget's disease of the breast, which is not necessarily associated with a mass. A number of dermatologic conditions can result in skin breakdown, but unlike Paget's disease, they are rarely confined to the nipple, nor are they uniformly indurated.

4. **Unilateral Nipple Retraction.** If symmetrically inverted, easily everted, and not associated with an underlying mass, this quite common condition is almost 100 per cent benign.

B. **Physical Examination.** A majority of women have normal palpable nodules scattered uniformly throughout the breasts. During each menstrual cycle, the breast changes in size and nodularity, with proliferation and engorgement occurring just prior to menses. Involution and regression begins with menstruation. The degree of cyclic proliferation and involution is not uniform throughout all areas of the breast. In response to the years of cyclic hormonal stimulation, most breasts develop areas that are to some degree nodular or irregular.

Many areas of nodularity that are felt immediately before and throughout menstruation may disappear five to seven days after menses stop. Suspicious areas should be reexamined when the breast is at its minimal volume, approximately five to seven days after menses. This is also the optimal period for self examination and mammography.

1. **Positions of Examination**
   a. Upright sitting, disrobed to the waist: thorough inspection is essential. The physician should listen to the patient, for she may be far more cognizant of subtle skin or tissue changes that are not readily obvious.
   b. Upright sitting with hands overhead, then with pressure applied with both hands on iliac crests: again the physician should search for skin changes as well as dimpling or flattening, retraction, or asymmetry of nipple position. Palpation should be begun quadrant-by-quadrant in concentric circles from the areola. Nipple compression to detect nipple discharge should be attempted in this position. Supraclavicular and axillary areas should be examined for masses or nodes in this position.
   c. Supine position with a small pillow under the shoulder of the side to be examined: the physician should repeat systematic examination while paying particular attention to the axillary tail of each breast (this is easily examined by placing the patient's ipsilateral hand behind her head).

Examination should be repeated again with her hand by her side to carefully compare each side.

2. If a Breast Lump Is Found

  a. Its *mobility* (encapsulated fibroadenomas move easily within the substance of the breast), *attachment* (degree of adherence to skin or nipple, causing dimpling, edema, or nipple retraction), and *fixation* (immobility of tumor when it invades the pectoralis or chest wall) should be described.

  b. The physician should note whether there is a *solitary nodule* or *multiple nodules*.

  c. *Consistency* should be noted. Benign lumps can be firm, soft, or cystic, while cancerous lesions are usually hard.

  d. *Size* and *shape* should be noted. Benign lumps usually assume regular well-defined borders, whereas malignant lumps tend to form irregular poorly defined surfaces.

  e. *Position* should be noted carefully by diagram to correlate later with other diagnostic imaging techniques.

  f. *Transillumination* is important. Benign lesions may appear clear or semiopaque, while malignant lesions always exhibit opacity to light.

3. Uncertain Findings. If there is uncertainty as to whether or not a mass exists, the patient should be examined at frequent intervals (perhaps at different times during the menstrual cycle). One author suggests that for an area of "thickness" found on examination a mild diuretic can be given (hydrochlorothiazide, 25 mg daily for three days) to decrease engorgement. This may eliminate or enhance an uncertain mass. Questionable areas should be considered in the context of the individual's particular risk factors. Further diagnostic work-

TABLE 49–2. CHARACTERISTICS OF COMMON BREAST MASSES*

CHARACTERISTICS	FIBROCYSTIC DISEASE	FIBROADENOMA	BREAST CANCER
Borders	Usually distinct	Distinct or ovoid	Often indistinct
Consistency	Rubbery	Hard	Hard
Response to menstrual cycle	Fluctuates	Rarely fluctuates	Rarely fluctuates
Fixation to underlying tissue	No	Usually movable	Yes
Tenderness	Yes	No	Rarely
Growth pattern	Stable over time	Stable over time	Progressive
Associated lymphadenopathy	No	No	Yes
Fluid aspirate	Clear, rarely bloody	None	Clear, often bloody
Mammogram	Benign disease	Benign	Highly diagnostic

*Adapted from Hatfield, H, Guthrie H: Breast cancer concepts. Am Family Physician 30:195–200, 1984.

up, if warranted, should proceed until a firm diagnosis is known.

Characteristics of common breast masses are outlined in Table 49–2.

RECOMMENDED DIAGNOSTIC APPROACH

Even the best physical examination cannot determine the histology of a lump in the breast. The detection of a suspicious mass should lead to a sampling technique that can produce a pathologic diagnosis.

A. **Evaluation Sequence.** There is no definite evaluation sequence for women with newly discovered breast lumps. The clinician, in collaboration with a surgeon, should consider obtaining mammograms, ultrasound of the breast, aspiration, or one of several types of biopsies.

1. *Laboratory Tests.* These tests are of little value prior to tissue diagnosis.

2. *Mammography*[1]
   a. Mammography offers an important confirmatory aid with approximately a 90 per cent diagnostic accuracy for whether a suspicious lesion is benign or malignant.
   b. Mammography can give information about occult satellite lesions in the same breast or clinically occult lesions in the contralateral breast.
   c. It can help localize small or clinically occult lesions for biopsy.
   d. A negative mammogram of a suspicious mass does not eliminate the possibility of intramammary cancer, especially in young women.
   e. A mammogram that is strongly positive in a patient with a negative biopsy requires immediate follow-up to be certain that the suspicious area has in fact been excised.

3. *Ultrasound.* Ultrasound may be helpful when combined with mammography for cyst localization or for differentiation between a cyst and a solid mass.

4. *Thermography, Computed Tomographic Scan, and Nuclear Magnetic Resonance.* In 1985, these are still considered experimental imaging procedures.

5. *Aspiration*
   a. Aspiration is easily performed with a 22-gauge needle and is an important tool to evaluate palpable cysts.
   b. Follow-up mammogram or ultrasound examination should be performed to rule out associated or residual tissue, and follow-up examination in four to five weeks should be done to check for reaccumulation of fluid.
   c. Cytology of the aspirated fluid is of little value, although bloody fluid or residual tissue following aspiration suggests malignancy.

6. *Biopsy.* Many physicians contend that any patient with an obvious mass needs tissue diagnosis, regardless of other clinical

TABLE 49–3. AMERICAN CANCER SOCIETY GUIDELINES FOR MAMMOGRAPHIC SCREENING OF ASYMPTOMATIC WOMEN

1. Baseline mammogram for all women at age 35 to 40 years
2. Mammogram at one- to two-year intervals from 40 to 49 years (greater frequency may be dictated by specific risk factors)
3. Annual mammogram for women 50 years or older

or mammographic findings. Although biopsy is usually performed at the discretion of the surgeon, several biopsy procedures are available:

a. **Needle Aspirate.** In some hands, when correlated with physical examination and mammography, fine needle aspiration has greater than 90 per cent accuracy for both malignant and benign lesions. Negative aspiration cytology should be followed by a procedure that yields more tissue for pathologic inspection.

b. **Percutaneous Biopsy.** This is usually an office procedure under local anesthetic. Core biopsy has a high yield for suspicious palpable masses. It is not indicated for small or occult (mammographically detected) lesions.

c. **Excisional Biopsy.** Most surgeons agree that the approach of diagnosis by frozen section followed by immediate mastectomy if cancer is found is outdated. This approach does not improve survival and excludes patients from decisions about their care. Studies have demonstrated that waiting two to three weeks between biopsy and definitive surgery has no effect on patient survival. Excisional biopsy on an ambulatory basis therefore becomes the technique of choice for small clinically occult lesions as well as presumptively benign nodules in women who are in specific risk categories.

B. **Breast Cancer Screening Programs.** The efficacy of mammography screening programs is still controversial. The last randomized trial of widespread mammography screening was conducted in the early 1960s by the Health Insurance Plan of New York. It showed a definite reduction in mortality in women over the age of 50 who were screened yearly by a careful physical examination and mammography (a 25 to 30 per cent reduction after 10 to 14 years when compared with "routine medical care"). The benefit of screening women under the age of 50 is still unsettled, but recent advances in mammography techniques and some preliminary data from cooperative studies have led the American Cancer Society to formulate guidelines for mammographic screening that should accompany a regular program of self- and physician examination (Table 49–3).

REFERENCES

1. Kopans DB, Meyer JE, Sadowsky N: Breast imaging. N Engl J Med 310:960–967, 1984.
A recent review of the newest radiographic imaging approaches.

2. Miller A, Abrahamson J, Boss J, Nash E: Rational and cost-effective management of the patient with a solid breast lump. Isr J Med Sci 17:905–910, 1981.

Takes the cost-containment approach without compromising good patient care.

3. Pash RM: Solitary breast nodule. *In* Eisman B (ed.): Prognosis of Surgical Disease. Philadelphia, W. B. Saunders Company, 1980.
4. Haagensen, Bodian, Haagensen: Breast Carcinoma Risk and Detection. Philadelphia, W. B. Saunders Company, 1981.

These last two references are the most recent textbooks on these topics.

50

HYPERCALCEMIA

By MITCHELL KARTON, M.D.

DEFINITION

Normal serum calcium values vary depending on the method of measurement, but generally total serum calcium (Ca) between 8.9 and 11 mg per 100 mL is considered normal. Calcium values greater than 11 mg per 100 mL (5.5 mEq per L) are considered hypercalcemic; values less than 8.9 mg per 100 mL (4.4 mEq per L) are hypocalcemic.

A. Approximately 40 per cent of total calcium is bound to serum proteins, and 80 to 90 per cent of this calcium is bound to albumin. The protein-bound fraction is in equilibrium with the other 60 per cent (the ultrafiltrable or diffusible calcium, which is 50 per cent ionized and 10 per cent complexed). The ionized fraction (normal values 4.5 to 5.5 mg per 100 mL [2.2 to 2.8 mEq per L]) is the biologically active form of calcium.

B. Variations in serum proteins alter measurements of total serum calcium proportionately; for example, a lowering of 0.8 to 0.9 mg Ca^{++} per 100 mL for each decrease of 1 g per 100 mL in serum albumin or an increase of 0.16 mg Ca^{++} per 100 mL for each increase of 1 g per 100 mL in serum total protein.

C. Changes in pH also affect protein-bound calcium. Each change of 0.1 pH correspondingly decreases or increases protein-bound calcium by 0.12 mg per 100 mL, respectively. Therefore, acidosis increases the ionized fraction of Ca^{++} and alkalosis decreases it.

D. Abnormally low serum magnesium (Mg^{++}) levels and elevations in serum potassium (K^+) potentiate the neurologic and cardiovascular effects of hypocalcemia. Mg^{++} and K^+ abnormalities must be corrected concomitantly with the correction of calcium levels.

EPIDEMIOLOGY AND GENERAL COMMENTS

Since the advent of automated biochemical screening procedures, hypercalcemia has been found more commonly than previously had been suspected.

A. **Causes of Hypercalcemia**
1. The most common cause of hypercalcemia is primary hyperparathyroidism (HPT), which accounts for approximately 50 per cent of all patients with hypercalcemia. The incidence of primary HPT is now ten times greater than was thought to be ten years ago. In women over 60 years old, screening studies have found 2 new cases per 1000 persons per year; the incidence of primary HPT in males is about one half this rate. Younger patients have a lower incidence, but females over the age of 40 still have an incidence of greater than 1 case per 1000 of the population at large.
2. The second most common cause of hypercalcemia is neoplastic disease, which accounts for about 35 per cent of all cases. Some individuals have estimated the annual incidence of hypercalcemia associated with malignancy to be 150 patients per 1-million population per year. Certain tumors such as squamous cell lung cancer may frequently appear with hypercalcemia (10 to 15 per cent; oat cell carcinoma is almost never associated with high Ca^{++}). Most series suggest that about 33 per cent of patients with advanced breast cancer develop hypercalcemia at some stage during the course of the disease.
3. Other causes include multiple myeloma (25 per cent of patients have Ca^{++} greater than 11.5 mg per cent at the time of diagnosis), sarcoidosis (high Ca^{++} is usually a manifestation of severely disseminated disease), adrenal insufficiency (transient hypercalcemia), and hyperthyroidism (minimal increase in serum calcium levels in 25 per cent of patients). Thiazide therapy has also become a recognizable source of curable hypercalcemia.
4. Vitamin D intoxication, milk-alkali syndrome, familial hypercalcemia of infancy, and hypercalcemia from immobilization (either in young patients who undergo rapid growth or in elderly patients with Paget's disease) are relatively rare causes of hypercalcemia.

DIFFERENTIAL DIAGNOSIS

A. **Hyperparathyroidism**
1. The triad of nephrolithiasis, metabolic bone disease, and hypercalcemia characterize HPT. The consequences of hypercalcemia account for most of the symptoms of HPT. Serum Ca^{++} is usually high, and serum $PO_4^=$ (phosphate) is usually low but may be normal, especially if renal failure is present.
2. The serum chloride-phosphate ratio has been said to be helpful

in differentiating between hyperparathyroid patients and those with other causes of hypercalcemia. If the ratio is greater than 33, it may well reflect the increased chloride or decreased phosphate, or both, owing to acidosis and the renal phosphate wasting of HPT. If the ratio is less than 30, then hypercalcemia is probably related to some other cause.

Sensitivity of the chloride-phosphate ratio is reported to be greater than 90 per cent. However, owing to the small variance of chloride values and the large variance of phosphorus values, the chloride-phosphate ratio is not as reliable as has been suggested.

Serum chloride alone is probably more helpful: levels are usually greater than 103 mEq per L in primary HPT and less than 98 mEq per L with hypercalcemia of malignancy. This is because patients with primary HPT have impaired HCO_3^- reabsorption in the proximal tubule with resulting HCO_3^- loss and renal tubular acidosis.

3. The corticosteroid suppression test may help differentiate primary HPT from myeloma, sarcoid, vitamin D intoxication, and some tumors. Patients with primary HPT have no hypocalcemic response to ten days of glucocorticoid administration.

4. Thiazide provocation tests may produce sustained hypercalcemia in patients with primary HPT and borderline elevation of serum Ca^{++} but not in normal persons (patients with vitamin D intoxication and metabolic bone disease may also have sustained increase in Ca^{++}).

5. Immunoassay for parathyroid hormone (PTH) is of increasing value in establishing the cause of hypercalcemia but not for distinguishing normal from abnormal subjects. When serum immunoreactive PTH (iPTH) is measured, plotted against serum Ca^{++} values, and compared with extensive groups of patients subjected to retrospective analysis, most patients with primary HPT and serum Ca^{++} above 12 per cent have unequivocally elevated iPTH, whereas most patients with hypercalcemia related to neoplasia have normal or undetectable iPTH levels. Patients with known malignancies, high Ca^{++}, and elevated levels of iPTH are far more likely to have coexistent primary HPT.

6. Finally, despite the availability of these tests, primary HPT is commonly diagnosed clinically because it is a chronic disease with evidence of the clinical triad noted above. Therefore, if isolated hypercalcemia is a recent discovery, without any historical symptomatology, a thorough search for causes other than primary HPT must be made.

B. **Malignancy.** There is no single test that can differentiate between hypercalcemia caused by primary HPT and hypercalcemia caused by malignancy. However, in addition to iPTH levels (discussed previously), elevated excretion of nephrogenous cyclic adenosine monophosphate (n-cAMP) may help differentiate hypercalcemia of malignancy associated with "PTH-like" humoral activity from both primary HPT and hypercalcemia of malignancy related to local bony involvement.

The most common solid tumors associated with hypercalcemia are lung cancer (squamous cell, not oat cell), hypernephroma, and breast cancer. Other solid tumors include squamous cell tumors of the head and neck, thyroid gland, ovary, and prostate. Myeloproliferative causes include myeloma, leukemia, lymphoma, and Hodgkin's disease. (With multiple myeloma bone scans often do not detect lytic lesions, and a marrow aspirate and serum and urine protein electrophoresis are still necessary for diagnosis.)

C. **Sarcoidosis.** Because hypercalcemia is indicative of widespread disease, the physician should look for pulmonary involvement, low to normal PTH levels, and abnormal pulmonary function tests; diagnosis must be made by biopsy of noncaseating granulomas.

D. **Thyrotoxicosis.** Hypercalcemia with a normal PTH is seen in approximately 25 per cent of hyperthyroid patients. The symptoms leading to medical evaluation are usually those of hyperthyroidism, not of hypercalcemia.

E. **Adrenal Insufficiency.** Transiently elevated calcium returns to normal with adrenal replacement therapy.

F. **Vitamin D Intoxication.** Vitamin D intoxication requires months of ingestion of greater than 100,000 units of D_2 or D_3 and is rare.

G. **Milk-Alkali Syndrome.** This syndrome has been rare since the introduction of nonabsorbable antacids.

CAUSES OF HYPERCALCEMIA

See Table 50–1.

HISTORY, SIGNS, AND SYMPTOMS

A. **Clinical Picture.** In addition to the specific findings of any particular disease causing an elevated calcium level, hypercalcemia causes a wide-ranging clinical picture involving many different organ systems. In the case of extreme hypercalcemia, the patient may have intractable nausea and vomiting, severe volume depletion, and obtundation with rapidly progressive renal failure and death. Even so, some patients with serum calcium concentrations as high as 14 mg per 100 mL may lack symptoms altogether.

The clinical picture of hypercalcemia is as follows:

1. *Gastrointestinal.* There are anorexia, constipation, nausea, vomiting, peptic ulcer pain, and acute pancreatitis.

2. *Genitourinary.* There are polyuria, polydipsia, renal insufficiency, calculi, and nephrocalcinosis.

3. *Neurologic.* Neurologic signs and symptoms include fatigue, muscle weakness, depressed tendon reflexes, disorientation, stupor, coma, and death.

4. *Psychiatric.* There may be apathy, depression, or psychotic behavior.

5. *Metastatic Calcification.* Ocular keratopathy, nephrocalcinosis, chondrocalcinosis, vascular calcification, and periarticular calcification occur.

TABLE 50–1. CAUSES OF HYPERCALCEMIA

Common
  Primary hyperparathyroidism, secondary hyperparathyroidism
  Malignancy
    Without metastases: in lung, kidney, or bone
    With metastases: in breast, lung, kidney, thyroid, prostate, ovary, head,
      and neck
  Multiple myeloma
  Sarcoidosis
  Hyperthyroidism (in some patients)
  Acute adrenal insufficiency
  Thiazides
Uncommon
  Hypervitaminoses D and A
  Milk-alkali (Burnett's) syndrome
  Leukemia, lymphoma, Hodgkin's disease
  Hypothyroidism
  Immobilization: in the young with rapid growth and in the old with
    Paget's disease
  Diuretic phase of acute renal failure
  Acromegaly
  Pheochromocytoma
  Berylliosis
  Pulmonary granulomatous disease (e.g., tuberculosis, coccidioidomycosis)
  Hypophosphatemia
  Hypercalcemia of infancy
  Iatrogenic causes

RECOMMENDED DIAGNOSTIC APPROACH

A. **History.** The history should be examined for chronicity versus
   acuteness of symptoms, medications, and symptoms consistent
   with malignancy, thyroid disease, sarcoidosis, and other diseases
   associated with hypercalcemia.
B. **Physical Examination.** The physician should look for signs of
   common causes of hypercalcemia, including the following areas:
   1. *General.* Evidence of cachexia and weight loss.
   2. *Eyes.* Nonspecific calcium deposits or exophthalmos.
   3. *Skin.* Soft tissue calcification or hyperpigmentation.
   4. *Neck.* Masses or lymphadenopathy (sarcoid, thyroid, metastatic
      disease, lymphoma).
   5. *Breast.* Masses.
   6. *Abdomen.* Hepatosplenomegaly, masses, or tumors.
   7. *Rectal.* Prostatic size and consistency.
   8. *Musculoskeletal.* Frontal bossing, joint effusions, and bone
      tenderness.

C. Laboratory Findings
1. ***General.*** These include calcium, phosphate, chloride, alkaline phosphatase, and PTH if necessary.
2. ***Other.*** Erythrocyte sedimentation rate (ESR) may be helpful for myeloma, malignancy, and tuberculosis and serum protein electrophoresis/urine immunoelectrophoresis for myeloma and increased globulins in sarcoidosis. Other tests may include thyroid function tests, acid phosphatase for prostatic disease, liver function tests for metastatic disease, A.M. cortisol and electrolytes for Addison's disease, and PFTs, skin tests, and sputum cultures as needed.

D. Other Diagnostic Procedures. These consist of chest x-rays; abdominal films or intravenous pyelogram for renal stones; mammography; hand x-rays for subperiosteal resorption, demineralization, and cysts; skull films for lytic lesions; bone scans for metastases; bone marrow aspirate (for myeloma or tuberculosis); and biopsy material (for malignancy or sarcoidosis).

REFERENCES

1. Habener JF, Gino VS: Parathyroid hormone radio-immunoassay. Ann Intern Med 91:782–785, 1979.

A thorough discussion of the parathyroid hormone radioimmunoassay, including a discussion of its use in helping to differentiate primary HPT from hypercalcemia caused by malignancy.

2. Mundy R: Clinical recognition and management of hypercalcemia in neoplastic disease. Internal Med 2:37–45, 1981.

A good discussion of evaluation and treatment, with critical commentary about the utility of various laboratory tests considered useful in differential diagnosis.

3. Palmer FJ, et al.: The chloride-phosphate ratio in hypercalcemia. Ann Intern Med 80:200–204, 1974.

This study examined the chloride-phosphate ratio in 52 hypercalcemic patients and clearly differentiated two groups of patients: those with primary HPT and those with hypercalcemia from other causes.

4. Stewart AF, et al.: Biochemical evaluation of patients with cancer-associated hypercalcemia. N Engl J Med 303:1377–1383, 1980.

This was one of the first good studies to demonstrate a biochemical distinction between cancer-associated hypercalcemia and primary HPT.

HYPOCALCEMIA

By MITCHELL KARTON, M.D.

DEFINITION

Hypocalcemia is defined as a total serum calcium concentration below 8.9 mg per dL. Further discussion of the relationship between serum calcium values and proteins, pH, and other electrolytes is included in the definition of hypercalcemia, *vide supra*.

EPIDEMIOLOGY AND GENERAL COMMENTS

A. **Causes of Hypocalcemia.** See Table 51–1.
   1. Hypocalcemia is most commonly associated with hypoalbuminemia; ionized calcium is normal, and no treatment is required.
   2. True hypocalcemia, which is characterized by a decrease in both total and ionized calcium, is usually symptomatic and caused by vitamin D deficiency (with or without frank malabsorption), acute pancreatitis, hyperphosphatemia (usually in the setting of acute or chronic renal failure), hypomagnesemia, hypoparathyroidism, pseudohypoparathyroidism and pseudopseudohypoparathyroidism, or renal tubular acidosis.
   3. Iatrogenic causes of true hypocalcemia include surgical removal of the parathyroid glands in thyroid or parathyroid surgery; radioactive iodine treatment for hyperthyroidism with radiation damage to the parathyroid glands; and intravenous phosphate infusions with formation of calcium-phosphate complexes and with 1,25 dihydroxycholecalciferol inhibition.
   4. Many medications may cause hypocalcemia: EDTA, phytate, and citrate—all complex calcium. Mithramycin inhibits bone resorption. Magnesium sulfate decreases parathyroid hormone secretion. Gentamicin causes renal wastage of magnesium and subsequent magnesium deficiency. Anticonvulsants cause increased degradation of vitamins D_2 and D_3.

DIFFERENTIAL DIAGNOSIS

A. **Hypoproteinemia.** As discussed earlier, hypoproteinemia causes a decreased total serum calcium level as a result of reduced protein binding; a normal serum ionized calcium level precludes symptoms of hypocalcemia.
B. **Hypoparathyroidism.** This disease should be considered in patients with symptomatic hypocalcemia, hyperphosphatemia, and

TABLE 51–1. CAUSES OF HYPOCALCEMIA

Hypoalbuminemia
Hypoparathyroidism
Pseudohypoparathyroidism
Vitamin D deficiency
  Nutritional
  Malabsorption
    Postsurgical
    Sprue
    Chronic pancreatitis
    Obstructive jaundice
    Biliary cirrhosis
    Cathartic ingestion
  Abnormal metabolism of vitamin D
    Renal disease
    Vitamin D–dependent rickets
    Hepatic dysfunction
Hyperphosphatemia: administered phosphate, renal disease, cytotoxic drugs
Acute pancreatitis
Hypomagnesemia
Postoperative: after thyroidectomy, after parathyroidectomy
Renal tubular acidosis
Medullary carcinoma of the thyroid
Medications
  Binders: EDTA, citrate, phytate
  Anticonvulsants
  Gentamicin
  Mithramycin
  Magnesium sulfate IV

---

normal renal function. Diagnosis is based on parathyroid hormone (PTH) assays (decreased or absent), urinary cyclic adenosine monophosphate (UcAMP) excretion (this increases ten- to 20-fold after PTH administration), and "N protein" (G unit) in erythrocyte membranes (normal) for diagnosis. Hypoparathyroidism may coexist with other autoimmune diseases such as Addison's disease, Hashimoto's thyroiditis, diabetes mellitus, and pernicious anemia.

C. **Pseudohypoparathyroidism.** Signs and symptoms are the same as for hypoparathyroidism, plus skeletal abnormalities (notably, short fourth and fifth metacarpals and metatarsals), short stature, and moon facies are found in patient or siblings. There is a female to male patient ratio of 2:1. There are normal PTH levels, little or no response of UcAMP to PTH, and decreased or absent "N protein."

D. **Malabsorption.** There is increased PTH with decreased vitamin D levels or other signs of malabsorption. Incidence is increased after small bowel disease, small bowel surgery, and in obstructive jaundice.

E. **Renal Failure.** Causes include increased PO_4^-, decreased Ca^{++}, chronic acidosis, and elevated blood-urea nitrogen (BUN) and creatinine. The physician should look for possible ectopic soft-tissue calcification secondary to hyperphosphatemia.

F. Acute Pancreatitis. The role of this condition as a cause of hypocalcemia is much debated but truly unknown. It is transient, however, occurring within the first 30 hours and improving after the acute episode.

G. Hypomagnesemia. Probably the main action is impairment of PTH secretion, causing secondary hypocalcemia. Hypomagnesemia is most common in alcoholics and others with chronically poor nutrition.

H. Postsurgical Hypocalcemia. This occurs in less than 5 per cent of postthyroidectomy patients, usually within 24 hours and especially after removal of a large goiter. Tetany occurs in two thirds of these patients, espccially in women. After parathyroidectomy, the serum calcium concentration drops an average of 3.0 mg per dL, usually between the second and fifth postoperative days.

I. Medication-Related Hypocalcemia. Patients receiving large amounts of blood by transfusion are especially vulnerable to citrate-induced complexing of calcium. Patients treated with radioactive iodine for hyperthyroidism suffer latent hypoparathyroidism almost 50 to 60 per cent of the time, but symptomatic hypocalcemia is extremely rare. Chronic epileptics may be susceptible if they are not treated with supplemental vitamins D_2 and D_3.

HISTORY, SIGNS, AND SYMPTOMS

A. In addition to the specific findings of any particular disease associated with a diminished serum calcium concentration, hypocalcemia causes five main categories of signs and symptoms.

1. Tetany. The clinical hallmark of hypocalcemia is tetany, in which there is a range of symptoms from circumoral paresthesias to stiff hands and feet to frank carpopedal spasm. On rare occasions the patient complains of laryngeal stridor.

    a. Chvostek's Sign. This consists of a twitch of the facial muscles (notably the angle of the mouth is drawn up) that is elicited by a sharp tap over the facial nerve in front of the ear. The sign may be positive in 10 per cent of normal adults.

    b. Trousseau's Sign. This is the induction of latent carpopedal spasm by reducing the circulation in the arm with a blood pressure cuff. It is rarely positive in normal adults.

2. Other Neurologic Signs. Other signs include cataracts, diminished deep tendon reflexes or areflexia, occasional papilledema, and possible seizures.

3. Mental Status Disturbances. These include irritability, confusion, memory loss, depression, delusions or hallucinations, seeming mental retardation, and mental instability.

4. Skin Disturbances. There may be dryness of skin and hair, alopecia, and brittle nails.

5. *Gastrointestinal.* The patient may complain of vague crampy abdominal pain with episodic vomiting and diarrhea.

RECOMMENDED DIAGNOSTIC APPROACH

A.* **History.** The examining physician should concentrate on dietary history with special reference to symptoms of malabsorption. In addition, note should be made of alcohol history, medications, and family history (stature, skeletal abnormalities, and multiple endocrine neoplasia [MEN] syndrome).
B. **Physical Examination.** Physical examination should cover the following:
   General: stature, facies
   Skin: ectopic calcifications, uremic frost, and alopecia
   Musculoskeletal: muscle wasting from malabsorption, short fourth and fifth metacarpals and metatarsals
   Neurologic: Chvostek's and Trousseau's signs and areflexia
C. **Laboratory Findings.** These should include serum albumin and total protein; $Ca^{++}/PO_4^=$, vitamin D; tests for malabsorption if necessary; PTH; amylase; magnesium; and renal function tests.
D. **Other.** Ultrasound should be used to assess the pancreas. Small bowel biopsy should be done in work-up of malabsorption. Hands and feet should be x-rayed.

REFERENCE

1. Juan D: Hypocalcemia: Differential diagnosis and mechanisms. Arch Intern Med 139:1166–1171, 1979.

A concise review of hypocalcemia that is especially helpful for its table charting the various causes, their proposed or known mechanisms, and clinical commentaries.

52

DIABETES MELLITUS*

By MICKEY S. EISENBERG, M.D., Ph.D

DEFINITION

Diabetes is a heterogeneous disease group consisting of disorders that share glucose intolerance in common.
The evidence in favor of this heterogeneity is overwhelming: there

---

*This chapter contains material modified from National Diabetes Data Group, NIH: Classification and diagnosis of diabetes mellitus and other categories of glucose intolerance. Diabetes 28:1039–1057, 1979. Reproduced with permission from the American Diabetes Association, Inc.

Text continued on page 399

TABLE 52–1. CLASSIFICATION OF DIABETES MELLITUS AND OTHER CATEGORIES OF GLUCOSE INTOLERANCE*

Class	Former Terminology	Associated Factors	Clinical Characteristics	Diagnostic Criteria
CLINICAL CLASSES **Diabetes mellitus (DM)** Insulin-dependent type (IDDM), Type I	Juvenile diabetes, juvenile-onset diabetes, juvenile-onset–type diabetes (JOD), ketosis-prone diabetes, brittle diabetes	Evidence regarding etiology suggests genetic and environmental or acquired factors, association with certain HLA types, and abnormal immune responses, including autoimmune reactions.	Persons in this subclass are dependent on injected insulin to prevent ketosis and to preserve life, although there may be preketotic, non-insulin–dependent phases in the natural history of the disease. In the preponderance of cases, onset is in youth, but IDDM may occur at any age. Characterized by insulinopenia. Islet cell antibodies are frequently present at diagnosis in this type.	Diagnosis of diabetes in adults should be based on: (1) unequivocal elevation of plasma glucose concentration together with the classical symptoms of diabetes or (2) elevated fasting plasma glucose concentration on more than one occasion
Non-insulin–dependent types (NIDDM), Type II 1. Nonobese NIDDM 2. Obese NIDDM	Adult-onset diabetes, maturity-onset diabetes, maturity-onset–type diabetes (MOD), ketosis-resistant diabetes, stable diabetes	There are probably multiple etiologies for this class, the common outcome being derangement of carbohydrate metabolism. Evidence on familial aggregation of diabetes implies genetic factors,	Persons in this subclass are not insulin-dependent or ketosis-prone, although they may use insulin for correction of symptomatic or persistent hyperglycemia and they can develop ketosis under	

	and this class includes diabetes presenting in children and adults in which autosomal dominant inheritance has been clearly established (formerly termed the MODY type, maturity-onset diabetes in the young). Environmental factors superimposed on genetic susceptibility are probably involved in the onset of the NIDDM types. Obesity is suspected as an etiologic factor and is recommended as a criterion for dividing NIDDM into two subclasses, according to the presence or absence of obesity.	special circumstances, such as episodes of infection or stress. Serum insulin levels may be normal, elevated, or depressed. In the preponderance of cases, onset is after age 40, but NIDDM is known to occur at all ages. About 60–90% of NIDDM subjects are obese and constitute a subtype of NIDDM: in these patients, glucose tolerance is often improved by weight loss. Hyperinsulinemia and insulin resistance characterize some patients in this subtype.	or (3) elevated plasma glucose concentration after an oral glucose challenge on more than one occasion Diagnosis of diabetes in children requires either (1) or (2) *and* (3).
Secondary diabetes	This subclass contains a variety of types of diabetes, in some of which the etiologic relationship is known (diabetes secondary to pancreatic disease, endocrine disease, or administration of	In addition to the presence of the specific condition or syndrome, diabetes mellitus is also present.	In order to place an individual in the subclass *Other types*, two diagnostic determinations must be made: the presence of diabetes (as described above) and the presence of the
Other types, including diabetes mellitus associated with certain conditions and syndromes: 1. Pancreatic disease 2. Hormonal 3. Drug- or chemical-induced			

Table 52–1 continued on following page

TABLE 52–1. CLASSIFICATION OF DIABETES MELLITUS AND OTHER CATEGORIES OF GLUCOSE INTOLERANCE *Continued*

CLASS	FORMER TERMINOLOGY	ASSOCIATED FACTORS	CLINICAL CHARACTERISTICS	DIAGNOSTIC CRITERIA
4. Insulin receptor abnormalities 5. Certain genetic syndromes 6. Other types		certain drugs). In others, an etiologic relationship is suspected because of a higher frequency of association of diabetes with a syndrome or condition (a number of the genetic syndromes).		associated condition or syndrome.
Impaired glucose tolerance (IGT) Nonobese IGT Obese IGT IGT associated with certain conditions and syndromes, which may be (1) pancreatic disease, (2) hormonal, (3) drug- or chemical-induced, (4) insulin receptor abnormalities, (5) certain genetic syndromes	Asymptomatic diabetes, chemical diabetes, subclinical diabetes, borderline diabetes, latent diabetes	Mild glucose intolerance in subjects in this class may be attributable to normal variation of glucose tolerance within a population. In some subjects, IGT may represent a stage in the development of NIDDM or IDDM, although the majority of persons with IGT remain in this class for many years or return to normal glucose tolerance.	Nondiagnostic fasting glucose levels and glucose intolerance of a degree between normal and diabetic. Some studies have shown increased prevalence of arterial disease symptoms and electrocardiographic abnormalities and increased susceptibility to atherosclerotic disease associated with known risk factors including hypertension, hyper-	Diagnosis is based on the oral glucose tolerance test after determining that fasting plasma glucose is <140 mg/dL.

		lipidemia, adiposity, and age. Clinically significant renal and retinal complications of diabetes are absent.	
Gestational diabetes (GDM)	Gestational diabetes	Glucose tolerance with onset during pregnancy is thought to be due to complex metabolic and hormonal changes, which are incompletely understood. Insulin resistance may be responsible in part for gestational diabetes.	Glucose intolerance that has its onset or recognition during pregnancy. Thus, diabetics who become pregnant are not included in this class. Associated with increased perinatal complications and with increased risk for progression to diabetes within 5–10 yr after parturition. Requires reclassification after pregnancy terminates in PrevAGT, DM, or IGT.
			Diagnosis is based on the oral glucose tolerance test.

	DESCRIPTION

STATISTICAL RISK CLASSES

Previous abnormality of glucose tolerance (PrevAGT)	Latent diabetes, prediabetes	This class is restricted to those persons who now have normal glucose tolerance but who have previously demonstrated diabetic hyperglycemia or impaired glucose tolerance either spontaneously or in response to an identifiable stimulus. Individuals who have been gestational diabetics and returned to normal glucose tolerance after parturition form an obvious subclass of PrevAGT. Another small but important group of individuals in this class are former obese diabetics whose

Table 52–1 continued on following page

397

TABLE 52–1. CLASSIFICATION OF DIABETES MELLITUS
AND OTHER CATEGORIES OF GLUCOSE INTOLERANCE* *Continued*

CLASS	FORMER TERMINOLOGY	ASSOCIATED FACTORS	CLINICAL CHARACTERISTICS	DIAGNOSTIC CRITERIA
			glucose tolerance has returned to normal after losing weight. Clinical studies have shown that many patients under acute metabolic stress due to trauma or injury experience transient hyperglycemia. Apart from studies of former gestational diabetics, there has been little systematic investigation of the later liability of persons who have exhibited glucose intolerance to develop diabetes. However, it is likely that this is increased and that there is utility in including all those with a history of glucose intolerance, now normal, in this separate class.	
Potential abnormality of glucose tolerance (PotAGT)	Prediabetes, potential diabetes		This class includes persons who have never exhibited abnormal glucose tolerance but who are at substantially increased risk for the development of diabetes. Individuals who are at increased risk for IDDM include (in decreasing order of risk): persons with islet cell antibodies; monozygotic twin of an IDDM diabetic; sibling of an IDDM diabetic, especially one with identical HLA haplotypes; offspring of an IDDM diabetic. Individuals who are at increased risk for NIDDM include (in decreasing order of risk): monozygotic twin of an NIDDM diabetic; first-degree relative of an NIDDM diabetic (sibling, parent, and offspring); mother of a neonate weighing more than 9 lb; obese individuals; members of racial or ethnic groups with a high prevalence of diabetes (a number of American Indian tribes). The degree of risk for any of these circumstances is not well established as yet.	

*Adapted, with permission, from the American Diabetes Association, Inc., from Diabetes 28:1039–1057, 1979.

are (1) more than 30 distinct, mostly rare, disorders in which glucose intolerance is a feature; (2) ethnic variability in prevalence and clinical features; (3) genetic heterogeneity in diabetic animal models; (4) clinical variability between thin, ketosis-prone, and insulin-resistant diabetes; (5) genetic and immunologic studies that show juvenile and adult-onset diabetes to be distinct entities; and (6) demonstration that a type of mild diabetes in young people, which is inherited in an autosomal dominant fashion, is clearly different from the classic acute-onset diabetes of juveniles.

CLASSIFICATION AND DIAGNOSIS

The types of diabetes and subtypes are identified in Table 52–1. Diagnostic criteria for diabetes in adults are shown in Table 52–2.

RECOMMENDED DIAGNOSTIC APPROACH

Diagnosis of diabetes should be based on (1) unequivocal elevation of plasma glucose (PG) concentration together with the classic symptoms of diabetes; or (2) elevated fasting plasma glucose concentration on more than one occasion; or (3) elevated PG concentration after an oral glucose challenge on more than one occasion.

Figure 52–1 is a flow diagram illustrating the set of measurements and decisions needed to classify an individual case.

The presence of such obvious diabetic symptoms as polyuria, polydipsia, ketonuria, and rapid weight loss, together with gross and unequivocal elevation of PG, is usually sufficient to make the diagnosis of diabetes. In the absence of these signs and symptoms, however, quantitative measurements of PG under carefully standardized conditions are the prescribed methods for making a clinical diagnosis of diabetes. These include measurement of the FPG concentration and, if FPG is not elevated, performance of the oral glucose tolerance test (OGTT). The PG levels considered to be diagnostic of diabetes are shown in Table 52–2.

The OGTT is not necessary if the fasting PG meets the criteria for diabetes shown in Table 52–2. Because of the reliance placed on the FPG level, it is essential that factors other than diabetes that elevate fasting blood glucose are carefully considered and are known to be absent in a subject.

The use of PG glucose levels in the fasting state or in response to an oral glucose challenge to establish a diagnosis of diabetes is associated with several well-recognized problems and limitations. These include a variety of metabolic disturbances or stresses, such as illness, trauma, pregnancy, endocrinopathies, and certain drugs that induce hyperglycemia. Physical inactivity or carbohydrate intake of less than 150 g per day for several days before the OGTT can produce abnormal glucose tolerance. Administration of the test in the afternoon

TABLE 52–2. DIAGNOSTIC CRITERIA*

Diabetes Mellitus in Nonpregnant Adults

Any one of the following are considered diagnostic of diabetes:

A. Presence of the classic symptoms of diabetes, such as polyuria, polydipsia, ketonuria, and rapid weight loss, together with gross and unequivocal elevation of plasma glucose.

B. Elevated fasting glucose concentration on more than one occasion:

> venous plasma ≥ 140 mg/dL (7.8 mmol/L)
> venous whole blood ≥ 120 mg/dL (6.7 mmol/L)
> capillary whole blood ≥ 120 mg/dL (6.7 mmol/L)

If the fasting glucose concentration meets these criteria, the OGTT is *not required.* Indeed, virtually all persons with FPG > 140 mg/dL exhibit an OGTT that meets or exceeds the criteria in C below.

C. Fasting glucose concentration less than that which is diagnostic of diabetes (B, above), but sustained elevated glucose concentration during the OGTT on more than one occasion. *Both* the 2-hr sample and some other sample taken between administration of the 75-g glucose dose and 2 hr later must meet the following criteria:

> venous plasma ≥ 200 mg/dL (11.1 mmol/L)
> venous whole blood ≥ 180 mg/dL (10.0 mmol/L)
> capillary whole blood ≥ 200 mg/dL (11.1 mmol/L)

Impaired Glucose Tolerance (IGT) in Nonpregnant Adults

Three criteria must be met: the fasting glucose concentration must be below the value that is diagnostic for diabetes; the glucose concentration two hours after a 75-g oral glucose challenge must be between normal and diabetic values; and a value between ½-hr, 1-hr, or 1.5-hr OGTT value later must be unequivocally elevated.

Fasting value:

> venous plasma < 140 mg/dL (7.8 mmol/L)
> venous whole blood < 120 mg/dL (6.7 mmol/L)
> capillary whole blood < 120 mg/dl (6.7 mmol/L)

½-hr, 1 hr, or 1.5 hr OGTT value:

> venous plasma ≥ 200 mg/dL (11.1 mmol/L)
> venous whole blood ≥ 180 mg/dL (10.0 mmol/L)
> capillary whole blood ≥ 200 mg/dL (11.1 mmol/L)

Table 52–2 continued on opposite page

TABLE 52–2. DIAGNOSTIC CRITERIA* *Continued*

2-hr OGTT value:
venous plasma of between 140 and 200 mg/dL
venous whole blood of between 120 and 180 mg/dL
capillary whole blood of between 140 and 200 mg/dL

Normal Glucose Levels in Nonpregnant Adults
Fasting value:
venous plasma < 115 mg/dL (6.4 mmol/L)
venous whole blood < 100 mg/dL (5.6 mmol/L)
capillary whole blood < 100 mg/dL (100 mmol/L)

2-hr OGTT value:
venous plasma < 140 mg/dL (7.8 mmol/L)
venous whole blood < 120 mg/dL (6.7 mmol/L)
capillary whole blood < 140 mg/dL (7.8 mmol/L)

OGTT values between ½-hr, 1-hr, or 1.5-hr OGTT value later:
venous plasma < 200 mg/dL (11.1 mmol/L)
venous whole blood < 180 mg/dL (10.0 mmol/L)
capillary whole blood < 200 mg/dL (11.1 mmol/L)

Glucose values above these concentrations but below the criteria for diabetes or IGT should be considered nondiagnostic for these conditions.

Gestational Diabetes
Two or more of the following values after a 100-g oral glucose challenge must be met or exceeded:

	venous plasma	venous whole blood	capillary whole blood
Fasting	105 mg/dL	90 mg/dL	90 mg/dL
1 hr	190 mg/dL	170 mg/dL	170 mg/dL
2 hr	165 mg/dL	145 mg/dL	145 mg/dL
3 hr	145 mg/dL	125 mg/dL	125 mg/dL

*Adapted, with permission, from the American Diabetes Association, Inc., from Diabetes 28:1039–1057, 1979.

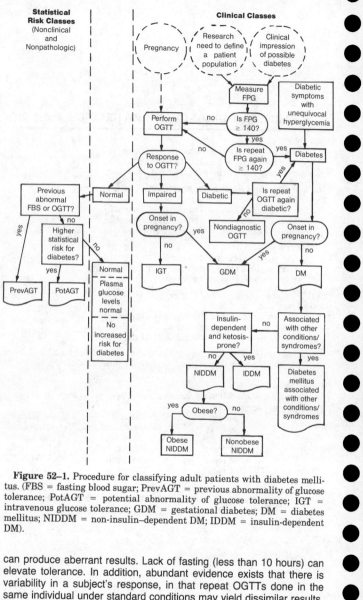

Figure 52–1. Procedure for classifying adult patients with diabetes mellitus. (FBS = fasting blood sugar; PrevAGT = previous abnormality of glucose tolerance; PotAGT = potential abnormality of glucose tolerance; IGT = intravenous glucose tolerance; GDM = gestational diabetes; DM = diabetes mellitus; NIDDM = non-insulin–dependent DM; IDDM = insulin-dependent DM).

can produce aberrant results. Lack of fasting (less than 10 hours) can elevate tolerance. In addition, abundant evidence exists that there is variability in a subject's response, in that repeat OGTTs done in the same individual under standard conditions may yield dissimilar results.

HYPOGLYCEMIA*

By EDWARD A. BENSON, M.D.

DEFINITION

Hypoglycemia is a symptomatic state that is produced by an abnormal depression of plasma glucose concentration. The symptoms and signs of hypoglycemia vary from subtle to dramatic. Some individuals experience symptoms when blood glucose level falls to just below normal (<60 mg per dL), whereas others may not become symptomatic until blood glucose is profoundly low (<30 mg per dL).

While true hypoglycemia is a rare condition, there is a popular belief, shared by many physicians, that a condition called "reactive" or "functional" hypoglycemia is common and frequently leads to fatigue, tension, inability to concentrate, depression, and other such dysphoric symptoms. Although this belief is almost certainly erroneous, "functional" hypoglycemia cannot simply be ignored, since many patients are convinced that their symptoms are a result of "low blood sugar."

CAUSES OF HYPOGLYCEMIA

A. **Postprandial Hypoglycemia.** The significance of hypoglycemia depends on the setting in which it occurs. Hypoglycemia following meals is common in patients who have had gastric surgery. In these patients, abnormally rapid gastric emptying stimulates the enteroinsular axis and causes an overshooting of insulin secretion followed by hypoglycemia one to four hours later. Such "reactive " hypoglycemia occurs rarely, if ever, in the absence of gastric surgery.

B. **Fasting Hypoglycemia.** Hypoglycemia that occurs in the fasting state always indicates the presence of a significant underlying disease (Table 53–1).

   1. *Exogenous Causes.* By far the most common and easily recognized cause of hypoglycemia is antidiabetic medication. Hypoglycemia is an ever-present risk for diabetics taking insulin or sulfonylureas. Spontaneous recovery from insulin- or sulfonylurea-induced hypoglycemia largely depends on an outpouring of counterregulatory hormones. Deficiencies in the release or action of these hormones may contribute to the recurrent hypoglycemia seen in some cases of "brittle" diabetes.

   Heavy alcohol consumption in the absence of food can also

---

*Adapted, with permission of authors and publisher, from Benson E, Fredlund P: Hypoglycemia. *In* Metz R, Larson E (eds.): Blue Book of Endocrinology. Philadelphia, W. B. Saunders Company, 1985.

TABLE 53–1. CAUSES OF FASTING HYPOGLYCEMIA

Endogenous
A. Hyperinsulinemia
    1. Insulin-secreting islet cell tumor
    2. "Autoimmune" hypoglycemia
B. Endocrine deficiencies
    1. Adrenal insufficiency
    2. Hypopituitarism
    3. Glucagon deficiency (rare)
C. Diffuse liver disease (inflammatory or neoplastic)
D. Tumor-associated hypoglycemia
    1. Large mesenchymal tumors
    2. Hepatoma
    3. Adrenal carcinoma
    4. Others: Gastrointestinal cancer, lymphomas, etc.
E. Other causes: Sepsis, chronic renal failure, antibodies to the insulin receptor, and congenital hepatic enzyme defects
Exogenous
A. Insulin and sulfonylureas (therapeutic and surreptitious)
B. Ethanol
C. Disopyramide
D. Pentamidine
E. ? Others

cause hypoglycemia by suppressing hepatic gluconeogenesis. Aspirin in children, disopyramide (Norpace), pentamidine, and perhaps a few other medications can cause hypoglycemia as well.

2. *Hyperinsulinemia.* The final common pathway for several causes of hypoglycemia is hyperinsulinemia, whether this is caused by an insulin-secreting islet cell tumor, therapeutic or surreptitious administration of insulin or sulfonylurea, or the unregulated release of insulin from circulating antibodies.

    a. Hypoglycemia from the surreptitious use of insulin or sulfonylurea hypoglycemic agents probably occurs with a frequency similar to that of insulin-secreting tumors.

        Surreptitious insulin administration can be detected in most cases by measuring insulin and C-peptide concentrations during hypoglycemia. Since commercial insulin contains no C-peptide, patients secretly injecting insulin have an elevated insulin level coupled with low or nondetectable C-peptide. In addition, the presence of insulin-binding antibodies in a patient's serum suggests exposure to exogenous insulin, although in rare cases insulin-binding autoimmune antibodies may arise in individuals never exposed to exogenous insulin.

    b. Hypoglycemia associated with insulin-binding autoimmune antibodies has only recently been recognized. Although the mechanism by which insulin antibodies produce hypoglycemia is uncertain, liberation of excessive amounts of insulin from a large pool of bound insulin during fasting, or potentiation of insulin effect by antibody aggregation, could explain the hypoglycemia.

Typical of both autoimmune hyoglycemia and surreptitious insulin injection are extraordinarily high concentrations of serum insulin. In autoimmune hypoglycemia, insulin antibodies interfere with the radioimmunoassay system, often giving rise to spuriously high results (insulin values in excess of 1000 μU per mL). Autoimmune hypoglycemia can be difficult to distinguish from surreptitious insulin administration. There is no laboratory test capable of differentiating between the two. Even close observation of the patient may fail to detect surreptitious administration of insulin.

A second autoimmune mechanism capable of producing hypoglycemia has been described in a few patients with antibodies to the insulin receptor. Although insulin receptor antibodies are usually associated with diabetes and severe insulin resistance, in some patients the insulinlike activity of the insulin receptor antibody predominates, and the patient manifests hypoglycemia rather than diabetes. The distinctive skin lesion acanthosis nigricans is often present in the antireceptor antibody syndrome, and its presence may be helpful diagnostically.

3. *Miscellaneous Causes*

a. Hypoglycemia can result from a deficiency of insulin counterregulatory hormones, as in adrenal insufficiency or hypopituitarism. Hypoglycemia as a result of a deficiency of glucagon has been reported but is rare. Diffuse liver disease such as fulminant hepatitis or advanced hepatocellular carcinoma can lead to hypoglycemia by compromising the liver's capacity for glycogenolysis and gluconeogenesis. Spontaneous hypoglycemia may occur in patients with chronic renal failure. The mechanism of hypoglycemia in this setting is uncertain, although it may be that the muscle wasting and malnutrition that sometimes accompanies azotemia may result in an inadequate supply of amino acid substrates for gluconeogenesis.

b. Several nonpancreatic tumors have been associated with hypoglycemia, with large mesenchymal tumors, hepatomas, and adrenal carcinomas accounting for about 75 per cent of reported cases. The mechanism of tumor-related hypoglycemia is unknown. Glucose consumption by the large mesenchymal tumors has been postulated, as has a defect in glycogenolysis associated with hepatomas and the elaboration of an insulinlike hormone (nonsuppressible insulinlike activity, or NSILA) by a variety of tumors.

c. Overwhelming sepsis may be accompanied by hypoglycemia. The prognosis in such cases is poor.

d. Artifactual hypoglycemia may be seen in conditions in which the cellular elements of blood are greatly increased, such as in chronic myelogenous leukemia and polycythemia vera.

SYMPTOMS AND SIGNS

A. **Autonomic Nervous System.** Hypoglycemia usually triggers a discharge of the autonomic nervous system, both parasympathetic and sympathetic, resulting in hunger, nervousness, tachycardia, diaphoresis, pallor, and tremulousness.

B. **Other Symptoms.** Other symptoms result from a lack of adequate glucose for the brain. The manifestations of neuroglycopenia are influenced by the state of the cerebral circulation as well as the rate of fall of blood glucose. Symptoms are diverse and include headache, lightheadedness, visual disturbances, irritability, lethargy, agitation, confusion, inappropriate behavior, stupor, convulsions, paralysis, and coma. Although these symptoms usually resolve when blood glucose concentration is returned to normal, permanent neurologic defects can follow severe or prolonged hypoglycemia. The cerebral cortex and cerebellum are most susceptible to the effects of hypoglycemia, while the midbrain and medulla are least vulnerable to permanent damage. Peripheral nerves can also be injured by repeated hypoglycemia, which can cause an irreversible neuropathy.

RECOMMENDED DIAGNOSTIC APPROACH

When the presence of hypoglycemia is obvious, the cause is often obvious as well, as for instance in alcohol abuse, fulminant hepatitis, Addison's disease, or malignancy.

The manifestations of hypoglycemia may be subtle, however, as in the patient who complains of "spells" brought on by missing a meal or by exercise and relieved by food. In such patients, the first diagnostic step is to verify that fasting hypoglycemia is present and then to document whether it is of the hyperinsulinemic or hypoinsulinemic category.

A. **Home Blood Glucose Testing.** For patients for whom the index of suspicion is low, home blood glucose testing with reagent strips can be useful in screening for hypoglycemia. A blood glucose level of less than 60 mg per dL during symptoms should prompt further investigation with an in-hospital fast. A laboratory blood glucose level measured after a 16-hour overnight fast can also be a useful "screening" test for patients considered less likely to have true hypoglycemia.

B. **In-Hospital Fast.** The definitive test for hypoglycemia is the carefully supervised in-hospital fast. The response of blood glucose to prolonged fasting and the correlation of symptoms with glucose and insulin levels usually provide sufficient information to establish a precise diagnosis.

The fast (allowing intake of only noncaloric fluids) is best begun in the morning, with breakfast omitted. Continuous intravenous access is maintained and 50 per cent dextrose kept available for possible emergency treatment of severe hypoglycemic symptoms. Blood samples for immediate glucose determination (estimated at the bedside by

**TABLE 53–2. IN-HOSPITAL FAST: SIGNIFICANCE OF
INSULIN AND C-PEPTIDE LEVELS DURING
HYPOGLYCEMIA**

INCREASED INSULIN AND C-PEPTIDE	INCREASED INSULIN AND DECREASED C-PEPTIDE	DECREASED INSULIN AND C-PEPTIDE
1. Insulinoma	1. Insulin administration	1. Tumor-associated hypoglycemia
2. Sulfonylurea	2. "Autoimmune" hypoglycemia*	2. Endocrine deficiencies
		3. Hepatic and renal failure

*Free C-peptide levels are suppressed, but because of the binding of endogenous proinsulin (containing the C-peptide sequence) to the circulating insulin antibody, total C-peptide level may be normal or even elevated.

glucose oxidase-impregnated strips and subsequently measured in the laboratory) and possible later insulin and C-peptide assays are collected every 4 hours or whenever symptoms of hypoglycemia occur. The fast is continued for 72 hours or until the patient has unequivocal symptoms of hypoglycemia and/or blood glucose falls below 40 mg per dL, whichever comes first. Although glucose concentration may occasionally fall below 35 mg per dL in normal women after 72 hours of fasting, the author terminates the test if the glucose concentration falls below 40 mg per dL. The author's experience suggests that a fasting blood glucose concentration below this level is virtually always pathologic. A ratio of immunoreactive insulin (in μU per mL) to glucose (in mg per dL) of more than 0.3 is highly suggestive of an insulin-secreting islet cell tumor, if it is assumed that other causes of hyperinsulinemia have been excluded. During hypoglycemia insulin concentration is usually greater than 6 μU per mL in patients with an insulinoma.

The in-hospital fast serves two purposes: (1) to confirm or exclude the diagnosis of fasting hypoglycemia and (2) to differentiate (by insulin and C-peptide measurement) between the various causes of hypoglycemia (Table 53–2).

"NONHYPOGLYCEMIA"

The term "nonhypoglycemia" describes the condition of patients who misattribute their symptoms to hypoglycemia. The notion that hypoglycemia or a "sugar imbalance" may be responsible for such chronic problems as loss of vitality, depression, allergies, and the like is understandably appealing to both patient and physician. The idea has been sustained in large part by inappropriate application of the glucose tolerance test. Impressively low blood glucose concentrations occur following a glucose load in many normal people (10 per cent of healthy individuals when given a glucose load have a blood glucose nadir below 47 mg per dL without experiencing symptoms). Despite this well-documented fact, the oral glucose tolerance test is often used to "confirm" an impression of hypoglycemia. The drop in glucose level that may occur during the course of the glucose tolerance test is rarely, if ever, duplicated following a normal meal. For this reason, the glucose tolerance test has little relevance to normal day-to-day glucose kinetics and no role in the evaluation of alleged hypoglycemia. A simple postmeal glucose determination, obtained during symptoms, is the most appropriate measurement and by its normal value supports the diagnosis of nonhypoglycemia. Since the symptoms of nonhypoglycemia are almost always "functional" or psychosomatic, the treatment must be designed accordingly. It may be tempting to advise dietary therapy, such as avoidance of simple sugars and frequent small feedings low in carbohydrate, but while such dietary measures may alleviate symptoms, it is debatable whether this is a result of a change in glucose dynamics or a placebo effect.

REFERENCES

1. Fajans SS, Floyd JC: Fasting hypoglycemia in adults. N Engl J Med 294:766–772, 1976.
2. Goldman J, Baldwin D, Rubenstein AH, et al.: Characterization of circulating insulin and proinsulin-binding antibodies in autoimmune hypoglycemia. J Clin Invest 63:1050–1059, 1979.
3. Selzer HS: Drug-induced hypoglycemia. Diabetes 21:955–966, 1972.
4. Service FJ (ed.): Hypoglycemia disorders. Boston, Hall Medical Publishers, 1983.
5. Service FJ, Dale AJD, Elveback LR, et al.: Insulinoma: Clinical and diagnostic features in 60 consecutive cases. Mayo Clin Proc 51:417–429, 1976.
6. Yager J, Young RT: Nonhypoglycemia is an epidemic condition. N Engl J Med 291:907, 1974.

54

ADRENAL GLAND DISEASES: CORTISOL EXCESS (CUSHING'S SYNDROME)*

By WILFRED Y. FUJIMOTO, M.D.

DEFINITION

A. **Excess Glucocorticoid.** Cushing's syndrome results from an excess of glucocorticoid, either exogenous or endogenous, the former occurring far more commonly than the latter. Endogenous

---

*Adapted, with permission of author and publisher, from Fujimoto WY: Disorders of glucocorticoid homeostasis. *In* Metz R, Larson E (eds.): Blue Book of Endocrinology. Philadelphia, W. B. Saunders Company, 1985.

overproduction of glucocorticoid occurs in a variety of conditions, all of which involve either a malfunction of one of the components of the homeostatic system of cortisol production (such as the hypothalamus or pituitary or adrenal cortex) or the introduction of ectopically produced adrenocorticotropic hormone (ACTH) into that system.

B. **Cushing's Syndrome Versus Cushing's Disease.** Conventionally, the term "Cushing's syndrome" has been applied to all clinical situations in which there is an excess of cortisol, whereas the term "Cushing's disease" has been restricted to Cushing's syndrome resulting from overproduction of ACTH from a pituitary tumor.

CAUSES OF ENDOGENOUS CUSHING'S SYNDROME

A. **Pituitary Cushing's Syndrome.** Overproduction of ACTH results in bilateral adrenal hypertrophy and overproduction of cortisol and, to a lesser extent, other adrenal steroids. Pituitary ACTH overproduction accounts for about two thirds of all cases of endogenous hypercortisolism. Pituitary Cushing's syndrome is usually caused by a pituitary adenoma, the majority of which are microadenomas. In a small number of cases, the adenomas are large enough to produce pressure on adjacent structures and erosion of bone in addition to the metabolic effects.

An important and as yet unresolved question relates to the role of the hypothalamus in the production of pituitary Cushing's syndrome. It is possible that the primary, or at least the initiating, disorder in patients with pituitary Cushing's syndrome is overproduction of corticotropin-releasing factor (CRF) by the hypothalamus. This possibility is strengthened by the fact that certain cases of Cushing's syndrome respond favorably to treatment with drugs that have either antiserotonin or dopaminergic activities. Furthermore, in up to 40 per cent of patients with pituitary Cushing's syndrome, no tumor is detectable on histologic examination of the pituitary gland.

Pituitary Cushing's syndrome occurs more frequently in females than in males, especially in women of child-bearing age, but although the majority of cases occur in adults, the condition may occur at any age.

B. **Adrenal Adenoma.** Cortisol-producing adenomas are usually unilateral and characteristically produce cortisol only. Thus, the clinical manifestations are those of pure glucocorticoid excess without any evidence of mineralocorticoid or sex steroid overproduction. Indeed, because the glucocorticoid excess turns off ACTH production, adrenal sex steroid production may actually be diminished. The female patients, in contrast to those with pituitary Cushing's syndrome, usually do not show excessive body hair or menstrual irregularities.

C. **Adrenocortical Carcinoma.** The great majority of adrenocortical cancers produce excessive quantities of all of the adrenal hormones, and in most of them androgens predominate. In adult males, the effects of excessive adrenal androgen may not be clinically apparent, and the tumor may appear metabolically silent. In females and male children, adrenal cancers characteristically produce a rapidly advancing Cushing's syndrome with conspicuous evidence of androgen excess that is usually manifested by rapidly progressive hirsutism. A few adrenal cancers produce estrogens, which, in males, cause feminization. In children, adrenal cancer is the most common cause of Cushing's syndrome. Adrenal cancer is almost invariably and rapidly fatal.

D. **Ectopic ACTH Production.** Ectopic Cushing's syndrome is largely a disease of men and most often occurs in patients with lung cancer, especially oat cell carcinomas. Elevated levels of circulating ACTH are measured by radioimmunoassay in many patients with lung cancer, and extracts of lung cancer usually contain immunoreactive ACTH. However, only a small fraction of patients with lung cancer show clinical evidence of hypercortisolism, probably because tumor ACTH, even when present in excess as determined by immunoassay, may be biologically inert. Other tumors that may produce clinically apparent Cushing's syndrome include thymoma, bronchial carcinoid, carcinoma of the pancreatic islet, medullary cancer of the thyroid, pheochromocytoma, and others. Almost one sixth of patients with Cushing's syndrome have ectopic ACTH production as the cause of the disorder.

Ectopic Cushing's syndrome usually lacks the somatic features of other Cushing's syndromes (striae, obesity with characteristic fat distribution, plethora, and hirsutism), since the patient does not survive long enough for them to become apparent. The predominant clinical features are profound weakness, hyperpigmentation, weight loss, and edema. The predominant metabolic findings are hypokalemic acidosis and hyperglycemia. In patients with the ectopic Cushing's syndrome, the underlying tumor is obvious, although in some cases manifestations of excessive ACTH production may be the initial clue to the presence of a tumor.

SIGNS AND SYMPTOMS

A. **Excess Cortisol Production.** The principal clinical manifestations of excess cortisol production are listed in Table 54–1. The predominant metabolic effect of cortisol is stimulation of gluconeogenesis, hence the term "glucocorticoid." The overall effect of gluconeogenesis is the production of increased amounts of glucose at the expense of protein anabolism. Many of the clinical manifestations of glucocorticoids can be explained by that gluconeogenic action, such as glucose intolerance, protein wasting manifested by muscle weakness, muscle laxity and wasting (abdominal protuberance, flat buttocks, shrunken thighs), loss of subcutaneous protein (thin skin, striae), loss of bone matrix (osteopenia), poor wound healing, and capillary fragility (ecchy-

TABLE 54–1. CLINICAL MANIFESTATIONS OF HYPERCORTISOLISM

Weight gain	Accumulation of adipose tissue, particularly centripetal (face, neck, trunk, limb girdles)
	Hyperphagia
Protein wasting	Thin skin
	Striae
	Capillary fragility (ecchymoses)
	Muscle wasting
	Muscle weakness
	Osteopenia (osteoporosis, hypercalciuria)
	Poor wound healing
	Growth retardation (children)
Carbohydrate intolerance	Impaired glucose utilization, hyperglycemia, insulin resistance
Mineralocorticoid effect of cortisol	Hypertension
	Hypokalemia
Depressed immunity	Increased susceptibility to infections
Other	Downy hirsutism
	Oligomenorrhea
	Plethora
	Erythrocytosis
	Personality changes

moses). The exact mechanism of some of the other manifestations of hypercortisolism such as increased appetite, centripetal accumulation of adipose tissue, plethora, and lanugo hair production are poorly understood.

B. **Cushing's Syndrome.** The clinical manifestations of Cushing's syndrome vary according to the cause. Thus, for instance, in ACTH excess the patient usually manifests not only the effects of glucocorticoid excess (Table 54–1) but usually also shows evidence of overproduction of androgens causing hirsutism, acne, and occasionally frank virilization. Other sources of variation arise depending on the duration and extent of the cortisol overproduction and also on the age, sex, and underlying state of health of the individual.

DIAGNOSIS

A. **Glucocorticoid Excess.** The physician should be alert to the possibility of Cushing's syndrome whenever any of the individual features of glucocorticoid excess (Table 54–1) are encountered, whether they occur alone or in any combination.

B. **Diagnostic Work-Up.** The diagnostic work-up is directed primarily at two questions: (1) Is there overproduction of glucocorticoid? and (2) If so, what is the source of that overproduction?

C. **"Overnight" Dexamethasone Suppression Test.** The customary first step in the work-up is a screening test known as the "overnight" dexamethasone suppression test. This test is suitable for the study of outpatients. The patient takes 1 mg of dexamethasone orally at about 11:30 P.M. before retiring. Plasma cortisol is measured the next morning at 8:00 A.M. The patient should omit all but essential medications during the day preceding the morning sample and should arrive at the laboratory in a calm and collected condition. A plasma cortisol level of 5 μg per dL or less indicates a negative test result and essentially excludes the possibility of Cushing's syndrome. False-negative tests are very rare. A plasma cortisol concentration greater than 5 μg per dL is considered a positive test result. False-positive tests may occur because of failure to take the dexamethasone at the proper time or because of accelerated metabolism of dexamethasone (caused by drugs such as barbiturates, Dilantin, or phenylbutazone that induce hepatic enzymes). Depressive illnesses and a variety of acute and chronic physical illnesses may be associated with abnormal false-positive results. Estrogen administration and obesity may also lead to false-positive results by raising cortisol binding protein.

D. **Urinary Free Cortisol.** A very useful test of cortisol overproduction is the measurement of urinary free cortisol over a 24-hour period. This test may be done before the results of the overnight dexamethasone suppression test have been obtained when the suspicion is high or may be ordered when the results of that test are positive. The 24-hour urine collection period should not include the time during which the dexamethasone suppression test is done. Urinary free cortisol reflects the free (unbound) cortisol concentration in plasma. This amount increases disproportionately when the total plasma cortisol exceeds the level of saturation of corticosteroid-binding globulin (about 20 μg per dL). Urinary free cortisol above 100 μg per day is indicative of excessive cortisol production. When the urinary free cortisol excretion rate is clearly diagnostic (above 200 μg per day), no further tests need be done to confirm the presence of hypercortisolism.

E. **"Formal" Dexamethasone Suppression Test.** When measurement of urinary free cortisol is equivocal, a test known as the "formal" dexamethasone suppression test is usually done. This test not only provides confirmation of the diagnosis of hypercortisolism but also provides a strong indication of the cause of the Cushing's syndrome. The test is performed as follows:

Day 1: baseline 24-hour urinary cortisol determination

Day 2: baseline 24-hour urinary cortisol determination

Day 3: administration of low-dose dexamethasone (0.5 mg every six hours) during collection of 24-hour urinary cortisol

Day 4: administration of low-dose dexamethasone again during collection of 24-hour urinary cortisol

Urinary cortisol excretion that does not suppress to less than 25 μg per 24 hours after low-dose dexamethasone administration is indicative of Cushing's syndrome.

Day 5: administration of high-dose dexamethasone (2.0 mg every six hours) during collection of 24-hour urinary cortisol

Day 6: administration of high-dose dexamethasone during collection of 24-hour urinary cortisol

Failure of the cortisol to be suppressed after high-dose dexamethasone administration is indicative of either adrenal Cushing's syndrome or ectopic Cushing's syndrome. Suppression of the 24-hour urinary cortisol excretion to about 50 per cent of baseline on the high dose in association with nonsuppression on the low dose is indicative of pituitary Cushing's syndrome. The urinary creatinine excretion should be measured in all samples to detect errors of collection. It is also worthwhile to measure urinary dehydroepiandrosterone or 17 ketosteroids on days one and two, since markedly elevated levels strongly suggest adrenal cancer and rule out adrenal adenoma as the cause of the Cushing's syndrome.

F. **Imaging Techiques.** The plasma ACTH assays and newer imaging techniques frequently obviate the need for the "formal" dexamethasone test. These imaging techniques are summarized in Table 54–2. Body imaging procedures are usually highly effective in detecting the tumor (pituitary, adrenal, or ectopic) that is responsible for almost all cases of Cushing's syndrome.

G. **Screening Procedure.** Frequently all that is necessary in coming to a definitive diagnosis is the following sequence:

1. Positive overnight dexamethasone screening test.
2. Elevated urinary free cortisol.
3. Plasma ACTH levels that are either abnormally low (as found in Cushing's syndrome secondary to adrenal adenomas or carcinomas) or high (as usually seen in ectopic Cushing's syndrome). In pituitary Cushing's syndrome the ACTH levels may not be strikingly elevated or may be normal.
4. If ACTH levels are low, adrenal imaging, especially an abdominal computed tomographic (CT) scan, shows a unilateral adrenal mass in adrenal adenoma or carcinoma. A tumor that is large enough can also be detected by ultrasound.
5. If ACTH levels are high but not strikingly elevated or normal,

TABLE 54–2. ANATOMIC LOCALIZATION TESTS

Pituitary Cushing's syndrome
  Visual fields
  Head CT scan

Adrenal Cushing's syndrome
  Abdominal CT scan
  Ultrasound
  Adrenal scintiscan
  Venography
  Adrenal vein cortisol
  Arteriography

Ectopic Cushing's syndrome
  Chest x-ray
  Abdominal CT scan
  Bronchogram
  Gastrointestinal x-ray

CT scan of the head should be done because of the possibility of pituitary Cushing's syndrome. The CT scan shows a pituitary tumor in 80 per cent of cases.

6. If ACTH levels are very high and ectopic Cushing's syndrome is suspected, chest x-rays should be done, and if these do not provide the answer, it will become necessary to search for other possible sites of the tumor.

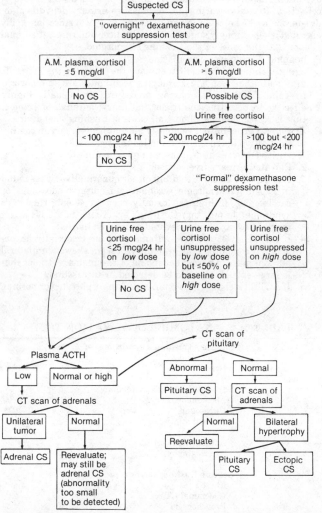

Figure 54–1. Diagnosis of Cushing's syndrome (CS). Exogenous glucocorticoids have been excluded.

Occasionally in the search for suspected adrenal adenoma, other procedures, including adrenal scintiscan, venography or arteriography, or sampling of adrenal venous blood for cortisol are necessary.

RECOMMENDED DIAGNOSTIC APPROACH

The recommended diagnostic approach is outlined in Figure 54–1.

REFERENCES

1. Gold EM: The Cushing syndrome: Changing view of diagnosis and treatment. Ann Intern Med 90:829–844, 1979.
2. Crapo L: Cushing's syndrome: A review of diagnostic tests. Metabolism 28:955–977, 1979.
3. Liddle GW: The adrenals. *In* Williams RH (ed.): Williams' Textbook of Endocrinology. W. B. Saunders Company, Philadelphia, pp. 249–276, 1981.
4. Krieger DT: Physiopathology of Cushing's disease. Endocrinol Rev 4:22–43, 1983.

55

ADRENAL GLAND DISEASES: GLUCOCORTICOID DEFICIENCY*

By WILFRED Y. FUJIMOTO, M.D.

DEFINITION

Glucocorticoid deficiency is caused by abnormalities in the components of the system controlling cortisol production: adrenocortical destruction, a defect in cortisol biosynthesis, or deficient pituitary adrenocorticotropic hormone (ACTH) secretion. The term "Addison's disease" has been applied to glucocorticoid deficiency caused by adrenocortical destruction. This condition is also referred to as primary adrenocortical insufficiency. Its incidence is the same in men and women. The disease may occur at any age. Secondary adrenocortical insufficiency is caused by ACTH deficiency and may be isolated or associated with deficiency of other pituitary hormones (hypopituitarism). This condition is seen more commonly as a consequence of the use of glucocorticoid medications.

---

*Adapted, with permission of author and publisher, from Fujimoto WY: Disorders of glucocorticoid homeostasis. *In* Metz R, Larson E (eds.): Blue Book of Endocrinology. Philadelphia, W. B. Saunders Company, 1985.

CAUSES OF GLUCOCORTICOID DEFICIENCY

A. **Primary Adrenocortical Insufficiency.** Known as Addison's disease, this condition is now most often caused by idiopathic adrenal atrophy. Since many patients with idiopathic adrenal atrophy have adrenal antibodies present in the sera (about 60 per cent), the disorder may be caused by autoimmune adrenalitis. Patients with idiopathic adrenal failure also have an increased risk of developing primary hypothyroidism, diabetes mellitus, idiopathic hypoparathyroidism, primary gonadal failure, or pernicious anemia as a result of autoimmune destruction of these other tissues. Addison's disease must be considered in the differential diagnosis of diseases characterized by weakness, weight loss, anorexia, and hypotension, especially if these symptoms occur in a patient who already has primary hypothyroidism, diabetes mellitus, idiopathic hypoparathyroidism, primary gonadal failure, or pernicious anemia. Formerly, infectious destruction of the adrenal glands, most often caused by tuberculosis, was the most frequent cause of primary adrenocortical insufficiency. Today it accounts for only about 20 per cent of all cases. Other causes of primary adrenocortical failure are systemic fungal diseases, metastatic tumor to the adrenals, amyloidosis, adrenal hemorrhage (from anticoagulant therapy, sepsis, or trauma), and adrenalectomy.

B. **Secondary Adrenocortical Insufficiency.** This is caused by deficient production of ACTH by the pituitary. The most common cause is suppression of ACTH secretion as a consequence of chronic glucocorticoid therapy for nonendocrine disease. ACTH deficiency may also arise from a primary pituitary or hypothalamic disorder. Secondary adrenocortical insufficiency should alert the physician to the possibility that ACTH deficiency may be either isolated or part of a deficiency of multiple pituitary hormones (hypopituitarism).

SIGNS AND SYMPTOMS

A. **Origin of Glucocorticoid Deficiency.** The clinical findings vary according to the origin of glucocorticoid deficiency. For example, in primary adrenocortical insufficiency there is combined glucocorticoid and mineralocortical deficiency (Table 55–1), while in secondary adrenocortical insufficiency mineralocorticoid production is unimpaired. In secondary adrenocortical insufficiency there may be clinical signs of deficiency of other pituitary hormones in addition to ACTH.

B. **Primary Adrenocortical Insufficiency.** In most cases primary adrenocortical insufficiency is gradual in evolution, and compensatory increases in ACTH and renin enable the adrenal glands to secrete enough cortisol and aldosterone in the absence of stress. When more than 90 per cent of the adrenal cortex has

TABLE 55–1. MANIFESTATIONS OF PRIMARY ADRENOCORTICAL INSUFFICIENCY

CORTISOL DEFICIENCY

Gastrointestinal: anorexia, nausea, vomiting, diarrhea, abdominal pain, weight loss

Mental: enervation, confusion, psychosis

Energy metabolism: impaired fat mobilization and utilization, decreased gluconeogenesis, liver glycogen depletion, hypoglycemia

Cardiovascular-renal: impaired "free water" clearance, impaired pressor response to catecholamines, hypotension

Pituitary: increased ACTH secretion, hyperpigmentation

Muscular: asthenia

ALDOSTERONE DEFICIENCY

Inability to conserve sodium: decreased extracellular fluid and blood volume, weight loss, decreased cardiac size and output, prerenal azotemia, increased renin production, weakness, hypotension, postural syncope, shock

Impaired renal secretion of potassium (K^+) and hydrogen (H^+): hyperkalemia, mild acidosis

been destroyed, compensation is inadequate and the patient has the clinical picture originally described by Addison.

C. **Acute Adrenal Insufficiency (Addisonian Crisis).** This condition is marked by nausea, vomiting, hypotension, abdominal pain, extreme muscle weakness, confusion, and ultimately shock. In the patient who becomes unexpectedly seriously ill without an obvious cause, acute adrenal failure must be considered.

D. **Chronic Adrenal Insufficiency.** This ranges from complete failure of adrenal hormone production to a minor impairment of adrenal reserve capacity.

1. Symptoms may be nonspecific and include weakness, weight loss, anorexia, and hypotension. Together these four nonspecific symptoms should make the physician consider a diagnosis of adrenal insufficiency. However, if any of these four features are absent, the patient probably does not have Addison's disease.

2. A major complaint is asthenia, both mental and physical. Patients lose weight but may not do so until adrenal failure is well advanced.

3. Anorexia, nausea, and constipation alternating with diarrhea are increasingly frequent complaints as the disease progresses. If adrenal crisis occurs, a patient may have abdominal pain and the findings of an acute abdominal condition.

4. Pigmentation of the skin is one of the classic signs that often leads to suspicion of primary adrenal insufficiency. Pigmentation is caused by increased melanin in the skin, particularly in regions normally pigmented and exposed to sunlight or pressure. Skin creases and scars acquired after the onset of adrenal insufficiency tend to be pigmented, while scars present before onset of primary adrenal failure remain unpigmented. Mucosal pigmentation of the mouth, conjunctiva, and

vagina may also occur. Pigmentation may precede other features of hypoadrenalism by many years and may be first appreciated by the patient as a better suntan that lasts longer than usual.

5. Vitiligo occurs in 10 to 20 per cent of patients with primary adrenal failure.
6. Hypotension is almost invariable, and postural dizziness may be a prominent symptom.
7. Hyponatremia, hyperkalemia, and azotemia are common.
8. The patient may give a history of slow recovery from illnesses.
9. Reactive and fasting hypoglycemia may occur.
10. Loss of body hair, reflecting loss of adrenal androgen production, may occur in women.

EFFECTS OF GLUCOCORTICOID DEFICIENCY

A. **Gluconeogenesis.** Since one of the predominant metabolic effects of glucocorticoids is to stimulate gluconeogenesis, deficiency of cortisol results in impairment of this metabolic process and is a cause of fasting hypoglycemia.
B. **Cardiovascular and Renal Effects.** Glucocorticoids have cardiovascular and renal effects, and deficiency of cortisol results in impaired ability for free water excretion, impaired pressor response to catecholamines, and hypotension.
C. **Other Effects.** Glucocorticoids have several other effects, including stimulation of appetite, hematopoiesis, fat deposition in certain anatomic sites, gastric acid production, and reduction of blood eosinophils. Therefore, deficiency of cortisol has the following effects: anorexia, mild anemia, weight loss, hypochlorhydria, and eosinophilia. Since there is impaired tolerance to stress when cortisol is deficient, these manifestations typically become more pronounced during times of stress.

DIAGNOSIS

A. **Adrenocortical Insufficiency.** If the clinical picture suggests a possibility of adrenocortical insufficiency, the diagnostic evaluation of the patient must be directed toward the following two points: (1) Is there inadequate production of glucocorticoid? and (2) Is endogenous ACTH low or high? (See Fig. 55–1.)
B. **ACTH Stimulation Test.** The customary first step in evaluation of a patient suspected to have adrenocortical insufficiency includes a short ACTH stimulation test. A blood sample is obtained for measurement of basal plasma level of cortisol. A portion of the sample is also set aside in case measurement of plasma ACTH concentration or aldosterone concentration is indicated after the results of this screening test are known. ACTH is then administered to the patient (synthetic α 1–24 ACTH, 0.25 mg) intramuscularly or intravenously, and blood samples are with-

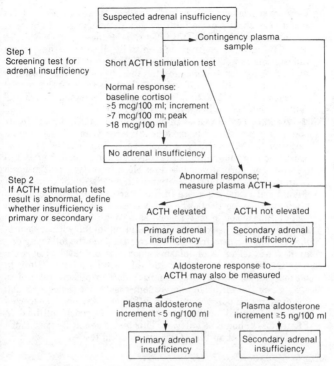

Figure 55–1. Diagnosis of adrenocortical insufficiency.

drawn at 30 and 60 minutes for measurement of plasma cortisol. An additional sample is saved for possible determination of plasma aldosterone levels at a later time. In this short ACTH stimulation test, a normal response is marked by a basal plasma cortisol level of at least 5 μg per 100 mL, an increment of >7 μg per 100 mL, and a maximal value of >18 μg per 100 mL. Cortisol fails to rise normally in both primary and secondary adrenocortical failure, and therefore this is an effective screening test. If the patient is suspected to be in Addisonian crisis and thus immediate administration of glucocorticoid is deemed essential, use of dexamethasone allows the ACTH test to be done while the dexamethasone is being given, since the latter does not interfere with subsequent measurements of plasma cortisol.

C. **Low Levels of Cortisol.** If low levels of cortisol are demonstrated, plasma ACTH should be measured in the sample that was set aside previously. Plasma aldosterone levels before and after stimulation can also be measured at this time. Low plasma cortisol levels with elevated plasma ACTH levels are found with primary adrenocortical insufficiency. In fully developed secondary adrenocortical failure, ACTH is low. However, since ACTH has a very short plasma half-life, if a patient is given glucocorticoids, the ACTH level will fall to the normal range within 15 to 30 minutes, even if it was initially elevated. The plasma aldosterone increment following ACTH stimulation is normally at least 5 ng per 100 mL greater than baseline. With primary adrenocortical failure, aldosterone also fails to show the normal increase after ACTH stimulation, whereas in secondary adrenal failure, aldosterone has a normal increase.

D. Metyrapone Test. In cases in which adrenocortical insufficiency is unlikely but should be excluded, the metyrapone test may be performed. Metyrapone is a competitive inhibitor of 11 β-hydroxylase and thus inhibits the conversion of 11-deoxycortisol to cortisol. The normal response to a block in cortisol biosynthesis is an increase in ACTH secretion with a consequent increase in steroid synthesis and a rise in the intermediate proximal to the block (11-deoxycortisol). The test is most conveniently performed by administration of metyrapone as a single dose (30 mg per kg of body weight) between 11 P.M. and midnight with measurement of plasma deoxycortisol and cortisol done the following day at 8 A.M. The 8 A.M. plasma deoxycortisol level rises from baseline levels of <3 μg per 100 mL to >7 μg per 100 mL in normal subjects (with a concomitant fall in plasma cortisol to <6 μg per 100 mL). The metyrapone test is not indicated when the diagnosis of adrenocortical insufficiency is strongly suspected from the clinical picture for which the approach outlined in Figure 55–1 should be followed. This test is generally used much less frequently than the ACTH stimulation test.

RECOMMENDED DIAGNOSTIC APPROACH

The recommended diagnostic approach is shown in Figure 55–1.

REFERENCES

1. Steinbeck AW, Theile HM: The adrenal cortex (excluding aldosteronism). Clin Endocrinol Metab 3:557–591, 1974.
2. Bayliss RIS: Adrenal cortex. Clin Endocrinol Metab 9:477–486, 1980.
3. Liddle GW: The adrenals. *In* Williams RH (ed.): Textbook of Endocrinology. Philadelphia, W. B. Saunders Company, 1981, pp. 281–288.

THYROID DISEASE

By MITCHELL KARTON, M.D.

INTRODUCTION

Production of thyroid hormone is the last step in a sequence of reactions beginning in the hypothalamus and ending in the thyroid gland. Under the influence of hypothalamic thyrotropin releasing hormone (TRH), the pituitary gland produces thyroid stimulating hormone (TSH), which stimulates the thyroid gland to produce and release thyroid hormone. Under normal conditions, when the level of thyroid hormone in the blood stream rises, the level of TSH falls; hence, the thyroid gland receives less stimulation and produces less hormone. When the peripheral level of thyroid hormone falls, TSH production increases, and hence so does production of thyroid hormone.

Hypo- and hyperthyroidism are functional abnormalities of thyroid metabolism that may result from a number of causes, incuding structural abnormalities of the thyroid gland itself. (See Tables 56–1 and 56–2.) The most common abnormality of thyroid structure

TABLE 56–1. CLASSIFICATION OF HYPOTHYROIDISM

Thyroid
A. *Thyroprivic (insufficient functional tissue)*
    Postablative: surgery or radioactive iodine
    Primary idiopathic
    Sporadic cretinism (aplasia/dysplasia)
    Endemic cretinism (often atrophic)
    Congenital TSH resistance
    Postradiation (lymphoma)

B. *Goitrous*
    Endemic iodine deficiency with or without goitrous cretinism
    Hashimoto's thyroiditis
    Defective hormone biosynthesis
      Iodide transport
      Organification defect
      Iodotyrosine coupling defect
      Iodotyrosine dehalogenase defect
      Abnormal iodoprotein secretion
    Goitrogens (rutabaga, white turnip, soy, cabbage)
    Maternally transmitted (iodides, antithyroid agents)
    Drug-elicited: lithium, para-aminosalicylic acid, phenylbutazone,
      iodides, propylthiouracil, methimazole, cobalt, resorcinol

Suprathyroid
A. *Hypothalamic*
B. *Pituitary*
    Tumor
    Necrosis (Sheehan's syndrome)
    Isolated TSH deficit (extremely rare)

TABLE 56–2. CLASSIFICATION OF THYROTOXICOSIS

Hyperthyroidism
  TSH hypersecretion (pituitary adenoma) (rare)
  Graves' disease
  Toxic multinodular goiter
  Toxic adenoma (uninodular goiter)
  Thyroid carcinoma
  Trophoblastic disease: hydatidiform mole, choriocarcinoma

Without hyperthyroidism
  Thyroiditis: pyogenic, subacute (de Quervain's), chronic painless with
    transient thyrotoxicosis
  Ectopic thyroid tissue: struma ovarii
  Thyrotoxicosis factitia
  Jod-Basedow phenomenon: iodine-induced

is the goiter, which is defined as an enlargement of the thyroid gland. A goiter may be either a diffuse or a nodular enlargement of the gland and may be associated with hypo-, hyper-, or euthyroid states. In hypothyroidism, a goiter occurs because the thyroid gland is overstimulated by excess TSH in an attempt to compensate for insufficient production of thyroid hormone. In hyperthyroidism, an enlarged gland overproduces thyroid hormone autonomously. A goiter also may be simple or nontoxic, that is, an enlarged thyroid gland that is neither associated with hypo- or hyperthyroidism, nor the result of inflammation or neoplasia. (See Table 56–3.)

THYROID FUNCTION TESTS

Thyroid function tests can be a source of great confusion, but they are the cornerstone of laboratory diagnosis in thyroid disease. The general practitioner need only be familiar with a few tests to evaluate almost all thyroid disease. (See Table 56–4.)

A. **Serum Free Triiodothyronine (T_3) and Free Thyroxine (T_4) Levels.** Greater than 99 per cent of both T_4 and T_3 is bound to serum carrier proteins and is inactive. Levels of free (active) hormone may be measured by radioimmunoassay. However, it is easier and less expensive to measure total T_4 (bound and unbound) and to use an indirect measurement of the T_4 free fraction known as the T_3 resin uptake test (RT_3U). The RT_3U measures the degree of saturation of the available T_4 binding sites on the major carrier protein thyroxine binding globulin (TBG). If TBG is increased (by medication or other illnesses) and thus produces abnormally high total T_4 measurements, but T_4 is normal, the RT_3U will be low, and the product of total $T_4 \times RT_3U$, known as the free thyroid index (FT_4I), will fall within the normal range, in a manner consistent with the patient's euthyroid clinical status. If, however, the patient is truly hyperthyroid, both the total T_4 and the RT_3U will be elevated, as will the FT_4I. The reverse of these situations occurs with lowered TBG in a euthy-

TABLE 56–3. GOITERS AND NODULES

DISEASE	GLAND	CLINICAL STATUS
Goitrous hypothyroidism	Smooth, diffusely enlarged	Hypothyroid
Hashimoto's disease	Pebbly, diffusely firm, mildly enlarged	Eu- or hypothyroid
Graves' disease	Smooth, diffusely enlarged	Hyperthyroid
Multinodular goiter	Large goiter, irregular with many nodules	Eu- or hyperthyroid
Adenoma	Solitary nodule	Eu- or hyperthyroid
Hemorrhage into preexistent nodule	Acute painful enlargement	Euthyroid
Subacute thyroiditis	Usually tender, finely nodular swelling	Hyperthyroid
Carcinoma	Usually single hard nodule or normal gland with regional adenopathy	Euthyroid

roid patient and with hypothyroidism. These relationships are displayed in Figure 56–1.

B. TSH. TSH stimulates all steps in hormone synthesis and secretion. It can be measured by radioimmunoassay. If a patient is hypothyroid, TSH will be elevated (except for those rare cases of hypothyroidism resulting from intrinsic pituitary or hypothalamic disease). TSH levels are also helpful for monitoring thyroid replacement in hypothyroidism: a normal level implies an adequate dose, but clinical status is the ultimate criterion.

C. TRH Stimulation Test. When a patient has sufficient or increased levels of thyroid hormone, the response of TSH secretion to administration of exogenous TRH is greatly diminished. This occurs in thyrotoxicosis, elderly patients, and in euthyroid Graves' disease with ophthalmopathy. In hypothyroid patients and premenopausal women in the preovulatory phase of the menstrual cycle, the TSH response is increased.

This test is useful in the following situations:

  1. Diagnosis of early or developing hyperthyroidism, when the total T_4 may still be within the normal range: There is a "blunted" response of TSH to exogenously administered TRH.

  2. Separation of pituitary from hypothalamic hypothyroidism, when both T_4 and TSH are below normal: If pituitary, TSH response is "blunted" or absent; if hypothalamic, TSH increases normally after TRH administration, but after an hour's delay, owing to the time needed for synthesis to occur.

  3. Diagnosis of euthyroid Graves' disease with ophthalmopathy: If the TSH response is decreased, the test is helpful; a normal response is nondiagnostic.

D. Radioactive Iodine Uptake (RAIU). This test involves giving the patient a dose of iodine-131 (^{131}I) and assessing radioactivity in

TABLE 56–4. THYROID FUNCTION TESTS

CONDITION	T_4 and T_3	R_3TU	FT_4I	TSH	RAIU	TRH STIMULATION
Hypothyroidism	Low	Low	Low	High*	Low or normal	Augmented response
Hyperthyroidism	High	High	High	Normal or low	High†	Blunted response
Euthyroid "sick" syndrome	Low‡	High	Low	Normal	Normal	Normal
Pregnancy, estrogens, acute liver disease, acute intermittent porphyria	High	Low	Normal	Normal	Normal	Normal
Androgens, hypoproteinemia, chronic liver disease, glucocorticoid excess	Low	High	Normal	Normal	Normal	Normal

*Pituitary or hypothalamic hypothyroidism is associated with a low or normal TSH.
†Thyrotoxicosis caused by thyroiditis or exogenous administration of thyroid hormone is associated with a low RAIU.
‡Reverse T_3 is elevated, except in certain cases of chronic renal disease in which T_3 is elevated and reverse T_3 normal.

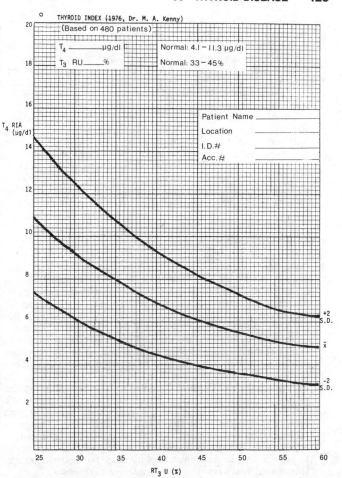

THYROID INDEX (1976, Dr. M. A. Kenny)

(Based on 480 patients)

T₄ ————— µg/dl   Normal: 4.I − II.3 µg/dl

T₃ RU ——— %   Normal: 33 − 45%

Patient Name _____

Location _____

I.D.# _____

Acc.# _____

T₄ RIA (µg/dl)

RT₃U (%)

+2 S.D.

x̄

-2 S.D.

Figure 56–1. "Normal" thyroid index based on measurement of T₄ RIA and RT₃U. (From the Laboratory Medicine Department of the University of Washington. Used with permission.)

the gland at selected time intervals (usually after 24 hours). If the patient is hyperthyroid, the gland overproduces hormone, and this is reflected in an increased uptake (usually greater than 30 per cent at 24 hours). If a patient is hypothyroid, the RAIU is low (usually less than 10 per cent at 24 hours).

Since the advent of reliable serum radioimmunoassays, the RAIU has diminished in importance as a diagnostic test. However, it is still helpful in differentiating between various causes of thyrotoxicosis. If the gland is overproducing thyroid hormone, the RAIU is increased. If the thyrotoxic state is the result of release of prestored hormone from an inflamed gland (as in thyroiditis) or of exogenous thyroid hormone administration, the RAIU is decreased.

E. **T_3 Suppression Test.** This test utilizes administration of exogenous hormone to suppress both the RAIU and the rate of hormone secretion. It is helpful for diagnosing early hyperthyroidism. However, it takes several days and may precipitate overt thyrotoxicosis, especially in the elderly. It has been supplanted by the TRH stimulation test.

F. **"Euthyroid Sick Syndrome."** Serious nonthyroidal illnesses, starvation, and the postsurgical state can produce a characteristic pattern of thyroidal functional abnormalities that must be differentiated from hypothyroidism: low T_3, low to normal T_4, increased RT_3U, increased reverse T_3, and normal TSH. Notable exceptions to this pattern are liver disease, which can be marked by elevations in T_4, T_3, and TSH, and renal disease, in which reverse T_3 may not be elevated.

HYPOTHYROIDISM

A. **Definition.** Hypothyroidism is characterized by insufficient production of thyroid hormone. In primary hypothyroidism the cause, whether structural or functional, lies with the gland itself. Secondary hypothyroidism is caused by intrinsic pituitary or hypothalamic disease resulting in insufficient stimulation of the thyroid gland. Myxedema consists of hypothyroidism plus deposition of hydrophilic mucopolysaccharides in the ground substance of the dermis and other tissues. Congenital hypothyroidism associated with myxedema, mental retardation, and other developmental abnormalities is called *cretinism.*

B. **Epidemiology and General Comments.** (A classification of the causes of hypothyroidism is listed in Table 56–1.) Primary hypothyroidism may be of the goitrous variety, resulting from excessive stimulation of the gland by TSH with inadequate compensatory production of thyroid hormone. Primary hypothyroidism may also simply involve the loss of enough thyroid tissue to provide an adequate amount of hormone for metabolic needs; this condition is known as *thyroprivic hypothyroidism.*

Hashimoto's thyroiditis, a chronic lymphocytic infiltration of the gland, is the most common cause of goitrous hypothyroidism in North American adults, especially middle-aged females. It is also the most common cause of sporadic goiter in children. In areas of the world that have iodine deficiency, *endemic goiter* and *goitrous cretinism* may be found more frequently. Congenital hypothyroidism can be found in 1 of 5000 births.

The most common cause of thyroprivic hypothyroidism is *post-ablative hypothyroidism,* which usually appears after treatment for Graves' disease. *Primary idiopathic hypothyroidism* may be part of an autoimmune constellation, and a careful search may reveal other endocrine insufficiencies or evidence of diseases such as pernicious anemia, lupus, rheumatoid arthritis, Sjögren's syndrome, or chronic active hepatitis.

Finally, pituitary and hypothalamic insufficiency account for less than 5 per cent of all cases of hypothyroidism.

C. History and Signs and Symptoms and Laboratory Findings

1. *Hypothyroidism (General).* In reviewing the history, the physician should ask specifically about prior thyroid disease and treatment, especially radioactive iodine or surgery and about goitrogenic drugs and foods. (See Table 56–1.)

The following list presents highlights of symptoms and signs in hypothyroidism according to the age of the patient:

a. **Neonatal.** There are persistent physiologic jaundice, a hoarse cry, somnolence, constipation, and feeding problems.

b. **Infant.** There are delayed achievement of developmental milestones; cretinous physicality (short stature, a broad nose, widely set eyes, a protruding tongue, and a protuberant abdomen with umbilical hernia); and mental retardation.

c. **Children.** Signs include mental retardation, short stature, delayed puberty, and poor school performance.

d. **Adult.** There is a nonspecific and insidious onset. The physician should look for neck scars or goiter. There may be a continuum of the following signs and symptoms:

1). Lethargy, cold intolerance, constipation, and menorrhagia or amenorrhea

2). Slowing of intellectual processes and motor activities, decreased appetite and weight gain, and bradycardia

3). Hair that becomes coarse and dry and then falls out, muscular stiffness, voice deepening with hoarseness, and diminished hearing

4.) Delay in relaxation time of deep-tendon reflexes, pale and cool doughy skin, flat expressionless facies, large heart with possible effusion, adynamic ileus, and psychiatric or cerebellar ataxia

5). Myxedematous coma with hypothermia and respiratory depression

e. **Laboratory Findings.** These include low T_4, low FT_4I, high TSH, low basal metabolism rate (BMR), and low RAIU. If a pituitary or hypothalamic cause is suspected, TSH will be normal or low; the TRH stimulation test differentiates between the causes (see the section on Thyroid Function Tests). Other laboratory abnormalities may include elevations of cholesterol, creatine phosphokinase, aspartate aminotransferase, and lactic acid dehydrogenase. Approximately 10 per cent of patients with idiopathic primary hypothyroidism have histamine-fast achlorhydria.

f. **Electrocardiogram (ECG).** The ECG may show bradycardia, low voltage, and inverted T waves.

g. **X-rays.** X-rays may show retarded bone age, epiphyseal dysgenesis, and delayed dental development in infants; delayed union of epiphyses in children; and large hearts because of effusions in adults.

2. Thyroiditis—Hashimoto's Disease

    a. History. The physician should ask about symptoms and family history of other autoimmune disorders such as pernicious anemia, Sjögren's syndrome, chronic active hepatitis, lupus, diabetes mellitus, Addison's disease, and occasionally Graves' disease.

    b. Physical Examination. There is goiter, usually with well delineated scalloped margins and a rubbery or pebblelike consistency. It is nontender, and the pyramidal lobe may be prominent.

    c. Laboratory Findings. These include normal T_4/T_3 with high TSH and slightly high RAIU in the early stages and low T_4, then low T_3, very high TSH, and low RAIU in the late stages. High titer antibodies directed against various thyroid antigens may be present, especially antithyroglobulin antibody and antimicrosomal antibody. Occasionally, but less frequently, they are present in Graves' disease and in primary idiopathic hypothyroidism as well. In adolescents with few clinical symptoms and low antibody titers, biopsy may be necessary to differentiate from diffuse nontoxic goiter.

THYROTOXICOSIS

A. Definition. Thyrotoxicosis denotes a clinical syndrome resulting from an excess of functioning thyroid hormone. There are a number of different causes of thyrotoxicosis, including hyperthyroidism, that is, sustained hyperfunctioning of the thyroid gland. However, not all thyrotoxic states are associated with hyperthyroidism. (See Table 56–2.)

The most important causes of thyrotoxicosis are the following:

    1. Graves' Disease. This is a disease of unknown origin that is characterized by the triad of hyperthyroidism with diffuse toxic goiter, ophthalmopathy, and dermopathy. These three manifestations of the disease are independent in appearance and natural history.

    2. Toxic Multinodular Goiter. Toxic multinodular goiter is defined as an enlarged thyroid gland with more than one region of excess growth with altered structure and function. No inflammation or neoplasia is present.

    3. Toxic Adenoma. Toxic adenomas are well encapsulated single nodules (occasionally two or three) functioning autonomously in the absence of TSH.

    4. Thyroiditis. Subacute thyroiditis (de Quervain's) is a temporary inflammation of the thyroid gland that is usually associated with an antecedent viral infection elsewhere in the body. Transient hyperthyroidism caused by leakage from the gland of excess preformed hormone characterizes both this condition and chronic painless thyroiditis with transient thyrotoxicosis (CT with TT).

5. *Thyroid Storm.* This is a syndrome of severe life-threatening thyrotoxicosis that is characterized by the abrupt onset of fever, hypotension with volume depletion, tachyarrhythmias, diarrhea, jaundice, and central nervous system abnormalities. The syndrome may rapidly progress to coma, shock, and death. Thyroid storm is now rarely seen but still may occur as a complication in incompletely treated hyperthyroid patients after surgery, infection, diabetic ketoacidosis, trauma, or as undiagnosed hyperthyroidism. Thyroid storm is diagnosed clinically; laboratory studies cannot differentiate it from chronic thyrotoxicosis.

B. **Epidemiology and General Comments**
1. *Graves' Disease.* This disease occurs primarily in the third or fourth decade and in women more frequently than men. There is a familial predisposition for Graves' disease, Hashimoto's disease, and pernicious anemia. The condition is associated with specific human leukocyte antigens.
2. *Toxic Multinodular Goiter.* This condition is primarily a disease of elderly patients. It often arises out of a long-standing simple goiter (both conditions involve attempted compensation for decreased efficiency of hormone synthesis, that is, increased TSH stimulates increased growth of the gland).
3. *Toxic Adenoma.* Toxic adenoma occurs in younger patients, in their thirties or forties. In contrast to Graves' disease, there is no ophthalmopathy or dermopathy, and the thyrotoxic symptoms are usually less severe.

C. **Clinical Assessment**
1. *Graves' Disease*
   a. **History.** Primary complaints include anxiety, restlessness, excessive sweating, heat intolerance, and insomnia. Other complaints include weight loss despite good appetite and hyperdefecation. Premenopausal females may complain of oligomenorrhea or amenorrhea. In older patients cardiac symptoms (palpitations, angina, dyspnea) or myopathic symptoms (weakness, especially proximal) may predominate over neurologic symptoms.
   b. **Physical Examination.** General signs include visible restlessness and "frightened facies." The skin is warm, moist, and velvety; the hair is silky and fine; alopecia is possible. The nails may be separated from the nail bed. The eyes stare, with widened palpebral fissure and lid lag. Cardiovascular signs include sinus tachycardia or atrial fibrillation, loud S1, systolic flow murmur, and possible cardiomegaly and congestive heart failure. Neurologic signs include hyperreflexia, fine tremor of fingers and tongue, and proximal muscle weakness. There is asymmetrically enlarged diffuse goiter, possibly lobular, and bruits are sometimes present over the thyroid gland.
      1). *Graves' Ophthalmopathy.* (This condition should be distinguished from reversible ocular signs of sympathetic overstimulation as listed above.) There is true exophthalmos with proptosis; ophthalmoplegia, first

with loss of superior temporal gaze and eventually all but downward gaze; and chemosis. Conjunctival and periorbital edema may lead to corneal ulceration and optic atrophy.

2). **Graves' Dermopathy.** (This condition may develop during thyrotoxicosis or after treatment.) There is pretibial myxedema that is notable for well-demarcated peau d'orange skin, pruritus, and hyperpigmentation over the dorsum of the legs and feet. Occasionally clubbing of fingers and toes is present (thyroid acropachy).

c. **Laboratory Findings.** These include high T_4/T_3, RT_3U, FT_4I, and RAIU. Long-acting thyroid stimulator findings (LATS) are present in 50 per cent of cases. Occasionally all are normal except for high T_3 and FT_3I. For confirmation of diagnosis in early thyrotoxicosis (such as euthyroid Graves' disease with ophthalmopathy), the TRH stimulation test should be used and note made of absent or "blunted" TSH response.

2. *Toxic Multinodular Goiter (MNG)*

a. **History.** Most commonly toxic MNG is asymptomatic and an incidental finding on physical examination. Symptoms of thyrotoxicosis occur less commonly than with Graves' disease; when they do, cardiac symptoms predominate. Complaints specifically referrable to the goiter may include dysphagia, stridor, dyspnea, and hoarseness; if hemorrhage into the gland occurs, acute painful neck enlargement may be the presenting sign.

b. **Physical Examination.** Signs of thyrotoxicosis, if present, are as described earlier. General examination shows signs of apathetic hyperthyroidism in the elderly, such as asthenia, emotional lability, muscle weakness, and wasting. In the head and neck there may be evidence of upper airway obstruction, hoarseness, and Horner's syndrome. In the thyroid there is goiter with multiple nodules. The consistency of nodules varies considerably within any one gland. Nodules are palpable when the gland is twice normal size and visible at three times normal size.

c. **Laboratory Findings.** Usually all laboratory results are within the normal range. If T_3 is in the upper range or normal, the physician should consider hyperthyroidism (T_3 level usually decreases with age). To confirm early disease, the TRH stimulation test should be used. Scans only confirm diagnosis of multinodularity, not thyrotoxicosis.

Neck x-rays may show punctate calcifications of medullary carcinoma or concentric calcifications of a benign nodule.

Barium swallow may show esophageal or tracheal displacement.

Pulmonary function tests may help evaluate clinical significance of stridor.

3. *Toxic Adenoma*

a. **History.** Often there is a long history of a neck lump. Symptoms of thyrotoxicosis usually are present only with nodules larger than 3 cm in size.

    b. **Physical Examination.** The thyroid has a smooth well defined mass that moves with the thyroid. There are no bruits over the gland.

    c. **Laboratory Findings.** Thyroid function tests remain normal until late, when T_4 and T_3 both increase. The radioactive iodine (RAI) scan shows a hot nodule with early uptake and no T_3 suppression (although early there may be some function in the rest of the gland).

4. Thyroiditis

    a. **Pyogenic Thyroiditis.** This condition is characterized by swelling, tenderness, erythema, and pain over the gland. Constitutional symptoms and signs of infection are usually present.

    b. **Subacute Thyroiditis.** This often follows an upper respiratory infection. Patients complain of pain over the thyroid and referred to the ear or jaw. The gland is usually painful and has tender nodularity on examination; however, occasionally there is no pain over the gland and referred pain and systemic malaise dominate the clinical picture. Key laboratory findings are an elevated erythrocyte sedimentation rate (ESR) and a depressed RAIU. Early thyroid function tests may be elevated owing to leakage of hormone, with transiently hypothyroid values later.

    c. CT with TT is characterized by a painless firm gland of normal or only slightly enlarged size. Laboratory tests show slightly elevated T_4/T_3 with low RAIU, normal or slightly elevated ESR, and absent or low antibody levels.

5. Solitary Nodules. (See Table 56–5.)

    a. **Epidemiology.** Approximately 70 per cent of thyroid nodules are "cold" on isotope scan. Only 10 per cent are hyperfunctioning thyrotoxic adenomas, suppressing function of the rest of the gland. "Cold" nodules are typically benign, but cancer occurs predominantly in "cold" nodules. Ten to 20 per cent of all "cold" nodules harbor malignancy.

TABLE 56–5. THYROID NODULES, RISK FACTORS FOR MALIGNANCY

	HIGHER RISK	LOWER RISK
Age	Younger than 30 Older than 65	Middle age
Sex	Male	Female
Consistency	Hard	Soft
Size	Enlarging	Shrinking
Radiation history	Yes	No
Adenopathy	Yes	No
Solitary	Yes	No*
Thyroid function tests	Normal	Hyper- or hypothyroid
RAI scan	Cold	Hot
Ultrasound	Solid	Cystic

*Multinodular glands in patients with a history of neck irradiation are still worrisome.

b. **Clinical Assessment**

   1). History. Risk factors for malignancy include male sex, age less than 30 or greater than 65, recent rapid growth of nodule, hoarseness, history of childhood head and neck radiation exposure, and family history of thyroid malignancy.

   2). Physical Examination. Risk factors for malignancy include firm and hard nodules, a nodule fixed to trachea or strap muscles, regional lymphadenopathy, and tracheal deviation.

   3). Laboratory Findings. Risk for malignancy may include normal thyroid function tests, a "cold" nodule on scan, and a solid (not cystic) nodule on ultrasound examination. Diagnosis of malignancy must be made by needle biopsy or surgery.

RECOMMENDED DIAGNOSTIC APPROACH

A. Hypothyroidism

1. A normal TSH rules out hypothyroidism.
2. Elevated TSH, low T_4, and low RT_3U (unless there is a pituitary or hypothalamic cause) rule in hypothyroidism.
   a. The TRH stimulation test is used to differentiate between pituitary and hypothalamic causes.
   b. Antibody titers are used to confirm Hashimoto's thyroiditis; if necessary, biopsy should be performed.

B. Thyrotoxicosis

1. Thyrotoxicosis is ruled out with a normal T_4 and RT_3U; a normal TSH is not helpful.
2. Thyrotoxicosis is ruled in with an elevated T_4 and RT_3U; a normal TSH is not helpful. Occasionally only T_3 is elevated.
   a. TRH stimulation is used to diagnose early thyrotoxicosis or euthyroid Graves' disease with ophthalmopathy while T_4 and RT_3U are still within the normal range.
   b. RAIU helps to differentiate between hyperthyroidism and thyrotoxicosis without hyperthyroidism.
   c. RAI scans help to locate functioning ectopic thyroid tissue; if normal, they are also helpful in the consideration of thyrotoxicosis factitia.

C. Solitary Nodules

1. Malignancy is ruled out with a "hot" nodule on RAI scan.
2. Malignancy is ruled in with positive biopsy results.

REFERENCES

1. De Groot LJ, et al.: Endocrinology. New York, Grune & Stratton, 1979.

This text offers a comprehensive section on thyroid disease, complete with its usual evaluation of laboratory testing, including indications, causes for false results, and so forth.

2. Harrison's Principles of Internal Medicine. 10th ed. New York, McGraw-Hill Book Company, 1983.
3. Werner, Ingbar: The Thyroid. 4th ed. New York, Harper & Row, 1978.

This remains the most complete textbook of thyroid metabolism and disease.

4. Williams R, et al.: Textbook of Endocrinology. 6th ed. Philadelphia, W. B. Saunders Company, 1981.
5. Beckers C: Thyroid nodules. Clin Endocrinol Metab 8:181, 1979.

A concise but thorough discussion of thyroid nodules.

6. Chopra IJ, et al.: Thyroid function in nonthyroidal illnesses. Ann Intern Med 98:946–957, 1983.

An excellent and up-to-date review of the topic, including discussion of treatment and prognosis.

7. Davis PJ, Davis FB: Hyperthyroidism in patients over the age of 60 years. Medicine 53:3, 1974.

This is the classic study of apathetic hyperthyroidism and thyrotoxicosis in older patients.

8. Stanbury JB, Wang C-A: Nontoxic goiter. Thyroid Today 4:3, 1981.

An excellent concise review of the topic, including etiology, diagnosis, management, and prognosis.

GASTROENTEROLOGY

57

ABDOMINAL PAIN

By MICHAEL KIMMEY, M.D.

GENERAL COMMENTS

A. Abdominal pain is one of the most common complaints patients bring to a physician. Approximately 5 per cent of emergency room visits are because of abdominal pain. Chronic abdominal pain is a frequent cause of patient suffering and physician frustration caused by diagnostic and therapeutic failures.

B. Diagnostic Principles

    1. Consideration should be given not only to the inciting painful stimulus but also to the patient's physiologic and psychologic response to the stimulus.

    2. Abdominal pain may be well localized if somatic afferent nerves (abdominal skin and wall musculature and parietal peritoneum) are stimulated, but they may be less well localized and referred to noninvolved parts of the body if visceral afferent nerves (abdominal organs) are stimulated.

    3. Repeated examinations of the patient over time are diagnostically valuable.

    4. Definitive diagnosis may not be reached in up to 40 per cent of cases of acute abdominal pain. The incidence of various causes of abdominal pain varies with the population studied.

DIFFERENTIAL DIAGNOSES

A. Multiple Classifications. There are multiple classifications of abdominal pain, including those based on pain duration (acute versus chronic), location, abruptness of onset, and pathogenesis (inflammatory, obstructive, or ischemic). These lists are useful insofar as they provide a framework for clinicians to structure the diagnostic and management approach to the patient. The causes of abdominal pain listed in Table 57–1 are arranged by location and rate of onset of pain, since these are two readily available historical features. It should be emphasized, however, that any classification of abdominal pain is a gross simplification, since exceptions to any categorization are frequent.

B. Diagnostic Clues in Selected Causes of Abdominal Pain

    1. The reader should see other sections of this book for clinical features of gastroenteritis, cholecystitis, pancreatitis, inflammatory bowel disease, nephrolithiasis, and pyelonephritis.

    2. *Appendicitis.* Patients with acute appendicitis have moderate to severe (95 per cent of cases) steady (60 per cent) pain that begins in the periumbilical region and then localizes to the right lower quadrant (75 per cent). Pain precedes other symptoms in over 90 per cent of patients. These symptoms include nausea (75 per cent), vomiting (60 per cent), and anorexia (75 per cent). Diarrhea is seen in 20 per cent of cases. Physical examination shows temperature greater than 38° C (45 per cent), rebound tenderness and guarding (70 to 80 per cent) usually in the right lower quadrant (65 per cent), and rectal tenderness (30 to 40 per cent). White blood cell count greater than 10,000 (90 per cent) with over 75 per cent neutrophils (80 per cent) is seen. Abnormal abdominal x-rays (appendicolith, localized ileus, increased right lower quadrant soft tissue density) are seen in about 50 per cent of patients but are not specific for appendicitis.

3. **Peptic Ulcer Disease.** Patients with gastric ulcer (GU) tend to be older and to have more pain that occurs sooner after meals and that is less likely to be relieved by antacids, in comparison with patients with duodenal ulcer (DU) and those with dyspepsia and no ulcer. Contrast radiography or endoscopy is needed to distinguish between these three entities. Epigastric pain (60 to 80 per cent of cases) that is relieved by antacids (40 to 80 per cent) and radiates to the back (20 to 30 per cent) is characteristic of ulcer patients. Anorexia (30 to 60 per cent), nausea (50 to 70 per cent), and vomiting (30 to 70 per cent) are common. Epigastric tenderness is present in 50 per cent of cases. Patients with perforated ulcers have the sudden onset of severe (95 per cent) steady (95 per cent) pain that often has a generalized distribution (50 per cent). Diminished bowel sounds (50 to 90 per cent), abdominal rigidity (80 per cent), and free subdiaphragmatic air on upright abdominal x-ray are characteristic of perforation.

4. **Bowel Obstruction.** Patients with small bowel obstructions have periumbilical (40 per cent), crampy (90 per cent), severe (60 per cent) abdominal pain that precedes vomiting (90 per cent). Eighty per cent of patients have a history of prior abdominal surgery. Physical examination reveals hyperperistaltic bowel sounds in 50 per cent of cases but diminished or absent sounds in 25 per cent. Abdominal distention is common but may be absent early in the illness. White blood cell counts greater than 10,000 (60 per cent) and dilated bowel loops with air-fluid levels on abdominal x-rays are useful findings but are not necessary for diagnosis.

5. **Diverticulitis.** Approximately 10 per cent of people in the United States have diverticula, and 10 to 20 per cent of these develop diverticulitis at some time in their lives. Patients with diverticulitis have pain that is steady (40 per cent) or cramping (30 per cent), of moderate severity (60 per cent), and located in the left lower quadrant (25 per cent) or generally in the lower half of the abdomen (35 per cent). Patients are generally elderly (70 per cent are over age 60) and may have nausea (50 per cent), vomiting (30 per cent), diarrhea (30 per cent), constipation (40 per cent), and rectal

TABLE 57–1. CAUSES OF ABDOMINAL PAIN GROUPED BY LOCATION AND RATE OF ONSET

	ONSET		
LOCATION AND DISORDER	Sudden	Rapid (minutes)	Gradual (hours)
Right upper quadrant (RUQ)			
1. Cholecystitis		**	*
2. Perforated duodenal ulcer	*		
3. Hepatitis			*
4. Hepatic congestion (vascular)			*
5. Perihepatitis (Fitz-Hugh–Curtis syndrome)			*
6. Retrocecal appendicitis		*	**
7. Pyelonephritis			*
8. Pneumonia			*
Epigastric (may also be RUQ or LUQ)			
1. Pancreatitis		*	**
2. Peptic ulcer		*	**
3. Gastritis		*	**
4. Myocardial infarction	*	**	
Left upper quadrant (LUQ)			
1. Splenic rupture or infarction	*		
2. Splenic enlargement			*
3. Colonic perforation (tumor, foreign body)	*		
4. Pyelonephritis			*
5. Pneumonia			*
Right lower quadrant (RLQ)			
1. Appendicitis		*	**
2. Mesenteric adenitis		*	**
3. Regional enteritis			*
4. Diverticulitis (cecal, Meckel's)		*	**

Table continued on opposite page

bleeding (25 per cent). Abdominal rebound, rigidity, and guarding are infrequent (30 per cent), and tenderness (20 per cent) or a mass (10 per cent) may be found on rectal examination. Leukocytosis is seen in over 90 per cent of cases, and results of proctosigmoidoscopy (done without preparation or air insufflation) are often abnormal.

6. *Vascular Diseases*
   a. **Abdominal Aortic Aneurysm (AAA).** Most patients with an AAA are asymptomatic, and 85 per cent are unaware of the presence of an aneurysm at the time of rupture. All patients with a ruptured or leaking aneurysm have pain that is felt either in the back (35 per cent), abdomen (30 per cent), or both the abdomen and back (35 per cent) that has been present over 24 hours in 50 per cent. A pulsatile abdominal mass is palpable in 90 per cent, and abdominal x-rays show an aneurysm in 75 per

TABLE 57–1. CAUSES OF ABDOMINAL PAIN GROUPED BY LOCATION AND RATE OF ONSET *Continued*

LOCATION AND DISORDER	ONSET		
	Sudden	Rapid (minutes)	Gradual (hours)
Left lower quadrant (LLQ)			
1. Diverticulitis (sigmoid)		*	**
2. Irritable bowel syndrome			*
RLQ or LLQ (depending on side involved)			
1. Ruptured ectopic pregnancy	**	*	*(before rupture)
2. Ruptured ovarian cyst	*		
3. Ovarian torsion		**	*
4. Salpingitis			*
5. Mittelschmerz		**	*
6. Ureteral calculi	*	**	*
7. Incarcerated inguinal hernia		**	*
8. Ruptured aortic aneurysm	**	*	*(before rupture)
Diffuse pain			
1. Gastroenteritis		*	**
2. Peritonitis	(see underlying cause)		
3. Early appendicitis		*	**
4. Intestinal obstruction		*(upper small bowel)	*(lower small bowel)
5. Intestinal infarction	*		
6. Diabetic ketoacidosis			*
7. Sickle cell crisis		**	*
8. Acute intermittent porphyria		*	**
9. Lead intoxication			*
10. Narcotic withdrawal			*

**Signifies a more common type of onset if mode of onset is variable.

cent of cases. Early diagnosis is crucial to successful surgical outcome.

b. **Intestinal Angina.** Intermittent dull or cramping mid-abdominal pain beginning 30 minutes after a meal and lasting for one to two hours is characteristic. Physical examination often reveals an abdominal bruit, but this is not diagnostically useful. Steatorrhea may be present. Definitive diagnosis requires angiography.

c. **Mesenteric Arterial Occlusion.** Severe midabdominal pain that is initially colicky, periumbilical, and with severity out of proportion to physical findings is seen in intestinal infarction. Over several hours pain becomes generalized, and systemic signs including fever and hypotension develop. Laboratory findings include metabolic acidosis, leukocytosis (often with white blood cell count greater than 30,000), and occasionally elevated amylase.

The same clinical findings in a patient with valvular heart disease or atrial fibrillation should suggest the presence of a superior mesenteric artery embolus, which may be amenable to surgical removal.

7. **Irritable Bowel Syndrome.** This syndrome is a benign intestinal motor disturbance that affects 15 to 20 per cent of the general population and is the most frequent cause for gastroenterologic consultation. Abdominal pain is of variable quality—usually lower abdominal, is relieved with defecation in 50 per cent of patients, but rarely awakens the patient at night. Frequently there is a history of both diarrhea and constipation, excessive flatulence, and mucus in stools. Results of laboratory and radiographic studies are normal.

8. **Lower Abdominal Pain in Women.** In addition to the usual causes of abdominal pain, special consideration must be given to disorders of the female reproductive system.

    a. **Ectopic Pregnancy.** Any woman of reproductive age who is not using oral contraceptives may have an ectopic pregnancy. Twenty-five per cent of patients with an ectopic pregnancy have a history of pelvic inflammatory disease. Other risk factors include prior ectopic pregnancy, IUD use, and prior tubal sterilization surgery (7 per cent of all ectopic pregnancies). Over 90 per cent of patients with an ectopic pregnancy have abdominal pain that initially is mild, crampy, and unilateral (75 per cent of cases). Pain may generalize and produce shoulder pain and orthostatic dizziness when the fallopian tube ruptures. Eighty-five per cent of patients have a history of a recently missed period, and 80 per cent have irregular, usually mild, vaginal bleeding. Pelvic examination may reveal cervical motion or adnexal tenderness, but a mass is often not found. A serum pregnancy test is positive in 95 per cent of cases, but urine pregnancy testing is only positive in 60 per cent. Ultrasound is helpful in stable patients with positive pregnancy test results to detect intrauterine pregnancies but may not visualize early ectopic pregnancies. Culdocentesis and laparoscopy are useful procedures when the diagnosis is unclear.

    b. **Ovarian Cysts.** Cysts commonly occur in mid to late cycle (follicular cysts) and in early pregnancy (corpus luteum cyst). They may rupture, causing acute severe low abdominal pain, often with peritoneal signs. White blood cells are usually not seen on cervical Gram's stain, and the pain resolves spontaneously over 6 to 24 hours. Cysts greater than 6 cm in size may undergo torsion. In this case pain does not resolve, and 80 per cent of patients have a palpable adnexal mass. Diagnostic laparoscopy should be used early if torsion is suspected.

    c. **Pelvic Inflammatory Disease (PID).** Lower abdominal pain (94 per cent of cases), increased vaginal discharge (55 per cent), temperature above 38° C (41 per cent), irregular vaginal bleeding (36 per cent), and right upper quadrant tenderness (30 per cent) are seen in women with pelvic inflammatory disease. Leukocytosis (50 per cent) and white blood cells on cervical Gram's stain are often seen. Since the clinical diagnosis of PID may be wrong in 35 per cent of cases, liberal use of diagnostic laparoscopy is encouraged.

CLINICAL MANIFESTATIONS

A. History
  1. *Character of Pain.* Severity, rate of onset, location, duration, frequency, radiation, and aggravating and alleviating factors should be sought.
      a. **Sudden Onset of Pain.** Sudden onset of pain that does not diminish should suggest perforated viscus, embolism, torsion, or hemorrhage.
      b. **Crampy Pain.** This suggests biliary colic, renal colic, intestinal obstruction, gastroenteritis, or ectopic pregnancy.
      c. **Severe Pain.** The most severe pains are seen with renal colic, intestinal infarction, dissecting aortic aneurysm, and perforated ulcer. Severe pain lasting greater than six hours usually indicates the presence of a condition requiring surgical management.
  2. *Associated Symptoms.* Associated symptoms relative to four basic systems should be sought.
      a. **Upper Digestive.** Symptoms are nausea, vomiting, anorexia, and bleeding.
      b. **Lower Digestive.** Symptoms are diarrhea, constipation, flatulence, bleeding, and stool color and caliber.
      c. **Urinary.** Symptoms are dysuria, frequent urination, and bleeding.
      d. **Gynecologic.** Symptoms are contraception, menstrual history, irregular bleeding, and discharge.
  3. *General Review of Systems.* This should cover potential sources of referred pain (myocardial or pulmonary) and metabolic causes (ketoacidosis or hyperlipidemia).
  4. *History.* A history of drug and alcohol use, prior abdominal surgery, concurrent medical problems including atherosclerotic disease, and family history of similar problems (porphyria, familial Mediterranean fever, or sickle cell anemia) should be sought.
B. Physical Examination
  1. *General Examination.* The physician should look for signs of increased autonomic activity (flushing, diaphoresis, tachycardia, or mydriasis), fever, postural hypotension, heart failure, and pneumonia.
  2. *Body Posture.* This may be revealing. Patients with renal, biliary, or intestinal colic move frequently, often in a writhing motion. Those with peritonitis lie quietly on their backs, often

with hips and knees flexed. Patients with pancreatitis prefer
a sitting posture, usually leaning forward.

3. *Abdominal Examination.* Abdominal examination must be
systematic and careful, with attention paid to the following:

   a. **Inspection.** Distention, dilated veins, an enlarged organ
   or mass, and visible peristalsis may be present.

   b. **Auscultation.** Bowel sounds (useful if absent or if high-
   pitched rushes are heard), bruits (present in the epigastric
   area of 20 per cent of normals), friction rubs, venous hums,
   and presence of a succussion splash should be evaluated.

   c. **Palpation.** The examining physician should begin with
   light touch with one finger before examining for deep
   tenderness, masses, and organomegaly. Local and remote
   rebound tenderness, involuntary guarding, and tenderness
   to light percussion signify underlying inflammation or
   peritonitis. Femoral and inguinal canals should be examined for hernias.

   d. **Percussion.** Liver and spleen sizes are estimated. Costovertebral angle tenderness should be noted.

   e. **Rectal Examination.** Rectal examination for a mass or
   tenderness is mandatory in all patients, as are pelvic
   examination in women and testicular examination in men.

LABORATORY EVALUATION

A. **Hematology.** The hematocrit is a useful index of bleeding.
However, the patient's state of hydration is important in the
interpretation of results. An elevated white blood cell count is a
useful indicator of the presence of an inflammatory disease;
however, a normal count does not eliminate any diagnostic
possibility. In general, the white blood cell differential is useful
only when a low or elevated total count is found. Screening
coagulation tests (prothrombin time and platelet count) are done
if bleeding or liver disease is suspected.

B. **Urinalysis.** This is an inexpensive, noninvasive, and valuable
screening test for urinary tract abnormalities. Urine specific
gravity is another indicator of intravascular volume status.
Inflammatory processes near the ureter (appendicitis) may produce pyuria.

C. **Electrolytes, Blood-Urea Nitrogen, and Creatinine.** These tests
are widely ordered and useful if renal disease or significant
vomiting or diarrhea are present.

D. **Amylase.** This test remains the most common screening test for
pancreatitis. Elevations may be caused by nonpancreatic disease,
usually from an elevated salivary isoenzyme. It should be noted
that 50 per cent of patients with acute alcohol intoxication have
an elevated total amylase level but that only about one fourth
of these have an elevated pancreatic isoenzyme level.

E. **Bilirubin.** Jaundice is detectable at bilirubin levels above 3 to 4
mg per dL. Bilirubin is most useful diagnostically in patients

with right upper quadrant pain who are not jaundiced but who have elevated bilirubin levels (1.5 to 4 mg per dL). Seven per cent of the population may have elevated bilirubin levels that are usually less than 5 mg per dL and primarily the unconjugated or indirect fraction (Gilbert's syndrome). This finding is not related to any abdominal pain that might be present.

F. **Serum Pregnancy Test.** Women of reproductive age with lower abdominal pain and irregular menstrual periods should have an ectopic pregnancy excluded, especially if unilateral adnexal tenderness is present.

G. **Abdominal X-Rays.** Significant abnormalities are not missed if this examination is limited to patients with moderate or severe abdominal tenderness and those with a high clinical suspicion of renal or biliary calculi, bowel obstruction, ischemia, or trauma.

H. **Other.** Chest x-ray, electrocardiogram, and measurement of liver enzymes may be useful in certain cases.

I. **Selected Clinical Settings.** Gastrointestinal endoscopy, radiographic contrast examination, ultrasound, computed tomography, biliary scintigraphy, and abdominal angiography are useful adjunctive measures in selected clinical settings.

RECOMMENDED DIAGNOSTIC APPROACH

A single diagnostic approach cannot be recommended in the evaluation of a given patient with abdominal pain. Laboratory and procedural investigation is different in each case and should be directed by the physician's diagnostic impressions after a complete and careful history and physical examination have been performed.

REFERENCES

1. Currie DJ: Abdominal Pain. Washington, Hemisphere Publishing Corporation, 1979.

   A comprehensive approach to patients is emphasized. Information available from the patient's history is nicely outlined.

2. Silen W: Cope's Early Diagnosis of the Acute Abdomen. 16th ed. New York, Oxford University Press, 1983.

   A recently rewritten classic monograph on the acute surgical abdomen.

3. Way LW: Abdominal pain. *In* Sleisenger MH, Fordtran JS (eds.): Gastrointestinal Disease. 3rd ed. Philadelphia, W. B. Saunders Company, 1983, pp. 207–221.

   A succinctly written chapter emphasizing diagnostic approaches.

4. Staniland R, Ditchburn J, de Dombal FT: Clinical presentation of acute abdomen: Study of 600 patients. Br Med J 3:393–398, 1972.

   Report of a series of patients admitted to a hospital with abdominal pain of less than one week's duration. Frequencies of diagnostic information are emphasized.

5. Brewer RJ, Golden GT, et al.: Abdominal pain: An analysis of 1000

consecutive cases in a university hospital emergency room. Am J Surg 131:219–223, 1976.

A review of diagnostic information available from patients in an emergency room setting.

6. Eisenberg RL, Heineken P, et al.: Evaluation of plain abdominal radiographs in the diagnosis of abdominal pain. Ann Intern Med 97:257–261, 1982.

Criteria for obtaining plain abdominal x-rays in patients with abdominal pain in an emergency room setting are developed.

58
ASCITES

By JAMES TALCOTT, M.D.

GENERAL COMMENTS

Ascites is always abnormal; its presence denotes disease. While a single item of history, physical examination, or laboratory data rarely seals a diagnosis, combinations of all of these items do. Every patient with new or acutely increasing ascites requires a diagnosis.

CAUSES OF ASCITES

Cancer and cirrhosis always predominate as the major causes of ascites in large series of patients.

A. **Causes Likely to Be Encountered by the Practicing Physician in the United States.** Listed in order of frequency, these are:
   1. Right-sided cardiac disease, most frequently tricuspid regurgitation and constrictive or restrictive cardiac disease
   2. Liver disease
   3. Nephrosis or dialysis
   4. Obstruction of the inferior vena cava or the hepatic vein
   5. Pancreatic pseudocyst
   6. Myxedema
   7. Traumatic interruption of an anatomic structure containing urine, bile, or pancreatic secretions

B. **Causes That Are Rare in Typical United States Practice But Common in Other Settings**
   1. Schistosomiasis
   2. Filariasis
   3. Kwashiorkor
   4. Hepatic veno-occlusive disease (after bone marrow transplantation)
   5. Graft-versus-host disease (after bone marrow transplantation)

PATHOPHYSIOLOGY

A. **Fluid Dynamics.** Fluid accumulates within the peritoneal cavity for two reasons: the accumulation rate exceeds the elimination rate (about 800 mL per day in healthy persons) or absorption is blocked, or both. Ascites may accumulate rapidly by crossing vessel walls or serosal surfaces, or it may leak directly into the peritoneum because of disrupted vessels or fluid-containing organs. Because fluid appears to be absorbed more rapidly than the protein within it, the composition of the ascitic fluid may vary at different stages in the same pathologic episode. The protein also increases from diuresis. Thus the protein content of ascites fluid is not as helpful diagnostically as the protein content of the pleural fluid. In addition, a single process such as cancer can cause ascites in different ways. It can irritate the peritoneal serosa directly, block lymphatics, and thus impede lymphatic drainage, or it can cause intrahepatic compression of portal or hepatic venules. The irritated peritoneum and blocked lymphatics tend to result in high-protein ascites, while compression of portal and hepatic venules produces a low-protein fluid that is indistinguishable from that in cirrhosis.

B. **Causes of the Pathophysiologic Processes**
1. *Increased Hydrostatic Pressure.* This is caused by right-sided heart failure, obstruction of the inferior vena cava, and obstruction of the hepatic vein (or venules in veno-occlusive disease).
2. *Obstruction of Lymphatics.* This is related to malignancy and infiltrating infection.
3. *Decreased Intravascular Oncotic Pressure.* This occurs in nephrosis, kwashiorkor, and severe liver dysfunction from all causes and possibly in protein-losing enteropathy.
4. *Increased Membrane Permeability.* This is related to primary or metastatic peritoneal malignancy, infection, systemic lupus erythematosus, foreign body irritation, and probably protein-losing enteropathy.
5. *Trauma.* Trauma can cause disruptions of ureters or blood, lymph, biliary, or pancreatic vessels (as in ruptured pancreatic pseudocyst).
6. *Unknown Mechanism.* The mechanism of fluid accumulation is unknown in myxedema, Whipple's disease, postrenal transplantation ascites, sarcoidosis, eosinophilic gastroenteritis, and allergic purpura.

SYMPTOMS AND SIGNS

A. **History.** The history should be explored in an attempt to determine the chronicity of the condition (although an astonishing number of patients report that they suddenly noticed a 2-L accumulation of ascites on the day they sought medical care) and to uncover some of the causes of ascites. These include alcohol abuse, past hepatitis, cancer (weight loss, fatigue, smoking, occupational exposure, or family history), infection (tuberculosis exposure, purified protein derivative status, or a travel history suggestive of schistosomiasis, filariasis, coccidioidosis, or histoplasmosis), renal disease (nephrosis, dialysis, or transplantation), or myxedema. Because ascites is frequently complicated by infection, pain and fever are important.

B. Physical Examination. Evaluation of ascites begins with determining its presence. Large amounts of ascites (1500 to 2000 cu cm) can often be detected by feeling a percussive wave cross the abdomen from one flank to the other with the ventral midline damped (fluid wave) or by a shift in the anterior limit of a flat percussed note when the patient shifts from the supine to the lateral decubitus position (shifting dullness). Smaller amounts (120 to 200 cu cm) may be detected by placing the patient in the elbow-knee position and moving the bell of a stethoscope across the lowest part of the abdomen. If tapping on the abdomen is muted and then heard clearly again as the bell is moved slowly away from the listening physician, this denotes a puddle of free ascitic fluid (the "puddle sign").

The general physical examination should direct special attention to the heart, the abdomen (feeling for enlarged organs and masses as well as documenting ascites), signs of liver failure (spider angiomata, testicular atrophy, jaundice, and so on), and deep tendon reflexes (for myxedema).

RECOMMENDED DIAGNOSTIC APPROACH

The clinician should use the following approach once the presence of ascites has been confirmed:

A. Routine Blood Studies. Routine blood studies may show anemia (from gastrointestinal bleeding or chronic inflammation), leukocytosis (from infection), or hyponatremia (from heart failure, cirrhosis, or nephrosis). Active liver disease may be demonstrated by elevated serum transaminases or alkaline phosphatase and liver dysfunction by abnormal bilirubin, albumin, or prothrombin time.

B. Urinalysis. Urinalysis may show albuminuria or an active sediment suggesting current renal disease.

C. Chest X-Ray. The chest x-ray reveals signs of congestive heart failure or serositis (pleural or pericardial effusions).

D. Paracentesis for Ascites Fluid. The most important laboratory examination is analysis of ascitic fluid. This can be safely obtained by inserting an 18- to 21-gauge needle through the anesthetized skin either in the midline 2 to 3 cm below the umbilicus, with the patient seated, or laterally 2 to 3 cm above the inguinal ligament, with the patient in the lateral decubitus position. If these two maneuvers fail, the "puddle pericentesis" with the patient in the elbow-knee position is usually successful. Occasionally, physicians resort to ultrasound to identify ascites and facilitate its sampling.

E. Analysis of the Ascitic Fluid. There continues to be a controversy about the most useful information to be obtained from ascitic fluid. Bloody or milky appearance suggests cancer and chylous ascites, respectively. Cell count and differential, protein, and glucose are universally considered helpful, as is culture and staining for bacterial and fungus and cytologic analysis. The ratios of serum to ascitic fluid measurements of protein and lactic acid dehydrogenase may be helpful, although not as useful as they are for pleural fluid analysis. Recently, it has been claimed that the gradient of protein concentration in serum and ascites reflects portal pressure. A difference of 1.0 g per 100 cc indicates portal hypertension rather than other causes of ascites. Detection of a significant amount of carcinoembryonic enzyme (CEA) is quite specific for malignancy and probably adds to cytology in detecting cancer. L-lactate levels in ascitic fluid, as in other body fluids, appears to be more sensitive than Gram's stain and substantially more specific for infection of ascitic fluid than the numbers of white blood cells or polymorphonuclear cells.

F. **Other Diagnostic Tests to Consider.** All tests are relatively expensive and some are invasive, but they can be helpful in specific situations.

1. *Percutaneous Liver Biopsy.* This is definitive for diagnosing hepatitis, cirrhosis, and neoplastic disease. Locating intrahepatic masses by an imaging test (see below) can improve diagnostic sensitivity in focal liver disease. Cirrhosis and neoplastic disease are notoriously unevenly distributed. Extensive disease in the right lobe of the liver is most suitable for percutaneous biopsy. CT scanning and ultrasound are useful in guiding the biopsy needle to small or deep lesions.

2. *Ultrasound.* This is the cheapest test for localizing intrahepatic masses and can document ascites or other intraperitoneal abnormalities as well.

3. *Computed Tomographic (CT) Scanning.* This technique is more expensive but more sensitive than ultrasound.

4. *Liver-Spleen Scanning.* This is less sensitive than CT scan for lesions smaller than 2 cm, but because uptake of radioactive colloid depends on adequate blood flow and active Kupfer cells, the scan additionally tests liver function. Shift of colloid to the spleen and bone marrow strongly suggests severe liver dysfunction (severe hepatitis, cirrhosis, or both).

5. *Percutaneous Liver Biopsy.* This may be falsely negative, since cirrhosis and malignant disease are notoriously unevenly distributed processes. Extensive disease in the right lobe of the liver is most suitable for percutaneous biospy. CT scanning and ultrasound are useful in guiding the biopsy needle to small or deep lesions.

6. *Laparoscopy.* The primary indication for laparoscopy is failure of percutaneous liver biospy. Prior laparotomy makes complete laparoscopic examination impossible about half of the time. Not only does laparoscopy increase the sensitivity of percutaneous biopsy, but visual appearance of the liver is useful in the diagnosis of cirrhosis. Laparoscopy is also very helpful in examining the peritoneum for malignant or granulomatous lesions.

7. *Laparotomy.* Laparotomy has little role in the diagnosis of ascites except for elaborate staging procedures for selected cancer treatment protocols.

REFERENCES

1. Conn HD: The diagnosis and examination of ascitic fluid. Lab Res Methods Biol Med 7:529–565, 1983.

An up-to-date review, emphasizing laboratory approach.

2. Bayor TD, et al.: Diagnostic value of ascite fluid lactic acid dehydrogenase, protein and WBC levels. Arch Intern Med 138:1103–1105, 1978.

A good review of the value of these tests.

3. Bar-Meir S, et al.: Analysis of ascite fluid in cirrhosis. Dig Dis Sci 24:136–144, 1979.

A review of the findings in cirrhotic patients.

---------------------59--------------------

CHRONIC DIARRHEA

By CHRISTINA M. SURAWICZ, M.D.

DEFINITION AND INITIAL APPROACH

A. **Definition.** The term "diarrhea" is used to describe either stool consistency or frequency. Subjectively, diarrhea is a change in stools: they are more frequent and more loose and watery. Organic diarrhea, that is, diarrhea with a structural cause, occurs at night as well as during the day; "functional" diarrhea (caused by a spastic colon) never wakes the patient up at night. Chronic diarrhea is diarrhea lasting more than one month.

B. **Documentation of Amount and Type of Chronic Diarrhea.** Because of the wide variation in patient definition of diarrhea, it is wise to document diarrhea by measuring *stool weight*. The normal stool weight is less than 200 g per 24 hours. More than 200 g of stool is by convention considered diarrhea. All stools from 8:00 A.M. one morning to 8.00 A.M. the next morning should be collected in a preweighed empty paint can. The patient should continue to eat and drink a normal diet. The can is then weighed, and the 24-hour stool weight can be determined. The contents of the can are then available for further study.

C. **Initial Approach.** The physician should analyze the contents of the can to classify the diarrhea as one of three types: fatty, watery, or bloody. Each type requires a different diagnostic approach.

   1. Stool Fat. A qualitative stool fat analysis is helpful if negative, because this excludes steatorrhea. Fat may be present in normal stools. An increased amount of fat in the stool is determined best by analysis of the 24-hour collection. More than 5 g per 24 hours indicates steatorrhea if the patient is eating an average diet.

2. **Gross or Occult Blood.** Gross blood can be detected by visual inspection and occult blood by the guaiac test or Hemoccult cards.

3. **Fecal Leukocytes.** The presence of sheets of leukocytes suggests bacterial dysentery, which usually causes an acute diarrhea. However, fecal leukocytes are not always present. Fecal leukocytes may be seen in the stool in inflammatory bowel disease, but their presence is not specific.

4. **Ova, Parasites, and Stool Culture.** These tests are best done on fresh specimens. The ova and parasites that can be seen are protozoal cysts or trophozoites and the ova or larva of helminths. Routine stool culture tests for *Salmonella* and *Shigella* species should be used. Most laboratories now also routinely culture for *Campylobacter* species, while special media are required for *Yersinia*.

FATTY DIARRHEA

There are two major causes of fatty diarrhea.

A. **Pancreatic Insufficiency.** Most often this is caused by recurrent episodes of acute or chronic pancreatitis. Keys to diagnosis include a history of abdominal pain (often alcohol-related); very marked steatorrhea (output can be over 40 g of fat per day); an abdominal flat plate that shows pancreatic calcification; or a therapeutic response to oral pancreatic enzyme replacement.

B. **Celiac Sprue.** This is a hereditary abnormality of small intestinal mucosa that is caused by gluten, a wheat protein. It may occur at any age. The key to diagnosis is a compatible small bowel biopsy and a positive response to a gluten-free diet.

BLOODY DIARRHEA

Blood in the stools must be investigated and often requires sigmoidoscopy and air contrast barium enema (BE) or colonoscopy. Upper gastrointestinal x-ray and endoscopy may also be needed. Colonoscopy reveals a lesion (a cancer, polyp, or unsuspected colitis) in 40 per cent of patients with hematochezia, even if sigmoidoscopy and BE are negative.

A. **Acute Self-Limited Colitis (ASLC).** ASLC is the most common cause of bloody diarrhea. Illness usually lasts less than two weeks. The most common causative organisms are *Campylobacter, Salmonella,* and *Shigella;* 40 to 60 per cent of patients are culture-negative. Keys to diagnosis are abrupt onset, exposure or travel, positive stool culture, and rapid spontaneous resolution.

B. **Idiopathic Inflammatory Bowel Disease (IIBD).** IIBD is a primary bowel disease that may have systemic manifestations (in eye, skin, joint, or other areas). The key to diagnosis is a clinical picture that varies with type and location of disease.

C. **Colon Cancer.** This condition may rarely be manifested as diarrhea. A change in bowel habit and weight loss are late clues to diagnosis. Rectal examination, sigmoidoscopy, barium enema, and colonoscopy are necessary for diagnosis.

D. **Massive Bleeding.** In elderly patients this is usually caused by right-sided colonic diverticulae or arteriovenous malformations. The key to diagnosis is painless bleeding.

WATERY DIARRHEA

Watery diarrhea has a multitude of causes. Some of the most common are medications, infections, milk intolerance, prior bowel surgery, and irritable bowel disease. Very rare causes are Zollinger-Ellison syndrome (gastrinoma), small bowel lymphoma, carcinoid, and other endocrine diseases.

The causes of chronic diarrhea are outlined in Table 59–1.

TABLE 59–1. CAUSES OF CHRONIC DIARRHEA

Drugs
A. Common
　　Laxative
　　Antacids
　　Ethanol
　　Coffee
　　Digitalis
　　Quinidine
　　Lactulose
　　Colchicine
　　Antibiotics
　　Neomycin
　　Chemotherapy
　　Antihypertensives
　　Alpha methyldopa
　　Propanolol
B. Uncommon
　　Excessive diuretics
　　Excessive opiates
　　Sorbitol (sugar-free gum)
　　Eye drops (anticholinesterase)
　　Cimetidine
　　Prostaglandins
Infections
A. Immunodeficiency syndrome
B. AIDS
C. Bacteria (usually cause acute, not chronic, diarrhea)
　　Campylobacter
　　Shigella
　　Salmonella
　　Yersinia
D. Parasites
　　Amebiasis (and sequelae)
　　Giardiasis
　　Coccidioidosis

Table continued on opposite page

RECOMMENDED DIAGNOSTIC APPROACH

The following is a recommended diagnostic approach for diarrhea that is chronic (lasting more than a month) and should not be followed for more acute self-limited episodes.

A. **History.** The physician should ask how much the patient eats (malabsorption should be suspected when the patient eats more than someone the same size but does not gain weight) and about night blindness, cramps (tetany), and easy bruisability. These result from the malabsorption of the fat-soluble vitamins A, D, and K. The physician should ask about medications (especially antacids and antibiotics), prior bowel surgery, recent travel (especially foreign), and exposure to others who have diarrhea. The patient should give a description of the stools; it should be remembered that floating stools may be an indicator of excess gas, not necessarily of excess fat. Patients who see fat globules in the toilet bowl water usually have pancreatic insufficiency (and severe fat malabsorption).

TABLE 59–1. CAUSES OF CHRONIC DIARRHEA *Continued*

D. Parasites *Continued*
  Cryptosporidiosis
  Helminthic infestation
  Trichuriasis (whipworm)
  Strongyloidiasis
  Capillariasis
  H. nana (dwarf tapeworm)
  Schistosomiasis (polyposis)
  Trichinosis (rare)
  Taenia species
Structural Causes
Inflammatory bowel disease
Prior gastric or intestinal surgery
Celiac sprue
Lactose intolerance
Pancreatic insufficiency
Gastrointestinal tumors
  Adenocarcinoma
  Lymphoma
Motility Problems
Irritable bowel syndrome
Scleroderma
Intestinal pseudo-obstruction
Amyloidosis
Metabolic and Endocrine Disorders
Zollinger-Ellison syndrome
Diabetes
Hyperthyroidism
Hypothyroidism
Medullary carcinoma of the thyroid gland
Addison's disease
Malignant carcinoid syndrome
Amyloidosis

B. **Evaluation of Stool.** Subsequent evaluation of the patient who has chronic diarrhea depends on whether the diarrhea is fatty, bloody, or watery. Therefore, the clinician should move early to the somewhat unattractive step (at least for the patient) of a 24-hour stool collection for fat and weight and to make sure that the patient is eating. A stool weight over 200 g per 24 hours confirms diarrhea.

1. *Chronic Bloody Diarrhea.* Gross or occult blood in a diarrheal stool should always be evaluated. This is usually caused by colonic disease, either infectious colitis or idiopathic inflammatory bowel disease (IIBD). Most infections are self-limited and resolve in less than four weeks. Stool cultures are diagnostic in 40 to 60 per cent of cases.

   a. A stool culture should be obtained for *Campylobacter, Salmonella, Shigella, Clostridium difficile,* and *Yersinia* and stool should be sent for *C. difficile* toxin determination if antibiotics have been taken recently. A positive toxin determination diagnoses pseudomembranous colitis. The physician should look for ova and parasites, especially *Entamoeba histolytica.* This can be excluded most definitively by ordering an ameba serology titer.

   b. If cultures are nondiagnostic and symptoms persist, sigmoidoscopy and rectal biopsy should be performed. Colitis is best diagnosed by sigmoidoscopy using either a rigid or a flexible instrument. Enemas or laxatives should not be used to prepare the patient because these products can damage the rectal mucosa and cause confusing artifacts. A tap-water enema can be used to cleanse the rectum.

   c. If the diagnosis is still unclear, an air contrast barium enema or colonoscopy, or both, should be done to evaluate the more proximal colon and differentiate ulcerative colitis from Crohn's disease. These tests also detect polyps and colon cancer, pseudomembranous colitis, and radiation damage.

2. *Chronic Watery Diarrhea.* This has a multitude of causes. Evaluation often depends on clues in the history or physical examination. The physician should ask about medications, alcohol consumption, milk intolerance, and prior bowel surgery.

   a. Stool culture and examination for ova and parasites should be done to exclude infectious causes. Amebic serology samples should be considered.

   b. Sigmoidoscopy and barium enema may diagnose unsuspected idiopathic inflammatory bowel disease, polyps, or cancers.

   c. If results of these procedures are normal, an upper gastrointestinal radiograph with small bowel follow-through should be used to diagnose prior gastric surgery, fistulae, or small bowel mucosal disease.

   d. If the radiograph appears normal, a lactose tolerance test should be used to diagnose lactose intolerance. This is best done by asking the patient to take 50 g of lactose in an 8-oz glass of water on an empty stomach. Cramps, gas, or diarrhea over the next four hours are suggestive of lactose intolerance.

   e. A small bowel biopsy should be considered to look for mucosal small bowel disease.

f. If the results of all of these procedures are normal, screening must be done for metabolic diseases such as carcinoid, Addison's disease (see Chapter 55), hyperthyroidism (see Chapter 56), and Zollinger-Ellison syndrome.

g. The last step in evaluation of a patient with chronic watery diarrhea is to hospitalize the patient and give intravenous fluids for 36 hours. If the patient still has diarrhea with no oral intake, the diarrhea is secretory, and the causes may be laxative abuse, pancreatic cholera, or other rare diseases such as disaccharidase deficiencies.

3. *Chronic Fatty Diarrhea.* A 24-hour stool fat content of greater than 5 g confirms fat malabsorption. Most commonly the cause is deficient luminal digestion of fat (pancreatic insufficiency with decreased enzyme output) or deficient absorption of fat caused by mucosal disease (celiac sprue). (See Chapter 64.)

a. A serum carotene determination should be used if the stool fat content is equivocal. The serum carotene and cholesterol levels are decreased in malabsorption. The decrease in carotene is very marked, down to 10 to 15 μg per 100 mL (normal serum carotene level is 50 to 300 μg per mL). A modest decrease in carotene may be caused by poor dietary intake of vegetables even without malabsorption.

b. A "protime" should be checked. Prothrombin time prolongation may be caused by malabsorption of fat-soluble vitamin K. This should be corrected with parenteral vitamin K administration.

c. A D-xylose test should not be done. The D-xylose test is attractive in theory because it should separate luminal from mucosal disease. However, in practice the results are affected by so many other factors such as gastric emptying and cardiac and renal function that it is not a reliable test in differential diagnosis of fat malabsorption.

REFERENCES

1. Phillips SF: Diarrhea: A current view of the pathophysiology. Gastroenterology 63:495, 1972.

This article explains the various mechanisms that result in diarrhea.

2. Read: Chronic diarrhea of unknown etiology. Gastroenterology 78:264, 1980.

Many of these patients had unsuspected laxative abuse.

3. Krejs GJ, Fordtran JS: Physiology and pathophysiology of ion and water movement in the human intestine. *In* Sleisenger MH, Fordtran JS: Gastrointestinal Disease. Philadelphia, W. B. Saunders Company, 1978.

A good overview of mechanisms of diarrhea; usefulness of measuring stool electrolytes is examined.

CONSTIPATION

By SHOBA KRISHNAMURTHY, M.D.

DEFINITION

Stool weight, size, and consistency can vary widely in normal people. Although normal stool frequencies range from three stools per day to three per week, constipation can be practically defined as the passage of less than three stools per week. It can be subjectively defined as small or hard stools or difficult passage of stools with abdominal discomfort and a feeling of incomplete evacuation. These subjective complaints are difficult to evaluate, and hence the objective definition is easier to apply and more practical.

There has been a widespread misconception for centuries that a daily stool is essential for a person's well-being. This has led many "normal" individuals to consider themselves to be constipated and even to abuse laxatives.

EPIDEMIOLOGY

Since constipation has different meanings to different people and can be caused by a wide variety of illnesses, it is difficult to find an accurate estimate of the prevalence of this symptom. A recent survey suggests that 6 per cent of individuals (20 per cent of elderly) not seeking medical care complain of constipation.

DIFFERENTIAL DIAGNOSIS

The most common cause of constipation in North America is an inadequate intake of dietary fiber (particularly in individuals on weight reduction diets). In practice, the amount of dietary fiber must be increased to 30 g per day before consideration is given to further diagnostic steps. Constipation can be caused by drugs (Table 60–1), metabolic and endocrine disorders (Table 60–2), gastrointestinal disorders (Table 60–3), and neurologic disorders (Table 60–4). In addition, lack of exercise, voluntary suppression of the urge to defecate, and prolonged travel are often considered causes of constipation. The role of these factors is unclear, however, because they have not been adequately studied. All of the conditions listed in the tables must be considered in the evaluation of anyone with constipation.

HISTORY, SIGNS, AND SYMPTOMS

Distinguishing features of several common disorders causing constipation include:
A. **Gastric and Small Bowel Obstruction and Emptying Disorders.**
   The most common cause of gastric outlet obstruction is peptic

TABLE 60–1. DRUGS THAT CAUSE CONSTIPATION

Analgesics	Bismuth
Anesthetic agents	Diuretics
Antacids (calcium and aluminum compounds)	Drugs for Parkinson's disease
Anticholinergics	Heavy metal poisoning (lead, arsenic, mercury, and phosphorus)
Anticonvulsants	
Antidepressants	
Antihypertensives	Monoamine oxidase inhibitors
Barium sulfate	

ulcer disease, and the two most common causes of gastroparesis (delayed emptying without mechanical obstruction) are post-surgical vagotomy and diabetes mellitus. The condition may be acute or chronic.

   1. Keys to Diagnosis. The diagnosis is indicated by predominant postprandial fullness and bloating, heartburn, nausea, vomiting, and upper abdominal distention associated with constipation.

B. Irritable Bowel Syndrome. This is the most common colonic disorder associated with constipation. Women with this condition outnumber men two to one. Onset usually occurs before age 35. The syndrome is characterized by disturbed motility, abdominal pain, and constipation alternating with diarrhea. A history of stress-induced symptoms is present in 50 per cent of cases. Seventy to 90 per cent of patients have abnormal psychologic features such as depression, anxiety, and panic-attack syndrome.

   1. Keys to Diagnosis. These include absence of weight loss, nocturnal abdominal pain, and hematochezia. There are no laboratory or radiologic abnormalities. (Depression could be associated with the weight loss.)

C. Diverticular Disease. Diverticular disease is present in 50 per cent of patients over 60 years old but symptomatic in only 20

TABLE 60–2. METABOLIC AND ENDOCRINE DISORDERS THAT CAUSE CONSTIPATION

Metabolic disorders
  Diabetes
  Porphyria
  Amyloidosis
  Uremia
  Hypokalemia

Endocrine disorders
  Panhypopituitarism
  Hypothyroidism
  Hypercalcemia
  Pheochromocytoma
  Pregnancy
  Glucagonoma

TABLE 60–3. DISORDERS OF THE GASTROINTESTINAL TRACT THAT CAUSE CONSTIPATION

Gastric emptying disorders
  Gastric outlet obstruction
  Gastroparesis

Small bowel obstruction

Colonic obstruction
Extraluminal
  Tumors
  Chronic volvulus
  Hernias
  Rectal prolapse

Luminal
  Tumors

| Strictures | { Benign | Infectious Inflammatory Ischemic colitis |
| | Malignant | |

Abnormalities of colonic motor function
  Irritable bowel syndrome
  Diverticular disease
  Segmental dilatation of the colon

Pseudo-obstruction
  Disorders of intestinal muscle
    Scleroderma
    Hollow visceral myopathy
  Disorders of myenteric nerves
    Visceral neuropathy
    Paraneoplastic neuropathy
    Chagas' disease

Hirschsprung's disease
Neuronal intestinal dysplasia

Rectal disorders (rectocele)
Anal problems (stenosis)

per cent. Symptoms are similar to those of irritable bowel syndrome. Diverticulitis and stricture formation are complications that can cause or worsen constipation.

D. Colonic Carcinoma. This diagnosis must be considered in every patient over 40 with a *recent* history of constipation.

  1. Keys to Diagnosis. These include recent onset, associated hematochezia, weight loss, anorexia and weakness, past history of colonic polyps, and family history of colonic cancer or polyposis.

**TABLE 60–4. NEUROLOGIC DISORDERS THAT CAUSE
CONSTIPATION**

Brain
    Parkinson's disease
    Tumors
    Cerebrovascular accidents

Other
    Trauma to splanchnic nerves
    Cauda equina tumor
    Meningocele
    Autonomic insufficiency
    Tabes dorsalis
    Multiple sclerosis
    Trauma to the medulla

E. **Hirschsprung's Disease.** This is an uncommon (1 in 5000 live births) familial disorder that is caused by absence of ganglion cells along a variable length of the distal colon. Spasticity of the affected segment behaves like an obstruction.
    1. *Keys to Diagnosis.* The patient is generally male with onset in childhood (infrequently in adult life). There is abdominal distention and an empty rectal ampulla on examination. Ganglion cells are absent on submucosal rectal biopsy.
F. **Neuromuscular Disorders.** These affect either the colonic muscle (scleroderma or visceral myopathy); or the colonic myenteric plexus (paraneoplastic neuropathy or sporadic or familial visceral neuropathy).
    1. *Keys to Diagnosis.* These include multiple gastrointestinal tract symptoms plus symptoms in other viscera such as dysphagia, abdominal distention, nausea, vomiting, and urinary symptoms. The constipation is chronic and responds poorly to laxatives.
G. **Metabolic and Endocrine Disorders.** Of the metabolic disorders in Table 60–2, diabetes is the major cause of constipation. Thirty per cent of diabetic patients without neuropathy and 80 to 90 per cent with peripheral and autonomic neuropathy are constipated. (Symptoms of neuropathy include orthostatic symptoms, numbness and burning in hands and feet, sexual dysfunction, urinary incontinence, and sweating disorders). Constipation is typically intermittent and alternates with diarrhea in 30 per cent of cases. Among endocrine disorders, hypothyroidism is the most common cause of constipation. Constipation may be the presenting symptom and can be associated with a megacolon. This is an important disorder to consider in the differential diagnosis because other symptoms of hypothyroidism may be absent. Thyroid replacement causes a dramatic improvement.
H. **Neurologic Disorders.** The exact frequency of constipation in these disorders is unknown, but it is a very commonly associated symptom. Ten per cent of patients with Parkinson's disease have megacolons, but a much higher number have constipation.

RECOMMENDED DIAGNOSTIC APPROACH

A. **History.** The physician should find out what the patient means by constipation. Many individuals who have normal bowel movements three to five times per week think they are constipated. The history should include a detailed account of drug intake and symptoms of metabolic, endocrine, neurologic, and gastrointestinal disease.

B. **Physical Examination.** The most frequent abnormalities will be detected in the neurologic examination.

C. **Routine Laboratory Tests.** These include (a) complete blood count, (b) stool for occult blood, (c) thyroid function tests, (d) blood-urea nitrogen (BUN), (e) serum electrolytes, and (f) fasting blood glucose.

D. **Fiber Diet.** If routine laboratory findings are normal, the patient should be put on a 30 g per day fiber diet. This can be done by having the patient take 1 cup of All Bran cereal or 2 tablespoons of Metamucil daily for 30 days. If constipation persists, work-up should be continued.

E. **Sigmoidoscopy.** The physician should look for anal fissure and rectal mass.

F. **Barium Enema.** The physician should look for (a) intraluminal mass or stricture, (b) narrowed distal segment (Hirschsprung's disease), (c) diverticula, (d) megacolon, and (e) elongated redundant colon.

G. **Rectal Biopsy.** Hirschsprung's disease and amyloidosis must be ruled out.

H. **Colonic Transit Time.** If the work-up described here reveals no abnormalities, the colonic transit time on a 30 g per day fiber diet should be measured by a radiopaque marker study. This test is also very useful if the patient's history is vague and inconsistent. The patient is given 20 radiopaque marker pieces (obtained from cutting a #12F nasogastric tube into 5-mm bits) which can be swallowed as such or after the pieces have been put into two empty capsules on day 0. Plain x-rays of the abdomen are obtained on days 2, 5, and 7. Normal results are passage of 80 per cent of markers by day 5 and of 100 per cent by day 7. This is an excellent way of confirming the patient's history, but an abnormal test result is not specific for any disorder. The test should begin the day after the patient has had a stool, and the patient should be instructed to avoid laxatives or enemas during the test.

I. **Other Methods.** If the results of the radiopaque marker study are abnormal but the rest of the work-up is normal and a neuromuscular disorder is suspected, the physician should consider (a) esophageal manometry to look for abnormal esophageal motor function, (b) upper gastrointestinal and small-bowel follow-through to look for retention or dilatation, or (c) an intravenous pyelogram to look for bladder dilatation or retention.

REFERENCES

1. Drossman DA, Sandler RS, et al.: Bowel pattern among subjects not seeking health care. Gastroenterology 83:529, 1982.

2. Devroede G: Constipation: Mechanisms and management. *In* Sleisenger MH, Fordtran JS (eds.): Gastrointestinal disease: Pathophysiology, diagnosis and management. Philadelphia, W. B. Saunders Company, 1983, pp. 288–308.

_____61_____

HEPATOMEGALY

By MICHAEL KIMMEY, M.D.

GENERAL COMMENTS

A. Usefulness of Physical Examination. Hepatomegaly is usually first detected by physical examination. However, anatomic variations of liver shape are frequent, and thus examination alone is not a sensitive or specific test of liver size. Imaging techniques, especially ultrasound, are more accurate but are currently not used to screen large populations for increased liver size. The prevalence of hepatomegaly in the general population is not known.

B. Physical Assessment of Liver Size. This is best accomplished by percussion in the right midclavicular or semilunar line, in which the normal span of dullness is 8 to 14 cm. Estimates of liver size increase if lighter percussion techniques are used. Liver size increases with height and weight, and males have larger livers than females. Falsely increased estimates of liver size are caused by: (1) depressed right hemidiaphragm (hyperinflated lungs), (2) subdiaphragmatic lesion (abscess or hematoma), (3) Riedel's lobe (anatomic variation with inferior projection of the right hepatic lobe). The liver edge is detectable more than 2 cm below the right costal margin with inspiration in 15 per cent of normal persons.

DIFFERENTIAL DIAGNOSIS

A. Vascular Congestion

1. Congestive Heart Failure. The liver is enlarged in over 95 per cent of patients with both acute and chronic right-sided heart failure. The liver edge is palpable over 5 cm below the costal margin in 50 per cent of patients. Liver enlargement with pure left-sided heart failure is unusual. Liver pulsation indicates the presence of tricuspid insufficiency.

2. Budd-Chiari Syndrome. Hepatomegaly is detected in 70 per cent of patients with hepatic venous occlusion. Ascites (90 per cent) and abdominal pain (60 per cent) are also usually seen in this rare syndrome.

3. *Veno-Occlusive Disease (VOD).* Approximately 70 per cent of symptomatic patients with VOD secondary to chemotherapy and radiation therapy have hepatomegaly.

B. **Inflammatory Conditions**

1. *Hepatitis.* All types of hepatitis involve diffuse hepatic inflammation and may be associated with hepatomegaly. The liver is uncommonly more than 3 to 5 cm larger than normal in viral hepatitis but is often tender. Two thirds of patients with subacute hepatic necrosis caused by hepatitis B or drugs have hepatomegaly.

C. **Alcoholic Liver Disease**

1. *Fatty Liver.* This is the most common type of liver pathology seen with alcohol ingestion. Most patients are asymptomatic. Liver tenderness from capsular distention is common.

2. *Alcoholic Hepatitis.* Liver biopsy is necessary to make this diagnosis with certainty. Ascites (70 per cent), jaundice (70 per cent), fever (50 per cent), splenomegaly (40 per cent), and encephalopathy (30 per cent) are variably seen.

3. *Cirrhosis.* Hepatomegaly is present in 75 to 95 per cent of cases but does not help distinguish between the various causes of cirrhosis. (See Chapter 63.) The liver may also be shrunken or have disproportionate enlargement of one lobe.

D. **Infiltrative Liver Disease**

1. *Fatty Liver.* Although most commonly this condition is caused by alcohol, it is also seen with inflammatory bowel disease (30 per cent of cases), obesity, postjejunoileal bypass, protein-calorie malnutrition, parenteral hyperalimentation, and Reye's syndrome in children. Liver enlargement in diabetic patients is caused by glycogen and fat deposition. Acute fatty liver of pregnancy is a rapidly progressive disorder occurring in the third trimester or immediately postpartum with an 80 per cent mortality.

2. *Amyloidosis.* Hepatomegaly is present in 50 per cent of patients with systemic amyloidosis.

3. *Hematologic Disorders.* Liver enlargement is found in approximately 50 per cent of patients with both acute and chronic leukemia at the time of diagnosis. Fifty per cent of patients with extramedullary hematopoiesis caused by agnogenic myeloid metaplasia have hepatomegaly. Hepatomegaly is seen in approximately 25 per cent of patients with non-Hodgkin's lymphoma, especially the lymphocytic type. Only about 10 per cent of patients with Hodgkin's disease have hepatomegaly, which may be due to multiple causes and should not be assumed to represent lymphomatous infiltration.

4. *Granulomatous Disorders.* Hepatic granulomas are seen in a wide variety of diseases. When they diffusely involve the liver, they may cause hepatomegaly. The most common cause of granulomatous liver enlargement is sarcoidosis. Hepatomegaly is seen at some time in the course of 20 per cent of patients with sarcoidosis.

5. *Iron Storage Disorders.* Hepatomegaly is present in 75 to 95

per cent of patients with hemochromatosis but less frequently in hemosiderosis related to alcoholic cirrhosis, thalassemia, and transfusional iron overload.

6. **Congenital Metabolic Defects.** Most of the disorders listed in Table 61–1 appear in infancy or early childhood. Gaucher's disease is caused by a lysosomal enzyme deficiency and may appear in the third decade with unexplained hepatosplenomegaly, especially in Ashkenazi Jews. In 5 per cent of patients with the Pi ZZ phenotype of alpha₁ antitrypsin deficiency, the disease appears in infancy with hepatomegaly and jaundice. In another 5 per cent it occurs in adulthood with cirrhosis and sometimes hepatomegaly. Coexistent emphysema is frequent in these patients.

E. **Biliary Obstruction.** Bile duct obstruction from common duct gallstones or carcinoma may cause moderate liver enlargement in addition to jaundice.

F. **Hepatic Tumors.** Metastatic tumors to the liver are 20 times more common than primary hepatocellular carcinoma in the United States. If metastases are large, they are often palpable as one or more nodules in the liver. Multiple small metastases may produce a diffusely enlarged liver. Symptoms or signs of the primary tumor are usually present. Ninety per cent of patients with primary hepatocellular carcinoma have hepatomegaly. Fifty per cent have ascites, and 30 per cent have an arterial bruit over the liver. A minority of patients with benign liver tumors have hepatomegaly.

G. **Cystic Liver Diseases.** Solitary cysts, whether parasitic or nonparasitic, may be palpable as a discrete nodule. Thirty per cent of patients with adult polycystic kidney disease also have multiple liver cysts, which expand with time and eventually produce nodular hepatomegaly.

CLINICAL MANIFESTATIONS

A. **History**
   1. **General.** Review of systems should include symptoms of congestive heart failure, malignancy, and infection.
   2. **Symptoms Referrable to Liver Dysfunction.** Such symptoms should be sought, including jaundice, ascites, gastrointestinal bleeding, and encephalopathy.
   3. **Other.** A history of alcohol consumption, drug or toxin exposure, foreign travel, and a family history of liver disease are important.

B. **Physical Examination**
   1. **General.** The physician should look for signs of congestive heart failure, malignancy, systemic infection, and signs of alcohol consumption (tremor, neuropathy, cerebellar dysfunction, or Dupuytren's contractures), and extrahepatic manifestations of liver disease (ascites, icterus, splenomegaly, palmar erythema, spider angiomas, gynecomastia, or testicular atrophy).

TABLE 61–1. CAUSES OF HEPATOMEGALY

Vascular congestion
A. Right-sided heart failure (common)
B. Budd-Chiari syndrome (rare)
C. Veno-occlusive disease (rare)
D. Tricuspid insufficiency (common)
E. Constrictive pericarditis (uncommon)

Inflammatory conditions
A. Hepatitis
   1. Viral (A, B, Non-A Non-B, cytomegalovirus (CMV), infectious mononucleosis) (common)
   2. Bacterial (rare)
   3. Parasitic (uncommon)
B. Abscess
   1. Bacterial (uncommon)
   2. Amoebic (uncommon)

Alcoholic liver disease
A. Fatty liver (common)
B. Alcoholic hepatitis (common)
C. Cirrhosis (common)

Infiltrative liver disease
A. Fatty liver (common)
B. Amyloidosis (rare)
C. Hematologic
   1. Leukemia (uncommon)
   2. Lymphoma (uncommon)
   3. Myeloid metaplasia (uncommon)
D. Granulomatous
   1. Sarcoidosis (uncommon)
   2. Bacterial (tuberculosis, leprosy, brucellosis, Q fever, syphilis) (uncommon)
   3. Parasites (schistosomiasis, toxocariasis) (uncommon)
   4. Viral (mononucleosis, CMV, psittacosis) (uncommon)
   5. Drugs or foreign substances (beryllium) (rare)
E. Iron storage disorder
   1. Hemochromatosis (uncommon)
   2. Hemosiderosis (alcohol, thalassemia, transfusional) (uncommon)
F. Congenital errors of metabolism
   1. Carbohydrate metabolism (hereditary fructose intolerance, galactosemia, glycogen storage disease) (rare)
   2. Protein metabolism (tyrosinemia) (rare)
   3. Lipid metabolism (Wolman's disease, cholesterol ester storage disease) (rare)
   4. Bile acid metabolism (rare)
   5. Lipoid storage disease (Niemann-Pick, Gaucher's) (rare)
   6. Miscellaneous (alpha$_1$-antitrypsin deficiency, cystic fibrosis) (rare)

Biliary obstruction
A. Carcinoma (pancreatic, ampullary, cholangiocarcinoma) (common)
B. Choledocholithiasis (common)

Hepatic tumors
A. Metastatic carcinoma (common)
B. Hepatocellular carcinoma (uncommon)
C. Benign liver tumors (adenoma, hyperplasia, hemangioma) (uncommon)

Cystic liver diseases
A. Parasitic *(Echinococcus)* (uncommon)
B. Nonparasitic (uncommon)
   1. Solitary (uncommon)
   2. Polycystic (uncommon)
C. Traumatic (uncommon)
D. Neoplastic (uncommon)

2. *The Liver.* The liver should be examined for:
   a. **Size.** Percussion in the midclavicular line is used.
   b. **Tenderness.** This is more likely with recent onset of hepatomegaly.
   c. **Nodularity.** Nodularity suggests tumor, macronodular cirrhosis, or polycystic disease.
   d. **Pulsation.** Pulsation is seen with tricuspid insufficiency.
   e. **Arterial Bruit.** This occurs in hepatocellular carcinoma or acute alcoholic hepatitis.
   f. **Venous Hum.** This may be caused by portal hypertension.
   g. **Friction Rub.** This may be related to perihepatitis, metastatic tumor, or recent liver biopsy.

LABORATORY STUDIES

A. Specific Tests
   1. *Screening.* Screening for hematologic, renal, and cardiac disease is often useful. (Complete blood count, creatinine level, and chest x-ray may be necessary.)
   2. *Biochemical Liver Tests.* These tests, including bilirubin, alanine aminotransferase (ALT), aspartate aminotransferase (AST), alkaline phosphatase, prothrombin time, and albumin yield some abnormality in most patients with significant hepatic disorders. These tests also help direct further evaluation based on their general pattern, either cholestatic or hepatocellular.
   3. *Serologic Tests.* Patients with abnormal liver enzymes and hepatomegaly should undergo serologic testing for viral hepatitis. If primary biliary cirrhosis or chronic active hepatitis is suspected on clinical grounds, testing for mitochondrial and smooth muscle antibodies is indicated.
   4. *Imaging Techniques*
      a. **Liver-Spleen Scan.** This study is frequently used as a screening test in patients with suspected hepatomegaly because of its widespread availability. It is roughly equivalent to ultrasound or computed tomography in detecting mass lesions (greater than 1 to 2 cm in size) but does not distinguish between the various types of lesions. Decreased parenchymal function may be detected by increased bone marrow isotope uptake.
      b. **Ultrasound.** In centers with technically good real-time ultrasonography, this is probably the imaging procedure of choice in the evaluation of hepatomegaly. Information obtained includes a qualitative estimate of liver size, extent and quality (cystic versus solid) of mass lesions, and the presence of biliary obstruction and cholelithiasis.
      c. **Computed Tomography (CT).** This technique is more expensive than ultrasound and the liver-spleen scan but provides the best evaluation of diffuse liver disease. Fatty infiltration and iron or glycogen deposition can be distinguished by their different CT densities. Ultrasound is

better than CT in defining cystic masses, but CT may detect more solid liver masses.

5. *Liver Biopsy.* Ultrasound or CT-directed biopsy of unexplained mass lesions usually provides a histologic diagnosis. Blind percutaneous liver biopsy should be performed in patients with unexplained diffuse hepatomegaly as well. Most diffuse liver diseases are safely diagnosed with this technique if the prothrombin time is prolonged less than 3 seconds and the platelet count is greater than 80,000.

RECOMMENDED DIAGNOSTIC APPROACH

A. Complete blood count, creatinine, prothrombin time, ALT or AST, alkaline phosphatase, bilirubin, and albumin values should be obtained.

B. If the results of these tests are normal and the examiner is confident that hepatomegaly is present, ultrasound or liver-spleen scan should be done to confirm liver enlargement and to look for mass lesions.

C. If ALT or AST are significantly elevated relative to alkaline phosphatase, a hepatitis screen should be done and other causes of hepatitis sought. Imaging techniques are usually unnecessary.

D. If alkaline phosphatase or 5'-nucleotidase levels are elevated out of proportion to the transaminases, ultrasound or CT should be done to rule out biliary obstruction and the presence of mass lesions.

E. Patients with unexplained diffuse parenchymal liver enlargement or unexplained mass lesions should undergo liver biopsy if clotting studies permit this.

REFERENCES

1. Zakim D, Boyer TD (eds.): Hepatology. Philadelphia, W. B. Saunders Company, 1982.

Several chapters pertain to various causes of hepatomegaly.

2. Sherlock S.: Diseases of the Liver and Biliary System. 6th ed. London, Blackwell Scientific Publications, 1981.

Several chapters are pertinent to various aspects of hepatomegaly.

3. Sapira JD, Williamson KL: How big is the normal liver? Arch Intern Med 139:971–973, 1979.

A comparison is made of ultrasound and physical examination in determining the liver size of 96 normal subjects.

4. Petasnick JP, Ram P, et al.: The relationship of computed tomography, gray-scale ultrasonography, and radionuclide imaging in the evaluation of hepatic masses. Sem Nucl Med 9:8–21, 1979.

The relative advantages of these three major hepatic imaging modalities in the detection of liver masses are outlined.

CIRRHOSIS

By MICHAEL KIMMEY, M.D.

DEFINITION

A. **Structural.** Cirrhosis is a derangement of liver architecture that is characterized by increased fibrous tissue together with nodular parenchymal regeneration. It is a common response by the liver to a variety of conditions that cause liver injury.

B. **Functional.** The disordered liver architecture is responsible for four distinct clinical syndromes, present individually or in combination:

1. *Hepatic Insufficiency.* This is characterized by jaundice, hypoalbuminemia, edema, and blood clotting abnormalities.

2. *Ascites.* This is the accumulation of excessive fluid volumes in the peritoneal cavity.

3. *Hepatic Encephalopathy.* This is an organic brain syndrome with fluctuating neurologic signs, asterixis, altered level of consciousness, and characteristic electroencephalographic (EEG) abnormalities.

4. *Portal Hypertension.* This is an elevated pressure in the portal venous system that leads to the development of portal-systemic venous collaterals. These collaterals, in the form of esophageal varices and hemorrhoids, are a frequent cause of gastrointestinal bleeding.

EPIDEMIOLOGY

A. **Prevalence.** Autopsy series show a prevalence of cirrhosis of 3 per cent in most populations but up to 10 per cent in chronic alcoholics in the United States.

B. **Mortality.** Cirrhosis is the fourth leading cause of death in men between ages 35 and 54 in the United States. It is the fifth leading cause of death in women of the same age group.

C. **Geographic Distribution.** There is a significant correlation between mortality for cirrhosis and alcohol consumption in European and North American countries. France and Italy have the highest per capita alcohol consumption and the highest mortality for cirrhosis. Residents of Finland and the Netherlands consume the least alcohol and have the lowest mortality from cirrhosis. Accurate data from China and Africa are not available; however, cirrhosis in these areas is most commonly related to chronic hepatitis B infection. All other causes of cirrhosis are much less frequent than alcoholic and postviral hepatitis.

DIFFERENTIAL DIAGNOSIS

A. Clinical. Patients with jaundice, ascites, and encephalopathy should have other causes of these disorders ruled out.

Portal hypertension may be caused by cirrhosis, but other causes should also be considered. These are best classified according to the site of pathology in relation to the hepatic sinusoids. Patients with presinusoidal portal hypertension have normal hepatocellular function and generally do not develop ascites. Patients with sinusoidal and postsinusoidal obstruction frequently have ascites and hepatocellular insufficiency. Cirrhosis is a sinusoidal disorder because the abnormal liver architecture disrupts the normal sinusoidal blood flow, leading to portal hypertension. Other causes of portal hypertension are listed in Table 62–1.

B. Etiologic. Table 62–2 lists most known causes of cirrhosis. Clues to the presence of the most common of these are given below. Greatest consideration should be given to the causes that have a treatable component. Although established cirrhosis is irreversible, removal or correction of the inciting agent or defect can halt progression of the disease in some cases.

C. Structural. The classification of cirrhosis based on the size of regenerative nodules is of historical interest but has limited clinical utility. Alcoholic cirrhosis is usually *micronodular*; however, it may also be *macronodular,* particularly late in the course. Cirrhosis following chronic hepatitis B may have nodules up to 5 cm in size and is often termed macronodular. Both small and large nodules can be seen in the same liver.

TABLE 62–1. CLASSIFICATION OF PORTAL HYPERTENSION

Presinusoidal
A. Extrahepatic
    Portal vein thrombosis (dehydration, oral contraceptives, hypercoagulable state)
    Malignant obstruction (pancreas, stomach, colon)
    Infection (peritonitis, neonatal)
    Congenital anomalies
B. Intrahepatic
    Schistosomiasis
    Toxins (vinyl chloride, arsenic, copper)
    Congenital hepatic fibrosis
    Sarcoidosis
    Myeloproliferative diseases (myelosclerosis, leukemia, Hodgkin's disease)
Sinusoidal
    Cirrhosis (all causes)
Postsinusoidal
    Hepatic vein occlusion (Budd-Chiari syndrome, congenital webs, tumors, hypercoagulable state, oral contraceptives)
    Veno-occlusive disease (chemotherapy, pyrrolizidine alkaloids)
    Constrictive pericarditis, cor pulmonale, congestive heart failure

TABLE 62–2. ETIOLOGY OF CIRRHOSIS

Alcohol		Common
Posthepatitis		Common
Type B		
Non-A non-B		
Autoimmune		
Metabolic		Rare
Wilson's disease		
Hemochromatosis		
Alpha$_1$ antitrypsin deficiency		
Galactosemia		
Glycogen storage disease (Type IV)		
Hereditary fructose intolerance		
Tyrosinosis		
Cystic fibrosis		
Prolonged cholestasis		Uncommon
Primary biliary cirrhosis		
Secondary biliary cirrhosis		
Cryptogenic		(Maybe up to 20% of cases)
Drug-induced		Uncommon
Methotrexate	(fibrosis and cirrhosis)	
Chlorpromazine	(biliary cirrhosis)	

Isoniazid
  Methyldopa
  Nitrofurantoin
	(chronic active hepatitis: may *not* progress to cirrhosis if drug is stopped)	

Congestive (tricuspid insufficiency, constrictive pericarditis, congestive heart failure)		

HISTORY

A. **Alcoholic Cirrhosis.** This is part of the spectrum of alcoholic liver disease (fatty liver, alcoholic hepatitis, and cirrhosis). All of these conditions may be seen in the same liver. There should be history of excessive alcohol consumption, generally of many years' duration. Other stigmata of chronic alcoholism may be present (peripheral neuropathy, congestive cardiomyopathy, cerebellar degeneration).

B. **Posthepatitc Cirrhosis.** This condition is also termed *postnecrotic cirrhosis*. It develops in patients who have had type B or non-A non-B hepatitis. It is not a sequelae of hepatitis A infection. Prior acute hepatitis may have occurred as recently as four years earlier, but generally chronic hepatitis is present for many years before cirrhosis develops. Risk factors (blood transfusion, intravenous drug abuse, and homosexuality) and serologic studies are useful, particularly in patients with no prior history of clinical hepatitis.

C. Autoimmune Chronic Active Hepatitis. This condition is seen primarily in females with other autoimmune manifestations (polyarthralgias, acne, erythema nodosum, and pericarditis). Laboratory findings include high serum globulins, antinuclear antibody (70 per cent of patients), and anti-smooth muscle antibody (80 per cent of patients).

D. Metabolic

   1. *Wilson's Disease.* This is an autosomal recessive disorder that is caused by a defect in copper metabolism and characterized by chronic liver disease (cirrhosis or chronic active hepatitis), hemolytic anemia, copper deposition in the cornea (Kayser-Fleischer rings), and central nervous system abnormalities (movement disorders and tremors). It should be excluded by laboratory evaluation in all patients with unexplained cirrhosis because it is treatable.

   2. *Hemochromatosis.* Hepatic parenchymal iron deposition causes hepatomegaly and eventually cirrhosis. Excessive iron may originate from multiple blood transfusions such as in the thalassemias or from inappropriately high intestinal iron absorption as seen in idiopathic hemochromatosis. The latter disease is an inherited defect that is also manifested by increased skin pigmentation, diabetes mellitus, congestive cardiomyopathy, arthritis, and hypogonadism.

   3. *Alpha$_1$ Antitrypsin Deficiency.* This is associated in some cases with cirrhosis and panacinar emphysema; however, deficient patients may also have normal livers and lungs.

   4. *Other Metabolic Disorders.* The other metabolic disorders in Table 62–2 occur primarily in neonates and young children.

E. Prolonged Cholestasis. Primary biliary cirrhosis is an immunologic disorder of small bile ducts that leads to cirrhosis. Pruritus, fatigue, hepatosplenomegaly, and xanthelasma may be seen early in the disease. Long-term extrahepatic bile duct obstruction caused by stones or stricture leads to secondary biliary cirrhosis.

F. Cryptogenic. No etiology is found for cirrhosis in up to 30 per cent of cases. Acute hepatitis is not seen in the course of cryptogenic cirrhosis.

SIGNS AND SYMPTOMS

The overall frequencies of various clinical findings in cirrhosis are listed in Table 62–3. These findings do not help distinguish between the various causes of cirrhosis.

LABORATORY EVALUATION

A. Biochemical Tests

   1. *Liver Enzymes.* Liver enzymes may be normal or elevated in cirrhosis. The degree of elevation does not correlate with the

TABLE 62-3. SYMPTOMS AND SIGNS IN CIRRHOSIS*

FINDING	INCIDENCE (PER CENT)
Hepatomegaly	72
Ascites	58
Jaundice	49
Weakness	43
Splenomegaly	40
Spider nevi	38
Anorexia	37
Encephalopathy	36
Abdominal pain	34
Nausea or vomiting	32
Hematemesis	28

*From Galambos.[1]

extent or activity of disease. Aspartate aminotransferase (AST) and alanine aminotransferase (ALT) reflect hepatocellular damage, while alkaline phosphatase and 5'-nucleotidase elevations are characteristic of cholestasis, as seen in biliary cirrhosis. Bilirubin elevations may be caused by decreased hepatic excretion or increased production as seen in hemolytic states.

2. *Serum Albumin and Prothrombin Times.* These parameters reflect hepatic synthetic function. Patients who have a prolonged prothrombin time that is not corrected after parenteral vitamin K administration have severe hepatocellular dysfunction and a higher mortality.

3. *Unexplained Cirrhosis.* Patients with unexplained cirrhosis should be screened for Wilson's disease and hemochromatosis, even if other symptoms of the disease are not present. Serum ceruloplasmin level is low (less than 20 mg per dL) in 96 per cent of patients with Wilson's disease. Decreased serum and elevated urinary copper levels are also seen but are not as sensitive as the ceruloplasmin level. Serum levels of iron, total iron binding capacity, and ferritin are all increased in hemochromatosis. The latter test is most useful in distinguishing between primary iron overload as seen in hemochromatosis and secondary liver iron deposition as seen in some cases of alcoholic cirrhosis.

B. Serology and Immunology

1. *Hepatitis B Surface Antigen.* Hepatitis B surface antigen and core antibody may indicate chronic hepatitis B infection. There are currently no serum markers for non-A non-B hepatitis infection.

2. *Elevations in Serum Gamma Globulins.* Elevations are frequently seen in cirrhosis. These are mainly caused by elevations of immunoglobulin A (IgA) in alcoholic cirrhosis, immunoglobulin M (IgM) in biliary cirrhosis, and immunoglobulin G (IgG) in cryptogenic cirrhosis and cirrhosis caused by chronic hepatitis.

3. *Autoantibodies.* Antinuclear antibodies (ANA) are seen in up

to 50 per cent of patients with cryptogenic cirrhosis. Antibodies to mitochondria (AMA) are seen in 90 per cent of patients with primary biliary cirrhosis. Antibodies to smooth muscle (SMA) are seen most frequently in patients with chronic active hepatitis but are present in up to 50 per cent of patients with cirrhosis.

C. **Liver Biopsy.** Patients with prothrombin times less than 3 seconds greater than control and platelet counts over 80,000 should have a percutaneous or laparoscopically directed needle liver biopsy if the cause of the liver disease is not clear. Characteristic morphologic features may be seen in cirrhosis caused by chronic active hepatitis, alcohol, alpha$_1$ antitrypsin deficiency, hemochromatosis, congestive heart failure, and in primary biliary cirrhosis. Tissue levels of copper and iron can be measured. Specific enzyme assays are available for some of the congenital metabolic defects.

RECOMMENDED DIAGNOSTIC APPROACH

A. History, physical examination, liver enzymes, bilirubin, albumin, and prothrombin time are used to screen for the presence of liver disease.

B. Hepatitis B serologies, immunologic tests, ceruloplasmin, serum iron and total iron-binding capacity, and ferritin levels suggest a cause in some cases.

C. If the diagnosis is not clear from this information, a liver biopsy should be done if blood clotting is adequate.

REFERENCES

1. Galambos JT: Cirrhosis. Philadelphia, W.B. Saunders Company, 1979.
   A thorough monograph on all aspects of cirrhosis.

2. Sherlock S: Diseases of the Liver and Biliary System. Oxford, Blackwell Scientific Publishing, 1981.
   Up-to-date discussion of liver diseases, including diagnosis and management.

3. Warnes TW: A new look at cirrhosis. J R Coll Physicians Lond 16:23–32, 1982.
   A recent review with extensive references.

63

MALABSORPTION

By MICHAEL KIMMEY, M.D.

DEFINITION

The syndrome of malabsorption is suggested by certain symptoms and signs and confirmed by laboratory testing. Symptoms may result from the inability to digest or absorb fat, protein, carbohydrate, minerals, or vitamins. The primary defect may be in the intraluminal preparation of the nutrient for absorption, in the absorption process itself, or in the transport of the nutrient away from the intestinal mucosa.

GENERAL COMMENTS

The incidence of malabsorption syndrome in the general population is unknown. Many patients have very mild symptoms that are attributed to psychologic influences and are not given the diagnosis of malabsorption until late in the course of illness, if at all. If symptoms and signs of malabsorption are present, laboratory testing should be done to define the nutrients involved and then to identify the underlying disease process so that specific treatment can be prescribed.

DIFFERENTIAL DIAGNOSIS

A. **Irritable Bowel Syndrome.** Patients with vague abdominal pain, fatigue, and alteration in bowel habits are frequently thought to have the irritable bowel syndrome. The physician must be alert to clues that suggest malabsorption in these patients. Weight loss, muscle wasting, and edema are symptoms of advanced malabsorption but may also be caused by poor nutrition, severe depression, and occult malignancy, which should be excluded.
B. **Various Causes of Maldigestion and Malabsorption.** Causes are listed in Table 63–1 according to the probable pathogenetic mechanism involved. A specific diagnosis is usually reached by considering the clinical manifestations and data from the selected laboratory tests described later.

CLINICAL MANIFESTATIONS

A. History
   1. **Weight Loss.** This may be absent in early malabsorption; however, with time weight loss usually becomes evident. Muscle wasting resulting from impaired protein metabolism may also be prominent.

Text continued on page 476

TABLE 63–1. CLASSIFICATION AND CLINICAL FINDINGS IN THE MALABSORPTION SYNDROME

CAUSE	HISTORY	PHYSICAL EXAM	FECAL FAT Normal <6 gm/d	LABORATORY TESTS D-XYLOSE	LABORATORY TESTS JEJUNAL BIOPSY	OTHER
I. INTRALUMINAL PANCREATIC ENZYME DEFICIENCY						
A. Chronic Pancreatitis	Recurrent episodes of acute pancreatitis, weight loss (95%), abdominal pain	Signs of weight loss Abdominal tenderness, edema/ascites (10%)	Abnormal (30-40 gm/d)	Normal	Normal	Abnormal Schilling (40%), abnormal triolein breath test (95%), abnormal secretin stimulation test
B. Pancreatic Resection	History of surgery	See above	See above	Normal	Normal	See above
C. Pancreatic carcinoma (40% after >80% of pancreas removed)	Abdominal pain, weight loss	Abdominal mass	See above	Normal	Normal	See above
D. Cystic Fibrosis (CF) (Accounts for 95% of cases of pancreatic insuff. in children; 80% of children with CF have pancreatic insufficiency.)	Recurrent respiratory tract symptoms (90%), oily stools; failure to thrive	Smaller than expected for age (wt & ht), pulmonary findings	Abnormal (20-30 gm/d)	Normal Normal Normal	Normal Normal Normal	Elevated sweat chloride (98%)
II. INTRALUMINAL BILE SALT DEFICIENCY						
A. Bile Duct Obstruction	Jaundice	Hepatomegaly	Abnormal (40 gm/d with complete obstruction, 15-20 gm/d with partial obstruction)	Normal	Normal	Elevated bilirubin, alkaline phosphatase

	Clinical Features	Physical Findings	Fecal Fat	D-Xylose	Other Tests
B. Hepatic Insufficiency (Generally chronic diseases, esp. cirrhosis; malabsorption may be due to neomycin therapy or pancreatic insufficiency; 5% of cirrhotic patients have symptomatic steatorrhea)	Weakness (40%), Encephalopathy (40%), Anorexia (40%), Abdominal pain (30%)	Hepatomegaly (70%) Ascites (60%), Jaundice	Abnormal (10-20 gm/d)	Normal	Prolonged prothrombin time, low albumin
C. Small Intestinal Bacterial Overgrowth (Blind loops, diverticuli, motor abnormalities, scleroderma, diabetes, pseudo-obstruction)	Prior surgery, abdominal pain and distention in pseudo-obstruction, arthritis/skin changes in scleroderma	Surgical scars, Findings of scleroderma or diabetes	Abnormal (15-20 gm/d)	May be abnormal due to bacterial xylose	Abnl Schilling, small bowel xray to R/O anatomic defects, Abnl bile acid breath test
D. Defective Ileal Bile Salt Absorption **1. Ileal Resection** (Generally greater than 100 cm to give symptoms)	Prior Surgery	Surgical scar	Abnormal (20-25 gm/d)	Normal	Abnl Schilling Abnl bile acid breath test, Gallstones (30%)
2. Ileitis	Diarrhea (90%), Abdominal Pain (80%)	Perianal Disease (20%), arthritis (20%)	Abnormal (15-20 gm/d)	Normal	May be Abnormal (granulomas) — Abnl Schilling, Abnl bile acid breath test, gallstones (30%)
III. SMALL INTESTINAL DISEASE **A. Mucosal Cellular Defects** **1. Disaccharidase Deficiency** Lactase - Common Maltase - Uncommon Sucrase - Rare	Diarrhea, flatulence, Pain after ingestion of involved sugar (usually milk)	Usually Normal	Normal	Normal	Abnormal sugar tolerance tests; Assay enzymes in jejunal biopsy
2. Abetalipoproteinemia (Rare childhood disease)	Failure to thrive Family history (autosomal recessive) Cardiac arrhythmias	Ataxia, nystagmus Retinitis pigmentosa, congestive heart failure	Abnormal (10-15 gm/d)	Normal	Characteristic lipid vacuoles; Normal villi, low cholesterol and triglyceride levels

Table 63-1 continued on following page

471

TABLE 63–1. CLASSIFICATION AND CLINICAL FINDINGS IN THE MALABSORPTION SYNDROME *Continued*

CAUSE	HISTORY	PHYSICAL EXAM	FECAL FAT Normal <6gm/d	LABORATORY TESTS D-XYLOSE	JEJUNAL BIOPSY	OTHER
B. Lymphatic Obstruction 1. Intestinal Lymphangiectasia (Unusual)	Progressive edema and anasarca beginning in first two decades	Edema Ascites	Abnormal (15–20 gm/d)	Normal	Characteristic dilated lacteals; may be patchy	Hypoproteinemia, Intestinal protein loss
2. Lymphoma – Malabsorption unusual with localized or secondary lymphoma; common with primary diffuse lymphoma	Abdominal pain, weight loss, ethnic history (Sephardic Jews, Arabs)	Clubbing, peripheral edema, Abdominal mass (10–20%)	Abnormal (30–40 mg/d)	Abnormal	Characteristic but patchy lesions seen in 50–70% of diffuse cases	Hypoproteinemia IgA heavy chains in serum (uncommon)
C. Other Small Intestinal Defects 1. Celiac Sprue (Gluten-sensitive enteropathy)	Typical malabsorption symptoms; extra-intestinal symptoms may be prominent. Childhood or adult onset.	Clubbing, edema, Dermatitis herpetiformis in a minority	Abnormal (25–30 gm/d)	Abnormal	Diffuse villous flattening with lymphocyte infiltration	Reversion to normal of jejunal biopsy after dietary gluten elimination

	Clinical Setting	Extraintestinal Manifestations	Steatorrhea	D-Xylose	Intestinal Biopsy	Diagnosis/Comments
2. Tropical Sprue	Prolonged (>1 yr) residence in tropical countries. Malabsorptive symptoms with prominent anorexia	Weight loss, glossitis (25%)	Abnormal (15-20 gm/d)	Abnormal	Abnormal; similar to celiac sprue	Clinical and biopsy response to folate and tetracycline therapy, megaloblastic anemia (95%), rule out parasites.
3. Whipple's Disease	Arthritis (75%), Fever (50%), CNS abnormalities (uncommon), recurrent pleuritis	Arthritis Lymphadenopathy Dementia, cranial nerve abnormalities (uncommon)	Abnormal (30-40 gm/d)	Abnormal	Characteristic PAS positive macrophages in lamina propria	Iron deficiency anemia, clinical and usually biopsy response to antibiotics
4. Eosinophilic Gastroenteritis	Food allergies, Abdominal pain Intermittent nausea and and vomiting, asthma, allergic rhinitis (50%)	Eczema Urticaria	Abnormal (10-15 gm/d)	Usually abnormal with mucosal disease	Patchy infiltration with eosinophils	Eosinophilia Hypoalbuminemia Negative intestinal parasites
5. Amyloidosis (Intestinal involvement in 70% systemic cases; malabsorption in 5%)	Abdominal pain, Abdominal distention, vomiting	Macroglossia (20%), hepatosplenomegaly, peripheral neuropathy, arthritis	Abnormal (10-15 gm/d)	Abnormal	Patchy amyloid deposition, especially in blood vessels	Abnormal rectal biopsy (80%), Thickened folds on x-rays
IV. MULTIPLE DEFECTS						
1. Zollinger-Ellison Syndrome	Peptic ulcer disease Diarrhea (30%)	Usually normal	Abnormal in 25% (15-20 gm/d)	Normal	Usually normal; patchy microulcers may be present	High serum gastrin

Table 63-1 continued on following page

473

TABLE 63-1. CLASSIFICATION AND CLINICAL FINDINGS IN THE MALABSORPTION SYNDROME *Continued*

CAUSE	HISTORY	PHYSICAL EXAM	FECAL FAT Normal <6gm/d	LABORATORY TESTS D-XYLOSE	JEJUNAL BIOPSY	OTHER
2. Post-gastrectomy	Prior gastric surgery (esp. Billroth II anastomosis)	Abdominal surgical scar	Abnormal (10-15 gm/d)	Normal	Normal	Iron deficiency anemia (50%), Osteomalacia (30%)
3. Radiation Enteritis	Prior abdominal radiation (>4000 rads), watery diarrhea, tenesmus	Usually normal	Abnormal (10-15 gm/d)	May be abnormal with small bowel involvement	Abnormal, although non-specific changes	Sigmoidoscopy may show proctitis; small intestinal x-ray: fistulas ulcers, strictures; bile acid breath test to R/O bacterial overgrowth
V. UNCERTAIN ETIOLOGY 1. Immunodeficiency	Recurrent intestinal infections	Usually normal	Abnormal (10-20 gm/d)	May be Abnormal	Abnormal: May show absence of plasma cells of nodular lymphoid hyperplasia	Hypogamma-globulinemia or isolated immunoglobulin deficiency
2. Carcinoid Syndrome	Cutaneous flushes (head and neck), episodic abdominal cramps and diarrhea, wheezing	Hepatomegaly, Tricuspid murmurs	May be abnormal (10-15 gm/d)	Usually Normal	Usually Normal	Increased urinary 5-hydroxyindoleacetic acid

3.	Parasitoses (Giardia lamblia, coccidia, strongyloides, cappillaria, and ancylostomiasis may produce malabsorption)	Loose, mucousy stools. Fever and headache with coccidiosis; borborygmi and abdominal distention with capillariasis	Usually normal	May be abnormal (10-15 gm/d)	Usually	Non-specific changes or may see Giardia oocysts	Stool for ova and parasites. Eosinophilia with strongyloides.
4.	Diabetes mellitus (Approx. 10% with diarrhea and 5% with steatorrhea)	Diarrhea often nocturnal. Renal, ocular, vascular disease often present.	Peripheral neuropathy; retinopathy; often signs of weight loss	Abnormal (20-25 gm/d)	May be normal or abnormal	Normal	Hyperglycemia, Abnormal bile acid breath test due to bacterial overgrowth in minority.
5.	Other endocrinopathies (hyperthyroidism, hypothyroidism, hypoadrenocorticism)	Findings of specific endocrinologic disorder		Abnormal (15-20 gm/d)	May be normal or abnormal	Normal	Specific hormone (or calcium) levels

R/O = rule out; Abnl = abnormal.

2. *Appetite.* Most patients with small intestinal disease have poor appetite and decreased food intake, often because food exacerbates abdominal pain and diarrhea.

Patients with pancreatic insufficiency may have hyperphagia and eat enormous quantities of food but lose weight. Patients with iron deficiency may have a peculiar craving, or pica, for clay or ice. Patients with lactase deficiency often deduce that dairy products exacerbate their symptoms.

3. *Stool Character and Frequency.* Bowel movements may be normal or increased in frequency. The earliest change is often a marked increase in the bulk of stools, which the patient may first notice because of difficulty in flushing the stool from the toilet. Oily rancid stools are found in advanced cases. Floating stools correlate with gas, not fat, content. Excessive flatulence may indicate carbohydrate malabsorption. Bloody stools are seen predominantly with inflammatory bowel disease, infection, and ischemia.

4. *Pain.* Most malabsorptive states are not accompanied by abdominal pain. Patients with Crohn's disease or radiation enteritis may have aching or cramping periumbilical or right lower quadrant pain. Back pain may be seen with chronic pancreatitis. Severe periumbilical pain not associated with food ingestion is present in many patients with intestinal lymphoma. Patients with vascular insufficiency of the intestine often have severe poorly localized pain that typically occurs 30 to 60 minutes after eating.

5. *Other Symptoms Potentially Caused by Malabsorption.* Bruising and easy bleeding may be signs of vitamin K malabsorption. Night blindness and dry eyes may signify vitamin A insufficiency. Bone pain, tetany, and paresthesias may be caused by abnormal calcium metabolism from vitamin D and calcium malabsorption. Malnutrition and weight loss may also lead to pituitary dysfunction, loss of libido, or amenorrhea.

6. *Prior Medical History and Other Factors.* Medical history (prior surgery, medications, alcohol use, ulcer disease, other medical problems such as arthritis and skin problems, and prior radiation), family history (cystic fibrosis, inflammatory bowel disease, and sprue), and ethnic background are all relevant and may provide etiologic clues.

B. Physical Examination
1. *Vital Signs.* Hypotension and tachycardia may be caused by volume depletion or simply by severe malnutrition. Fever usually indicates the presence of infection or tumor.

2. *Abdominal Examination.* Abdominal distention may be caused by ascites or excessive intestinal gas. Bowel sounds may be hyperperistaltic, normal, or decreased and are not diagnostically helpful. Hepatosplenomegaly may be seen with amyloidosis and occasionally with lymphoma. Abdominal masses may be felt in Crohn's disease, carcinoma, diverticulitis, and lymphoma. Significant abdominal tenderness is unusual in most diseases that are manifested by malabsorption.

3. *General Physical Examination*
   a. **Signs of Malabsorption.** These include muscle wasting, edema, Trousseau's and Chvostek's signs, skeletal deformities, bruises and purpura, glossitis, peripheral neuropathy, and clubbing.
   b. **Signs Suggestive of Underlying Cause.** These include thickened skin, especially over the fingers (scleroderma); grouped vesicles, especially on extensor skin surfaces consistent with dermatitis herpetiformis (gluten-sensitive enteropathy); wheezing (eosinophilic gastroenteritis or carcinoid syndrome); urticaria and flushing (systemic mastocytosis); cataracts, retinopathy, and neuropathy (diabetes mellitus); arthritis (inflammatory bowel disease, Whipple's disease, amyloidosis, and hypogammaglobulinemia); and signs of hypo- and hyperthyroidism.

LABORATORY EVALUATION

A. **Specific Tests**
   1. *Routine Tests.* Routine tests that are often used for screening include:
      a. Hematocrit with indices (macrocytosis due to folate or vitamin B_{12} deficiency; microcytosis from iron deficiency)
      b. Electrolytes (severe diarrhea or laxative abuse)
      c. Prothrombin time (vitamin K malabsorption or liver disease)
      d. Calcium (vitamin D or calcium malabsorption; hypoparathyroidism)
      e. Albumin (protein malabsorption, protein loss, or liver disease)
      f. Erythrocyte sedimentation rate (inflammatory bowel disease, lymphoma)
      g. Vitamin B_{12} and folate levels (useful to determine the cause of macrocytic anemia)
      h. Cholesterol (low in fat malabsorption)
   2. *Fecal Fat Determination*
      a. **Qualitative.** Staining of a smear made from a routine stool specimen with Sudan stain and acetic acid provides a qualitative estimate of steatorrhea. The number and size of fat droplets correlate fairly well with results of quantitative fat determination in adults who excrete greater than 12 to 15 g of fat per day. False-negative results are seen with low-fat diets, in children, and in mild degrees of steatorrhea (6 to 12 g of fecal fat per day).
      b. **Quantitative.** The patient is placed on a standard diet containing 80 to 100 g of fat per day. After two days stool collection is begun and continued for 72 hours. Collection can be facilitated by using a paint can that is kept sealed between uses. Excretion of greater than 6 g of fat per 24 hours is abnormal (two standard deviations above the mean). Since normal fat digestion and absorption involve

all phases of the digestive process, this test provides the most sensitive evaluation of the overall process. Fecal fat quantitation does not distinguish between the various causes of malabsorption, and if results are abnormal further testing should be done to define the specific defect present. Potential errors and disadvantages of the test include: (1) inadequate stool collection; (2) the necessity of patient cooperation; (3) a defined, usually unsupervised diet over a five-day period; (4) stool collection and analysis are unpleasant; (5) laxatives such as mineral oil and castor oil cause falsely elevated values; and (6) a normal test result does not exclude malabsorption of substances other than fat (such as carbohydrates and vitamins).

3. **D-Xylose Test.** D-xylose is a five-carbon sugar that is absorbed in the duodenum and proximal jejunum, is not metabolized by man, and is excreted unchanged in the urine. The test is performed by having the patient drink a solution of 25 g of the sugar in 500 cu ml of water. A plasma specimen one hour after ingestion should be greater than 20 mg per dL, or urine collected for five hours should contain over 4 g of xylose. Low xylose concentrations are seen with inadequate intestinal absorption caused by a decreased absorptive surface (in celiac sprue or intestinal resection) and infiltrative intestinal diseases if these are extensive (regional enteritis, lymphoma, or amyloid). Bacterial overgrowth states may give low values because of bacterial metabolism of the xylose. Falsely low urine, but not serum, values are seen with massive ascites and decreased renal function.

4. **Breath Tests**

   a. **Triolein Breath Test.** The triglyceride triolein, labeled with carbon-14, is ingested by the patient. If normal digestion and absorption are present, the triolein is metabolized with release of carbon-14–labeled carbon dioxide ($^{14}CO_2$), which can be measured in the expired breath. Nonobese patients with steatorrhea exhale less $^{14}CO_2$ than nonobese patients without steatorrhea. Results correlate well with quantitative fecal fat determination (100 per cent sensitivity, 96 per cent specificity). False-positive results are seen in 25 per cent of obese patients, and potentially in situations of delayed gastric emptying and obstructive pulmonary disease. Although currently not widely available, this test may eventually become a more usable test for fat malabsorption than quantitative fecal fat determination. The specific defect causing fat malabsorption is not defined by this test.

   b. **Bile Acid Breath Test.** Orally ingested conjugated bile acids labeled with ^{14}C-glycine normally undergo enterohepatic circulation with minimal deconjugation. In the presence of small intestinal bacterial overgrowth or ileal dysfunction or resection, bile acids are deconjugated, and when the glycine is metabolized, $^{14}CO_2$ is released and measured in the exhaled breath. When compared with small intestinal cultures, the bile acid breath test detects bacterial overgrowth with a sensitivity of 70 per cent and a specificity of 90 per cent. This test is most useful when the pretest probability of bacterial overgrowth is intermediate, such as in diarrhea or steatorrhea of unknown cause, diabetes with diarrhea, and scleroderma. Ileal dysfunction is best detected when both breath and stool $^{14}CO_2$ are measured. The latter procedure is cumbersome, and hence the Schilling test is more widely used to detect ileal dysfunction.

5. *Schilling Test.* Several recent modifications make this classic test of vitamin B_{12} absorption even more useful. Cobalt-57–labeled vitamin B_{12} (^{57}Co B_{12}) bound to intrinsic factor can be given to the patient together with cobalt-58–labeled B_{12} unbound to intrinsic factor. If intrinsic factor is absent (as in pernicious anemia or after gastrectomy), only ^{57}Co can be found in the urine; if nutritional B_{12} deficiency is present, both isotopes can be recovered; if ileal dysfunction or bacterial overgrowth are present, neither isotope can be recovered. The test result is corrected to normal after antibiotic therapy for bacterial overgrowth. The test result is abnormal in diffuse ileal diseases such as regional enteritis and after greater than 100 cm of ileum has been resected. Since pancreatic enzymes are needed to degrade a gastric juice protein that inhibits intrinsic factor binding to B_{12}, the Schilling test can also be used as a test for pancreatic insufficiency. Abnormal Schilling test results that become normal when the B_{12} is given along with pancreatic enzymes are seen in about 40 per cent of patients with pancreatic insufficiency.

6. *Small Intestinal Biopsy.* Peroral suction biopsy of the small intestinal mucosa is a safe procedure that provides useful diagnostic information in patients with evidence of intestinal malabsorption. Biopsy findings are usually diagnostic in celiac sprue, immunodeficiency, Whipple's disease, and abetalipoproteinemia. Small intestinal biopsy may be diagnostic in other diseases with a patchy distribution, including amyloidosis, systemic mastocytosis, eosinophilic enteritis, lymphoma, parasitic infestation, intestinal lymphangiectasia, and radiation enteritis. Nonspecific or normal findings are usually found in regional enteritis, tropical sprue, and conditions of bacterial overgrowth.

7. *Small Intestinal X-Rays.* This noninvasive test is most useful in defining abnormal anatomic details, including diverticula, congenital anomalies, enteroenteric fistulas, and postsurgical changes. Nonspecific abnormalities such as delayed transit time, thickened mucosa, and small bowel dilatation may be seen in other diseases of malabsorption. This test is frequently done early in the diagnostic evaluation because it is easy and noninvasive; however, it is rarely sufficient by itself in yielding the underlying diagnosis.

8. *Pancreatic Function Tests.* Duodenal intubation with aspiration of contents after a test meal or intravenous secretin

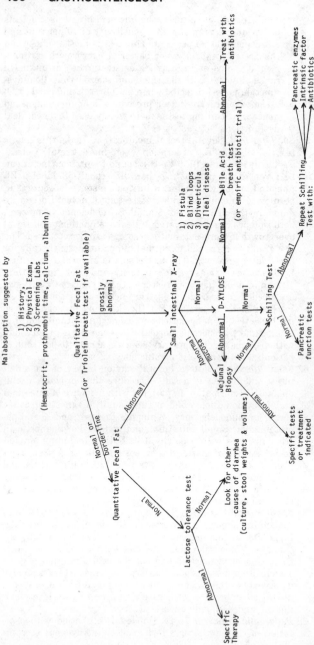

Figure 63–1. Diagnostic evaluation of malabsorption.

and pancreozymin provides the most commonly used test of pancreatic function. Duodenal contents are assayed for volume, bicarbonate, and pancreatic enzymes. The test is cumbersome and, because of the large pancreatic reserve, requires greater than 75 per cent of pancreatic function to be lost before results are abnormal. Imaging procedures such as ultrasound, computed tomography, endoscopic retrograde cholangiopancreatography, and the clinical response to oral pancreatic enzyme supplementation are also used in the evaluation of pancreatic insufficiency.

RECOMMENDED DIAGNOSTIC APPROACH

A. The history, physical examination, and screening laboratory tests (hematocrit, prothrombin time, calcium, and albumin) suggest which patients should undergo specific laboratory testing.
B. A diagnostic principle is to first define specific nutrient malabsorption (fecal fat, d-xylose, Schilling, and carbohydrate tolerance tests) and then to proceed to evaluation of the specific cause of the malabsorption defect (jejunal biopsy, pancreatic function tests, bile acid breath test, and small intestinal x-ray). A flow sheet is outlined in Figure 63–1. The outlined sequence of tests will necessarily be modified if the clinical findings in an individual patient are suggestive of a specific diagnosis.

REFERENCES

1. Greenberger NJ, Isselbacher KJ: Disorders of absorption. *In* Petersdorf RG, et al. (eds.): Harrison's Principles of Internal Medicine. 10th ed. New York, McGraw-Hill, 1983, pp. 1720–1738.

A clearly written overall review of the subject.

2. Gray GM: Maldigestion and malabsorption: Clinical manifestations and specific diagnosis. *In* Sleisenger MH, Fordtran JS (eds.): Gastrointestinal Disease. 3rd ed. Philadelphia, W.B. Saunders Company, 1983, pp. 227–256.

A good review of diagnostic approach and specific tests. Other chapters are referred to for information on specific diseases.

3. Sleisenger MH, Brandborg LL: Malabsorption. *In* Smith LH (ed.): Major Problems in Internal Medicine. Vol. 13. Philadelphia, W.B. Saunders Company, 1977.

A detailed monograph on the subject that emphasizes aspects of pathophysiology.

4. Newcomer AD, Hofmann AF, DiMagno EP, et al.: Triolein breath test. A sensitive and specific test for fat malabsorption. Gastroenterology 76:6–13, 1979.

This breath test compares favorably with fecal fat determination in most situations.

PANCREATITIS

By MICHAEL KIMMEY, M.D.

DEFINITION

A. Acute Pancreatitis

1. Acute pancreatitis is defined clinically by the combination of specific symptoms (most commonly abdominal pain), signs, and laboratory findings (especially hyperamylasemia)—in the absence of other known causes of these findings. Specific laboratory tests such as pancreatic isoamylase and pancreatic selective lipase may eventually allow a more precise definition of acute pancreatitis; however, these tests currently are not widely available.

2. A clinical diagnosis of pancreatitis can be considered definite if all of the following factors are present:

   a. A known risk factor (e.g., alcoholism or gallstones) for pancreatitis

   b. A compatible physical examination

   c. The presence of signs of inflammation (fever, tachycardia, or leukocytosis)

   d. Compatible radiologic studies (abdominal x-ray or ultrasound)

   e. An elevated amylase or lipase level

   f. No other explanation for these findings

If amylase or lipase levels are not elevated but the other factors exist, a diagnosis of pancreatitis can be considered probable. If only risk factors and compatible physical findings are present, pancreatitis is possible.

B. Chronic Pancreatitis. Chronic pancreatitis is also usually diagnosed clinically and is characterized by recurrent abdominal pain. A history of previous episodes of acute pancreatitis is often obtained. Pancreatic functional impairment causing malabsorption and hyperglycemia are important additional findings in chronic pancreatitis. The presence of risk factors (such as alcoholism) and laboratory confirmation of malabsorption are the most useful diagnostic features.

C. Pathology. Pancreatitis may also be defined pathologically. Interstitial edema, leukocytic infiltration, and, if severe, acinar cell disruption with necrosis and hemorrhage are seen histologically in patients with acute pancreatitis. Chronic pancreatitis is characterized by fibrosis, reduced numbers of acini, and ductal calcification. Histologic information is usually not obtained, since biopsy of the pancreas is contraindicated when inflammation is present.

EPIDEMIOLOGY

A. Acute Pancreatitis. The annual incidence of acute pancreatitis is approximately 10 to 30 per 100,000 people. Countries with a higher alcohol consumption have a higher incidence of acute pancreatitis. The numbers of male and female patients are approximately equal.

B. **Chronic Pancreatitis.** The incidence of chronic pancreatitis in the general population is unknown. Estimates vary from 3.5 to 27 per 100,000 population per year. Males exceed females by a ratio of three to one.

DIFFERENTIAL DIAGNOSIS

A. **Other Causes of Abdominal Pain.** Other causes should be considered in patients with abdominal pain.
  1. *Acute Pain.* Peptic ulcer disease, gastritis, cholecystitis, reflux esophagitis, bowel infarction, dissecting aortic aneurysm, and myocardial infarction are the most frequent diagnostic considerations.
  2. *Chronic Pain*
     a. Differential diagnostic considerations in the patient with chronic pancreatitis include other causes of abdominal pain and malabsorption. In addition, pancreatic pseudocyst, abscess, and carcinoma should be considered.
     b. **Hyperamylasemia.** There are numerous causes of hyperamylasemia other than pancreatitis (see Table 64-1).

TABLE 64-1. CAUSES OF HYPERAMYLASEMIA

Pancreatic disease
A. Acute pancreatitis (65-75%)*
B. Chronic pancreatitis
C. Pseudocyst
D. Carcinoma
Disorders of nonpancreatic origin (mechanism known)
A. Renal insufficiency (uncommon; rarely over twice normal)
B. Tumor (lung, ovary, thymoma, prostate)
C. Salivary gland lesions
  1. Mumps (80%)
  2. Calculus
  3. Drugs (phenylbutazone)
D. Macroamylasemia
Diseases of complex origin (mechanism uncertain)
A. Intra-abdominal diseases other than pancreatitis
  1. Perforated peptic ulcer (0-6%)
  2. Intestinal obstruction (20%)
  3. Ruptured ectopic pregnancy
  4. Mesenteric infarction (30%)
  5. Peritonitis (70%)
  6. Acute appendicitis
B. Cerebral trauma
C. Burns and traumatic shock
D. Diabetic ketoacidosis
E. Pneumonia
F. Total parenteral nutrition

*Figures in parentheses refer to the incidence of elevated serum amylase in the specific condition.

B. Causes of Acute Pancreatitis. (See Table 64–2.)

1. ***Alcohol.*** A history of prolonged excessive alcohol consumption is usual. Recurrent episodes and the development of chronic pancreatitis are common. Alcohol is the cause of 50 to 60 per cent of cases of acute pancreatitis in the United States, especially in urban populations.

2. ***Gallstones.*** This is the most common cause of acute pancreatitis in populations with low alcohol consumption (70 per cent of cases in Israel). Recurrence is seen in 50 per cent of patients if the stones are not surgically removed. Chronic pancreatitis rarely develops. Some patients have very high amylase levels

TABLE 64–2. CAUSES OF PANCREATITIS

Acute pancreatitis
A. Alcohol ⎫
B. Gallstones ⎬ 90% of cases
C. Idiopathic ⎭
D. Trauma
E. Postsurgical
F. Drugs
G. Metabolic
   1. Hypertriglyceridemia
   2. Hypercalcemia
H. Hereditary
 I. Ductal manipulation
J. Ductal obstruction
   1. Crohn's disease
   2. Duodenal diverticulum
   3. Pancreatic divisum
   4. Annular pancreas
   5. Afferent loop obstruction (postgastrojejunostomy)
K. Infection
   1. Mumps
   2. Coxsackievirus B
   3. *Mycoplasma* pneumonia
   4. Hepatitis B
   5. *Ascaris lumbricoides*
   6. *Clonorchis sinensis*
L. Miscellaneous
   1. Pregnancy (90% from gallstones)
   2. Penetrating duodenal ulcer
   3. Vasculitis
      a. Systemic lupus erythematosus
      b. Thrombotic thrombocytopenic purpura
      c. Henoch-Schönlein purpura
Chronic pancreatitis
A. Alcohol (75% of cases)
B. Tropical diseases
C. Metabolic
   1. Hypertriglyceridemia
   2. Hypercalcemia
D. Hereditary
E. Traumatic
F. Pancreatic divisum
G. Idiopathic

that seem out of proportion to the degree of pain or illness. Common duct stones are found in only one third of cases, but ultrasound detects coexistent gallbladder stones in over 90 per cent of these patients.

3. **Idiopathic.** No known cause is found in 10 to 20 per cent of cases. Recurrence is seen in about one quarter of patients.

4. **Abdominal Trauma.** Direct or penetrating blows to the epigastrium, often caused by hitting an automobile steering wheel, can cause acute pancreatitis (3 to 5 per cent of cases) and are the most common cause of acute pancreatitis in children. Pseudocysts (2 to 10 per cent) and chronic pancreatitis (3 per cent) may develop. Hyperamylasemia is seen acutely in only 25 per cent of cases of blunt trauma-induced pancreatitis.

5. **Postsurgical.** Postsurgical pancreatitis is seen after surgery near the pancreas (0.8 per cent after gastrectomy, 0.2 to 0.4 per cent of biliary tract surgery). This condition is difficult to diagnose (hyperamylasemia is too nonspecific postoperatively) and has a high mortality (25 to 40 per cent). It also may be seen after cardiopulmonary bypass, perhaps secondary to prolonged ischemia. Pancreatitis after renal transplantation (2 to 7 per cent) is often late (50 per cent after six months) and has a multifactorial origin (drugs, infection, and metabolic conditions).

6. **Drug-Related Pancreatitis.** A definite association has been established between pancreatitis and the use of azathioprine, estrogens (including oral contraceptives), furosemide, sulfonamides, tetracycline, thiazide diuretics, and valproic acid. Associations with other drugs have not been proved. Corticosteroids have not been conclusively shown to be associated with pancreatitis.

7. **Metabolic Disorders**
   a. **Hypertriglyceridemia.** Patients with familial hypertriglyceridemia (usually Frederickson types IV and V) who develop triglyceride levels greater than 2000 mg per dL (often associated with alcohol ingestion, untreated diabetes mellitus, or estrogen therapy) may develop pancreatitis. Amylase levels may be artifactually low. The serum is grossly lipemic with these levels of triglycerides.
   b. **Hypercalcemia.** The incidence of pancreatitis in patients with hyperparathyroidism is probably not significantly greater than in the general population. However, isolated cases of pancreatitis have been reported with other causes of hypercalcemia.

8. **Pancreatic Duct Manipulation.** Hyperamylasemia is seen in up to 50 per cent of patients after endoscopic retrograde cholangiopancreatography. However, only 3 per cent develop clinical pancreatitis.

C. **Causes of Chronic Pancreatitis**
   1. About 75 per cent of cases of chronic pancreatitis are caused by alcohol consumption. Heavy prolonged alcohol use is the rule in these cases. Gallstones rarely cause chronic pancrea-

titis. Several other causes of acute pancreatitis may also lead to chronic disease and are listed in Table 64–2. Approximately 25 per cent of cases remain idiopathic.

CLINICAL MANIFESTATIONS

A. History
  1. The frequencies of various historical and physical findings in patients with acute or chronic pancreatitis are listed in Table 64–3. The presence of risk factors that suggest the cause should be ascertained (see Table 64–1).
  2. Patients with acute pancreatitis usually have a gradual onset of epigastric (70 per cent) continuous (85 per cent) pain that

TABLE 64–3. CLINICAL FINDINGS IN PANCREATITIS*

Acute pancreatitis
A. Symptoms
  1. Abdominal pain (98%)
  2. Vomiting (50%)
  3. Hematemesis (2%)
  4. Mental confusion (25%)
B. Signs
  1. Fever (80%)
  2. Hypertension (40%)
  3. Hypotension (25%)
  4. Abdominal distention (60%)
  5. Pleural effusion (15%)
  6. Ascites (2%)
  7. Grey-Turner's sign (1%)
  8. Cullen's sign (1%)
  9. Necrotic skin nodules (1%)
Chronic pancreatitis
A. Symptoms
  1. Abdominal pain (90%)
  2. Weight loss (95%)
  3. Gastrointestinal bleeding (10%)
B. Signs
  1. Jaundice (25%)
  2. Ascites (2%)
  3. Palpable abdominal mass (5%)
Pseudocyst
A. Symptoms
  1. Abdominal pain (95%)
  2. Nausea or vomiting (60%)
  3. Weight loss greater than 10 pounds (50%)
B. Signs
  1. Fever (20%)
  2. Abdominal mass (50%)
  3. Abdominal tenderness (70%)
  4. Ascites (20%)
  5. Jaundice (10%)

*Figures in parentheses refer to the frequency of the specific finding in patients with definite pancreatitis.

may radiate to the back (30 per cent). Food may exacerbate symptoms, but patients are generally anorectic or vomiting. Factors associated with increased mortality include hypotension, massive fluid requirements, respiratory failure, and hypocalcemia.

3. Over 90 per cent of patients with chronic pancreatitis have abdominal pain. This pain varies from mild continuous epigastric pain that is exacerbated by eating to an intermittent excruciating deep boring type of pain that may radiate to the back. Approximately one third of patients are addicted to narcotics. Steatorrhea and symptoms of glucose intolerance are common. The patients often assume a sitting posture with forward flexion at the waist to reduce pain.

B. Complications of Pancreatitis

1. *Pancreatic Pseudocysts.* These collections of fluid and necrotic debris develop between one and four weeks after an episode of acute pancreatitis in about 5 per cent of cases. A pseudocyst should be suspected if a palpable mass is found on abdominal examination (50 per cent are pseudocysts) and if clinical pancreatitis or hyperamylasemia do not resolve within one week. Clinical features of pseudocysts are listed in Table 64–3.

2. *Pancreatic Abscess.* Abscesses occur in 3 to 10 per cent of cases of acute pancreatitis, especially postsurgical and clinically severe cases. An abscess should be suspected in patients with persistent fever, tachycardia, leukocytosis, and signs of toxicity, especially if deterioration occurs after a period of initial improvement.

LABORATORY EVALUATION

A. Expected Findings

1. *Miscellaneous.* Hematocrit may be elevated as a result of hemoconcentration or decreased secondary to blood loss. Leukocytosis (15,000 to 24,000) is frequent. Hyperglycemia (25 per cent), hypocalcemia (25 per cent), hypertriglyceridemia (10 to 20 per cent), hyperbilirubinemia (10 per cent with bilirubin >4 mg/dl), elevated liver enzymes (60 per cent of gallstone-associated but only 10 per cent of alcohol-associated pancreatitis), and hypoxemia (25 per cent with PO_2 <60) are seen in acute pancreatitis.

2. *Amylase.* The utility of total serum amylase activity in the diagnosis of pancreatitis has been overrated. Approximately 75 per cent of patients with acute pancreatitis have an elevated total amylase level that occurs within 24 hours of onset and returns to normal within three to five days. Severe pancreatitis may be present with a normal serum amylase level. Since 60 per cent of the normal total serum amylase has a salivary gland origin, it is not surprising that many cases with an elevated total amylase concentration are caused

by nonpancreatic disorders. Up to 50 per cent of unselected acutely intoxicated patients may have an elevated total amylase level, but fewer than 20 per cent of these have elevated pancreatic isoamylase levels. Retrospective studies have shown that numerous diagnostic errors occur in this setting because of too much reliance on the total amylase level. Urinary amylase and ratios of amylase to creatinine clearance are nonspecific and add little to the diagnosis.

3. **Lipase.** Serum lipase levels are elevated in about 70 per cent of patients with acute pancreatitis and may be elevated when the serum amylase is normal. New lipase assays may be as specific as pancreatic isoamylase determinations for the diagnosis of pancreatitis.

4. **Pancreatic Function Tests.** Serum amylase and lipase activities are usually normal in chronic pancreatitis. Diagnosis often depends on the demonstration of loss of exocrine function. The secretin stimulation test is the most sensitive test and may give the only abnormal finding in patients with abdominal pain caused by chronic pancreatitis. Approximately 75 per cent of pancreatic function must be lost before the secretin test result is abnormal. Increased stool fat is seen after 90 per cent of pancreatic function has been lost. An abnormal Schilling test result that is corrected by oral administration of pancreatic extract is found in 40 per cent of patients with chronic pancreatitis.

5. **Radiologic Tests.** Plain abdominal x-rays are abnormal (colonic dilatation, obscured psoas margins, small intestinal ileus, increased separation of stomach from colon, pleural effusion, or pancreatic calcification) in 40 to 50 per cent of patients with acute pancreatitis. Pancreatic calcification is seen in about 30 per cent of patients with chronic pancreatitis and generally signifies far advanced disease.

Ultrasound is a very useful diagnostic modality in the management of patients with pancreatitis. It detects pseudocysts (90 per cent accuracy), abscesses, the presence of gallstones, and pancreatic calcifications. If excessive bowel gas is present, computed tomography is a better diagnostic modality. The latter also is better to detect small pancreatic fluid collections and interstitial edema.

6. **Endoscopic Retrograde Cholangiopancreatography (ERCP).** This procedure provides an outline of the pancreatic duct. It is contraindicated in patients with acute pancreatitis and may be dangerous if a pseudocyst is present. It is less sensitive than the secretin test for detecting chronic pancreatitis and is most useful in defining the appropriate approach if surgery is being considered.

RECOMMENDED DIAGNOSTIC APPROACH

A. **Acute Pancreatitis.** Patients with a history and physical examination compatible with acute pancreatitis should have laboratory testing including complete blood count (CBC), glucose, electrolytes, calcium, and amylase. If isoamylases and lipase are available, they should be used to confirm the diagnosis. Abdominal x-rays should be done if pain is severe, primarily to rule out other pathology. Patients without a history of alcohol ingestion should undergo abdominal ultrasonography for the detection of gallstones. Ultrasound is also useful later in the course of illness if a pseudocyst or abscess is suspected.

B. Chronic Pancreatitis. Patients with a history and physical examination compatible with chronic pancreatitis should be tested for hyperglycemia, fat malabsorption (qualitative or quantitative stool fat), and pancreatic calcification on abdominal x-ray. If the diagnosis is still in question, a secretin test, if available, should be performed. If not, a Schilling's test with and without pancreatic extract should be done. Endoscopic retrograde cholangiopancreatography is useful in patients for whom surgery is contemplated or if the diagnosis is unclear and the presence of pancreatic structural anomalies (annular pancreas, pancreatic divisum) is suspected.

REFERENCES

1. Brooks FP: Diseases of the exocrine pancreas. *In* Smith LH (ed.): Major Problems in Internal Medicine. Vol. 20. Philadelphia, W.B. Saunders Company, 1980.

A comprehensive monograph on acute and chronic pancreatitis.

2. Toskes PP, Greenberger NJ: Pancreatitis. Disease-a-Month 29:1–81, 1983.

The best current review of pancreatitis.

3. Soergel KH. Acute pancreatitis. *In* Sleisenger MH, Fordtran JS (eds.): Gastrointestinal Disease. 3rd ed. Philadelphia, W.B. Saunders Company, 1983, pp. 1452–1485.

4. Grendell JH, Cello JP: Chronic pancreatitis. *In* Sleisenger MH, Fordtran JS (eds.): Gastrointestinal Disease. 3rd ed. Philadelphia, W.B. Saunders Company, 1983, pp. 1485–1514.

5. Salt WB, Schenker S: Amylase—its clinical significance: A Review of the literature. Medicine 55:269–288, 1976.

A complete list of causes of elevated amylase with an extensive bibliography.

6. Koehler DR, Eckfeldt JH, Levitt MD: Diagnostic value of routine isoamylase assay of hyperamylasemic serum. Gastroenterology 83:887–890, 1982.

A retrospective study showing the utility of isoamylases in the diagnosis of acute pancreatitis.

7. Bloch RS, Weaver DW, Bouwman DL: Acute alcohol intoxication: Significance of the amylase level. Ann Emerg Med 12:294–296, 1983.

Elevated amylase values in intoxicated patients are frequently caused by the salivary isoenzyme.

GALLBLADDER DISEASE

By ANDREW K. DIEHL, M.D.

DEFINITIONS

Most gallbladder diseases are related to gallstones. They range in severity from asymptomatic cholelithiasis (which may remain undiscovered throughout life) to gallbladder cancer (which frequently is lethal within a year of diagnosis). "Silent gallstones" may be discovered during the work-up of gastrointestinal symptoms caused by other conditions. Roughly one quarter of persons with asymptomatic cholelithiasis eventually develop biliary symptoms. Biliary colic is an attack of right upper quadrant abdominal pain caused by the impaction of a gallstone in the gallbladder infundibulum or in the cystic or common ducts. Acute cholecystitis is characterized by prolonged biliary pain, vomiting, and fever and is associated with severe inflammation of the gallbladder wall. Approximately 95 per cent of attacks are related to cholelithiasis. Approximately 80 per cent of patients with gallbladder cancer have coexisting gallstones.

A. Criteria for Diagnosis

  1. The diagnosis of gallbladder disease is suggested by clinical symptoms and confirmed by radiologic tests. Cholelithiasis usually presents with right upper abdominal or epigastric pain. Gallstones may be demonstrated by oral cholecystography or by ultrasonography. Acute cholecystitis can be distinguished from other causes of abdominal pain with cholescintigraphy (nuclear imaging with technetium-99m iminodiacetic acid derivatives). Failure of the gallbladder to be visualized on cholescintigraphy is indicative of cystic duct obstruction. Cancer of the gallbladder has a nonspecific clinical picture. Radiologic tests cannot reliably detect gallbladder cancer, and the diagnosis is usually made at surgery.

EPIDEMIOLOGY

A. Incidence.
Gallbladder disease is very common. About 6 per cent of adult white women under age 50 years and 15 per cent over age 50 have clinically recognized gallbladder disease; for adult men, the corresponding figures are 1 and 6 per cent. Many more persons with gallstones go undiagnosed. Nearly 500,000 cholecystectomies are done annually in the United States.

B. Risk Factors for Cholesterol Gallstones.
These include female gender, increasing age, obesity, increasing parity, family history, and disease of the terminal ileum. Exogenous estrogen use has been inconsistently associated with gallstones. Recently, low high-density lipoprotein (HDL) cholesterol levels have been associated with cholelithiasis, and ethanol use may reduce the risk of cholesterol gallstone formation.

C. **Risk Factors for Pigment Gallstones.** About 30 per cent of persons with cholelithiasis have pigment gallstones. Risk factors for pigment stones include chronic hemolysis, alcoholic cirrhosis, biliary infection, and age.

D. **Major Ethnic Differences.** At highest risk are native Americans (Eskimos and American Indians); Pima Indian women have a gallstone prevalence of 70 per cent by age 30. Mexican-American women have a prevalence 1.5 to 2 times that of non-Hispanic whites. In contrast, blacks have a reduced rate of gallstone disease.

E. **Gallbladder Cancer.** Gallbladder cancer is strongly related to gallstones and shares most of the same risk factors. Seventy per cent of patients are over age 60. Persons with calcified gallbladder walls or with gallstones 3 cm or larger may have an elevated risk for cancer.

CLINICAL MANIFESTATIONS

A. **"Silent Gallstones."** These are by definition asymptomatic. They may be found incidentally at laparotomy or during the work-up of gastrointestinal symptoms related to other causes.

B. **Nonspecific Symptoms.** Several studies have found that nonspecific symptoms such as indigestion, heartburn, flatulence, and fatty food intolerance are found no more frequently in persons with gallstones than in persons with normal gallbladders.

C. **Biliary Colic.** Biliary colic is usually a severe constant pain that in a minority of patients (10 per cent) fluctuates in intensity. In 30 per cent the pain is maximal at onset, while in 32 per cent maximal intensity is reached within an hour and in the remainder after several hours. Approximately 50 per cent of attacks last 15 minutes to 2 hours, with the other half lasting longer. Pain involves the epigastrium (65 per cent of cases) and the right hypochondrium (50 per cent) and radiates to the right scapula in one third of cases.

D. **Acute Cholecystitis.** When cystic duct obstruction is prolonged, biliary colic can progress to acute cholecystitis. In addition to the symptoms listed earlier, patients with acute cholecystitis may have vomiting (80 per cent) or jaundice (25 per cent). Such symptoms may indicate passage of a gallstone into the common duct. Physical examination reveals fever and right upper quadrant tenderness, and Murphy's sign (tenderness halting inspiration during palpation over the gallbladder) is present in 27 per cent. A distended gallbladder is palpable in one third of cases. Leukocytosis is usually present.

E. **Obstruction Caused by Stones.** In 15 per cent of patients stones pass from the gallbladder to the common duct, in which they can cause obstruction. In such circumstances marked elevations of serum bilirubin and alkaline phosphatase may occur. If stones pass through the common duct, the serum amylase level may become elevated with or without associated pancreatitis. About half of patients with choledocholithiasis develop ascending cholangitis or pancreatitis.

F. **Gallbladder Cancer.** The clinical picture of gallbladder cancer is nonspecific. Common features are abdominal pain (76 per cent), jaundice (38 per cent), nausea and vomiting (32 per cent), and weight loss (39 per cent). Sixteen per cent have presentations that mimic acute cholecystitis.

G. **Differential Diagnosis.** The differential diagnosis of right upper abdominal pain includes pancreatitis, hepatitis, rib fractures, pleurisy, and duodenal ulcer. Unusual causes of right upper quadrant pain include hepatic abscess, Fitz-Hugh-Curtis syndrome, renal stones, and acute appendicitis.

LABORATORY STUDIES

A. **Blood Tests.** In asymptomatic cholelithiasis, serum chemistries (including tests of liver function) are normal. During acute cholecystitis serum transaminase levels may be normal or may rise to two to four times normal. Alkaline phosphatase may double or triple, and the bilirubin level may reach 4 mg per dL. High levels of bilirubin or alkaline phosphatase suggest obstruction of the common bile duct. The leukocyte count is usually mildly elevated in acute cholecystitis (up to 15,000 per cu mm) with a shift to the left. Patients with biliary colic without acute cholecystitis have normal white blood cell counts. No blood test or combination of blood tests is sensitive or specific for gallbladder disease.

B. **Plain Abdominal Radiographs.** About three quarters of gallstones are composed of cholesterol and are radiolucent. Not all pigment stones can be identified on plain radiographs. Hence the sensitivity of the kidney, ureter and bladder (KUB) radiograph is low (about 15 per cent).

C. **Oral Cholecystography (OCG).** This test is very useful for the diagnosis of cholelithiasis in patients who are not jaundiced. Its sensitivity is 90 to 95 per cent, and its specificity is greater than 99 per cent. However, OCG has limitations. Approximately 20 to 25 per cent of studies show nonvisualization of the gallbladder after a single dose of contrast material and require a second administration. Nonvisualization may be caused by prolonged fasting, malabsorption, vomiting, diarrhea, liver disease, or failure to take contrast material. If these causes can be excluded, a nonvisualized gallbladder after two doses indicates a 90 per cent probability of cholelithiasis (this is the predictive value of nonvisualization).

D. **Ultrasonography (US).** Gray-scale and real-time US have supplanted OCG as the initial diagnostic test for gallstones in some centers. US has an accuracy comparable with OCG and is comfortable to the patient, rapidly performed, uses no contrast material, and does not depend on liver or gallbladder function. Stones as small as 1 mm in diameter can be visualized. Only 1 per cent of US studies are technically inadequate. With real-time US, sensitivity is 90 to 95 per cent and specificity is 94 to 98 per cent.

E. **Computed Tomography (CT).** CT offers no advantages over OCG or US for the diagnosis of gallstones and is more expensive.

F. **Cholangiography.** Although US can be used to diagnose dilated biliary ducts, both it and CT have poor sensitivities for the diagnosis of common duct stones. Transhepatic or endoscopic cholangiography provides direct opacification of the biliary tree and facilitates the diagnosis of choledocholithiasis.

G. **Tests for Acute Cholecystitis.** Neither OCG nor US is reliable in distinguishing acute cholelithiasis from other causes of severe upper abdominal pain, although they may support the diagnosis. In acute cholecystitis, the OCG does not visualize. US may reveal gallstones, but obstruction of the cystic duct cannot be confirmed. However, focal tenderness over the gallbladder elicited by the radiologist's examining transducer ("sonographic Murphy's sign") strongly suggests acute cholecystitis. Nuclear technetium scanning (cholescintigraphy) has a sensitivity of 95 per cent and a specificity of 94 per cent for acute cholecystitis. Cholescintigraphy may be of particular value when cholecystitis is only one of several diagnoses being considered and may distinguish acute cholecystitis from pancreatitis. It is more expensive than US.

H. **Tests for Gallbladder Cancer.** Despite progress in diagnostic technology, gallbladder cancer is only infrequently recognized prior to surgical exploration and pathologic studies.

RECOMMENDED DIAGNOSTIC APPROACH

A. **Nonspecific Complaints.** Patients with nonspecific complaints such as indigestion, belching, and fatty food intolerance are not at special risk for gallbladder disease and should not receive tests.

B. **Biliary Colic.** Patients with biliary colic should be followed up with either OCG or US (preferably real-time). If the gallbladder does not visualize on OCG, the presence of gallstones should be confirmed by US.

C. **Acute Cholecystitis.** If acute cholecystitis is suspected in a patient not known to have gallstones, technetium cholescintigraphy or US should be performed. If cholelithiasis has been demonstrated previously in a patient with the clinical picture of acute cholecystitis, cholescintigraphy may be unnecessary unless pancreatitis is also a strong consideration. A white blood count and differential count and serum amylase, bilirubin, and alkaline phosphatase determinations are indicated.

D. **Choledocholithiasis.** If choledocholithiasis is suspected, the patient should be investigated with transhepatic cholangiography or endoscopic retrograde cholangiography.

REFERENCES

1. Berman MD, Carey MC: Biliary tract stones and associated diseases. *In* Stein JH (ed.): Internal Medicine. Boston, Little, Brown & Company, 1983, pp. 227–238.

2. Berk RN, Leopold GR, Fordtran JS: Imaging of the gallbladder. Adv Intern Med 28:387–408, 1983.
3. Krook PM, Allen FH, Bush WH Jr, Malmer G, MacLean MD: Comparison of real-time cholecystosonography and oral cholecystography. Radiology 135:145–148, 1980.
4. Krishnamurthy GT: Acute cholecystitis: The diagnostic role for current imaging tests. West J Med 137:87–94, 1982.

66

IDIOPATHIC INFLAMMATORY BOWEL DISEASE

By CHRISTINA M. SURAWICZ, M.D.

DEFINITION AND GENERAL COMMENTS

There are two types of idiopathic inflammatory bowel disease (IIBD): ulcerative colitis and Crohn's disease. These two diseases are distinct from specific inflammatory bowel diseases, in which a cause can be identified, such as infection, ischemia, or antibiotics.

A. **Ulcerative Colitis.** Ulcerative colitis is a diffuse mucosal inflammation involving the entire length of the colon, including the rectum. The term "ulcerative proctitis" refers to ulcerative colitis that is limited to the distal 10 cm of rectum, with no progression to the rest of the colon over a one-year period.

B. **Crohn's Disease.** (Other names are granulomatous ileocolitis, regional enteritis, and segmental colitis.) Crohn's disease is a segmental and transmural inflammation that can involve any part of the gastrointestinal tract from the mouth to the anus. Fistulae frequently form between the bowel and adjacent organs or between segments of bowel. There are three common conditions: Crohn's colitis (27 per cent of cases; solely colonic involvement), isolated Crohn's disease of the small intestine (28 per cent; also called regional enteritis), and Crohn's ileocolitis (41 per cent; the colon and ileum—usually the terminal ileum—are both involved). Isolated anorectal Crohn's disease occurs in 4 per cent of patients.

C. **Epidemiology.** Both ulcerative colitis and Crohn's disease appear most often in the second through the fourth decades of life. A second peak time of incidence, although less frequent, is in the 60s. Jews have a higher prevalence of idiopathic inflammatory bowel disease than the general population.

D. **Etiology.** No known cause exists for either ulcerative colitis or Crohn's disease. Currently most investigators consider idiopathic inflammatory bowel disease as either an immunologic disease or a disease caused by an infectious agent.

SYMPTOMS AND SIGNS

See Table 66–1.

A. Ulcerative Colitis. The most common symptoms are bloody diarrhea, tenesmus, and crampy abdominal pain. Weight loss, anorexia, fever, nausea, and vomiting may also be present.

B. Crohn's Disease. The symptoms are often the same as in ulcerative colitis. Diarrhea is frequent. Abdominal pain occurs in 55 to 65 per cent of people diagnosed as having Crohn's disease and malnutrition in 12 to 22 per cent. Fever, nausea and vomiting, and anorexia may also be prominent symptoms. Growth retardation may occur in 3 to 5 per cent of children with inflammatory bowel disease.

C. Complications. (See Table 66–2.) Many extraintestinal manifestations occur in both ulcerative colitis and Crohn's disease.

 1. *Arthritis Associated with IIBD.* One of two types of arthritis can occur in association with idiopathic inflammatory bowel disease. This occurs in up to 25 per cent of patients.

 a. In the ankylosing spondylitis type, human leukocyte antigen B27 is often positive. The arthritic flares are unrelated to exacerbations of bowel disease.

 b. The second type is peripheral monoarticular arthritis of the large joints, in which arthritic flares are associated with exacerbation of bowel disease.

 2. *Skin.* Complications include aphthous ulcers in the mouth (5 to 10 per cent), erythema nodosum (3 per cent), and pyoderma gangrenosum (1 to 4 per cent).

 3. *Eye.* Iritis occurs in 5 to 10 per cent of cases.

 4. *Hepatic Problems.* These include pericholangitis, fatty liver, chronic active hepatitis, cirrhosis, and sclerosing cholangitis and occur in 7 per cent of cases.

 5. *Cancer.* A colonic adenocarcinoma can occur, often after more than seven years of disease. It may be multifocal. Dysplasia evident on colonic biopsy is a precursor of cancer.

 6. *Complications in Crohn's Disease.* Some complications occur with Crohn's disease but not with ulcerative colitis. For example, cholesterol gallstones (from bile salt malabsorption) occur in 30 per cent of cases, as well as oxalate renal stones (from fat malabsorption), amyloidosis, and right hydrone-

TABLE 66–1. COMPARISON OF ULCERATIVE COLITIS AND CROHN'S DISEASE

FEATURES	ULCERATIVE COLITIS	CROHN'S DISEASE
Distribution	Colon, diffuse	Entire gastrointestinal tract, segmental, skip areas
Inflammation	Superficial	Transmural
Ulcers	Microscopic	Macroscopic
Strictures	Rare	Common
Rectal sparing	Almost never	Common
Fistulae	Never	Can occur

TABLE 66–2. COMPLICATIONS OF CROHN'S DISEASE BY SITE OF INVOLVEMENT*

	SMALL INTESTINAL DISEASE	ILEOCOLITIS	COLITIS
Rectal bleeding	10	22	46
Rectal fistula	5	21	19
Intestinal obstruction	35	44	17
Internal and cutaneous fistulae	17	34	16
Perianal fistula	14	38	36

*Numbers represent per cent of patients with confirmed Crohn's disease.

phrosis (secondary to an obstruction by a right lower quadrant mass).

PHYSICAL EXAMINATION

A. **General Physical Examination.** Abdominal tenderness, especially in the left lower quadrant or right lower quadrant (with ileocecal involvement in Crohn's disease), is particularly common. Aphthous mouth ulcers are frequent but nonspecific. Some findings strongly suggest Crohn's disease, including right lower quadrant mass (ileocecal involvement) and perianal fistulae (however, fissures or abscesses can occur in ulcerative colitis or in normals). Splenomegaly and clubbing of the nails each occur in 10 per cent of patients.
B. **Rectal Examination.** A nodular rectal mucosa suggests Crohn's disease. Occult blood is often present.
C. **Sigmoidoscopy.** Laxatives in suppository form or enemas should be avoided prior to sigmoidoscopy because they damage the mucosa and cause confusing artifacts.
   1. *Ulcerative Colitis.* In ulcerative colitis the rectum is almost always diffusely involved. Early changes are mucosal edema, in which individual vessels are less visible, or friability, in which the bowel mucosa bleeds spontaneously or when wiped. In more severe cases, there is loss of normal mucosa. Pseudopolyps are islands of normal mucosa surrounded by ulceration; they look like polyps but are only inflamed colonic mucosa.
   2. *Crohn's Disease.* Often the rectum may be normal. Aphthous ulcers may be present, or there may be discrete linear ulcers with normal surrounding mucosa. The mucosal involvement is usually not diffuse.

DIAGNOSTIC TESTING IN INFLAMMATORY BOWEL DISEASE

A. **Laboratory Studies**
   1. *Anemia.* Anemia is common, often microcytic and hypochromic as a result of iron deficiency or chronic disease. In

Crohn's disease the anemia may be macrocytic, owing to a lack of vitamin B_{12}. The white blood cell count may be increased, especially if the patient is severely ill.

2. *Hypokalemia and Hypoalbuminemia.* Hypokalemia occurs when the patient has severe diarrhea. Hypoalbuminemia can occur as a result of albumin loss from the intestines.

3. *Erythrocyte Sedimentation Rate (ESR).* The ESR may be increased, although this is a nonspecific finding.

4. *Superinfection.* Superinfection can occur, usually with *Salmonella.* The physician should look for ova and parasites, send serum for serology to rule out the presence of ameba, and send stool for *Clostridium difficile* toxin determination to rule out pseudomembranous colitis. Stool Hemoccult or guaiac tests are often positive. Stool fat is increased only in Crohn's disease and then only if malabsorption from small intestinal disease is present.

B. **Barium Enema.** A barium enema is indicated if sigmoidoscopy is equivocal or if the extent of disease needs to be documented.

1. *In Ulcerative Colitis.* The barium enema can be normal in mild disease, but diffuse colonic involvement with shallow ulceration is common. In chronic disease a loss of the haustral pattern in the transverse colon or the appearance of a shortened smooth colon can occur on barium enema examination.

2. *In Crohn's Disease.* The barium enema shows skip areas and nondiffuse involvement with discrete ulcers or fistulae. The terminal ileum is contracted or stenosed (string sign). The barium enema can be normal in isolated small intestinal disease.

C. **Colonoscopy.** This method is useful to diagnose the presence of disease, to differentiate ulcerative colitis from Crohn's disease, to assess severity, and to screen ulcerative colitis patients for precancerous dysplasia.

1. *In Ulcerative Colitis.* The findings are the same as in sigmoidoscopy, with diffuse involvement and superficial erosions and friability. Discrete ulcers are rare; the rectum is usually involved.

2. *In Crohn's Disease.* The findings are similar to the findings on sigmoidoscopy, with focal or segmental involvement. Aphthous or linear ulcers with normal surrounding mucosa are classic.

D. **Rectal Biopsy.** This is indicated in most cases and probably is best done by a gastroenterologist. The rectal biopsy can distinguish between ulcerative colitis and Crohn's disease.

1. *Ulcerative Colitis.* The typical biopsy appearance of ulcerative colitis is diffuse mucosal inflammation, with increased numbers of acute and chronic inflammatory cells in the lamina propria and crypt abscesses. Crypt architecture is distorted, and crypt atrophy may be present, even in acute ulcerative colitis.

2. *Crohn's Disease.* The diagnostic hallmark of Crohn's disease is the epithelioid granuloma. This can be seen in up to 30 per cent of rectal biopsies. Epithelioid granulomas are occasionally seen in homosexual men who have proctitis from *Chla-*

mydia trachomatis infection. Diagnostic granulomas can be found in biopsies from normal mucosa. Crypt architecture may be either normal or abnormal in Crohn's disease. Finally, rectal biopsy can diagnose dysplasia, which may indicate development of colon cancer in either ulcerative colitis or Crohn's disease.

DIFFERENTIAL DIAGNOSIS

The following diseases should be considered as alternative diagnoses in patients suspected of having idiopathic inflammatory bowel disease.

A. **Infectious Colitis.** This has a short self-limited course (less than four weeks). Often there has been antecedent foreign travel.
   1. *Bacterial.* Forty to 60 per cent of patients have stool cultures that are positive for *Campylobacter, Salmonella, Shigella, Escherichia coli* (0157), or *Yersinia.*
   2. *Parasitic.* Infection with amebae or schistosomiasis (from endemic areas) is possible.
   3. *In Homosexual Men.* Homosexual men may have other pathogens such as *Gonococcus, Chlamydia trachomatis,* or herpes.

B. **Ischemic Colitis.** This usually occurs in older patients and occasionally in young adults. Splenic flexure involvement is common (watershed area). No good diagnostic methods exist. Sigmoidoscopy should be done.

C. **Pseudomembranous Colitis.** This is often associated with recent use of antibiotics. *Clostridium difficile* organisms and toxin are detected in the stool. Diagnostic pseudomembranes are observed at sigmoidoscopy.

D. **Cancer.** A mass lesion can be detected by proctoscopy, barium enema examination, or colonoscopy.

E. **Radiation Colitis.** This condition occurs after radiation therapy.

RECOMMENDED DIAGNOSTIC APPROACH

A. The following approach is recommended:
   1. The physician should take a good history and do a thorough physical examination with a rectal examination and guaiac test of the stool. Complete blood count, electrolytes and erythrocyte sedimentation rate should be obtained.
   2. If the stool has blood in it the following tests are necessary:
      a. A stool sample should be sent for culture and sensitivity tests (*Campylobacter, Salmonella, Shigella, Yersinia*) and examination for ova and parasites (especially amebae).
      b. Amebic serologies should be done for patients with chronic diarrhea.
      c. Stool should be sent for *C. difficile* culture and toxin to rule out pseudomembranous colitis.

    d. Male homosexuals should have tests done for gonorrhea, *Chlamydia,* syphilis, and herpes virus infection.

3. If cultures are negative, sigmoidoscopy, either rigid or flexible, should be performed without a bowel preparation. A rectal biopsy should be considered, even if the mucosa is normal, to look for evidence of Crohn's disease.

4. If results of sigmoidoscopy are normal or equivocal, barium enema or colonoscopy should be considered plus an upper gastrointestinal series with small bowel follow-through to evaluate the ileum.

REFERENCES

1. Farmer RG, Hawk WA, Turnbull RB: Clinical patterns in Crohn's disease: A statistical study of 615 cases. Gastroenterology 68:627–635, 1975.

Reviews the frequency of the different types of Crohn's disease (colitis, ileocolitis, and isolated small intestinal disease).

2. Kirsner JB, Shorter RG: Recent developments in "nonspecific" inflammatory bowel disease. N Engl J Med 306:775–785, 837–848, 1982.

A good review of most of the recent research; a good background.

3. Surauch CM, Belic L: Rectal biopsy helps to distinguish acute self-limited colitis from idiopathic inflammatory bowel disease. Gastroenterology 86:104–113, 1984.

An excellent discussion of the value of the rectal biopsy in acutely ill patients.

HEMATOLOGY

67

ANEMIA

By RICHARD O. CUMMINS, M.D.

GENERAL COMMENTS

This chapter presents a practical and simplified approach to the diagnosis of the causes of anemia. Few areas of medicine are better suited to systematic diagnostic probing. The clinician, in the interests of time and diagnostic economy, should select the many available tests in an orderly manner.

A. Definition. Anemia is defined as a reduction in red cell mass, measured by a decrease in the concentration of red blood cells or hemoglobin in the peripheral blood, or by both. The clinician most frequently encounters anemia when a patient has a low hematocrit or hemoglobin concentration:

NORMAL RANGES	ADULT MALE	ANEMIA	ADULT FEMALE	ANEMIA
Hematocrit (%)	47 ± 5	<42	42 ± 5	<37
Hemoglobin (g/dL)	16 ± 2	<14	14 ± 2	<12

B. Diagnostic Approaches. Once the anemia has been recognized, one of two approaches has traditionally been recommended. This chapter recommends a combination of these two approaches:

1. *Dynamic Approach.* The clinician must consider whether the anemia is the result of acute blood loss, decreased production, or increased destruction.

    a. **Acute Blood Loss.** The clinician should always ask whether the low hematocrit and hemoglobin are caused by acute blood loss. The physician should measure postural blood pressure changes, check for gastrointestinal bleeding, examine for acute coagulation problems, and consider the need for immediate volume resuscitation.

    b. **Decreased Production.** This is the most frequent cause of anemia.

    c. **Increased Destruction.** This is a diverse but much less frequent group of causes.

2. *Morphologic Approach.* The other approach starts with a review of the red cell indices and bases the diagnostic approach on the size of the red blood cells (mean corpuscular volume, MCV) and the color (mean corpuscular hemoglobin concentration, MCHC). With automated systems, the MCHC

is evaluated by an electronic counter and is generally not reliable. The MCV is the most clinically useful value:

	MCV U^3 (Normal range = 87 ± 7)
Microcytic	< 80 U^3
Macrocytic	>100 U^3
Normocytic	80–100 U^3

HISTORY, SYMPTOMS, AND PHYSICAL FINDINGS

A. **Comment.** The physician must remember that the signs and symptoms of anemia are not simply related to the degree of the anemia but are also the product of its chronicity, the rapidity with which it develops, and the symptoms of any underlying diseases that might be causing or contributing to the anemia.
B. **Subjective Symptoms**
   1. *Symptoms Related to Cardiovascular and Respiratory Function.* Most are due to the cardiovascular and respiratory changes that occur to compensate for the decrease in the red cell mass.
      a. If there has been rapid development of the anemia, there are marked symptoms of hypovolemia and hypoxia. (Early in its course anemia produces increased heart rate, increased diastolic blood pressure, and normal or slightly decreased systolic blood pressure; more severe anemia produces a 25 per cent increase in heart rate, decreased diastolic blood pressure, and a sharp drop in systolic blood pressure.)
      b. If underlying vascular disease is present, anemia may precipitate symptoms of angina, claudication, or cerebral ischemia.
      c. Hemoglobin concentration less than 7.5 g per dL leads to an increase in heart rate and stroke volume that may cause palpitations, pounding pulse, and a hyperdynamic state.
      d. Symptoms and signs of congestive heart failure may develop even in patients who have no underlying vascular disease.
   2. *Other.* Other symptoms include dizziness, headaches, syncope, tinnitus, increased cold sensitivity, indigestion, nausea, and even abdominal pain.
   3. *Fatigue and Weakness.* Although anemia is often associated with fatigue and weakness, it only rarely explains these symptoms when they are the primary complaints.
   4. *Medical History.* The physician should ask about chronic illnesses (involving the liver and kidney), medications, operations (splenectomy or heart valve prostheses), and foreign travel (malaria).

C. Physical Findings

1. *Pallor.* Pallor is the most common finding, but it is affected by so many other factors such as skin thickness and texture, blood flow to the skin, melanin concentration, and jaundice that it is almost useless as an indication. As a guideline, if skin creases are as pale as the surrounding skin, the hemoglobin concentration is less than 7 g per dL.

2. *Other.* Other findings include increased heart rate, wide pulse pressure, dynamic precordium, systolic ejection murmurs, and splenomegaly.

3. *Underlying Diseases.* Often the physical findings are dominated by the disease that is causing the anemia rather than by the anemia itself, as with arthritic changes, hepatomegaly, lymphadenopathy, jaundice, dark urine, and the physical changes of various endocrinopathies.

4. *Platelets and Coagulation Factors.* Acute and chronic causes that lead to anemia may also affect platelets and coagulation factors so that petechiae, hemorrhages under the skin and mucous membranes, and gastrointestinal bleeding may occur.

EPIDEMIOLOGY

A. **Race and Ethnic Groups.** This feature can supply some diagnostic direction.

1. *Blacks.* Sickle cell disease is common among blacks.

2. *Scandinavians.* Pernicious anemia occurs often in Scandinavians.

3. *Asians.* Thalassemias are common in Asians.

4. *Family History.* There are several congenital abnormalities of the red cell membrane that lead to hemolytic anemia (spherocytosis).

5. *Italy and the Mediterranean.* Thalassemia is common in this area.

B. **Sex**

1. *Female.* Menstruating women are chronically close to an iron-deficient state.

2. *Male.* Occult gastrointestinal blood loss is the most frequent cause of anemia in men.

RECOMMENDED DIAGNOSTIC APPROACH

(See Tables 67–1 to 67–6.)

This chapter does not supply the details of all the tests needed to confirm a specific diagnosis (such as to determine which cause of malabsorption produced the B_{12}-deficiency anemia). Instead it takes the clinician reasonably far down initial diagnostic pathways. Many end points in the tables still need to be pursued (such as the immunohemolytic anemias). The tables encourage clinicians to readily pursue even minor decreases in hematocrit and hemoglobin but to do so systematically and economically.

A. **Overview.** It must always be remembered that several processes can be intermixed. For example, patients with anemia, regardless of the cause, can develop gastrointestinal bleeding to further drop the red cell mass. A woman with hypothyroidism and an anemia of endocrine failure can still develop iron deficiency anemia from the menorrhagia of the hypothyroidism.

B. **Step One: Think Again of Acute Blood Loss.** The physician should recheck blood pressures, stool for blood, and consider placing a nasogastric tube. Acute blood loss may cause equal decreases in red cell mass and plasma volume, so the hematocrit may be only mildly decreased. In addition, some of the later recommended tests may be misleading.

1. *Early Blood Loss.* This causes increased reticulocytosis until iron stores are lost; only then does the reticulocyte count decrease.

2. *Macrocytic Anemia.* Macrocytic anemia may be present with early blood loss as more young large red blood cells exit the marrow (MCV > 100 U³).

3. *Blood-Urea Nitrogen (BUN).* BUN may increase because of decreased renal blood flow from the blood loss and digested blood proteins from gastrointestinal bleeding. This falsely suggests anemia caused by uremia.

4. *Extravasated Blood.* Blood extravasated into tissues (as after femoral fracture) can cause increased unconjugated bilirubin as hemoglobin breaks down, thus falsely suggesting hemolytic anemias.

C. **Step Two: Get the Reticulocyte Count.** The reticulocyte count is the single most useful test, from which the overall diagnostic approach branches. The physician should use the corrected reticulocyte index (reticulocyte production index, RPI):

$$\text{reticulocyte index} = \text{reticulocyte \%} \times \left[\frac{\text{patient's hematocrit}}{45 \text{ ("normal" hematocrit)}} \right] {}^{*}$$

$$\times \frac{1}{(1.5 \text{ to } 3)} {}^{\dagger}$$

D. **Step Three: Get Red Blood Cell Indexes.** Very precise measurements of these indexes are now widely available with automated red blood cell counting devices. The mean red cell volume (MCV) is the most useful measurement and broadly classifies the anemias as microcytic, macrocytic, or normocytic.

---

*This corrects for the reduction in the circulating red blood cell mass.

†This corrects for the premature entrance of reticulocytes into the circulation, which then take two to three days to lose the staining reticulum (normally it takes one day). Clinicians should always make this correction if normoblasts are noted in the peripheral smear.

E. **Step Four: Examine the Peripheral Smear.** Clinicians should develop the ability to examine the peripheral smear. Laboratory technicians prepare the stained smear to count the leukocytes and often fail to evaluate the red blood cells. Sometimes diagnostic red blood cell changes are noted. (See Table 67–6).

1. *Anisocytosis.* Red blood cells have variation in size. This is noted in hemolytic anemias and hypersplenism.

2. *Spherocytes.* These are spherical red blood cells that appear solid without the normal central pallor.

3. *Elliptocytes (Ovalocytes).* These are red blood cells that have an elliptical, oval, or cigar shape. The normal value is <1 per cent; patients with microcytic and macrocytic anemias have up to 10 per cent, while patients with hereditary elliptocytosis have > 20 per cent.

4. *Stomatocytes.* These are red blood cells with a slitlike central area rather than the normal round central pallor. They are noted in alcoholic cirrhosis, general liver disease, acute alcoholism, and as a hereditary problem.

5. *Target Cells.* The red blood cell looks like a target, with hemoglobin deposited in the center forming the target. Target cells are noted in chronic disease and the hemoglobinopathies.

6. *Teardrop Cells.* The red blood cells look like typical teardrops. These are noted in myelophthisis and the thalassemias.

7. *Acanthocytes (Spur Cells).* These are red blood cells with thorny projections on the surface, like underwater mines. They are noted in traumatic or hypersplenic hemolysis, liver and kidney disease, and abetalipoproteinemia.

8. *Fragmented Red Blood Cells.* These suggest intravascular coagulation, hemolytic transfusion reactions, and hemolysis caused by cardiac prostheses or vascular disease.

9. *Sickle Cells.* These appear, as the name suggests, with pointed ends on crescent-shaped red blood cells. They are noted in sickle cell anemia, both homozygous and heterozygous.

10. *Poikilocytosis.* This is a general term for variations in the shape of red blood cells. It is noted in leukemia, toxic states, hemoglobinopathies, microangiopathic anemia, macrocytic anemias, extramedullary hematopoiesis, and all anemias with accelerated erythrocyte production.

F. **Step Five: Refer to the Tables.** At this point in the diagnostic approach, the clinician knows the hematocrit, the hemoglobin, the reticulocyte count, abnormalities on the peripheral smear, and the red blood cell indexes. A quick reference to Table 67–1 should allow the clinician to classify the anemia into one of four categories. These categories determine the next steps in the diagnostic work-up:

1. *Decreased Production or Microcytic Anemias.* Iron studies are done. See Table 67–2 for further work-up.

2. *Decreased Production or Macrocytic Anemias.* Serum folate and vitamin B_{12} levels are ordered. See Table 67–3 for further work-up.

3. *Decreased Production or Normocytic Anemia.* Bone marrow aspirate and biopsy are performed. The reader should note from

Text continued on page 511

TABLE 67–1. INITIAL STEPS AND CLASSIFICATIONS IN THE DIAGNOSTIC APPROACH TO ANEMIA

```
Sex ─── Male ──── yes ── Hct < 42%
                          and
                          Hgb < 14?
         │                           ──── yes ── Anemia
         └── Female ── yes ── Hct < 37%        │
                              and               │
                              Hgb < 12?         │
                                                ▼
                                          Step 1
                                          Evaluate for ── yes ── Treat appropriately
                                          acute blood loss
                                                │
                                                │ no
                                                ▼
                                          Step 2
                                          Reticulocyte
                                          production
                                          index
                                          ╱        ╲
                              Decreased          Increased
                              or normal
                                ╱                    ╲
                        Step 4                    Obtain serum ── Decreased ── Probable ── To
                        Obtain RBC                haptoglobin               hemolytic    Table 68–5
                        indexes                                             anemia
                          │
                          │
                        Step 3
                        Examine
                        peripheral
                        smear
```

MCV < 80
MCHC < 32 ── Decreased production/ microcytic anemia ── To Table 68–2

MCV > 100
MCHC: 32–36 ── Decreased production/ macrocytic anemias ── To Table 68–3

MCV: 80–100
MCHC: 32–36 ── Decreased production/ normocytic anemias ── To Table 68–4

TABLE 67–2. DIAGNOSTIC APPROACH TO DECREASED PRODUCTION AND MICROCYTIC ANEMIAS

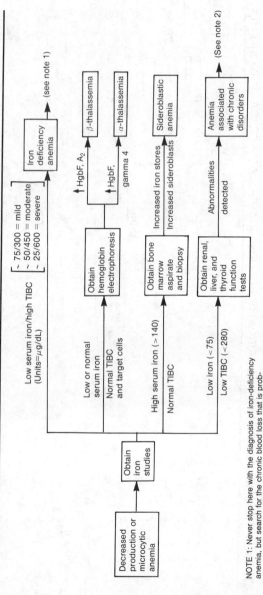

NOTE 1: Never stop here with the diagnosis of iron-deficiency anemia, but search for the chronic blood loss that is probably causing the anemia (menstruation or benign or malignant gastrointestinal disorders).

NOTE 2: More often these diseases are normocytic rather than microcytic. See Table 67–4 for more detail.

TABLE 67–3. DIAGNOSTIC APPROACH TO DECREASED PRODUCTION AND MACROCYTIC ANEMIAS

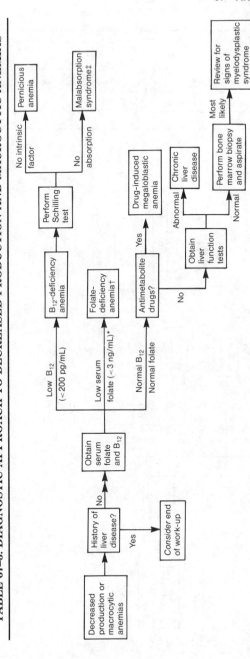

*If hospitalization or other means has improved the patient's diet for several days before serum folate is determined, measure RBC folate levels instead, since RBC levels more accurately reflect prehospital folate state.

†Once folate-deficiency anemia is diagnosed, further work-up is needed to determine the cause. Possibilities include poor intake, malabsorption, increased requirements, and impaired metabolism.

‡See Chapter on Malabsorption Syndromes.

TABLE 67–4. DIAGNOSTIC APPROACH TO DECREASED PRODUCTION AND NORMOCYTIC ANEMIAS

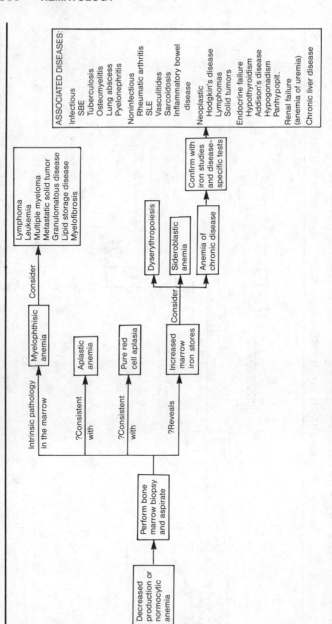

TABLE 67–5. DIAGNOSTIC APPROACH TO PROBABLE HEMOLYTIC ANEMIAS (INCREASED RETICULOCYTES WITH DECREASED HAPTOGLOBIN)

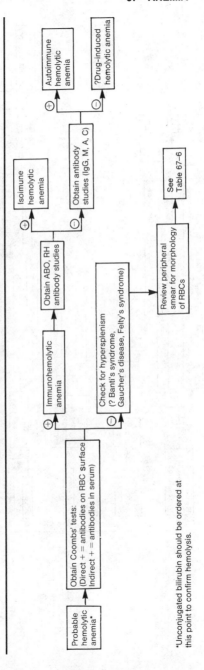

*Unconjugated bilirubin should be ordered at this point to confirm hemolysis.

TABLE 67–6. EVALUATION OF HEMOLYTIC ANEMIAS BY REVIEW OF PERIPHERAL SMEAR

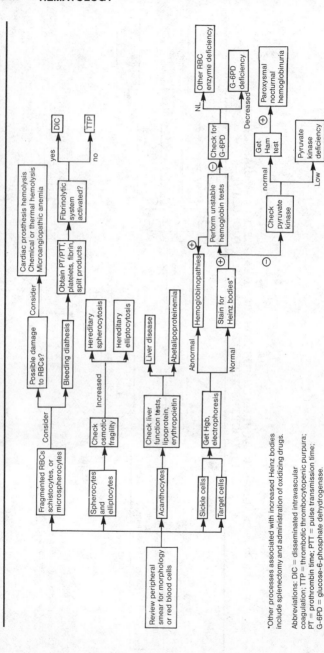

*Other processes associated with increased Heinz bodies include splenectomy and administration of oxidizing drugs.

Abbreviations: DIC = disseminated intravascular coagulation; TTP = thrombotic thrombocytopenic purpura; PT = prothrombin time; PTT = pulse transmission time; G-6PD = glucose-6-phosphate dehydrogenase.

the tables that bone marrow aspirates and biopsies are not required in all work-ups for anemia. See Table 67–4.

4. **Increased Destruction.** The red blood cell indexes are usually normocytic, and the peripheral smear may have already shown diagnostic abnormalities. The next step is to obtain both a serum haptoglobin level, which documents the presence of hemolysis, and the Coombs' antiglobulin test. See Table 67–4 for further work-up.

G. **Subsequent Steps.** Tables 67–5 and 67–6 guide the clinician to a diagnosis for most anemias encountered in general medicine. Further work-up and confirmatory steps should be determined in consultation with hematologists and other specialists.

REFERENCES

1. Liu PI: Diagnostic tests for erythrocytic disorders. *In* Liu PI (ed.): The Blue Book of Diagnostic Tests. Philadelphia, W. B. Saunders Company, in press.

An excellent new work, with tables that were modified to provide the diagnostic approach tables for this chapter.

2. Bunn HF: Anemia. *In* Petersdorf RG, Adams RD, Braunwald E, Isselbacher KJ, Martin JB, Wilson JD (eds.): Harrison's Principles of Internal Medicine. 10th ed. New York, McGraw-Hill, 1983, pp. 282–292.

A thoughtful general chapter for the clinician.

3. Henry JB (ed.): Clinical Diagnosis and Management by Laboratory Methods. 17th ed. Philadelphia, W. B. Saunders Company, 1983.

An up-to-date discussion of laboratory methods used to evaluate patients with anemia.

68

LEUKEMIAS

By DAVID H. BOLDT, M.D.

DEFINITION

A. **General.** Leukemias are malignant disorders characterized by uncontrolled proliferation of bone marrow cells. An important hallmark of leukemias is maturation arrest. This means that the leukemia cells have morphologic, cytochemical, or other features that allow them to be classified as immature blood cell precursors arrested at certain stages of differentiation. Clinical findings in leukemia result from tendencies of the malignant cells to accumulate in bone marrow and peripheral blood and to infiltrate organs. Although there are many subtypes of leukemias, four prototypes are considered here: acute nonlymphocytic leukemia (ANLL), acute lymphocytic leukemia (ALL), chronic myelocytic leukemia (CML), and chronic lymphocytic leukemia (CLL).

The prompt and precise diagnosis of leukemia, especially acute leukemia, is essential. In the past two decades great progress has been made in management of these devastating illnesses. Given optimal current therapy more than half of children with ALL will be long-term survivors and probably will be cured. The majority (75 per cent) of patients with ANLL will achieve temporary remissions of the disease, and 15 to 20 per cent may be long-term (five year) survivors. Emerging new therapies such as bone marrow transplantation may soon improve these results. For these reasons it is imperative that an experienced hematologist participate in the early evaluation and management of all patients with suspected diagnoses of leukemia.

B. **Criteria for Diagnosis.** Diagnosis of leukemia, although frequently inferred from clinical and peripheral blood findings, requires bone marrow examination. Frequently, sophisticated cytochemical, cytogenetic, and cell surface marker analyses also are required for precise diagnosis and classification.

1. *ANLL.* ANLL is diagnosed when bone marrow is infiltrated by ≥30 per cent myeloblasts. The presence in blast cells of Auer rods is pathognomonic for ANLL. Auer rods may be observed with diligent searching in about half the cases. Cytochemical features of myeloblasts useful in diagnosis include positive staining for peroxidase, Sudan black B, and specific or nonspecific esterases. Myeloblasts are negative when stained by periodic acid-Schiff (PAS) reagent. ANLL can be divided into six subtypes (designated M1 to M6) based on morphologic and cytochemical features of the blast cells according to the French-American-British (FAB) classification. To date, the FAB classification has not been useful in assessment of prognosis or choice of therapy. Subtype M3, acute promyelocytic leukemia (5 per cent of ANLL), in which leukemia cells are hypergranular with morphologic features of promyelocytes, is noteworthy because of the frequent occurrence of disseminated intravascular coagulation and associated bleeding diathesis.

2. *ALL.* ALL is diagnosed when bone marrow is infiltrated by ≥30 per cent lymphoblasts. Lymphoblasts may display coarse granular PAS positively, but they are negative by other cytochemical tests, including Sudan black B, peroxidase, and esterases. They are usually (> 90 per cent) positive for the enzyme terminal deoxynucleotidyl transferase (TDT) and may express lymphocyte differentiation markers. Most notable is the presence of the common ALL antigen (CALLA) on surfaces of lymphoblasts in 50 to 75 per cent of all patients. FAB classification of ALL denotes three subtypes, termed L1 to L3, and does have prognostic utility.

3. *CML.* CML differs from other leukemias in that diagnosis is not based on identification of a predominance of one specific cell type in bone marrow or blood. Typically, CML is mani-

fested by the peripheral blood and bone marrow showing
excessive granulocyte production. Leukocytosis is profound
(average white blood cell count [WBC] is 75,000). All stages
of granulocyte development from blast to mature polymorphonuclear leukocyte are expanded in bone marrow and all are
present in peripheral blood. Confirmatory findings include
splenomegaly, a decreased leukocyte alkaline phosphatase
(LAP) score in peripheral cells, and basophilia. The diagnosis
of CML is established conclusively by demonstrating the
Philadelphia chromosome in bone marrow cells. However, 10
to 15 per cent of patients have characteristic clinical and
laboratory findings but lack the Philadelphia chromosome.
4. **CLL.** CLL is diagnosed by documenting an absolute peripheral
blood lymphocytosis ≥15,000 per μL and lymphocytic marrow
infiltration of ≥40 per cent. CLL cells have morphologic
characteristics of mature small lymphocytes. In 95 per cent
of cases the lymphocytes have monoclonal B cell surface
markers, that is, surface immunoglobulin with all kappa or
all lambda light chains. In 5 per cent of cases T cell surface
markers can be found.

EPIDEMIOLOGY

A. **Demographic Features**
1. **ANLL.** ANLL represents 40 per cent of all leukemias. It occurs
in all age groups but is predominantly a disease of adults.
Whereas 85 per cent of acute leukemias in individuals over
age 25 are ANLL, only 18 per cent in younger individuals
are ANLL. There is a slight predominance of ANLL in males.
2. **ALL.** ALL makes up 20 per cent of all leukemias and is the
predominant leukemia of children. Its incidence peaks between ages two and six. Only 15 per cent of adult acute
leukemias are ALL. There is a slight predominance of ALL
in males.
3. **CML.** CML makes up 15 per cent of all leukemias. Median
age of onset is the fourth decade. There is no apparent
predilection by sex.
4. **CLL.** CLL represents 25 per cent of all leukemias in the
Western hemisphere. It is uncommon in oriental populations.
Median age of onset is the sixth and seventh decades. CLL
does not occur in children and adolescents and is increasingly
rare below the age of 35. There is a 2:1 male-to-female
predominance.
B. **Etiologic Considerations**
1. **Associated Factors.** Although recent evidence strongly links
an RNA retrovirus, human T cell leukemia virus (HTLV), to
the development of one uncommon type of leukemia, adult T
cell leukemia, in general the cause of leukemia is unknown.
A variety of factors, including heredity, ionizing radiation,
drugs and chemicals, and other hematologic disorders are
associated with development of leukemia in some instances.

2. *In Siblings.* Siblings of patients with leukemia have an increased risk (approximately fourfold) of developing the disease. This risk is particularly striking in the case of identical twins, in which there is a 20 per cent concordance of ALL under age ten. Certain hereditary diseases such as trisomy 21, Bloom's syndrome, Fanconi's anemia, and ataxia-telangiectasia are associated with increased risk of leukemia.

3. *Ionizing Radiation.* Ionizing radiation is a well-documented leukemogenic agent in man. Japanese survivors of atomic bombings have manifested dose-related increased incidences of ANLL, ALL, and CML but not of CLL. Exposure to therapeutic x-rays also carries a markedly increased risk of leukemia (for radiologists working in the era before adequate shielding; patients with ankylosing spondylitis treated with spinal radiation; and individuals who received thymic irradiation during infancy). The incidence of radiation-induced leukemia appears to peak at five to seven years after exposure, but increased incidence rates may be maintained for over two decades.

4. *Drugs and Chemicals.* Drugs and chemicals associated with increased incidences of leukemia include benzene, toluene, cancer chemotherapeutic agents, chloramphenicol, and phenylbutazone. The most common type of associated leukemia has been ANLL. It is likely that the increased incidence of ANLL now recognized in patients treated for Hodgkin's disease (as high as 5 to 10 per cent of patients surviving after combination chemotherapy), multiple myeloma (actuarial risk as high as 20 per cent five years after diagnosis), and polycythemia vera (15 per cent) may represent therapy-associated leukemia.

5. *Association with Certain Hematologic Diseases.* Certain hematologic diseases are associated with high risk for subsequent development of leukemia. These include refractory anemia with excess blast cells (30 per cent), myeloproliferative syndromes (15 per cent), acquired sideroblastic anemia (5 to 10 per cent), and aplastic anemia (5 per cent).

CLINICAL MANIFESTATIONS

A. Acute Leukemias

1. *Bone Marrow Failure.* Patients with acute leukemias most commonly have signs and symptoms of bone marrow failure. Bone marrow infiltration by leukemia cells leads to decreased or absent production of normal blood cells. Therefore, patients develop the following conditions:

   a. **Anemia.** Anemia occurs in 98 per cent of cases. Characteristic clinical findings include easy fatigability, weakness, orthostasis, and pallor.

   b. **Granulocytopenia.** This occurs in 75 per cent of cases. About one third of patients with acute leukemia have elevated total WBC, one third have normal WBC, and one third have low WBC. Because in patients with normal or high WBC blasts usually make up the majority of the cells, absolute granulocytopenia is seen in most patients. Patients with granulocytopenia, especially with absolute granulocyte counts <500 per µL, are susceptible to infection. These individuals may have fever and signs referrable to local or systemic infection.

c. **Thrombocytopenia.** Thrombocytopenia occurs in 80 to 90 per cent of cases. Characteristic clinical findings include petechiae, purpura, and mucous membrane bleeding. Individuals with platelet counts <20,000 per µL are at risk for developing spontaneous intracranial hemorrhage.

2. *Organ Infiltration.* Signs and symptoms also occur because of organ infiltration by leukemia cells. Leukemia cells can infiltrate virtually any tissue. Clinical findings seen commonly in acute leukemias because of organ infiltration include hepatosplenomegaly and lymphadenopathy (70 per cent of ALL patients; 30 to 40 per cent of ANLL); nodular skin lesions (5 per cent of ALL; 10 per cent of ANLL); bone pain and arthralgias (50 per cent of ALL); gingival hypertrophy (characteristic of monocytic ANLL variants); and headaches, blurred vision, papilledema, seizures, or cranial nerve dysfunction caused by meningeal leukemia (5 to 10 per cent of ALL; 1 per cent of ANLL).

3. *Disseminated Intravascular Coagulation (DIC).* DIC is seen frequently in association with the acute promyelocytic variant of ANLL.

4. *Time Course.* In most patients with acute leukemia, the time course of illness is short, progressing rapidly over days to weeks. By contrast, in elderly patients disease onset may be more insidious, occurring over many months, with the so-called "smoldering" acute leukemia.

B. **Chronic Leukemias**

1. *Insidious Onset.* Unlike acute leukemias, chronic leukemias are most likely to develop insidiously. As a result the diagnosis of CML or CLL may be made incidentally during evaluation of unrelated complaints or during routine medical examinations (30 per cent of CLL and 10 per cent of CML diagnoses may be incidental).

2. *Nonspecific Complaints.* Patients with CML frequently have nonspecific complaints such as easy fatigability, fever, and weight loss. An enlarged spleen is found in 90 per cent of patients and frequently may produce symptoms such as left upper quadrant pain or early satiety. Bone pain is a frequent complaint (30 to 40 per cent of cases), and sternal tenderness can often be elicited. Infection is not a problem because mature granulocytes are present in markedly increased numbers. Platelets are usually normal or increased in numbers, and bleeding is uncommon despite platelet dysfunction in most patients.

3. *Clinical Course of CML.* The clinical course of CML is unique among all the leukemias. Following a median three to four years of stable disease, virtually all patients enter a phase of

accelerated leukemia activity. This phase has been termed *blast crisis, metamorphosis,* or *transformation.* The clinical picture may resemble acute leukemia or, alternatively, progressive bone marrow failure may ensue. Therapy for CML in the accelerated phase is ineffective, and median survival from onset of this stage is six to eight months.

4. **Clinical Features of CLL.** Clinical features most commonly reflect organ involvement by leukemia cells. The Rai staging system provides a useful clinical framework for assessing prognosis. An outline of this classification follows:

Stage 0: peripheral blood ($\geq$15,000 per μL) and bone marrow lymphocytosis ($\geq$40 per cent); median survival 12.5 years; 20 per cent of patients

Stage I: above lymphocytosis plus lymphadenopathy; median survival 6 to 8 years; 25 per cent of patients

Stage II: above lymphocytosis plus splenomegaly $\pm$ lymphadenopathy; median survival 4 to 5 years; 25 per cent of patients

Stages III and IV: above lymphocytosis $\pm$ lymphadenopathy $\pm$ splenomegaly but with anemia (hemoglobin <12 g per cent) and/or thrombocytopenia (platelets <100,000 per μL); median survival 1.5 years; 30 per cent of patients

5. **Immunologic Phenomena in CLL.** CLL is unique in its association with a variety of immunologic phenomena. These include hypogammaglobulinemia (50 per cent of cases), autoimmune hemolytic anemia (10 to 25 per cent), and immune thrombocytopenia.

DIFFERENTIAL DIAGNOSIS

A. **Leukemia vs. Leukemoid Reactions.** The myeloid leukemias (ANLL and CML) must be distinguished from exuberant reactive leukocytoses termed *leukemoid reactions.* Leukemoid reactions are caused most commonly by infections or malignancies and less commonly by immunologic diseases. Total leukocyte counts >50,000 per μL or blasts in the peripheral blood, or both, strongly suggest leukemia. Features that favor a diagnosis of CML include low LAP score, basophilia, and elevated serum vitamin B_{12} levels. Bone marrow morphology and cytogenetics are diagnostic.

B. **Leukemia vs. Other Malignancies.** Metastatic carcinoma or myelofibrosis invading bone marrow may provoke a leukoerythroblastic peripheral blood picture with anemia, leukocytosis, immature leukocytes, and nucleated erythrocytes. Clinically affected patients may experience weight loss and fatigue similar to those of leukemia patients. Definitive diagnosis is established by bone marrow biopsy. Rarely a leukoerythroblastic picture may be produced by infection in the bone marrow.

C. **ALL vs. Benign Causes of Lymphocytosis and Lymphadenopathy.** A number of diseases of childhood and adolescence involve peripheral blood lymphocytosis with or without lymphadenopathy and must be distinguished from ALL. Careful examination of peripheral smears usually distinguishes atypical lymphocytes from the lymphoblasts of ALL. In other cases the occurrence of characteristic serologic findings is diagnostic. Differential diagnosis includes consideration of infectious mononucleosis, cytomegalovirus infection, toxoplasmosis, acute infectious lymphocytosis, other viral infections, immunologic disorders such as lupus erythematosus, and juvenile rheumatoid arthritis.

D. CLL vs. Other Lymphoid Malignancies. In middle-aged to elderly adults a peripheral blood lymphocytosis in which the cells resemble normal mature lymphocytes is considered CLL until proved otherwise. The chief consideration of differential diagnosis is to distinguish CLL from other lymphoid malignancies such as hairy cell leukemia, lymphosarcoma cell leukemia, Waldenström's macroglobulinemia, and the Sézary syndrome.

E. Leukemia vs. Other Hematologic Disorders. In as many as 50 per cent of patients with ALL, leukemia may appear as pancytopenia with few or no blasts in the peripheral blood. In this situation leukemia must be differentiated from other hematologic causes of pancytopenia. Disorders include aplastic anemia, myelofibrosis, refractory anemia with excess blasts, sideroblastic anemia, and deficiencies of vitamin B_{12} or folic acid. Bone marrow examination should be readily diagnostic.

LABORATORY TESTS

A. Complete Blood Count, Platelets, and Examination of Peripheral Smear

B. Bone Marrow Aspiration and Biopsy. Cytogenetic analysis should be included. Cultures should be performed when infection is considered possible.

C. Cytochemical Tests on Blood or Bone Marrow Smears. These include:

1. Peroxidase: ANLL
2. Sudan black B: ANLL
3. Specific and nonspecific enterases: ANLL
4. Periodic acid–Schiff: ALL
5. Terminal deoxynucleotidyl transferase (TDT): ALL
6. Leukocyte alkaline phosphatase: CML

D. Surface Markers and Other Specialized Tests

1. Lymphocyte markers: common ALL antigen (CALLA) and T and B cell markers
2. Myeloid differentiation antigens
3. Lysozyme
4. DNA restriction enzyme analyses

E. Blood Chemistry and Miscellaneous Laboratory Tests
   1. Metabolic Derangements. A variety of metabolic derangements may occur in association with leukemia. These include

hyperuricemia, hyperkalemia, hypokalemia, hypercalcemia, hypocalcemia, and hypophosphatemia.

2. *Coagulation Screen for DIC.* Prothrombin time, partial thromboplastin time, thrombin time, fibrinogen, and fibrinogen-fibrin degradation products should be examined.

3. *CLL*
   a. Serum protein electrophoresis indicates hypogammaglobulinemia. There is a monoclonal spike in 15 per cent of cases.
   b. Coombs' test is used to evaluate autoimmune hemolytic anemia.
   c. Reticulocyte count also is used to study autoimmune hemolytic anemia.

4. *Lumbar Puncture in ALL.* This is used to evaluate meningeal leukemia.

RECOMMENDED DIAGNOSTIC APPROACH

As a general rule, the critical diagnostic decisions are first to diagnose acute leukemia and second to differentiate ALL from ANLL. This is because therapy must be instituted promptly, and the managements and prognoses for these two leukemias are quite different.

A. **Morphology.** Careful morphologic assessment of peripheral blood smears and bone marrow preparations establishes a diagnosis of acute leukemia in virtually all cases, but the differentiation between ALL and ANLL may be more difficult.

B. **Morphologically Undifferentiated Acute Leukemia.** Approximately 25 to 30 per cent of acute leukemia cases remain morphologically undifferentiated even after review by experienced hematologists. Therefore, additional tests are needed to distinguish between ALL and ANLL.

1. *Cytochemistry Including TDT Determination.* Ninety per cent of ALL is positive for TDT and only 10 per cent for ANLL. Most undifferentiated acute leukemias are resolved by cytochemical tests.

2. *Serum or Urine Lysozyme.* This is positive in monocytic variants of ANLL.

3. *Analysis for CALLA.* This is positive in 50 to 75 per cent of ALL and negative in ANLL; availability is limited.

4. *Analyses for Expression of Other Lymphoid or Myeloid Differentiation Antigens.* Availability is limited.

5. *DNA Restriction Endonuclease Analyses.* These are available for research only.

C. **Diagnosis of Chronic Leukemias.** This does not have the same urgency as diagnosis of acute leukemias. Nonetheless, precise diagnosis should be made promptly. The differentiation of CLL from other lymphoid leukemias is beyond the scope of this manual. Differentiation of CML from leukemoid reactions is a frequently encountered clinical problem and is discussed earlier under Differential Diagnosis. The presence of the Philadelphia chromosome is diagnostic of CML.

REFERENCES

1. Boggs DR, Wintrobe MM, Cartwright GR: The acute leukemias: Analysis of 322 cases and review of the literature. Medicine 41:163–225, 1962.
2. Gallo RC, et al.: Association of the human type C retrovirus with a subset of adult T-cell cancers. Cancer Res 43:3892–3899, 1983.
3. Gehan EA, Smith TL, Freireich EJ, Bodey G, Rodriguez V, Speer J, McCredie K: Prognostic factors in acute leukemia. Semin Oncol 3:271–282, 1976.
4. Henderson ES: Acute leukemia—general considerations. *In* Williams WJ, Beutler E, Erslev AJ, Lichtman MA (eds.): Hematology. 3rd ed. New York, McGraw-Hill, 1983, pp. 221–239.
5. Koeffler HP, Golde DW: Chronic myelogenous leukemia—new concepts. N Engl J Med 304:1201–1209, 1269–1274, 1981.
6. Korsmeyer SJ, et al.: Immunoglobulin gene rearrangement and cell surface antigen expression in acute lymphocytic leukemias of T cell and B cell precursor origins. J Clin Invest 71:301–313, 1983.
7. Rai KR, Sawitsky A, Cronkite EP, Chanana AD, Levy RN, Pasternack BS: Clinical staging of chronic lymphocytic leukemia. Blood 46:219–234, 1975.
8. Shaw MT: The cytochemistry of acute leukemia: A diagnostic and prognostic evaluation. Semin Oncol 3:219–228, 1976.
9. Sweet DL Jr, Golomb HM, Ultmann JE: The clinical features of chronic lymphocytic leukemia. Clin Haematol 6:185–202, 1977.

69

LYMPHOMAS

By DAVID H. BOLDT, M.D.

DEFINITION

A. **General.** Lymphomas are malignant disorders that are characterized by uncontrolled proliferation of lymphocytes, lymphocyte precursors, or certain other cell types normally involved in immune reactions. There are two large groups of lymphomas: Hodgkin's disease (HD) and non-Hodgkin's lymphoma (NHL). HD and NHL share similarities in clinical picture and natural history, but there are key differences between them that bear on therapy and prognosis. Therefore both recognition and accurate classification of lymphomas are essential to the proper management of patients with these disorders.

B. **Diagnostic Criteria.** Precise classification of lymphomas can only be achieved by microscopic examination of nodal tissue. Architectural features that permit accurate lymphoma typing require an intact lymph node so that excisional biopsy generally should be performed. It is important to perform biopsy of representative nodes from anatomic areas in which extraneous processes are least likely to confuse the pathologic interpretation. For example, reactive hyperplasia often is present in lymph nodes from inguinal and femoral regions. Therefore, biopsy at these sites should be avoided. Also, it should be noted that whereas the diagnosis of lymphoma can be made by examination of biopsy samples from nonlymphoid tissues, these specimens usually do not contain the histopathologic features necessary for precise lymphoma typing.

1. Diagnosis of HD requires demonstration of Reed-Sternberg cells in the appropriate cellular milieu. In HD, Reed-Sternberg cells are present in a setting of pleomorphic cellular infiltrates consisting of lymphocytes, plasma cells, histiocytes, eosinophils, and variable amounts of fibrosis. The Reed-Sternberg cell is believed to be the malignant cell of HD. Recent evidence suggests that the Reed-Sternberg cell is closely related to the dendritic cell, a type of cell that is present in normal lymphoid follicles and that is responsible for processing and presentation of antigen to lymphocytes during initiation of immune responses. In HD, Reed-Sternberg cells may be inconspicuous, and diligent search may be required for their identification.

2. Diagnosis of NHL is made when lymph nodes show replacement of normal architecture by relatively uniform populations of lymphoid cells. This nodal infiltration may display either a diffuse or a nodular pattern. Reed-Sternberg cells are not present.

C. **Classification.** Both HD and NHL are divided into subtypes based on histopathologic features. These subtypes are important because they have both prognostic and therapeutic implications.

1. Four subclasses of HD are recognized. They are:
   a. Lymphocyte predominance (10 to 15 per cent of cases), with the most favorable prognosis
   b. Nodular sclerosis (30 to 40 per cent), with an intermediate prognosis
   c. Mixed cellularity (30 per cent), with an intermediate prognosis
   d. Lymphocyte depletion (5 to 15 per cent), with the least favorable prognosis

2. Classification of NHL is in a state of flux. Detailed discussion of histopathology is beyond the scope of this manual. Two classifications that are widely used are the *Rappaport Classification* and the *NCI Working Group Classification*. Both classifications facilitate identification of favorable and unfavorable histologic subtypes. This differentiation is most critical in terms of planning appropriate management and assessing prognosis.
   a. Favorable histologic NHL subtypes are characterized by indolent disease courses (median survival seven to eight years) and high rates of responsiveness to therapy (80 to 85 per cent). Paradoxically, although favorable NHL may be controlled by therapy for prolonged periods of time, it is seldom, if ever, cured.
   b. Unfavorable histologic NHL subtypes pursue aggressive disease courses (median survival of untreated patients less

than one year), but approximately 50 per cent of cases may be curable if they are treated aggressively with appropriate chemotherapy.

3. Most cases of NHL are of B lymphocyte origin (75 per cent). The so-called "cutaneous" lymphomas—mycosis fungoides and Sézary syndrome—usually originate from T lymphocytes. Less than 1 per cent of all lymphomas are derived from macrophages. The term "histiocytic lymphoma" is a misnomer, since the malignant cells in this disorder are activated lymphocytes or immunoblasts.

EPIDEMIOLOGY

A. **Demographic Features**
   1. HD represents 1 per cent of human malignancies. It may occur at any age but displays a unique bimodal age-specific incidence curve. One peak occurs between ages 15 and 35 years and a second after age 50. Overall the incidence is higher in males, but in the 15 to 35 year age range it is identical in both sexes. Favorable histologic subtypes are more prevalent in young patients. Unfavorable subtypes are more prevalent in older patients.
   2. NHL makes up 2 to 3 per cent of human malignancies. It may occur at any age, but incidence peaks between ages 40 and 60. There is no sex predilection.
B. **Etiologic Considerations**
   1. *Viruses.* Viruses are strongly implicated as causes of at least two human lymphomas: Epstein-Barr (EB) virus in Burkitt's lymphoma and human T cell leukemia virus (HTLV) in adult T cell leukemia-lymphoma. Sporadic reports of geographic clustering of HD and its bimodal incidence pattern suggest the possibility of an infectious cause, but supportive data do not exist.
   2. *Disorders of Immunoregulation.* Both inherited (severe combined immunodeficiency disease, Wiskott-Aldrich syndrome, ataxia-telangiectasia, and others) and acquired (drug-induced immunosuppression as in renal transplant recipients, acquired immunodeficiency syndrome [AIDS]) immunodeficiency syndromes are associated with increased incidences of malignant lymphomas. Risks range from 40 to 100 times those expected in renal transplant recipients to 10,000 times those expected in patients with hereditary immunodeficiency diseases. AIDS that appears to be caused by HTLV infection has been associated with development of lymphomas in 5 per cent of affected subjects. Besides immunodeficiency diseases, certain autoimmune diseases are associated with increased incidences of development of lymphomas.
   3. *Hereditary Factors.* A three- to sevenfold increase of HD has been noted in siblings and close relatives of affected patients. An association exists between HD and human leukocyte antigen (HLA) types A1, B1, B6, and B15.

CLINICAL MANIFESTATIONS

A. **Lymphadenopathy.** The majority of patients with lymphomas
first seek medical attention because of lymphadenopathy (90 per
cent of HD; 67 per cent of NHL). In HD adenopathy is most
likely to be localized and central in location (mediastinal adenopathy in up to 60 per cent), whereas in NHL it is most likely
to occur at multiple sites and to be peripheral in location
(epitrochlear, popliteal, or mesenteric nodes; Peyer's patches;
and Waldeyer's ring). In both HD and NHL cervical adenopathy
is the most common site of nodal involvement (60 to 70 per cent).

B. **Constitutional Symptoms.** These are prominent features of both
HD and NHL. Fever, sweats, and weight loss are present in 20
to 25 per cent of patients at diagnosis. In a minority of this
group constitutional symptoms may occur in the absence of
detectable lymphadenopathy. Therefore, lymphomas must always be considered in the differential diagnosis of fever of
unknown origin. HD may also occur with pruritus (10 to 15 per
cent of cases) or with a peculiar alcohol pain syndrome in which
pain occurs in involved lymph nodes shortly after alcohol ingestion.

C. **Extranodal Disease.** A major difference between HD and NHL
involves occurrence of extranodal disease. Fewer than 1 per cent
of HD patients have extranodal primary sites, and only 10 per
cent have disease widely disseminated to visceral sites (most
commonly liver, bone marrow, lung, and pleura). By contrast,
25 per cent of NHL occurs with extranodal primary sites and 50
to 60 per cent of patients have disease disseminated to viscera.
The liver (20 to 50 per cent of patients) and bone marrow (30 to
50 per cent) are the most common sites of involvement and are
involved most frequently in favorable histologic subtypes. Gastrointestinal involvement is present initially in 15 per cent of
NHL and is important to document because of its association
with gastrointestinal bleeding and perforation. Central nervous
system involvement is uncommon at examination but should be
carefully excluded in patients with unfavorable subtypes of NHL
because it ultimately develops in 15 to 20 per cent of these
individuals.

DIFFERENTIAL DIAGNOSIS

A. **Differential Diagnosis of Lymphadenopathy**
   1. *Infections.* These can be bacterial, mycobacterial, fungal,
      viral, or parasitic.
   2. *Immunologic Diseases.* These include collagen vascular dis-
      eases, sarcoidosis, serum sickness, and drug reactions.
   3. *Malignancies.* Malignancies include lymphoma and meta-
      static carcinoma.
   4. *Miscellaneous or of Unknown Cause.* Angioimmunoblastic
      lymphadenopathy, dermatopathic lymphadenopathy, and be-
      nign lymphadenopathy syndrome (pre-AIDS) should be con-
      sidered in the differential diagnosis.

B. **Diagnostic Considerations**
1. The likelihood that lymphadenopathy is malignant increases with age. Diagnostic lymph node biopsy specimens are malignant in 20 per cent of patients younger than 30 years and in 60 per cent of those older than 50. Among young patients malignant nodes are two to three times more likely to be lymphoma than carcinoma. In older patients the situation is exactly reversed.
2. The likelihood that lymph node biopsy will reveal a malignancy is two thirds for supraclavicular and one third for cervical, axillary, or inguinal adenopathy.
3. The consistency of lymph nodes on palpation may be helpful in differential diagnosis. Nodes containing lymphoma are "rubbery," whereas those involved by carcinoma are rock-hard. Tender warm erythematous nodes associated with fluctuance or lymphangitic streaking are characteristic of regional infections.
4. The presence of nodal tenderness alone or fluctuation in size of lymph nodes over weeks to months is not a reliable sign by which to assess whether lymphadenopathy is benign or malignant.

RECOMMENDED DIAGNOSTIC APPROACH

A. **Regional Lymphadenopathy**
1. *Chest X-Ray.* If hilar or mediastinal adenopathy is present, the physician should proceed to lymph node biopsy.
2. *Supraclavicular Area.* Biopsy should be done.
3. *Cervical Area*
   a. Evaluation and treatment should be done for local infections of the oropharynx, ear, and face.
   b. If there is a history of sore throat, culture should be done for *Streptococcus* and *Gonococcus* (if there has been recent oral-genital contact). Evaluation for infectious mononucleosis syndromes (EB virus, toxoplasmosis, or cytomegalovirus) should be performed as discussed in Chapter 42.
   c. If results of these measures (3a and b) are negative and nodes persist for two weeks, or if the patient's condition is deteriorating, the physician should proceed to lymph node biopsy.
4. *Axillary Area*
   a. Evaluation should be done for local trauma or infections of hands and arms.
   b. Breast examination is performed in women.
   c. If these measures (4a and b) are negative and nodes persist for two weeks, or if the patient's condition is deteriorating, the physician should proceed to lymph node biopsy.
5. *Inguinal Area*
   a. Evaluation is done for local trauma or infections of feet and legs.

    b. The perineal area is examined for lesions of herpes simplex type 2, lymphogranuloma venereum, syphilis, and other infections.

    c. Lymphogranuloma venereum complement fixation titers, if appropriate, are studied.

    d. If these measures (5a, b, and c) are negative and nodes persist for two weeks, or if the patient's condition is deteriorating, the physician should proceed to lymph node biopsy.

B. Generalized Lymphadenopathy

1. Chest x-ray is done. If hilar or mediastinal adenopathy is present, the physician should proceed to lymph node biopsy.
2. If the patient is taking phenytoin, hydralazine, or allopurinol, the physician should order drug use discontinued and make observations.
3. Evaluation is done for infectious mononucleosis syndrome.
4. Blood cultures, purified protein derivative skin test results, and fungal and collagen vascular disease serologies are obtained.
5. If these measures are negative, or if the patient's condition is deteriorating, lymph node biopsy should be done.

C. Principles of Lymph Node Biopsy.
Lymph node biopsy should be undertaken with careful planning to maximize the amount of diagnostic information obtained. Considerations for optimal processing of node biopsies are as follows:

1. Excisional biopsy is done of an intact lymph node including the capsule (see earlier discussion of Diagnostic Criteria).
2. The node is bisected and smears and cultures are obtained for bacteria, mycobacteria, and fungi.
3. Lymph node imprints are prepared.
4. Frozen section is performed to determine the need for further specimens and types of special studies to be initiated.

    a. If frozen section shows carcinoma in a male, the specimen is placed in formalin for routine permanent sections. In a female, part of the fresh node should be processed for steroid receptor studies if breast carcinoma is possible.

    b. If undifferentiated malignancy is evident on frozen section, part of the specimen should be placed in glutaraldehyde for electron microscopy, and part should be processed for lymphocyte marker studies.

    c. If frozen section shows reactive hyperplasia or another nondiagnostic process, and if malignancy is strongly suspected, a second node biopsy should be carried out. Up to 25 per cent of patients with documented lymphoma may require multiple biopsies to establish a diagnosis.

5. The remaining specimen is placed in fixative for routine permanent sections.
6. The average yield for lymph node biopsies in establishing diagnosis is 60 per cent. Follow-up studies of patients with nondiagnostic lymph node biopsies reveal that half will develop either a malignancy or a collagen vascular disease within the ensuing decade.

D. Staging Evaluation in Lymphomas.
When lymph node biopsy reveals lymphoma, staging evaluation should be undertaken to

determine the extent of disease involvement. Stage of disease for either HD or NHL may be assessed by means of the *Ann Arbor staging classification*:

STAGE	EXTENT OF DISEASE
I	Single lymph node region (I) or single extralymphatic site (IE)
II	Two or more lymph node regions on same side of diaphragm (II) or single extralymphatic site plus one or more lymph node regions on same side of diaphragm (IIE)
III	Lymph node regions on both sides of diaphragm alone (III) or plus single extralymphatic site (IIIE), the spleen (IIIS), or both (IIISE)
IV	Diffuse or disseminated involvement of extralymphatic organs
A category	No symptoms; denotes favorable prognosis
B category	Unexplained weight loss ≥10% of body weight; unexplained fever ≥38°C; night sweats; denote unfavorable prognosis

1. In HD prognosis relates directly to Ann Arbor stage, and precise staging is critical for designing optimal therapy. Staging evaluation may require a variety of clinical, laboratory, x-ray, and surgical procedures designed to provide maximal information about disease extent. As a general rule, decisions about which tests should be performed during staging are individualized and are based on the extent to which results will influence management of each patient.

2. In NHL prognosis does not relate so clearly to Ann Arbor stage, and treatment options are usually based on histologic subtype (favorable vs. unfavorable) rather than anatomic extent of disease. Therefore, in NHL staging evaluation is less aggressive than in HD and is used primarily to document response to therapy or disease progression.

REFERENCES

1. Boldt DH: Lymphadenopathy or splenomegaly *In* Stein JH (ed.): Internal Medicine. Boston, Little, Brown & Company, 1983, pp. 1518–1523.
2. Fauci AS, Macher AM, Longo DL, Lane HC, Rook AH, Masur H, Gelmann EP: Acquired immunodeficiency syndrome: Epidemiologic, clinical, immunologic, and therapeutic considerations. Ann Intern Med 100:92–106, 1984.
3. Greenfield S, Jordan MC: The clinical investigation of lymphadenopathy in primary care practice. JAMA 240:1388–1393, 1978.
4. Kaplan HS: Hodgkin's Disease. 2nd ed. Cambridge, Harvard University Press, 1980.
5. Lester EP, Ultmann JE: Non-Hodgkin's lymphoma. *In* Williams WJ, Beutler E, Erslev AJ, Lichtman MA (eds.) Hematology. 3rd ed. New York, McGraw-Hill, 1983, pp. 1035–1056.
6. Lee YT, Terry R, Lukes RJ: Biopsy of peripheral lymph nodes. Am Surg 48:536–539, 1982.

RHEUMATOLOGY

ARTHRALGIAS AND MYALGIAS

By RICHARD DEYO, M.D., M.P.H.

DEFINITIONS AND EPIDEMIOLOGY

A. **Arthritis or Joint Pain.** Arthralgia refers to joint or periarticular
   pain in the absence of signs of inflammation or joint deformity.
   In the terminology of most patients, "arthritis" is a term for
   such musculoskeletal pain, rather than the medically understood
   synovial inflammation. Myalgia refers to muscle pain that may
   reflect an inflammatory process. Most patients complaining of
   "arthritis" do not actually have significant rheumatic disease.
   The various conditions that cause arthralgia or myalgia in the
   absence of actual joint disease will be referred to here as forms
   of nonarticular rheumatism.

B. **Incidence.** Data from the National Ambulatory Medical Care
   Survey show that musculoskeletal complaints are second only to
   respiratory complaints as a cause for visits to office-based physicians in the United States. Furthermore, nonarticular rheumatism is the single largest diagnostic category of these visits.
   Roughly half of all patients with arthritic complaints in family
   practice prove to have nonarticular rheumatism (tendinitis,
   bursitis, myalgias, and low-back pain). These same conditions
   constitute nearly half of all diagnoses in community-based rheumatology practices. In primary care settings, another 30 to 40
   per cent of patients have osteoarthritis, leaving only 10 to 15
   per cent of musculoskeletal complaints attributable to rheumatoid and other forms of arthritis.

C. **Definitions.** Many of the conditions listed in Table 70–1 are
   familiar to most clinicians or are self-explanatory. For some
   readers, however, definitions may be helpful.
   1. *Fibrositis.* This term is misleading in the sense that no actual
      inflammatory lesion has been found. It is actually a "pain
      amplification disorder." The clinical characteristics are de-
      scribed in Table 70–2.
   2. *Somatization Disorder.* This condition, sometimes called *Bri-
      quet's syndrome,* often includes arthralgias as a prominent
      symptom. This psychiatric disorder is a distinct syndrome,
      although it is similar to hypochondriasis and hysteria. Cri-
      teria for this diagnosis have been set forth by the American
      Psychiatric Association in their *Diagnostic & Statistical Man-
      ual of Mental Disorders* (DSM-III; see Table 70–2). It almost
      always occurs in women, and symptoms usually begin before
      age 30.
   3. *Polymyalgia Rheumatica.* This is a syndrome of limb-girdle
      pain in the elderly. Although clinical signs of joint inflam-

TABLE 70–1. FORMS OF PAINFUL NONARTICULAR RHEUMATISM

GENERALIZED	UPPER EXTREMITY	LOWER EXTREMITY	BACK OR TRUNK
Fibrositis	Shoulder	Foot	Lumbar strain
Somatization disorder (also called Briquet's syndrome)	Calcific tendinitis	Metatarsalgia	Costochondritis
Myalgia in influenza or other viral infections	Bicipital tendinitis	Heel bursitis, tendinitis, periostitis	
	Rotator cuff tears	Achilles tendinitis	
Rare but more serious:	"Frozen shoulder" or adhesive capsulitis	Plantar fasciitis	
Polymyalgia rheumatica		Leg	
Polymyositis, dermatomyositis	Arm	Trochanteric bursitis	
	Tennis elbow or lateral epicondylitis	Anserine bursitis	
	Olecranon bursitis	Prepatellar bursitis	
	de Quervain's tendinitis	Fascia lata fasciitis	
	Carpal tunnel syndrome	Leg cramp	
		"Shin splints"	

TABLE 70–2. PROPOSED DIAGNOSTIC CRITERIA FOR GENERALIZED FORMS OF NONARTICULAR RHEUMATISM

Polymyalgia rheumatica[4]
1. Pain in neck, shoulders, and pelvic girdle that persists for at least a month. Morning stiffness is common and marked. No muscle atrophy or weakness.
2. Patient ≥55 years of age.
3. ESR >50 mm/hr.
4. Relief of symptoms within four days with administration of as little as 10 mg of prednisone daily.

Fibrositis[2]
1. Widespread aching of more than 3 months' duration.
2. Local tenderness of 12 of 14 specified sites.
3. Skin roll tenderness over upper scapular region.
4. Disturbed sleep with morning fatigue and stiffness.
5. Normal ESR, rheumatoid factor, antinuclear antibody, muscle enzymes, aspartate transaminase (SGOT), and sacroiliac films.

Somatization disorder[8]
Women must have at least 14 and men at least 12 of the following 37 unexplained symptoms:

Sickly: the patient believes he or she has been sickly for a good part of life.
Conversion or pseudoneurologic symptoms: dysphagia, loss of voice, deafness, double vision, blurred vision, blindness, fainting or loss of consciousness, memory loss, seizures, difficulty walking, paralysis or muscle weakness, urinary retention, or difficulty urinating.
Gastrointestinal symptoms: abdominal pain, nausea, vomiting spells, bloating, diarrhea, intolerance of a variety of foods.
Female reproductive symptoms: excessively painful menstruation, menstrual irregularity, excessive bleeding, severe vomiting throughout pregnancy or causing hospitalization during pregnancy.
Psychosexual symptoms: sexual indifference, lack of pleasure during intercourse, dyspareunia.
Pain: in back, joints, extremities, genital area, or elsewhere, except headaches or dysuria.
Cardiopulmonary symptoms: dyspnea, palpitations, chest pain, dizziness.

mation are lacking and results of muscle biopsy are normal, there is laboratory evidence of an inflammatory process (elevated erythrocyte sedimentation rate and abnormal joint scintigrams in some patients). This condition is sometimes associated with a true inflammatory vasculitis known as *giant cell arteritis* or *temporal arteritis.*

4. **de Quervain's Tendinitis.** This condition, also known as *stenosing tenosynovitis,* refers to pain at the radial aspect of the wrist, sometimes with swelling. This is a tendinitis of the extensor pollicis brevis and abductor pollicis longus and usually is related to trauma.

5. **"Shin Splints."** This term is used to refer to pain over the anteromedial aspect of the mid or distal tibia. It is thought to be caused by strain or minimal tears of periosteum, interosseous membrane, muscle belly, or muscle-tendon junction.

This most often occurs from overuse in walking or running and must be distinguished from stress fractures, which may also occur with overuse.

6. **Lumbar Strain.** This term refers to low-back pain of uncertain origin. Evidence of herniated disc or structural bony lesions is absent, and a more precise diagnosis is usually impossible. Many innervated structures in the back may be the actual source of pain, including several ligaments, the facet joints, vertebral periosteum, and paravertebral muscles.

7. **Carpal Tunnel Syndrome.** This is an entrapment neuropathy of the median nerve. It is most often caused by an idiopathic flexor tenosynovitis but may be secondary to obesity, acromegaly, myxedema, amyloidosis, local edema, diabetes mellitus, or rheumatoid arthritis.

8. **Calcific Tendinitis.** The tendons of the supra- and infraspinatus muscles (part of the rotator cuff) may calcify with aging or trauma. Although this process is most often asymptomatic (and occasionally seen as an incidental x-ray finding), it may lead to inflammation and pain in the subdeltoid bursa. The terms "subdeltoid bursitis" and "subacromial bursitis" are commonly used for this syndrome, but the primary inflammation occurs in the rotator cuff tendons, and the bursa becomes secondarily inflamed.

DIFFERENTIAL DIAGNOSIS

A. **Body Region.** Table 70–1 gives a list of various forms of nonarticular rheumatism according to body region. There are no data on incidence or prevalence of most of these individual syndromes because such detailed data are rarely collected in larger surveys and because precise diagnosis is often impossible. As suggested previously, these syndromes are very common in the aggregate. It is estimated that somatization disorder may occur in nearly 2 per cent of women.

B. **Low-Back Pain.** Low-back pain is thought to occur in nearly 80 per cent of all adults at some time in their lives, although a minority of these seek medical care. Of those who do, nearly 80 per cent have idiopathic low-back pain which is often called lumbar strain.

C. **Causes of Myalgia and Arthralgia.** The serious causes of myalgia or arthralgia listed in Table 70–1 are quite rare. The incidence of polymyositis and dermatomyositis is estimated at 1 in 280,000 per year among the general population. Most cases occur between ages 30 and 60. *Polymyalgia rheumatica* is a disease almost exclusively of patients over age 50, and in this age range the annual incidence is about 54 per 100,000.

D. **Other Causes.** Depending on the clinical picture, other causes of soft tissue pain may need to be considered. These include venous thrombosis, muscle hematomas, and reflex sympathetic dystrophies.

HISTORY AND PHYSICAL EXAMINATION

A. **Reliance on History and Physical Examination.** The diagnosis of most of the conditions in Table 70–1 is made by the history and physical examination alone. Indeed, the absence of abnormal laboratory or radiologic findings is characteristic of most of these conditions.

B. **Nonarticular Rheumatism.** These conditions tend to affect areas adjacent to the large joints. Involvement of fingers and toes often suggests a true arthritic disorder.

C. **Identification of Minor Conditions.** The history and physical examination should quickly establish the duration of the complaint, any associated symptoms or signs of systemic illness (such as fever, weight loss, or rash), the recent occurrence of serious trauma, or any associated neurologic problems. Figure 70–1 provides an algorithm that shows that if symptoms are of brief duration and the findings listed here are absent, serious illness is unlikely and laboratory investigation at the initial visit is unlikely to be helpful. For the rare patient in this category

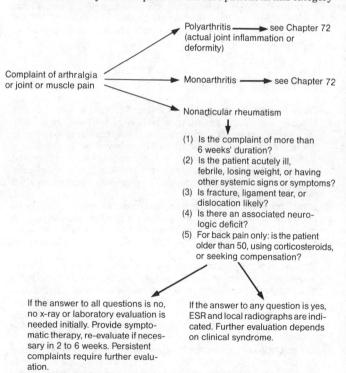

Complaint of arthralgia or joint or muscle pain

Polyarthritis (actual joint inflammation or deformity) ——→ see Chapter 72

Monoarthritis ——→ see Chapter 72

Nonarticular rheumatism

(1) Is the complaint of more than 6 weeks' duration?
(2) Is the patient acutely ill, febrile, losing weight, or having other systemic signs or symptoms?
(3) Is fracture, ligament tear, or dislocation likely?
(4) Is there an associated neurologic deficit?
(5) For back pain only: is the patient older than 50, using corticosteroids, or seeking compensation?

If the answer to all questions is no, no x-ray or laboratory evaluation is needed initially. Provide symptomatic therapy, re-evaluate if necessary in 2 to 6 weeks. Persistent complaints require further evaluation.

If the answer to any question is yes, ESR and local radiographs are indicated. Further evaluation depends on clinical syndrome.

Figure 70–1. Approach to evaluation of arthralgia and myalgia pain. (Modified from Fries JF, Mitchell DM.[1])

who proves to have a significant rheumatic disease, it is unlikely that a therapeutic opportunity will be lost by a delay of weeks for observation.

D. **Generalized Disorders.** Table 70–2 lists diagnostic criteria that have been proposed for polymyalgia rheumatica, fibrositis, and somatization disorder, which has also been called Briquet's syndrome. An understanding of these conditions is still evolving, and these criteria may change. Myalgias caused by viral illness are usually associated with a variety of other influenzalike upper respiratory symptoms. Polymyositis most often presents with actual muscle weakness (92 per cent of cases). About 25 per cent of patients have myalgias, and about 25 per cent have arthralgias at the time of presentation. In patients with dermatomyositis, all of these symptoms are less likely to be seen at presentation, but 93 per cent have cutaneous signs.

E. **Local Conditions**

  1. The Shoulder. The lesions discussed are often characterized by recurrent exacerbations and symptoms related to activity.

   a. **Calcific Tendinitis.** Pain is often acute in onset and may be related to trauma. Night pain is prominent, and pain is aggravated by nearly any shoulder motion. Radiation to the neck or down the arm may occur.

   b. **Bicipital Tendinitis.** There is tenderness of the biceps tendon within its groove, and pain is well localized. Pain is accentuated by resisted supination of the forearm, with the elbow flexed at 90 degrees.

   c. **Rotator Cuff Tears.** There is a wide spectrum of severity of these tears. Mild syndromes may be difficult to definitely diagnose. A complete tear results in inability to abduct the shoulder, although it can be held in abduction once it is passively elevated to 90 degrees or more (by deltoid muscle action).

   d. **Frozen Shoulder.** There is usually a history of a period of inactivity of the shoulder that is often caused by stroke, trauma, tendinitis, or myocardial infarction. Marked reduction of passive range of motion is characteristic, especially when rotation is tested. Pain is dull, aching, and anterior or lateral in location. Tenderness is usually not prominent.

  2. The Arm

   a. **Tennis Elbow.** There is pain over the lateral epicondyle. It is aggravated by grasping, wrist extension, or arm supination and is often seen in athletes, plumbers, gardeners, carpenters, and dentists. Physical examination shows point tenderness over the lateral epicondyle and normal range of joint motion. Resisted pronation is often quite painful.

   b. **Olecranon Bursitis.** This superficial bursa may become inflamed secondary to trauma, gout, infection, or rheumatoid arthritis. Visible swelling occurs, and aspiration should be performed.

   c. **de Quervain's Tendinitis.** There is often a history of repetitive joint use such as in peeling vegetables or knitting. Pain at the radial aspect of the wrist as a result of this condition must be distinguished from osteoarthritis, which also occurs commonly at this site. The Finkelstein test distinguishes between the two. The patient's thumb is folded into the palm, with the remaining fingers flexed over the thumb. The examiner then gently moves the wrist in an ulnar direction and the involved tendons are stretched. This maneuver causes an acute exacerbation of pain if there is tendinitis.

d. **Carpal Tunnel Syndrome.** There is pain, paresthesia, and numbness in the median nerve distribution. Discomfort often occurs at night. Light percussion at the wrist (Tinel's sign) and forced wrist flexion (Phalen's sign) may reproduce symptoms. In long-term cases there is wasting and weakness of the thenar muscles.

3. The Foot and Leg

a. **Overuse Syndromes.** Several of the conditions listed in Table 70–1 for the lower extremity are commonly related to overuse. New sports activities, running, jumping, or other exercise may underlie plantar fasciitis, Achilles tendinitis, and shin splints. An unusually intense workout and rapid change in exercise routine are often part of the history. Plantar fasciitis causes heel or foot pain with the onset of weight-bearing after rest, and each step is painful. Achilles tendinitis causes burning in the back of the heel, which often occurs early in running or after awakening from sleep and which may improve during a run or with daily activities. The tendon itself is tender and when chronic may have a nodule or swelling. Fascia lata fasciitis causes pain in the lateral aspect of the thigh, with tender points along the fascial band. Shin splints are characterized by pain in the lower anteromedial tibial area. Examination reveals only tenderness in this area.

b. **Metatarsalgia.** This is pain at the ball of the foot, which is sometimes caused by pes cavus, shortened Achilles tendon, or rheumatoid arthritis.

c. **Heel Pain.** Heel pain may result from bursitis, tendinitis, periostitis, spurs, or plantar fasciitis. Trauma or inflammatory arthritis may be causal (as in Reiter's syndrome and rheumatoid arthritis). Examination is nonspecific.

d. **Trochanteric Bursitis.** This causes lateral hip pain (over the greater trochanter of the femur), which is sometimes acute and usually worse at night. There is point tenderness on physical examination.

e. **Anserine Bursitis.** The anserine bursa lies at the inferomedial aspect of the knee in the area of the medial tibial collateral ligament. Bursitis here is often associated with osteoarthritis and is often worse at night. The patient may sleep with a pillow between the thighs. Point tenderness is greater than in uncomplicated osteoarthritis.

f. **Prepatellar Bursitis.** This usually results from trauma caused by repeated kneeling (often seen in nuns, carpenters, carpet layers, and plumbers). There may be warmth and tenderness, and if an effusion is present it should be aspirated and examined.

g. **Leg Cramps.** Leg cramps are common and rarely caused by metabolic derangements. There may be a family history or a history of prolonged squatting, kneeling, or standing on concrete floors.

4. Back and Trunk

a. **Lumbar Strain.** This term is applied to low-back pain without a specific cause. There may be some radiation of pain to the legs but no neurologic deficits. Straight leg raising to less than 60 degrees implies some nerve root irritation (but not necessarily a herniated disc). Many traditional tests for specific causes (such as muscle spasm by examination and tests for sacroiliac disease) are unreliable.

b. **Costochondritis.** This causes pain and tenderness of the anterior chest wall, which may radiate, mimicking intrathoracic or abdominal disease. Palpation of the thoracic cage elicits tenderness. If there is actual swelling over costal cartilage, the term "Tietze's syndrome" is applied.

LABORATORY STUDIES AND X-RAYS

A. **Normal X-Ray and Laboratory Results.** Most of the syndromes are characterized by normal x-ray and laboratory findings. Excessive use of x-rays and serologic or other tests may lead to false-positive results, excessive concern, patient dependency, erroneous diagnostic labeling, and ill-advised therapy.

B. **Serious Inflammatory Conditions.** An elevated ESR (erythrocyte sedimentation rate) is characteristic of polymyalgia rheumatica, and the test should be performed in patients over age 55 in whom suggestive symptoms persist for a month. Muscle weakness or rash suggesting an inflammatory myopathy should prompt ESR and muscle enzyme (creatine kinase and aldolase) determinations.

C. **Carpal Tunnel Syndrome.** The carpal tunnel syndrome can be confirmed by testing nerve conduction velocity.

D. **Olecranon and Prepatellar Bursitis with Effusions.** These conditions should prompt aspiration and fluid examination.

E. **Laboratory Testing for Patients with Low-Back Pain.** Such testing is controversial, but the suggestions in Figure 70–1 are supported by many experts. In selected cases the ESR and lumbar spine films are a useful screen for rare causes of back pain such as multiple myeloma, osteomyelitis, or metastatic cancer.

RECOMMENDED DIAGNOSTIC APPROACH

See Figure 70–1.

REFERENCES

1. Fries JF, Mitchell DM: Joint pain or arthritis. JAMA 235:199–203, 1976.
   An approach to initial evaluation, emphasizing the distinction between arthritis and arthralgia.

2. Smythe HA: "Fibrositis" as a disorder of pain modulation. Clin Rheum Dis 5:823–832, 1979.
   Clinical features and therapy of fibrositis; proposed diagnostic criteria are included.

3. Spitzer WO, Harth M, Goldsmith CH, et al.: The arthritic complaint in primary care: Prevalence, related disability, and costs. J Rheumatol 3:88–99, 1976.
   Prevalence of various diagnoses in primary care; nonarticular rheumatism was the most common diagnostic category.

4. Healey LA: Polymyalgia rheumatica. *In* McCarty DJ (ed.): Arthritis and Allied Conditions, a Textbook of Rheumatology. 9th ed. Philadelphia, Lea & Febiger, 1979, pp. 681–684.
   A clinical review, including diagnostic criteria.

5. Rodnan GP, Schumacher HR (eds.): Primer on the Rheumatic Diseases. 8th ed. Atlanta, The Arthritis Foundation, 1983.
   Helpful, concise chapters that discuss the many forms of nonarticular rheumatism.

6. James SL, Bates BT, Osternig LR: Injuries to runners. Am J Sports Med 6:40–50, 1978.
   Diagnosis and treatment of the common overuse syndromes.

7. Goroll AH, May LA, Mulley AG (eds.): Primary Care Medicine. Philadelphia, J. B. Lippincott Company, 1981.
   Practical chapters for the nonspecialist on various forms of nonarticular rheumatism, including treatment and indications for referral.

8. American Psychiatric Association: Diagnostic & Statistical Manual of Mental Disorders (DSM-III). 3rd ed. American Psychiatric Association, Washington, D.C., 1980.

71

POLYARTHRITIS

By THOMAS D. KOEPSELL, M.D., M.P.H.

DEFINITION

The term "polyarthritis" refers to the clinical syndrome of pain and signs of inflammation or internal injury that are present simultaneously in two or more joints. General signs of arthritis include joint tenderness to palpation, synovial effusion, pain on joint motion, restricted range of motion, and crepitus or "grating" on joint

TABLE 71–1. DISEASES THAT CAN INVOLVE POLYARTHRITIS

Degenerative joint disease
Rheumatoid arthritis
Systemic lupus erythematosus
  Idiopathic
  Drug-induced
Ankylosing spondylitis
Psoriatic arthritis
Reiter's syndrome
Arthritis associated with inflammatory bowel disease
Progressive systemic sclerosis (scleroderma)
Polyarteritis nodosa
Rheumatic fever
Virus-associated arthritis (hepatitis B, rubella, other)
Hemophilia
Sickle cell disease
Polymyositis
Sarcoidosis
Hemochromatosis
Amyloidosis
Gonococcal arthritis
Serum sickness
Dermatomyositis
Mixed connective tissue disease
Behçet's syndrome
Arthritis associated with malignancy
Gout
Pseudogout

motion. An acutely inflamed joint also exhibits increased warmth and erythema over the joint. These signs help to distinguish arthritis from polyarthralgias (which occur in many systemic illnesses) and from such periarticular problems as bursitis, tendinitis, and cellulitis, none of which are considered here.

An exhaustive differential diagnosis of polyarthritis would be very lengthy. Table 71–1 lists most of the disease processes that can cause this syndrome. Attention is focused on six diseases that satisfy the following criteria: (1) they are relatively common; (2) polyarthritis is the usual pattern of joint involvement; and (3) they are either primarily joint diseases or systemic diseases that may not be clinically obvious otherwise. These six diseases are degenerative joint disease (DJD), rheumatoid arthritis (RA), systemic lupus erythematosus (SLE), ankylosing spondylitis (AS), psoriatic arthritis, and Reiter's syndrome.

EPIDEMIOLOGY

Table 71–2 shows the estimated prevalence of each disease and, when known, its pattern of occurrence by age, sex, race, and other characteristics. Overall, DJD is many times more common than any other cause of polyarthritis and affects a majority of elderly individuals to some degree. Since DJD can also be caused by almost any

TABLE 71–2. EPIDEMIOLOGIC CHARACTERISTICS OF SELECTED POLYARTHRITIDES

FEATURE	DEGENERATIVE JOINT DISEASE	RHEUMATOID ARTHRITIS	SYSTEMIC LUPUS ERYTHEMATOSUS	ANKYLOSING SPONDYLITIS	PSORIATIC ARTHRITIS	REITER'S SYNDROME
Prevalence	35–40%	10–30/1000	0.1–1.0/1000	1–10/1000	0.2–1.4/1000	1/1000
Age	Steady increase with age	Steady increase with age	Peaks in 2nd to 4th decades	Peaks at ages 15–30	Peaks at ages 15–45	Peaks at ages 15–45
Sex	Before age 45: slight male excess; after age 45: slight female excess	Females predominate 2–3:1	Females predominate 8–9:1	Males predominate 2–10:1	No marked predominance in either sex	Males predominate 15–60:1 (except postenteric form, for which there is no predominance of either sex)
Race	Little variation	Little variation	Blacks at about threefold higher risk	Blacks at about 1/4 the risk of whites	?	?
Other high-risk groups	Obesity?	HLA-DR4	HLA-DR2 and HLA-DR3; positive family history	HLA-B27; selected Indian tribes (Haida, Pima, others)	HLA-B27	HLA-B27

HLA = human leukocyte antigen.

other form of arthritis, its existence in a younger person should at least raise suspicions of a coexisting joint disease.

Marked differences in patterns of occurrence by age and sex are useful diagnostically. Both DJD and RA become increasingly frequent with advancing age, while the remaining four diseases occur predominantly in younger adults. Ankylosing spondylitis and Reiter's syndrome are much more common in men, while SLE is equally strikingly more common in women. The risk of RA is increased two- to threefold in women. Modest sex differences in DJD prevalence reverse at around the age of menopause.

Except for DJD, each of the diseases is known to be associated with certain HLA types. However, the cost and low specificity of HLA type determinations argue against their routine use as diagnostic tests.

HISTORY

Table 71–3 describes the symptomatology of these six diseases. All can occur with abrupt or gradual onset, but only in Reiter's syndrome is an acute onset more common. Peripheral joint involvement in the spondyloarthropathies (AS, psoriatic arthritis, and Reiter's syndrome) is usually asymmetric, while RA and SLE are usually symmetric. Generalized DJD is typically symmetric; DJD secondary to previous trauma or arthritis can be symmetric or not, depending on the primary mechanism of damage.

As shown in Table 71–3, there are differences in characteristic patterns of joint involvement. In the hand DJD usually affects the DIP joints and the first carpometacarpal joint. RA usually affects the MCP joints and wrists, sparing the DIP joints. In general, AS primarily affects the axial skeleton, psoriatic arthritis the hands and feet, and Reiter's syndrome the joints of the lower extremities.

Morning stiffness is most characteristic of RA but is also found more rarely in other polyarthritides. In RA, however, morning stiffness often persists for more than half an hour.

DJD has no important extra-articular symptoms. The other five diseases do, as shown. It should be noted, however, that most of them are relatively infrequent.

PHYSICAL SIGNS

The characteristic signs of arthritis, as described earlier, are seen in all six diseases. The symmetry and pattern of joint involvement (see History) are of great value in differential diagnosis. In addition, at least for patients with moderately advanced disease, many of the causes of polyarthritis have fairly specific joint deformities, as shown in Table 71–4.

A number of valuable clues to the cause of polyarthritis in a particular patient can come from the general physical examination, since each disease except DJD is associated with certain extra-

TABLE 71-3. TYPICAL SYMPTOMS OF SELECTED POLYARTHRITIDES

Feature	Degenerative Joint Disease (DJD)	Rheumatoid Arthritis	Systemic Lupus Erythematosus	Ankylosing Spondylitis	Psoriatic Arthritis	Reiter's Syndrome
Onset	Gradual (generalized DJD in postmenopausal women may be abrupt in onset)	Gradual (80%) or acute (20%)	Usually gradual	Usually gradual	Gradual or acute	Usually acute
Symmetry	Primary DJD: usually symmetric; secondary DJD: symmetric or asymmetric	Symmetric (80%)	Symmetric (over 80%)	Affects axial skeleton; usually affects peripheral joints asymmetrically	Asymmetric (80%)	Asymmetric (95%)
Joints commonly affected	DIP, knees, hips, spine, 1st CMC, 1st MTP	MCP, wrists, elbows, knees, shoulders, hips	PIP, MCP, knees, wrists, ankles, elbows	Spine, sacroiliac, costovertebral, sternoclavicular, manubriosternal joints, hips, knees, shoulders	Hand and foot joints, axial skeleton, sacroiliac joints	Knees, sacroiliac joints, ankles, feet

Morning stiffness	20–30%, usually for less than 0.5 hour	90–100%, often for more than 0.5 hour	20%, usually of short duration	Common	15%?	
Extra-articular symptoms	Usually none, although other systemic diseases can predispose to DJD	Anorexia, weight loss, dry eyes or mucous membranes, symptoms of vasculitis or neuropathy	Photosensitivity (17–41%), seizures or psychosis (16–20%), myalgias or weakness (33%), Raynaud's disease (19–44%), pleurisy (60–70%); can be associated with use of certain drugs (hydralazine, procainamide)	Iritis (25%)	Hyperkeratotic skin lesions on extensor surfaces (95%)	Urethritis, eye discomfort (60%), heel pain (57%), back pain (70%); possible prior episode of diarrhea

MTP = metatarsal-phalangeal joint; DIP = distal interphalangeal joint; MCP = metacarpophalangeal joint; PIP = proximal interphalangeal joint; CMC = carpometacarpal joint.

TABLE 71-4. PHYSICAL SIGNS OF SELECTED POLYARTHRITIDES

FEATURE	DEGENERATIVE JOINT DISEASE	RHEUMATOID ARTHRITIS	SYSTEMIC LUPUS ERYTHEMATOSUS	ANKYLOSING SPONDYLITIS	PSORIATIC ARTHRITIS	REITER'S SYNDROME
Symmetry Joints commonly affected	See Table 71-3					
Deformities	Heberden's nodes (at distal interphalangeal joint); Bouchard's nodes (at proximal interphalangeal joint); bony overgrowth at joint margins	Ulnar deviation at MCPs, wrists; swan-neck and boutonniere deformities; lateral deviation at MTPs, hallux valgus, cock-up toes	Rare; in advanced disease: ulnar deviation, swan-neck deformities, subluxation as in RA	Loss of lumbar lordosis	"Sausage digits"	Rare
Extra-articular signs	None	Subcutaneous nodules on extensor surfaces; purpura, digital infarcts or ulcers; pleural or pericardial effusions; carpal tunnel syndrome; neuropathy; pulmonary fibrosis	Butterfly-shaped facial rash (40–64%), mucosal ulcers (15–36%), discoid lupus (20–30%), alopecia (40–70%)	Iritis (25%), aortic regurgitation murmur (rare)	Hyperkeratotic skin lesions on extensor surfaces (95%), nail changes (30%)	Urethritis or cervicitis (85%), circinate balanitis (34%), keratodermia blennorrhagica (20%), asymptomatic oral lesions (24%), conjunctivitis

MCP = metacarpophalangeal joint; MTP = metatarsal-phalangeal joint.

articular signs. Rheumatoid nodules over extensor surfaces or signs of rheumatoid vasculitis favor RA. Particularly in a younger woman, dermatologic and mucosal manifestations of SLE should be sought. The cardiac and ophthalmologic examinations can occasionally support a diagnosis of AS. Psoriatic arthritis can be associated with only mild skin disease, and a careful examination of skin over extensor surfaces and the scalp is in order. Classically, Reiter's syndrome includes urethritis (or cervicitis) and conjunctivitis, which may be mild or asymptomatic.

LABORATORY STUDIES

Table 71–5 shows the main blood test and x-ray findings most characterisic of these six polyarthritides. The erythrocyte sedimentation rate (ESR), although it is inexpensive, is of little differential diagnostic value because it is elevated in all of the inflammatory polyarthritides and because of the frequency of elevated ESRs in the elderly, who are most prone to have DJD. A positive rheumatoid factor test result, particularly if the titer exceeds 1:160 (on the latex fixation method) favors RA; however, as Table 71–5 shows, it is neither perfectly sensitive nor specific for RA. The antinuclear antibody (ANA) test is highly sensitive for SLE; however, false-positive results (generally at low titers) are encountered in normals and in persons with other arthritides increasingly with advancing age. Antibodies to native (double-stranded) DNA are virtually specific for SLE, although they are less sensitive than the ANA test.

An x-ray of the joint(s) that are most frequently clinically affected is among the most valuable tests for differential diagnosis, provided the disease process has been chronic enough (lasting at least a few weeks) to cause radiographic joint changes. Typical findings are shown in Table 71–5. Hand films generally show characteristic joint abnormalities in DJD, RA, and psoriatic arthritis. Normal sacroiliac joints on x-ray essentially rule out AS; however, sacroiliac x-rays show abnormality in 20 to 25 per cent of patients with other spondyloarthropathies.

With rare exceptions, arthrocentesis is indicated for differential diagnosis of polyarthritis. Usual findings in six polyarthritides are shown in Table 71–6. Turbidity generally correlates with leukocyte count and is visibly increased in any of the inflammatory arthritides (RA and the spondyloarthropathies); it is generally low in DJD and SLE. Forcing a little synovial fluid from the syringe also permits a gross evaluation of viscosity which is low in the inflammatory arthritides—the fluid is nearly water-thin because of loss of hyaluronic acid. Most of the leukocytes in an inflammatory effusion are polymorphonuclear neutrophils (PMNs). Culture of joint fluid is always warranted, since patients with an underlying noninfectious arthritis are thought to be at increased risk for septic arthritis, and because signs of infection may be subtle. Joint fluid hemolytic complement is often low in RA and SLE (presumably owing to consumption of complement by immune complexes), normal in DJD, and high in some patients with AS or Reiter's syndrome; however,

TABLE 71–5. LABORATORY FEATURES OF SELECTED POLYARTHRITIDES

Feature	Degenerative Joint Disease	Rheumatoid Arthritis	Systemic Lupus Erythematosus	Ankylosing Spondylitis	Psoriatic Arthritis	Reiter's Syndrome
Erythrocyte sedimentation rate	Usually normal: under 20 mm/hr (59%), 20–40 mm/hr (34%)	Usually elevated (85%)	Usually elevated	Usually elevated	Usually elevated in acute phase	Usually elevated in acute phase
Rheumatoid factor	Normal for age (5–20% positive, usually at low titer)	70–90% positive, usually at 1:160 or greater (Latex)	20–40%	1–6%	1–15%	3–6%
Antinuclear antibody (ANA)	Normal for age	15–50% positive, usually at low titers	99–100% positive	Normal for age	Normal for age	Normal for age
Anti-double-stranded DNA	Negative	Negative	80–90%	Negative	Negative	Negative
HLA-B27	6–8%	10%	6–10%?	90–95%	20% (50% with sacroiliitis)	75–80%
X-ray	Joint space loss, sclerosis, new bone formation, cysts	Symmetric erosion without new bone formation, osteoporosis, deformities (see Table 71–4)	Soft-tissue swelling; late: juxta-articular osteoporosis, deformities	Ankylosis, sacroiliitis (99–100%), asymmetric peripheral arthropathy with sclerosis	Resorption of distal phalangeal tufts, sacroiliitis (25%), "pencil-in-cup" (25%), periostitis (25%)	Sacroiliitis (20%), plantar spurs, erosion at calcaneal insertion of Achilles tendon
Other		Normocytic-normochromic anemia	LE cells (48–97%), false-+ syphilis test (8–26%), leukopenia (40–47%)			

HLA = human leukocyte antigen; LE = lupus erythematosus.

TABLE 71-6. TYPICAL JOINT FLUID FINDINGS IN SELECTED POLYARTHRITIDES

FEATURE	DEGENERATIVE JOINT DISEASE	RHEUMATOID ARTHRITIS	SYSTEMIC LUPUS ERYTHEMATOSUS	ANKYLOSING SPONDYLITIS	PSORIATIC ARTHRITIS	REITER'S SYNDROME
Appearance	Clear	Turbid	Usually clear	Turbid or translucent	Turbid or translucent	Turbid or translucent
Viscosity	Usually normal (high)	Low	High	Low	Low	Low
Leukocyte count	Under 2000/mm^3 (93%)	Under 2500 (6%), 2500–25,000 (67%), 25,000–50,000 (23%), over 50,000 (4%)	1000–5000, usually under 3000	5000–50,000, average about 7000	2000–100,000	2000–100,000
Per cent PMNs	Usually under 30%	Usually over 60%	Usually under 20%	Usually over 40%	Usually over 50%	Usually over 50%
Culture	Negative	Negative	Negative	Negative	Negative	Negative
Other		Low complement	LE cells	Normal to increased complement		Normal to increased complement

this test is neither particularly sensitive nor specific to a particular disease and should probably not be regarded as a first-line test. Gout and pseudogout are more commonly monoarthritides than polyarthritides; however, routine examination of joint fluid for characteristic crystals of these diseases is easily performed and prevents missing an atypical picture.

RECOMMENDED DIAGNOSTIC APPROACH

First, the physician should take maximal advantage of clues provided by the history and physical examination and be alert to the possibility of other nonrheumatologic diseases that can cause polyarthritis, such as inflammatory bowel disease or a bleeding disorder. The physician should ask about the chronicity and symmetry of joint symptoms, the pattern of joint involvement, and the degree of morning stiffness. Extra-articular symptoms can be especially valuable for diagnosis of SLE, psoriatic arthritis, and Reiter's syndrome (see Table 71–3).

When performing the physical examination, the physician should watch for signs of acute inflammation and joint effusions (which suggest that the joint should be tapped) or chronic inflammation, such as boggy synovial thickening at the joint margins (which suggest that a joint x-ray may be diagnostic). The pattern of symmetry and joint involvement should be noted for comparison with Table 71–3. The hands should be examined closely for deformities. During the general physical examination, the extra-articular clues listed in Table 71–4 should be sought for diagnoses high on the list of differential diagnoses. In most instances, the history and physical examination alone can lead to an accurate provisional diagnosis.

If the history or physical examination suggests an arthritic process that has been chronic (lasting at least weeks), an x-ray of the joint(s) most affected clinically is indicated. If DJD, RA, or psoriasis is a strong possibility, hand x-rays can be diagnostic. If AS is suggested by, for example, back pain in a younger man, x-rays of the lower back and sacroiliac joints should confirm the diagnosis. Reiter's syndrome is usually too acute to cause x-ray changes in an affected joint, but heel films may show erosion at the insertion of the Achilles tendon, which supports the diagnosis.

In general, if the physical examination reveals an effusion in a large joint, arthrocentesis is indicated. The volume, viscosity, and turbidity of fluid should be noted, and a leukocyte count and differential, culture of the fluid, and examination for crystals should be ordered. The findings should be compared with the information in Table 71–6.

A rheumatoid factor determination is useful to help confirm a diagnosis of RA or to help distinguish RA from SLE, if the physician remains aware of its imperfect sensitivity and specificity. For SLE the diagnosis is essentially ruled out by a negative ANA; a positive anti–double-stranded DNA rules it in.

REFERENCES

1. Spiegel RM (ed.): Practical Rheumatology. New York, John Wiley & Sons, 1983.
   A recent textbook, with emphasis on practical diagnosis.

2. Beary JF III, Christian CL, Sculco TP: Manual of rheumatology and outpatient orthopedic diseases. Boston, Little, Brown & Company, 1981.

An excellent and useful handbook.

3. Getter RA: A Practical Handbook of Joint Fluid Analysis. Philadelphia, Lea & Febiger, 1984.

A practical reference to use when interpreting joint fluids.

4. Moskowitz RW, Howell DS, Goldberg VM, Mankin JH: Osteoarthritis—diagnosis and management. Philadelphia, W. B. Saunders Company, 1984.

The most up-to-date textbook now available.

72

ARTHRITIS ASSOCIATED WITH SPONDYLITIS

By RICHARD O. CUMMINS, M.D., M.P.H.

DEFINITIONS, EPIDEMIOLOGY, AND CRITERIA FOR DIAGNOSIS

A. **Definition.** The spondylarthropathies are a group of connective tissue disorders interrelated by several key features.
  1. *Spondylitis.* This is an inflammation of the vertebral bodies. The condition manifests itself almost invariably in the following two ways:
    a. **Clinically.** Low-back pain is present.
    b. **Radiographically.** There are radiographic findings of sacroiliitis (see later discussion).
  2. *Seronegativity.* Rheumatoid factor in the serum and rheumatoid nodules clinically are virtually never found. This accounts for the alternative term "seronegative arthropathies."
  3. *HLA-B27 Association.* The familial nature and clinical overlap of these disorders was well known before HLA-B27 was discovered as a genetic marker. HLA-B27 has more utility for epidemiologic and clinical studies than as a diagnostic test.
B. **Disorders Included in the Spondylarthropathies**
  1. *Ankylosing Spondylitis*
  2. *Reiter's Syndrome*
  3. *Psoriatic Arthritis*
  4. *Arthritis Associated with Inflammatory Bowel Disease*
  5. *Reactive Spondylarthropathies.* These occur in association

with nongonococcal urethritis, certain strains of *Shigella, Yersinia, Salmonella,* and *Campylobacter.*

C. Epidemiology. See Chapter 71.

D. Criteria for Diagnosis. The key aspect of the diagnostic criteria for these diseases is whether or not radiographic evidence of bilateral spondylitis (which can range from possible to definite) is required in addition to the clinical features.

   1. Ankylosing Spondylitis. International conferences have declared the diagnostic criteria as:

   a. Low-back pain present for over three months and not relieved by rest

   b. Pain and stiffness in the thoracic cage

   c. Limited chest expansion

   d. Limited motion in the lumbar spine

   e. Evidence of iritis, either past or present

   f. Bilateral radiographic sacroiliitis

   g. Radiographic syndesmophytosis

Diagnosis can be made if four of the five clinical criteria are present or if bilateral sacroiliitis is present on x-ray *and* one of the five clinical criteria is present.

   2. Reiter's Syndrome. Reiter's syndrome is characterized by any three of the following features, manifested during the same episode of illness (appearance may be asynchronous) *or* arthritis plus any one of the other features if it is characteristic (so-called "incomplete" Reiter's syndrome):

   a. Arthritis

   b. Urethritis

   c. Conjunctivitis

   d. Balanitis

   e. Keratodermia blennorrhagica.

   3. Psoriatic Arthritis. It is mandatory that clinically apparent psoriasis of skin or nails be present, plus arthritis in at least one joint. In addition, two or more of the following supportive criteria must also be present (two suggest possible, four probable, and six definite disease):

   a. Distal interphalangeal inflammatory arthritis

   b. "Sausage digits"

   c. Absence of subcutaneous nodules

   d. Negative rheumatoid factor

   e. Inflammatory synovial fluid with normal or increased complement and no crystals or infection

   f. Synovial biopsy without granulomas or tumor

   g. Erosive arthritis or arthritis that radiographically is not erosive osteoarthritis

   h. Spinal radiographs that show sacroiliitis, syndesmophytes, or paravertebral ossification

   4. Arthritis Associated with Inflammatory Bowel Disease. This is characterized by the presence of chronic ulcerative colitis, Crohn's disease, Whipple's disease, Behçet's syndrome, or various forms of bacilliary dysentery plus a simultaneous or closely associated peripheral joint arthritis or ankylosing spondylitis.

KEY CLINICAL AND LABORATORY FEATURES

A. **Ankylosing Spondylitis.** Early findings are described rather than an advanced case.
   1. *Pain.* There is morning back pain and stiffness that improves with exercise. In addition, pain may occur in the hips, buttocks, and shoulders. Onset is insidious rather than acute, occurring over a period of weeks or months and usually in men under the age of 40.
   2. *Limited Forward Flexion.* This is measured objectively by the modified Schober test: a 10-cm vertical line is measured upward, along the vertebrae, from the level of the posterior iliac spines. The patient is asked to bend forward, and the amount of distraction of the line is measured; more than 5 cm is considered normal.
   3. *Joint Involvement.* The spondylitis is the key, but in 20 per cent of patients an asymmetric arthropathy occurs in the knees, hips, ankles, and less commonly in the shoulders and arms.
   4. *Associated Findings.* These are seen early in many patients.
      a. **Symptoms from Enthesopathic Aspects of the Disease (Pain at the Sight of Tendon Insertion).** These include Achilles tendinitis, plantar fasciitis, iliac crest pain, and pleuritic chest pain caused by inflammation at the insertion of the costovertebral and costosternal muscles.
      b. **Anterior Syndesmophytes.** This occurs in 20 to 30 per cent of patients.
B. **Reiter's Syndrome.** The sequence of the classic Reiter's triad is symptoms of urethritis and conjunctivitis followed one to three weeks later by arthritis.
   1. *Urethritis.* Urethral discharge is usually scant and clear and may be present only in the morning.
   2. *Ulcerations on the Penis.* These ulcerations begin as vesicles on the glans and sometimes on the shaft and scrotum. The lesions may become confluent, producing a large serpiginous patch on the glans that is called *cincinate balanitis.*
   3. *Conjunctivitis.* Conjunctivitis is brief, bilateral, and nonpurulent.
   4. *Iritis (Anterior Iritis or Iridocyclitis).* A common ocular problem; this should be distinguished clinically from conjunctivitis because treatment is different.
   5. *Ulceration in the Mouth.* The ulceration is present anywhere in the mouth, such as cheek, tongue, palate, and pharynx. The ulcerations start as small vesicles, but a key feature is their painlessness (unlike herpetic and aphthous ulcers).
   6. *Keratoderma blennorrhagicum.* This is a late manifestation, beginning one to two months after the urethritis, that occurs in 10 to 30 per cent of patients with Reiter's syndrome. It begins on the feet as small papules or vesicles that become confluent, eventually becoming indistinguishable from pustular psoriasis.

7. **Arthritis.** Classically Reiter's syndrome causes an abrupt asymmetric oligoarthritis of the heels and ankles ("lover's heels"). Knees and hips are next most commonly affected. Inflammation and effusion are present.

8. **Radiographic Findings.** Two notable findings in Reiter's syndrome are calcaneal spurs and the formation of syndesmophytes from close to the middle vertebrae rather than from the margin.

C. **Psoriatic Arthritis.** Occasionally the psoriasis may follow a puzzling case of arthritis (15 per cent of the time), but simultaneous onset is rare.

1. **Classic Clinical Features.** These consist of distal interphalangeal arthritis with characteristic onycholysis and nail ridging and pitting.

2. **"Sausage Digits."** This condition is caused by swelling and inflammation of the interphalangeal joints in the fingers.

3. **Oligoarthritis.** Seventy per cent of the time psoriatic arthritis is a mild oligoarthritis of the small joints of the hands and feet. The psoriasis may be minimal and present only on the scalp.

4. **Arthritis Mutilans.** This is a severe destructive arthritis that occurs rarely and causes destruction of the interphalangeal joints and a severe widespread ankylosis of the spine.

5. **Radiographic Findings.** A characteristic finding in Reiter's syndrome is the "pencil-in-cup" deformity that results from erosion of the tufts of the distal phalanges (the "pencil") and a cuplike erosion of the distal end of the middle phalanx. If this process progresses, "telescoped" fingers may develop. Like psoriatic arthritis, syndesmophytes often form nonmarginally from the spine.

D. **Arthritis Associated with Inflammatory Bowel Disease.** There are two patterns of joint involvement with inflammatory bowel disease:

1. **Spondylitis.** This pattern is indistinguishable from ankylosing spondylitis except for the lack of male predominance.

2. **Peripheral Arthritis.** This typically affects a single joint in the leg, most frequently the knee or ankle, with gradual asymmetric extension to two or three other joints.

RECOMMENDED DIAGNOSTIC APPROACH

A. **Suggestive Symptoms.** Typically the clinician suspects one of the spondylarthropathies when a patient has symptoms of spondylitis, primarily low-back pain, that are unrelieved by rest and last for more than three months. In this situation the following approach is recommended:

1. **History Review.** The physician should search for the clinical features noted previously for the various spondylarthropathies,

in particular histories of past psoriasis, eye problems, inflammatory bowel disease, lower urinary tract symptoms, recent diarrhea, oral or genital ulcers, and a positive family history.

2. **Physical Examination.** The physician should concentrate on evidence of limited lumbar motion (Schober's test) or thoracic cage movement. Skin and nail changes of psoriasis and eye signs of conjunctivitis and iritis should be sought. Examination should be made for "sausage digits," keratoderma blennorrhagica, genital and oral lesions, and subcutaneous nodules.

3. *Laboratory Tests*
   a. **Complete Blood Count and Sedimentation Rate**
   b. **Rheumatoid Factor, Venereal Disease Serology, Antinuclear Antibody, and Serum Complement.** These measurements should be considered.
   c. **HLA-B27.** This is rarely of diagnostic value for individual patients except when the clinical and radiographic features are somewhat suggestive but still borderline, such as with one month of back pain and *unilateral* sacroiliitis. The reader should refer to Khan and Khan for an excellent discussion of the usefulness of HLA-B27 in diagnostic testing.
   d. **Synovial Fluid.** Synovial fluid should be examined if possible, particularly if a single joint is involved. (See Table 71–6, Examination of Synovial Fluid.)

4. *Radiography*
   a. **Single Posteroanterior View of the Pelvis.** This is useful when spondylitis is suspected.
   b. **Radiographs of the Spine.** These should be ordered to look for ankylosis and syndesmophyte formation.
   c. **Radiographs of the Peripheral Joints.** These radiographs, particularly of the fingers, are helpful and may display the diagnostic findings seen in Reiter's syndrome.

REFERENCES

1. McCarty DJ (ed.): Arthritis and Allied Conditions. 9th ed. Philadelphia, Lea & Febiger, 1979.

One of the two major textbooks on rheumatology, this has been considered a definitive work since 1940, valuable for its efforts to establish criteria for the diagnosis of rheumatic diseases.

2. Gilliland BC, Mannik M: Ankylosing spondylitis and Reiter's syndrome, psoriatic arthritis, arthritis associated with gastrointestinal diseases, and Behçet's syndrome. *In* Petersdorf RG, Adams RD, Braunwald E, et al. (eds.): Harrison's Principles of Internal Medicine. New York, McGraw-Hill, 1983.

Contains reviews for the nonspecialist.

3. Khan MA, Khan MK: Diagnostic value of HLA-B27 testing in ankylosing spondylitis and Reiter's syndrome. Ann Intern Med 94:70–76, 1982.

Discusses proper application of the B-27 test in clinical medicine. This test is poor for screening asymptomatic patients and most useful for the diagnostically uncertain case that has some suggestive findings but is not a definite case.

4. Caline A: The spondylarthropathies. *In* Rubenstein E, Federman DD (eds.): Scientific American Medicine. New York, Scientific American 15:III–8, 1980.
A marvelously illustrated and tabulated chapter.

5. Rodman GP, Schumacker HR, Zvaifler JN (eds.): Primer on the Rheumatic Diseases. 8th ed. Atlanta, Arthritis Foundation, 1983.
An excellent source of information.

_____73_____

DEGENERATIVE JOINT DISEASE

By THOMAS D. KOEPSELL, M.D., M.P.H.

DEFINITION AND DIAGNOSTIC CRITERIA

A. Degenerative Joint Disease (DJD). DJD, also termed *osteoarthritis* or *osteoarthrosis,* is a very common chronic joint disorder that is initiated by erosion and fragmentation of articular cartilage. The remaining pathologic features of DJD follow from the cartilage degeneration.

Three factors that contribute to the cartilage lesion appear to be loss and biochemical alteration of proteoglycans in ground substance, mechanical or inflammatory damage resulting from "wear and tear" or prior joint disease, and the very limited ability of hyaline cartilage to repair itself. As cartilage deteriorates, there is sclerosis of subchondral bone and bony overgrowth at the joint margins, with resulting loss of normal joint architecture. The inflammatory response is much less prominent in DJD than in most other joint diseases, leading some authors to shun the term "osteoarthritis" altogether. Nonetheless, the mechanical joint changes and the cartilage fragments and crystals released into joint fluid in advanced disease can cause a synovitis that at least partially accounts for joint pain. Moreover, anti-inflammatory drugs often ameliorate DJD symptoms, providing indirect evidence of an inflammatory component.

DJD is commonly termed *secondary* if the involved joint(s) are known to have experienced prior trauma, arthritis, or severe mechanical stress. DJD is termed *primary* if no such pre-existing lesion can be identified. Secondary DJD commonly involves one or a few joints; primary DJD tends to be polyarticular with certain characteristic patterns of joint involvement, although symptoms in a single joint may predominate. Both forms are increasingly prevalent with advancing age.

B. Criteria for Diagnosis
  1. X-Ray Appearance. There are no universally accepted diagnostic criteria for DJD. However, the diagnosis of DJD is

usually based on x-ray appearance of the affected joint(s). A standard atlas of joint radiographs has been developed for use in epidemiologic studies, which defines stages of DJD for the most commonly affected joints on the basis of the characteristic radiographic features.

2. **Associated Clinical Findings.** The clinician must expect to find x-ray evidence of DJD in many older patients even if another disease process is responsible for the patient's current joint complaints. A (sole) diagnosis of DJD is therefore made more tenable by certain normal clinical findings, namely, the absence of heat, redness, and soft tissue swelling around the joint, the absence of a prominent effusion, and the absence of systemic signs and symptoms.

EPIDEMIOLOGY

A. **Prevalence.** X-rays of a national sample of adults in the United States from 1960 to 1962 provided the age- and sex-specific prevalence rates for DJD of the hands and feet, as shown in Table 73–1. These and other data show that (1) DJD prevalence increases very strikingly with age in both sexes, affecting a large majority of elderly adults; (2) DJD is more common in men than in women before about age 50; and (3) after age 50 (the approximate age of menopause) DJD is more frequent in women.

B. **Asymptomatic DJD.** Although the frequency of joint pain correlates positively with the degree of radiographic joint abnormality, a majority of the DJD that is detectable on x-ray surveys of population samples is asymptomatic. In the survey noted earlier, even among examinees with severe hip DJD evident on x-ray, 43 per cent reported no hip symptoms, and the same pattern of results has been found for other joints.

C. **"Wear and Tear."** Much of the evidence implicating "wear and tear" as a cause of DJD in humans comes from epidemiologic studies:

1. **Occupational Studies.** Many of these studies show high rates of DJD in joints heavily used at work, such as fingers of

TABLE 73–1. PREVALENCE BY AGE AND SEX OF DJD OF THE HANDS AND FEET IN UNITED STATES ADULTS

	PREVALENCE (Per Cent)	
AGE (Years)	*Males*	*Females*
18–24	7.2	1.6
25–34	13.6	6.2
35–44	30.2	19.6
45–54	47.0	46.3
55–64	63.2	75.2
65–74	75.8	84.7
75–79	80.9	89.8

cotton pickers, knees of football players, and ankles and feet of ballet dancers.

2. **Handedness.** DJD is more likely to develop in the right hand in right-handed persons.

3. **Obesity.** Obesity is associated with DJD, particularly of the weight-bearing joints (although debate continues as to whether this association is causal).

D. **Prior Joint Disease.** The risk of DJD is increased in persons with prior joint disease of almost any kind, including those with congenital, inflammatory, infectious, traumatic, or other causes.

E. **Hereditary Factors.** Family and twin studies suggest a strong hereditary component to the syndrome of generalized DJD with bony enlargement of the DIP joints, which chiefly affects women.

CLINICAL PICTURE

A. **History**
1. **Pattern of Joint Involvement.** Because certain joints are common sites of DJD and others are not, the pattern of joint involvement is useful diagnostically. The following approximate ranking, from frequently involved to rarely involved, is based on the prevalence of DJD in each joint in epidemiologic surveys: distal interphalangeal (DIP), knee, first metatarsophalangeal, first carpometacarpal, lumbar spine, proximal interphalangeal (PIP), hip, metacarpophalangeal, cervical spine, tarsal, sacroiliac, wrist, shoulder, elbow, and lateral metatarsophalangeal joints.

2. **Joint Pain.** This is the most common initial complaint but in fact affects only a minority of radiographically affected joints. Classically, it is made worse by use of the joint (as in weight-bearing on the hip or knee), becomes worse as the day wears on, and is relieved by rest. Pain at rest can occur in advanced disease, presumably as a result of synovitis or capsular swelling.

3. **Morning Stiffness ("Gelling").** Such stiffness, which lasts less than half an hour and is ameliorated by joint use, has been said to be typical of DJD. However, studies show that only 20 to 30 per cent of joints with moderate to advanced DJD exhibit morning stiffness, which has a prevalence only slightly above that found in radiographically normal joints. Hence the low sensitivity and specificity of this symptom make its diagnostic usefulness questionable. However, some studies do show morning stiffness to be more common in advanced disease.

4. **Pre-Existing Joint Lesions.** A wide variety of joint injuries, of which the most common are listed in Table 73–2, are risk factors for later development of DJD. Particularly for DJD confined to a particular joint or joint group, a history of one or more such pre-existing joint lesions is consistent with secondary DJD.

B. **Physical Signs.** Very little quantitative information is available

TABLE 73–2. SOME PRE-EXISTING CONDITIONS THOUGHT TO PREDISPOSE TO SECONDARY DJD

Previous joint disease or injury
Trauma
Infectious arthritis
Aseptic necrosis
Menisectomy (knee)
Intra-articular steroids
Rheumatoid arthritis
Gout
Pseudogout
Spondyloarthropathy
Congenital hip dysplasia
Neuropathic joint (Charcot's arthritis)
Endocrine or metabolic disease
Diabetes mellitus
Paget's disease
Hyperparathyroidism
Acromegaly
Ochronosis
Hemochromatosis
Wilson's disease
Homocystinuria
Other
Hemophilia
Sickle cell disease
Many heritable syndromes: mucopolysaccharidoses, Ehlers-Danlos
   syndrome, Marfan's syndrome, multiple epiphyseal dysplasia, and
   others

as to the frequency of various physical signs by joint and severity of DJD. However, the findings most commonly cited as typical are:

1. **Decreased Range of Motion.** This occurs with pain at the extremes of this range.
2. **Osteophytes.** Osteophytes are palpable as painless bony enlargement adjacent to the joint. At the DIP joints these are called *Heberden's nodes*; at the PIP joints they are called *Bouchard's nodes*.
3. **Crepitus or "Grating" Sensations.** These are palpable over the joint with movement.
4. **Tenderness Along the Joint Margin.** As noted earlier, DJD alone does not usually produce an acute inflammatory response. Hence a joint that is painful solely as a result of DJD normally exhibits little or no soft tissue swelling, redness, or heat. Effusions are relatively rare in DJD, except for modest effusions at the knee.

C. **Laboratory Abnormalities**
  1. **Joint Fluid.** Joint fluid that is obtained from a joint with DJD has the following characteristics:
     a. It is clear, viscous, and does not clot.
     b. The total cell count is:
        <500 cells per cu mm in about 52 per cent of cases
        <1000 cells per cu mm in about 86 per cent of cases

<2000 cells per cu mm in about 93 per cent of cases

<5000 cells per cu mm in nearly all cases

Counts of up to about 15,000 cells per cu mm have been reported in active synovitis.

c. Mononuclear cells predominate in joint fluid. The absolute polymorphonuclear neutrophil (PMN) cell count is:

<500 PMNs per cu mm in about 96 per cent of cases

<1000 PMNs per cu mm in nearly all cases

d. The joint fluid protein concentration is nearly always <3 g per dL in primary DJD but can be up to about 5 g per dL in secondary DJD.

e. Microscopic examination shows fibrin and debris but generally no crystals. However, DJD can occur secondary to crystal-induced arthropathies.

2. *Extra-Articular Manifestations.* DJD has no important extra-articular manifestations. Hence the erythrocyte sedimentation rate, rheumatoid factor, and other peripheral blood tests are unaffected by DJD. These tests may be elevated in older individuals for various reasons, and DJD prevalence increases with age, so that noncausal associations between DJD and blood test abnormalities may be expected on this basis.

D. **X-ray Findings.** The characteristic x-ray findings of DJD are outlined as follows:

1. *Osteophytes at the Joint Margins or Ligamentous Attachments*
2. *Narrowing of the Joint Space*
3. *Sclerosis of Subchondral Bone*
4. *Cystic Areas with Sclerotic Walls in Subchondral Bone*

Periarticular ossicles, especially at the PIP and DIP joints, are also common. Advanced DJD can produce changes in the shape of bone ends adjacent to the joint.

The order in which these findings develop varies by joint. An atlas of standard radiographs illustrates the usual progression of abnormalities for commonly affected joints.

RECOMMENDED DIAGNOSTIC APPROACH

A. **X-ray of the Suspect Joint.** This should be the usual method to document DJD. Compatible history and physical findings alone (if they indicate no acute inflammation) are probably sufficient evidence in a person with known DJD in other joints.

B. **Arthrocentesis.** Arthrocentesis with analysis of joint fluid for appearance, cell count and differential, protein, crystals, and appropriate cultures should be performed if an effusion is present or if the joint is swollen, red, or warm.

REFERENCES

1. The epidemiology of chronic rheumatism. *In* Atlas of Standard Radiographs of Arthritis. Vol. II. Philadelphia, FA Davis Company, 1963.
2. National Center for Health Statistics: Osteoarthritis in Adults by Selected

Demographic Characteristics, United States, 1960–1962. Vital and Health Statistics, Series 11, No. 20, 1966.

3. Kelsey JL: The Epidemiology of Musculoskeletal Conditions. New York, Oxford University Press, 1983.

4. Acheson RM, Chan Y-K, Clemett AR: New Haven survey of joint diseases. XII. Distribution of symptoms of osteoarthrosis in the hands with reference to handedness. Ann Rheum Dis 29:275–286, 1970.

5. Kellgren JH, Lawrence JS: Osteo-arthrosis and disk degeneration in an urban population. Ann Rheum Dis 17:388–397, 1958.

6. Lawrence JS, Bremner JM, Bier F: Osteoarthrosis. Prevalence in the population and relationship between symptoms and x-ray changes. Ann Rheum Dis 25:1–24, 1966.

7. O'Brien WM, Clemett AR, Acheson RM: Symptoms and pattern of osteoarthrosis in the hand in the New Haven survey of joint disease. Chap. 55. In Bennett PH, Wood PHN (eds.): Population Studies of the Rheumatic Diseases. International Congress Series No. 148. Amsterdam, Excerpta Medica Foundation, 1968.

8. Ropes MW, Bauer W: Synovial Fluid Changes in Joint Disease. Cambridge, Harvard University Press, 1953.

9. Moll JMH: Investigation of osteoarthrosis. Clin Rheum Dis 2:587–613, 1976.

10. Moskowitz RW: Clinical and laboratory findings in osteoarthritis. Chap. 75. In McCarty DJ (ed.): Arthritis and Allied Conditions. 9th ed. Philadelphia, Lea & Febiger, 1979.

74

PROGRESSIVE SYSTEMIC SCLEROSIS (SCLERODERMA) PLUS MIXED CONNECTIVE TISSUE DISEASE AND THE CREST SYNDROME

By RICHARD O. CUMMINS, M.D., M.P.H.

DEFINITION AND CRITERIA FOR DIAGNOSIS

A. **Definition.** These are multisystem disorders of connective tissue, in which immunologic mechanisms play the major etiologic role. The clinical hallmark and unifying feature of these syndromes is *scleroderma*, which properly refers only to the fibrotic and degenerative changes of the skin. A better picture emerges if the clinician thinks in terms of the syndromes that feature scleroderma, which include the following:

1. *Progressive Systemic Sclerosis (PSS).* This is a diffuse scleroderma.

2. *The "CREST" Variant of PSS.* C = calcinosis; R = Raynaud's phenomenon; E = esophageal dysmotility; S = sclerodactyly; and T = telangiectasias.

3. *Mixed Connective Tissue Disease (MCTD).* This is an admix-

ture of the clinical features of PSS, systemic lupus erythematosus, and polymyositis.

    a. PSS. This involves mainly Raynaud's phenomenon, esophageal hypomotility, pulmonary diffusion abnormalities, scleroderma, and telangiectasias.

    b. Systemic Lupus Erythematosus. This is manifested mainly as arthritis and skin rash.

    c. Polymyositis. There is mainly the inflammatory myopathy with myalgias, proximal muscle weakness, and elevated muscle enzymes.

  4. *Overlap Syndromes.* There are admixtures of clinical features similar to MCTD but less well defined.

  5. *Chemically Induced Scleroderma.* This includes polyvinylchloride disease; pentazocine-, trichloroethylene-, and bleomycin-induced fibrosis; and scleroderma associated with carbidopa and L-5-hydroxytryptophan.

  6. *Localized (Focal) Scleroderma.* This term applies to a skin condition only and does not include the internal fibrosis of PSS.

B. Epidemiology. More often these diseases occur in black middle-aged women.

C. Criteria for Diagnosis of PSS.

  1. *Required.* There must be sclerodermatous skin changes and tight firm skin that may precede other involvement by years.

  2. *Required.* There must be signs of fibrotic involvement of some other organ, notably the gastrointestinal tract, lungs, heart, and kidney.

  3. *Recommended.* Tests for antinuclear antibodies (ANA) should be positive. (See Chap. 76, Table 76–1.)

    a. ANA Test. The ANA test is positive in 40 to 80 per cent of patients with PSS; the nuclear immunofluorescence pattern is almost always speckled.

    b. Specific Antinuclear Antibodies. At least four antinuclear antibodies have been identified in patients with PSS.

      1). High titers to the nuclear ribonucleoprotein (RNP) are most frequently associated with the clinical features of mixed connective tissue disease.

      2). High titers to the protein bound to centromere DNA are usually associated with the CREST syndrome.

KEY CLINICAL FEATURES OF PSS

    As noted earlier, the diagnosis of PSS is based on clinical features, and laboratory data are supportive.

A. Skin Changes (Scleroderma)

  1. *Early: the Edematous Phase.* This involves symmetric painless pitting edema of hands and fingers ("sausage digits"). This phase lasts a few weeks to several months.

  2. *Later: the Indurative Phase.* In this phase the edema is gradually replaced by the thickening, hardening, and tightening of the skin of the fingers, hands, face, trunk, and later the feet and legs. These changes were the reason that the name "scleroderma" was first given to PSS.

B. **Raynaud's Phenomenon.** This occurs in 90 to 98 per cent of patients with PSS, and may antedate all other features.

C. **Joint Problems.** The majority of PSS patients complain of joint pain and stiffness, but a frank arthritis with multiple joints symmetrically affected is uncommon.

   1. *Tuft Erosion.* X-rays occasionally show distal tuft erosion with soft tissue atrophy and calcinosis in subcutaneous tissues.

   2. *CREST Syndrome.* This bone erosion and calcinosis are much more common in the CREST syndrome.

D. **Esophageal Dysfunction.** As noted, signs of fibrotic changes in other organs are required for the diagnosis of PSS. Esophageal dysfunction is the most common of these signs of internal involvement.

   1. *Symptoms.* Symptoms include mainly dysphagia and the pain of peptic esophagitis and esophageal reflux. The lower two thirds of the esophagus lose peristaltic waves and become atonic and dilate as PSS progresses. Even when there are no symptoms, roentgenographic abnormalities of the esophagus are present in over 75 per cent of patients.

E. **Pulmonary Problems.** PSS clinically causes interstitial bibasilar *pulmonary fibrosis* (linear, nodular, or diffuse densities in reticular or honeycomb pattern). Evidence of this is found postmortem in virtually all patients.

   1. *Exertional Dyspnea.* This is the most frequent symptom.

   2. *Severe Pulmonary Arterial Hypertension.* Such hypertension with calcinosis of the arteries is a classic finding in the CREST syndrome.

F. **Cardiac Problems.** PSS typically causes a myocardial fibrosis with a resultant cardiomyopathy and left-sided failure.

   1. *Conduction Abnormalities.* This is the most frequent cardiac problem.

   2. *Right-Sided Failure.* Right-sided failure caused by lung disease also occurs as well as pericarditis and pericardial effusion.

G. **Gastrointestinal Problems.** As in the esophagus, hypomotility is the cardinal abnormality, leading to cramps, bloating, recurrent diarrhea, and an overgrowth of small intestinal bacteria that produces a typical malabsorption syndrome.

   1. *Unique "PSS-sacculations."* These occur in the large intestine as muscularis atrophy leads to characteristic wide-mouthed diverticula.

H. **Renal Problems.** As in other connective tissue diseases, when PSS causes death, the majority of the time it does so by renal failure.

   1. *Typical Pattern.* In PSS there is the sudden occurrence of severe malignant hypertension in a patient whose condition is apparently stable; progressive and irreversible renal failure follows rapidly.

2. *Prediction of Which PSS Patients Will Develop Renal Failure.*
Prediction is difficult, although chronic pericardial effusion
or the development of a microangiopathic hemolytic anemia
is said to be an antecedent sign.

DIFFERENTIAL DIAGNOSIS

A. **Clinical Pattern.** As in systemic lupus erythematosus, it is the
combination of clinical findings, often unfolded serially over
time, that leads to the diagnosis of PSS. The classic skin changes,
combined with Raynaud's phenomenon and other visceral problems, secure the diagnosis. There are variations such as the
CREST variant and mixed connective tissue disease that should
be considered.

Because of the "unfolding" nature of PSS, its differential diagnosis
becomes the differential diagnosis of each of its clinical manifestations. If patients have unexplained cardiomyopathy, heart block,
dysphagia, pulmonary fibrosis, or malabsorption syndrome, they
must be evaluated appropriately for these problems. (The reader
should see the relevant chapters in this book.) The clinician, however, should ask whether the problem could be early PSS prior to
or without cutaneous involvement.

B. **Raynaud's Phenonemon as a Prominent Sign.** PSS must always
be considered, as well as other causes of Raynaud's phenomenon,
including cold agglutinin disease, cryoglobulinemia, vinyl chloride exposure, reflex sympathetic dystrophies, thoracic outlet
syndromes, and posttraumatic fibrosis.

C. **Arthralgia or Arthritis as a Prominent Sign.** The differential
diagnosis involves a list of the causes of polyarticular arthritis
(see Chap. 71), although rheumatoid arthritis and SLE have the
most similarities to PSS.

RECOMMENDED DIAGNOSTIC APPROACH

A. **Sclerodermalike Skin Changes**
1. *Connective-Tissue or Immunologic Disease.* The physician
should look for evidence of such disease.
a. **ANA Test with Nuclear Immunofluorescence.** (See
Chap. 76, Table 76–1.) If test results are positive, more
specific antinuclear antibodies should be examined.
b. **Complete Blood Count.** The physician should look for
anemia, especially microangiopathic and hemolytic anemia,
and lymphopenia.
c. **ESR, Rheumatoid Factor, and Serum Complement.**
ESR is often elevated; rheumatoid factor is present in 25 per
cent of PSS patients; and serum complement is seldom
decreased.
2. *Evidence of Other Organ Involvement*
a. **Chest Radiograph.** Basilar pulmonary fibrosis and cardiac
enlargement may be present and minimally symptomatic.

   b. **Electrocardiogram.** The physician should look for conduction abnormalities.
   c. **Blood-Urea Nitrogen, Creatinine, Urinalysis for Casts, Hematuria, and Proteinuria.** The physician should look for renal damage.
   d. **Barium Swallow with Small Bowel Follow-Through.** Abnormalities with esophageal and small bowel motility are so common in patients with PSS that this radiographic procedure should be performed whenever the diagnosis of PSS is considered seriously, even in people with no gastrointestinal symptoms.
   3. *Rare Conditions That Cause Sclerodermalike Skin Lesions.* These include scleredema, scleromyxedema, and primary amyloidosis. A dermatology consultation with skin biopsy may be required to distinguish these conditions.
B. **Visceral Involvement.** For the patient with evidence of visceral involvement, the following approach is recommended:
   1. *Organ System Involvement.* The diagnostic approach here should be guided by the organ system affected. The reader should refer to related chapters on interstitial lung disease, congestive heart failure, and malabsorption.
   2. *Tests.* The tests recommended under Sclerodermalike Skin Changes should be added during the work-up as the possibility of PSS increases.

REFERENCES

1. Progressive systemic sclerosis and related disorders; Mixed connective tissue disease. *In* Rodman GP, Schumacker R, Zuaifler JN (eds.): Primer on the Rheumatic Diseases. 8th ed. Atlanta, Arthritis Foundation, 1983, pp. 59–66.
An excellent publication that should always be initially consulted to review the rheumatologic diseases.

2. Gilliland BC, Mannik M: Progressive systemic sclerosis (diffuse scleroderma). *In* Petersdorf RG, Adams PD, Braunwald E, Bselbacker KJ, Martin JB, Wilson JD (eds.): Harrison's Principles of Internal Medicine. 10th ed. New York, McGraw-Hill, 1983, pp. 2002–2006.
A good review for the general clinician.

3. LeRoy BC: Scleroderma (systemic sclerosis). *In* Kelly WN, et al. (eds.): Textbook of Rheumatology. Philadelphia, W.B. Saunders Company, 1981, pp. 1211–1230.
A review for the more specialized clinician.

SARCOIDOSIS

By PATRICIA SATO, M.D.

DEFINITION AND CRITERIA FOR DIAGNOSIS

A. Definition. In 1975 the Seventh International Conference on Sarcoidosis defined the disorder as "a multisystem granulomatous disorder of unknown etiology, most commonly affecting young adults and presenting most frequently with bilateral hilar lymphadenopathy, pulmonary infiltrates, skin or eye lesions." Several other organ systems may be involved, most commonly peripheral lymph nodes, liver, spleen, mucous membranes, parotid glands, phalangeal bones, muscles, heart, and nervous system.

B. Criteria for Diagnosis. The diagnosis is established most firmly when the following four criteria are met:

1. Histologic evidence of noncaseating epithelioid-cell granulomas in more than one organ system
2. Consistent clinical findings in more than one organ system (see later discussion)
3. Consistent findings on the chest roentgenogram (see later discussion)
4. Exclusion of infectious or neoplastic processes that may simulate sarcoidosis

EPIDEMIOLOGY

The disease occurs throughout the world but more commonly in temperate areas. The average age of onset is between 20 and 35, but sarcoidosis has been diagnosed at as early as one year and as late as 80 years of age. Blacks are affected 10 to 20 times more frequently than whites, and women are affected more commonly than men, particularly among blacks. The clinical course of the disease is benign in the majority of patients. Severe pulmonary fibrosis develops in 10 to 20 per cent of patients. The fatality rate attributable to sarcoidosis is 5 to 10 per cent.

HISTOLOGY AND IMMUNOLOGY

A. Histology. Multiple noncaseating granulomas are the characteristic histologic finding in sarcoidosis. The granuloma consists of a central collection of epithelioid cells and multinucleated giant cells surrounded by lymphocytes. These granulomas are nonspecific and may be found in other diseases such as mycobacterial or fungal infections, lymphoma, foreign body reactions, berylliosis, leprosy, and in regional lymph nodes associated with neoplastic or inflammatory reactions.

B. **Immunology.** Abnormalities in the immune system are well recognized in sarcoidosis. Patients exhibit hyporeactivity to skin tests that measure type IV cell-mediated reactions. This anergy does not prevent tuberculin skin reactivity in patients with active tuberculosis. The pulmonary parenchyma in patients with sarcoidosis has abundant T lymphocytes, but the peripheral circulation shows lymphopenia with decreased T cell number and function. If bronchoalveolar lavage (BAL) is performed in patients with sarcoid, the fluid recovered contains T cells that are increased in number and function. These findings from BAL may prove useful in assessing disease activity. The number of circulating B lymphocytes is normal or high, and antibody production is preserved or increased. Circulating immune complexes have been recovered in some patients, but there has been no demonstrable correlation between these complexes and disease activity. Despite the depression of cell-mediated immunity, sarcoid patients do not appear to be predisposed to infections or to development of cancer.

SIGNS AND SYMPTOMS

A. **History.** The history seldom leads clinicians to suspect sarcoidosis because about 50 per cent of the patients are asymptomatic when the disease is first diagnosed. The diagnosis is most frequently made when asymptomatic people are found to have an abnormal chest x-ray on a screening examination and are then referred for evaluation. Several series, however, show that nearly 90 per cent of patients with sarcoidosis have symptoms at some time during the course of the disease. The most common symptoms are cough and dyspnea that reflect the almost universal pulmonary involvement. Patients also complain of nonspecific constitutional symptoms such as weight loss, fatigue, malaise, weakness, and occasionally fever. Additional complaints are related to the various organ systems involved and may include arthralgia, arthritis, skin lesions, and eye pain.

B. **Physical Examination.** The findings on physical examination vary but are related to the most commonly involved organ systems: the lungs, lymph nodes, skin, and eyes.

1. *The Lungs.* Tachypnea, rales, and occasionally wheezing are the most frequent pulmonary symptoms.

2. *Lymph Nodes.* Lymphadenopathy should be carefully sought. It may be generalized or localized to one region and most commonly involves the supraclavicular, epitrochlear, axillary, inguinal, and auricular nodes.

3. *Skin.* The dermatologic manifestations are variable and multiple. Specific lesions of noncaseating granulomas may be found in old scars or traumatized areas of skin. Erythema nodosum is a common but nonspecific finding that occurs in conjunction with bilateral hilar adenopathy, arthritis, or

uveitis. Macules, papules, and plaques may also occur. Lupus pernio, a deep plaquelike lesion, may cause disfiguring lesions of the nose, cheeks, or ears.

4. **Eyes.** Ophthalmologic findings may be acute or chronic and can include keratoconjunctivitis, conjunctival follicles, iridocyclitis, and chorioretinitis. Ocular involvement is a specific indication for intraocular steroid therapy.

5. **Other.** Other findings include hepatosplenomegaly, arthritis in the small joints, and rarely manifestations of cardiac involvement (heart blocks or arrhythmias) or neurologic involvement (cranial nerve palsies, seizures, or peripheral neuropathies). Table 75–1 lists the frequency of involvement of different organ systems.

LABORATORY STUDIES AND THE CHEST X-RAY

A. Laboratory Studies

1. **Hypercalcemia.** One important abnormality seen in only 10 per cent of cases is hypercalcemia. The mechanism for this is abnormal sensitivity to vitamin D. Patients also have increased levels of 1,25-dihydroxy vitamin D, an active metabolite. As a result, sarcoid patients have enhanced intestinal absorption of calcium that results in hypercalcemia and hypercalciuria. Prednisone readily reverses the hypercalcemia.

2. **Serum Angiotensin Converting Enzyme (ACE).** The activity of this enzyme is elevated in more than half of patients with active disease. Levels fall toward normal with spontaneous remissions or with steroid therapy. ACE may be increased in other granulomatous disorders, and not all patients with sarcoid have elevated levels. Despite their lack of sensitivity or specificity, ACE levels can support other diagnostic data or help assess disease activity in individual patients.

TABLE 75–1. FREQUENCY OF ORGAN INVOLVEMENT IN SARCOIDOSIS

Organ	Per Cent
Lungs	95–100
Lymph nodes	73
Skin	32
Eye	21
Liver	21
Spleen	18
Bone	14
Salivary glands	6
Joints	6
Heart	5
Nervous system	5
Kidneys	4
Nose and mouth	3
Lacrimal glands	3

3. *Gallium Scan.* Sarcoid granulomas take up gallium and accumulate the marker in lymph nodes, lung tissue, and other extrapulmonary sites. Many authorities consider this technique used in conjunction with ACE levels to be very specific for diagnosis. Its use is not universally favored, however, and long-term efficacy remains to be established.

B. **Pulmonary Function Tests.** The most common findings on pulmonary function testing are decreased vital capacity, total lung capacity, and other volume measurements that reflect the usual restrictive pattern. The diffusing capacity for carbon monoxide is typically reduced, as is lung compliance. An obstructive pattern may be found with bronchial involvement or in end-stage disease. Arterial blood gases typically show a decreased PaO_2 with a widened alveolar to arterial oxygen difference. Evaluation of pulmonary function tests (PFTs) cannot predict the patient's course or response to therapy but may detect changes in disease severity and aid in clinical decision-making.

C. **Chest Roentgenogram.** Ninety per cent of patients with sarcoidosis have radiologic evidence of involvement with parenchymal infiltrates or lymph node enlargement, or both. The following radiographic staging classification has been established to aid in disease description:

1. *Stage I.* This stage is characterized by bilateral hilar adenopathy with or without enlarged paratracheal nodes. The lung fields are clear. Despite the normal appearance, biopsy of lung tissue yields granulomas in virtually all cases. Fifty per cent of all patients have this appearance on chest x-ray. Prognosis is good in this group, since 80 per cent show regression of the enlarged glands by two years. Ten per cent remain in this stage and the other 10 per cent progress to Stage II.

2. *Stage II.* One fourth of patients appear for examination in this stage with bilateral hilar adenopathy and symmetric but diffuse parenchymal involvement. The parenchymal pattern ranges from a fine reticular pattern to a more nodular one. As in Stage I, most patients have spontaneous remission of the illness, and approximately one third have persistent or progressive disease.

3. *Stage III.* This stage is characterized by diffuse parenchymal involvement without lymph node enlargement. Approximately 15 per cent of patients have this appearance on chest x-ray. Fibrosis may be present with decreased lung volumes and evidence of honeycombing. These patients tend to be the most symptomatic, with respiratory symptoms of cough and dyspnea, and may progress to respiratory failure.

RECOMMENDED DIAGNOSTIC APPROACH

The manifestations of sarcoidosis are so variable that the diagnosis is often a matter of exclusion.

A. **Abnormal Chest Roentgenogram.** To evaluate a patient who has an abnormal chest roentgenogram suggestive of one of the stages of sarcoidosis, the physician should evaluate the following:

1. **Physical Examination.** Evidence of multisystem involvement should be sought, in particular of the lymph nodes, skin, eyes, and central nervous system. Ophthalmology consultation to look for ocular involvement is mandatory because such involvement is an indication for steroid therapy.

2. **Serum Calcium.** Serum calcium should be determined. Severe hypercalcemia is another indication for steroid therapy.

3. **Electrocardiogram.** Conduction system abnormalities and evidence of myocardial sarcoidosis should be sought.

4. **Pulmonary Function Tests.** Progressive pulmonary impairment also requires steroids.

5. **Skin Tests.** Skin tests should be done to evaluate possible tuberculosis and anergy.

6. **Gallium Scan and Serum Angiotensin Converting Enzyme Level.** In centers in which the facilities are available, a gallium scan and measurement of serum angiotensin converting enzyme level should be performed. These results may offer strong evidence for the diagnosis.

7. **Kveim Test.** This is another diagnostic test that is well known but rarely used. A suspension of known sarcoid spleen is injected intradermally. A positive reaction yields a typical noncaseating granuloma at the injection site in four to eight weeks. Major problems with the test are availability of the suspension, its standardization, and the length of time required for diagnosis. Because of these problems the Kveim test is rarely used in clinical practice in the United States.

8. **Biopsy.** The presence of noncaseating granulomas on biopsy is required for a confirmed diagnosis. (See comments below.)

B. **Comments on Biopsy**

1. **Occasionally Unnecessary.** There are some clinical pictures that are so distinctive that some authors consider a biopsy unnecessary. The picture of acute sarcoidosis with bilateral hilar adenopathy, erythema nodosum, uveitis, and arthritis is one such example. Asymptomatic bilateral hilar adenopathy with negative findings at physical examination is another. This remains a controversial issue; most clinicians decide in favor of histologic confirmation.

2. **Biopsy Site.** The choice of biopsy site should be governed by the expected yield and the potential complications of the procedure. If any palpable lymph nodes or cutaneous lesions are present, biopsy of these areas can be easily performed with little morbidity. Random biopsy of minor salivary glands, lacrimal glands, or enlarged parotid glands can also be done in experienced hands. If these tests are unavailable, transbronchial lung biopsy is a very effective and safe procedure. Its efficacy varies with the radiographic stage. Stage I disease yields granulomas on transbronchial biopsy 60 per cent of the time. With Stage II and III disease the biopsy is positive in 80 to 95 per cent of patients eventually shown to have sarcoidosis.

TABLE 75–2. YIELD RATES FOR BIOPSY SITES

BIOPSY SITE	PER CENT YIELD
Open lung biopsy	100
Mediastinoscopy	90–100
Transbronchial biopsy	
Stage I	60
Stages II and III	80–95
Liver	70
Blind scalene node	50–80
Skin	35
Conjunctiva with follicles	25
Minor salivary glands	60

If further diagnostic procedures are needed, biopsy by means of mediastinoscopy or liver biopsy should be performed. Open lung biopsy is almost never needed to make a diagnosis, but its yield is essentially 100 per cent. Table 75–2 lists biopsy sites with their expected yields.

REFERENCES

1. Transactions of the New York Academy of Sciences: Seventh International Conference on Sarcoidosis and other Granulomatous Disorders. Ann NY Acad Sci 278:1, 1975.

The most recent consensus definition of sarcoidosis.

2. Mayock RL, Bertrand P, Morrison LE, Scott JH: Manifestations of sarcoidosis. Am J Med 35:67, 1963.

A classic description of the major clinical features. Still useful.

3. Nosal A, Schleissner LA, Mishkin FS, Lieberman J: Angiotensin-1-converting enzyme and gallium scan in noninvasive evaluation of sarcoidosis. Ann Intern Med 90:328, 1979.

A new combined diagnostic test that may eliminate the need for some biopsies.

4. Winterbauer RH, Belic N, Moores KD: A clinical interpretation of bilateral hilar adenopathy. Ann Intern Med 78:65, 1973.

An extremely useful review of the causes of bilateral hilar adenopathy. Sarcoid and lymphoma top the list.

5. DeRemee RA: The roentgenographic staging of sarcoidosis. Chest 83:128, 1983.

An essential review, since so much of the evaluation and prognosis of patients with sarcoidosis depends on the roentgenographic stages.

SYSTEMIC LUPUS ERYTHEMATOSUS

By RICHARD O. CUMMINS, M.D., M.P.H.

DEFINITION AND CRITERIA FOR DIAGNOSIS

A. **Definition.** Systemic lupus erythematosus (SLE) is a chronic multisystem disease of inflammatory nature and unknown cause. Immunologic mechanisms, particularly antigen-antibody immune complex formation, appear to produce the tissue injury.
B. **Epidemiology.** This is primarily a disease of 20- to 40-year-old women, most often black.
C. **Criteria for Diagnosis**
   1. *Required Criteria That Are Hallmarks of the Disease.* Antibodies to components of the cell nucleus are present.
      a. There are positive antinuclear antibodies with immunofluorescence in a peripheral pattern (most common) or occasionally a speckled or diffuse pattern. (See Table 76–1.)
      b. More specifically, there can be positive antibodies to double-stranded native DNA or other nuclear antigen such as Sm, ribonucleoprotein, or nucleoprotein. These antibodies are present in only 25 to 75 per cent of SLE patients and therefore have limited sensitivity. However, because they are rare in diseases other than SLE, a positive test result is virtually diagnostic.
   2. *Clinical and Laboratory Evidence.* Involvement of other organ systems, either serially or simultaneously, must also be observed (see later discussion of Signs That Indicate SLE).

KEY CLINICAL AND LABORATORY EVIDENCE OF MULTISYSTEM INVOLVEMENT IN SLE

The usual pattern of appearance of SLE is a gradual "unfolding" in a series of episodes. It is the combination, over time, of the clinical and laboratory abnormalities that eventually leads to the correct diagnosis.
A. **Signs That Indicate SLE.** Three or four of the following findings (presented in order of frequency in patients with SLE) combined with positive antinuclear antibodies confirm the diagnosis of SLE:
   1. *Joint Involvement.* There is joint involvement in over 95 per cent of cases. It may precede findings in other systems by years. The hands at the proximal interphalangeal, metacarpophalangeal, and wrist joints are most commonly affected. The arthritis is strikingly symmetric and nonerosive on x-ray.

TABLE 76–1. USE OF ANTINUCLEAR ANTIBODIES IN THE DIAGNOSIS OF RHEUMATOLOGIC DISEASES

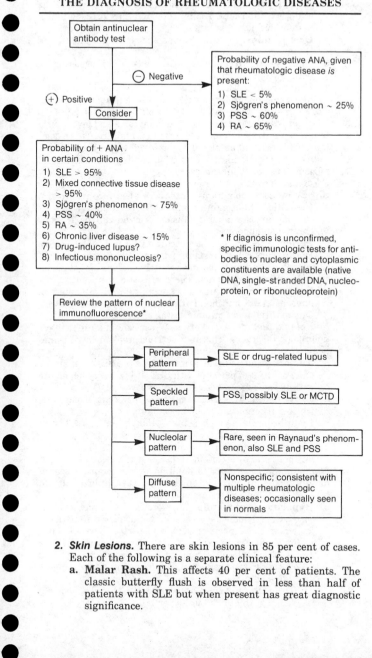

2. *Skin Lesions.* There are skin lesions in 85 per cent of cases. Each of the following is a separate clinical feature:

   a. **Malar Rash.** This affects 40 per cent of patients. The classic butterfly flush is observed in less than half of patients with SLE but when present has great diagnostic significance.

  b. **Discoid Rash.** There is discoid rash in 15 per cent of cases. It can occur over the chest and arms as well as the scalp, ear, and face. Again, this sign may precede multisystem findings by years.
  c. **Oral Lesions.** Painless lesions appear in the mouth and throat.
  d. **Photosensitivity.** Sun exposure leads to a diffuse eruption with erythema and acute edema.
  e. **Other Signs.** These include patchy alopecia, purpura, hives, angioneurotic edema, and Raynaud's phenomenon.
3. *Renal Disorder.* This affects 50 to 60 per cent of patients. Disorders can range from minimal hematuria and proteinuria to the nephrotic syndrome and total renal failure. This causes most SLE-related deaths. Diagnosis of lupus nephritis is indicated by proteinuria of over 0.5 g per day, hematuria, and various types of cellular casts.
4. *Serositis.* Serositis is present in 50 to 75 per cent of cases. SLE produces predominantly three serosal surface syndromes:
  a. **Pleuritis.** This condition affects 50 per cent of cases. It can appear as a pleural effusion, friction rub, or acute or chronic pneumonitis.
  b. **Pericarditis.** Pericarditis occurs in 25 per cent of cases. It can vary from a small friction rub to electrocardiographic abnormalities and a massive pericardial effusion.
  c. **Abdominal Problems.** These affect 50 per cent of patients. Recurrent pain is common as well as anorexia, nausea, and vomiting. Patients also experience ascites, pancreatitis, and a protein-losing enteropathy.
5. *Neurologic Disorders.* Twenty to 50 per cent of patients have neurologic disorders. This is a serious problem in SLE and has many manifestations, including:
  a. **Anemia.** Anemia (hemoglobin < 11 g per dL) occurs in 70 to 80 per cent of patients with SLE. It is usually hemolytic with normocytic indices and reticulocytosis.
  b. **Leukopenia.** This affects 50 to 60 per cent of patients; white cell count is < 4000 per cu mm.
  c. **Lymphopenia.** Lymphopenia (<1500 lymphocytes per cu mm on two or more measurements) may occur.
  d. **Thrombocytopenia.** Thrombocytopenia (<100,000 platelets per cu mm) occurs in 15 per cent of cases.
6. *Immunologic Disorders.* In addition to the requisite search for antibodies to nuclear constituents, the clinician should look for the following immunologic problems:
  a. **Hypocomplementemia.** This occurs in 75 per cent of cases. Complement levels should be measured in patients for whom a diagnosis of SLE is suspected. Low measurements confirm active disease. Complement decreases as a result of activation by immune complexes; it is helpful to follow therapeutic response. The following measurements should be obtained:
    1). Total Hemolytic Complement (CH$_{50}$): The normal range is 150 to 250 units per mL.

      2). **Serum Complement** C_3. The normal range is 55 to 120 mg per dL.

      3). **Serum Complement** C_4. The normal range is 20 to 50 mg per dL.

  b. **Hypergammaglobulinemia.** Hypergammaglobulinemia of >1.5 g per dL occurs in 60 to 77 per cent of patients with SLE. Elevations occur when disease is active.

  c. **Rheumatoid Factors.** Tests are positive in 20 per cent of cases. Titers are usually lower than for rheumatoid arthritis.

  d. **Biologic False-Positive Test for Syphilis.** This sometimes occurs before the clinical onset of SLE.

DIFFERENTIAL DIAGNOSIS

As noted, SLE most often appears as a series of clinical manifestations frequently separated in time. Few clinicians would fail to think of SLE when confronted with a young woman with symmetric arthritis and a butterfly flush over the malar eminence. However, if SLE occurs with involvement of only one system as described earlier, the differential diagnosis becomes the differential diagnosis of that problem, for example, hemolytic anemia, psychosis, or a positive venereal disease reaction level.

A. **Arthritis with Involvement of Some Other System.** This situation poses the most common problem for the clinician in the differential diagnosis of lupus. The clinician should consider the several other connective tissue disorders that are manifested in this way, including:

  1. *Rheumatoid Arthritis.* This is the most frequent initial diagnosis made in patients with early lupus. The key is that rheumatoid arthritis lacks the skin, brain, and renal involvement seen in lupus.

  2. *Scleroderma.* Clinical and immunologic differences distinguish SLE from scleroderma. The key is a lack of sclerodermatous skin changes in SLE.

  3. *Sjögren's Syndrome.* Serologic findings are key diagnostic distinctions if Sjögren's syndrome is associated with rheumatoid arthritis. Sjögren's syndrome with SLE can occur.

  4. *Mixed Connective Tissue Disease.* This condition may well be a variation of SLE rather than a separate disorder. The key is that SLE lacks the sclerodermatous skin changes observed in mixed connective tissue disease.

RECOMMENDED DIAGNOSTIC APPROACH

A. Suspected Diagnosis of SLE

  1. The physician should screen with antinuclear antibody (ANA) tests (see Table 76–1). If positive results are obtained, the following measures are used:

    a. Specific nuclear antibody tests are done.

   b. Activity of disease is measured with sedimentation rate and serum complement levels.
   c. History, physical examination, and laboratory findings are reviewed for confirmation of multisystem involvement.
B. Other System Involvement. The physician must establish whether or not and to what degree other systems are affected.
   1. Radiographs
      a. Affected Joints. Erosions are rarely seen.
      b. Chest X-Ray. Pleural and cardiac effusions or pneumonitis are sought.
   2. Laboratory Findings
      a. Renal Function. Blood-urea nitrogen, creatinine concentration, urinalysis for hematuria, and protein (longer collection if positive), microscopy for casts and red blood cells should be analyzed.
      b. Hematologic Function. Hematocrit, hemoglobin, RBC indices, reticulocyte count, white blood count and differential, and platelets should be studied.
      c. Immunologic Function. Gammaglobulin levels, rheumatoid factor, and venereal disease reaction level are analyzed.
   3. Electrocardiogram. Evidence of pericarditis is the most frequent abnormality.

REFERENCES

1. Systemic lupus erythematosus. *In* Rodman GP, Schumacker R, Zuaifler NJ (eds): Primer on the Rheumatic Diseases. 8th ed. Atlanta, Arthritis Foundation, 1983, pp. 49–59.

An excellent publication that attempts to provide consensus definitions for all rheumatologic disorders.

2. Dubois EL (ed.): Lupus Erythematosus. 2nd ed. Los Angeles, University of Southern California Press, 1974.

This is considered by many to be the definitive textbook about SLE.

3. Notman DD, et al.: Profiles of antinuclear antibodies in systemic rheumatic diseases. Ann Intern Med 83:464, 1975.

A helpful introductory review of a rapidly changing field.

COMA

By ARTHUR KELLERMANN, M.D., M.P.H.

DEFINITION

Coma can be defined as a sleeplike unresponsiveness from which a patient cannot be aroused. The comatose individual lacks all awareness of self or environment. Coma must be distinguished from similar but distinct clinical conditions such as a vegetative state (awake but unaware) and the locked-in syndrome (awake and aware but unable to respond).

Coma is a symptom, not a disease. It is a manifestation of some severe underlying pathologic process. Other clinical terms such as "lethargy," "obtundation," and "stupor" represent a continuum of disorders involving the *level* of consciousness, the most severe of which is coma. Delirium and related alterations in the *content* of consciousness are discussed separately (see Chapter 78).

PATHOPHYSIOLOGY

A. **Structural and Physiologic Derangements.** Coma can result from a wide variety of structural and physiologic derangements (see Table 77–1). These processes produce either bilateral dysfunction of the cerebral hemispheres or impairment of the reticular activating system (RAS), which is located along the central core of the brain stem and diencephalon.

B. **Causes of Coma.** Causes can be grouped into three general categories:

   1. *Supratentorial Mass Lesions.* These lesions cause increased intracranial pressure and compress or displace the diencephalon and brain stem RAS against unyielding dural and bony structures.

   2. *Subtentorial Lesions.* These lesions in the posterior fossa or brain stem either ablate or directly compress the RAS.

   3. *Diffuse, Toxic, and Metabolic Processes.* These processes widely damage or impair neuronal function.

C. **Psychogenic Coma and Coma Following Prolonged Seizure Activity.** These can be considered special cases. Psychogenic coma has no currently known organic basis, while coma that follows prolonged seizure activity is often a cause or consequence of metabolic derangement.

Grouping the causes of coma into these three major categories is useful in the initial evaluation and treatment of coma and helps to guide subsequent diagnostic tests and therapy.

TABLE 77–1. COMA OF UNKNOWN CAUSE*

	Per Cent
Diffuse causes	50–65
Toxic (drugs, poisons)	25–50
Anoxic ischemia	3–5
Infectious (meningitis, encephalitis)	3–5
Hypoglycemia	3–5
Hepatic coma	3–5
Subarachnoid hemorrhage	2–4
Hyperosmolarity	less than 3
Hyponatremia	less than 3
Other endocrine disorders (Addison's hypopituitarism, myxedema)	less than 3
Hypercalcemia	less than 3
Uremia	less than 3
Postictal (seizures)	less than 3
Disorder of temperature regulation	less than 3
Nutritional deficiencies	less than 1
Hypercarbia	less than 1
Structural causes	35–50
Supratentorial	25–30
Hemorrhage	
Intracerebral	8–10
Subdural	3–5
Epidural	less than 1
Pituitary apoplexy	less than 1
Trauma (contusion or occult)	less than 3
Infarction (massive)	less than 3
Infectious (abscess)	less than 3
Tumor	
Primary	less than 1
Metastatic	less than 3
Subtentorial (common)	10–15
Infarction	
Pontine or brain stem	8–10
Cerebellar	less than 3
Extra- or subdural	less than 1
Hemorrhage	
Pontine or brain stem	2–4
Cerebellar	less than 3
Tumor	less than 1
Abscess	less than 1
Demyelination	less than 1
Basilar migraine	less than 1

*Following identification of obvious trauma, drug ingestion, and postarrest anoxia.

EPIDEMIOLOGY

A. **Incidence.** Coma and related disorders of consciousness are commonly encountered problems in hospital emergency wards and may account for 3 per cent or more of all hospital admissions.

B. **Patient Groups.** Considerable variation exists between different patient groups and institutions on the incidence, causes, and prognosis of coma.

C. **Drugs and Poisons.** Drugs and poisons are the single most common cause of coma of unknown origin even after known cases of self-poisoning have been excluded (Table 77–1). Ethanol and barbiturates remain the most common causes of drug-induced coma in the United States.

D. **Head Injury.** Following exclusion of "obvious head injuries" (such as from high-speed vehicular accidents and penetrating wounds), closed head trauma and its sequelae (epidural and subdural hematomas) remain a common cause of coma of unknown origin (4 to 6 per cent).

SUGGESTED MANAGEMENT

A. **Stabilization.** The key to management is stabilization, which must accompany initial evaluation of the comatose patient. Immediate management is directed toward correcting remedial causes of permanent brain damage and prevention of complications of coma such as aspiration and respiratory arrest.

1. *Cerebral Function.* Cerebral function and in fact survival require provision of the essential elements of brain metabolism. An adequate airway and respiratory exchange must be ensured. If any question exists, the patient should be intubated and ventilation-assisted. The airway of a comatose patient must be protected by a cuffed endotracheal tube prior to any attempts at gastric aspiration or lavage.

2. *Cardiac Output and Blood Pressure.* These must be adequate for cerebral perfusion. Aggressive hemodynamic support may be necessary. Cardiac arrythmias are frequently associated with coma, so the patient should be monitored continuously during transport and evaluation. Hypotension is rarely caused by intracranial lesions.

3. *Glucose.* Glucose (25 to 50 grams) should be provided intravenously (25 to 50 mL of a 50 per cent solution) after blood has been drawn for necessary metabolic studies (see later discussion). If a bedside blood glucose determination (Dextrostix) can be made, it should precede administration of hypertonic glucose. If not, the danger of untreated hypoglycemia outweighs the risk of slightly worsening a hyperosmolar coma. Transient improvement does not indicate a diagnosis of hypoglycemia, since the hyperosmolar glucose can briefly lower elevated intracranial pressure.

4. *Wernicke's Encephalopathy.* This is a rare cause of coma but can be precipitated by a carbohydrate load in a nutritionally deprived individual. Intravenous thiamine, 100 mg, should therefore be administered immediately before or after glucose, and a second dose of 100 mg should be given intramuscularly.

5. *Cervical Spine.* If any question of head trauma exists, the cervical spine should be immobilized until adequate radiographic evaluation is completed.

6. *Small Pupils.* If coma is associated with small pupils, naloxone 0.8 mg (2 mL) may be administered as a therapeutic trial. Naloxone specifically antagonizes opiates, but some transient increase in arousal may be noted in other sedative hypnotic intoxications.

7. *The Comatose Patient.* No comatose patient should be left alone. Risks of apnea, aspiration, arrhythmias, seizures, and sudden circulatory collapse mandate constant observation and care until the diagnosis is certain and definitive management has been established.

B. **Evaluation Following Initial Stabilization.** This should narrow the diagnostic possibilities to one of the three major diagnostic groups outlined earlier. A directed history and physical examination guide the subsequent choice and urgency of specific laboratory tests, diagnostic procedures, and immediate medical or surgical therapy.

The three major causes of coma in the United States (trauma, overdose, and postarrest ischemia) often are obvious on admission to the emergency ward. The skilled examiner still proceeds with a careful objective evaluation. Things are not always as "obvious" as they appear. The motor vehicle accident may have been preceded by hypoglycemic coma, the alcoholic may have an acute subdural hematoma, and the cardiac arrest may have been precipitated by an intracranial bleed or an overdose of tricyclic antidepressants.

1. *History.* Information should be obtained from all available sources, including family, friends, bystanders, ambulance personnel, and so forth.

   a. **Onset**

      1). Sudden onset suggests drug overdose, trauma, or intracranial bleed. In older persons brain stem or cerebellar hemorrhage or infarction must also be excluded.

      2). A more gradual onset suggests an evolving toxic or metabolic encephalopathy, brain tumor, or chronic subdural hematoma.

   b. **Associated Symptoms**

      1). Headache or recent history of head trauma (no matter how trivial) suggests a supratentorial mass lesion. Asymmetric motor or sensory complaints are supportive.

      2). An occipital headache, especially if it is associated with vertigo, ataxia, diplopia, or vomiting, suggests a subtentorial lesion.

      3). Confusion, disorientation, and somnolence preceding coma suggest a toxic or metabolic cause. Motor findings are usually symmetric, although old focal pathology can be unmasked by an evolving process.

   c. **Associated Medical Problems**

      1). A history of a previous seizure disorder or liver, renal, or endocrine disease may be important. Patients may be wearing a medical alert tag or carrying a card in a wallet or purse.

   d. **Surroundings**
      1). Circumstances at the time of discovery may provide valuable clues, such as pill bottles, drug paraphernalia, evidence of a struggle, or a cold room and suggest potential diagnoses.
   e. **Medications**
      1). All drugs prescribed to the patient as well as those to which he or she may have had access should be reviewed.
2. *Directed General Physical Examination*
   a. **General Observation of the Patient.** The patient should be observed undisturbed for several moments. Body position, spontaneous movements, and respiratory rate and pattern should be noted. Comatose patients with acute hemiplegia may lie with the affected leg externally rotated. Myoclonic jerks and tremor may suggest a toxic or metabolic cause. Jacksonian or generalized seizures should be noted and aggressively treated.
   b. **Skull Palpation.** The physician should carefully inspect and palpate the skull for lacerations, hematomas, edema, or skull depressions.
   c. **Hemorrhage and Ecchymoses.** The physician should search for subconjunctival hemorrhages, sharply demarcated periorbital ecchymoses ("raccoon sign"), mastoid ecchymoses (Battle's sign), and blood in the external auditory canal or hemotympanum. If drum perforation is suspected, caloric stimulation should be deferred.
   d. **Cerebrospinal Fluid (CSF) Rhinorrhea or Otorrhea.** CSF rhinorrhea or otorrhea appears as a clear watery discharge. A positive test for glucose in the fluid is nonspecific and unhelpful. CSF mixed with blood may separate when placed on filter paper. This "rim sign" is strongly suggestive of a basilar skull fracture. If it is present, caloric stimulation should be deferred.
   e. **Mouth and Facial Bones.** The mouth and facial bones should be examined and palpated. Loose teeth should be removed to prevent aspiration. Tongue lacerations, especially laterally, are suggestive of recent seizure activity. The patient's breath should be noted for the odor of ketones, alcohol, paraldehyde, and uremic or hepatic fetor.
   f. **Evidence of Fracture or Soft Tissue Injury.** The remainder of the body should be examined for evidence of fractures or soft tissue injury. Breath sounds should be symmetric and confirm good ventilatory exchange. Pneumothorax should be excluded.
   g. **Core Temperature.** Core temperature should be checked with a rectal temperature probe. Disordered thermoregulation can cause coma and requires urgent treatment.
   h. **Skin.** Skin should be inspected for needle tracks, abscesses, stigmata of chronic liver disease, petechiae, purpura, and evidence of prolonged pressure injury.

        i. Nuchal Rigidity. Once cervical trauma has been excluded, the neck should be flexed to detect nuchal rigidity.

        j. Optic Fundi. The optic fundi must be examined to detect papilledema (which develops after several hours of increased intracranial pressure), optic neuritis (suggesting methanol intoxication), retinal artery spasm, and subhyaloid hemorrhage (often associated with subarachnoid bleeds). Mydriatic agents should be avoided, since their use obscures subsequent determination and monitoring of pupillary reflexes. Changes in pupillary responses are more sensitive then papilledema for detection of increasing intracranial pressure.

3. Directed Neurologic Examination. Evaluation of the following five neurologic functions provides invaluable information on the level of neurologic impairment (see Table 77–2). This information, combined with the short-term clinical course, should provide an initial presumptive diagnosis and guide further laboratory evaluation.

a. Level of Consciousness

    1). By definition, the patient is unresponsive in coma. Subsequent improvement in level of consciousness as well as patterns of speech serve as good measures of clinical improvement after a patient has regained consciousness.

b. Pupillary Responses

    1). Normal pupillary function implies that the midbrain and third cranial nerves are intact.

    2). Symmetric or diffuse diencephalic processes produce small reactive pupils.

    3). Preservation of the pupillary light reflex in the presence of other signs of brain stem impairment strongly supports a toxic or metabolic cause of the coma. Abnormal pupillary reflexes are uncommon (less than 5 per cent of cases) in hepatic and other metabolic encephalopathies.

    4). Mild anisocoria with intact bilateral reactivity is most likely congenital. Asymmetric reactivity suggests an acute structural process.

TABLE 77–2. ANATOMIC LOCALIZATION OF NEUROLOGIC SIGNS

Examination Findings	Neuroanatomic Substrate
Cognition	Cortex
Conscious behaviors	Cortex and reticular activating system
Pupils	Midbrain
Extraocular movements (oculocephalic response)	Brainstem (midbrain to medulla)
Motor responses	Pons or medulla (if flaccid)
Respiration	Medulla (if ataxic)

5). Enlarging supratentorial mass lesions can produce uncal herniation. Subsequent compression of the peripheral pupilloconstrictor fibers of the third cranial nerve produces a dilated unresponsive pupil on the same side as the lesion.

6). Midbrain damage can produce midposition and unreactive pupils. Severe hypothermia and barbiturate intoxication can also produce midposition unreactive pupils, simulating brain death.

7). Pontine bleeds or infarction can produce small to pinpoint pupils. The pupillary light reflex is generally preserved when the eyes are examined with a magnifying glass. Small to pinpoint pupils can also be seen with opiate or anticholinesterase intoxication.

8). Dilated unreactive pupils are often seen after an agonal release of norepinephrine following anoxia or ischemia. Atropine, scopolamine, and glutethimide intoxication can also produce dilated pupils that are unreactive to light.

c. **Oculocephalic Responses**

1). The doll's eye reflex becomes evident with loss of consciousness and release of voluntary control from the frontal gaze centers. (Evaluation should be delayed until cervical spine injury is excluded.)

2). A normal symmetric response indicates that the tegmentum of the midbrain, pons, and medulla is largely structurally intact. Loss of the oculocephalic response suggests brain stem dysfunction and a greater risk for subsequent respiratory arrest.

3). Asymmetric responses are more commonly seen with structural than with metabolic lesions.

4). Cold calorics (irrigation of the external auditory canal with 50 cu cm of ice water while elevating the head at 30 degrees) is a more potent stimulus for eye deviation than the oculocephalic reflex. Observed abnormalities have the same pathophysiologic significance.

5). Cortical mass lesions may produce ipsilateral conjugate deviation of the eyes, which can be overcome with the doll's eye maneuver or caloric stimulation.

6). Brain stem lesions produce contralateral conjugate deviation of the eyes. Since the pontine centers for gaze are affected, maneuvers and calorics do not reverse the deviation.

7). If deviation is associated with hemiplegia, the eyes tend to look *away* from cortical hemiplegia but *toward* pontine brain stem hemiplegia.

8). Deep metabolic coma and midbrain lesions produce midline immobile eyes. Eyes directed straight ahead have no localizing value.

9). Except for mild divergence, disconjugate deviation points to a brain stem lesion.

10). Fast nystagmus opposite the side of cold caloric stimulation is diagnostic of psychogenic unresponsiveness.

d. **Motor Responses**

1). Abnormal responses should be described and noted. Use of diagnostic labels such as "decorticate" and "decerebrate" are potentially confusing and neuroanatomically inaccurate.

2). Abduction to a noxious stimulus is not observed in withdrawal reflexes and represents purposeful movement.

3). Abnormal but symmetric motor responses may be seen in midline structural or toxic and metabolic coma and have no localizing value.

4). Asymmetric motor responses at any level suggest a structural cause of coma.

5). Previously occult focal motor deficits may be unmasked by toxic or metabolic impairment.

6). Abnormal posturing may be subtle and intermittent or produced only by noxious stimulation.

7). An upper extremity flexor and lower extremity extensor response implies cortical or high diencephalic dysfunction.

8). An upper extremity extensor and lower extremity extensor response is seen in deep diencephalic or brain stem impairment. Even slight upper extremity extension or pronation is consistent with this response.

9). Flaccidity appears with progressive involvement of pons or medulla and is also seen with acute spinal cord injury.

10). Asymmetric resting muscle tone, deep tendon reflexes, or Babinski's reflexes suggest a structural lesion. Bilateral upgoing toes are commonly seen in toxic and metabolic coma.

e. **Respiratory Patterns**

1). Several characteristic patterns of respiration are believed to have approximate neuroanatomic locations.

2). In acute brain injury, breathing abnormalities are common and diverse. Gross irregular (ataxic) respirations appear to correlate with medullary involvement, especially when associated with hypercapnea. Ataxic respirations frequently precede sudden respiratory arrest.

3). Central neurogenic hyperventilation is sometimes associated with midbrain lesions, and inspiratory pauses (apneustic) breathing have been reported with pontine damage.

4). Periodic (Cheyne-Stokes) respirations are a nonspecific finding associated with cortical and high diencephalic dysfunction. Sedative hypnotics, metabolic encephalopathies, congestive heart failure, and cerebrovascular disease can also produce this respiratory pattern.

f. **Clinical Course**

1). Rostral-caudal progression of neurologic dysfunction is characteristic of supratentorial mass lesions and toxic and metabolic encephalopathy. Midline mass lesions or bilateral lesions may produce few or no focal signs. Laterally placed lesions may demonstrate focal signs early in the clinical course that are masked by progressive pressure and damage to lower brain centers. Thus, structural lesions can mimic toxic metabolic coma.

2). Absence of an orderly rostral-caudal progression, especially with impaired oculovestibular and pupillary responses, suggests a subtentorial structural lesion.

3). Toxic encephalopathies can mimic subtentorial lesions. (For example, opiate overdose can cause small pupils and apnea resembling medullary damage, while anticholinesterase poisoning can cause coma, small pupils, extraocular palsy, and a flaccid quadriparesis similar in pattern to pontine hemorrhage.)

4). When confronted with obvious clinical deterioration, measures to treat potential increased intracranial pressure (including hyperventilation and administration of mannitol) may be initiated prior to definitive diagnostic tests.

The typical clinical features for general diagnostic categories are summarized in Table 77–3.

4. **Laboratory Evaluation.** Immediate laboratory tests that should be obtained in the initial evaluation of coma include:

a. **Serum Electrolytes, Glucose, Blood Urea-Nitrogen, Creatinine, and Measured Serum Osmolality.** Observation of an "osmolar gap" (measured osmolality greater than calculated osmolarity) suggests an additional significant solute such as ethanol or methanol.

b. **Arterial Blood Gas**
   1). Hypoxemia must be corrected immediately.
   2). Hypercarbia may warn of impending respiratory arrest.
   3). Spontaneous hypocarbia (CO_2 less than 30 mm Hg) is associated with a worse prognosis.
   4). A terra cotta color of the blood sample may suggest methemoglobinemia or sulfhemoglobinemia.
   5). The cherry red color described for carboxyhemoglobinemia (carbon monoxide poisoning) is infrequently seen and not clinically useful.
   6). A difference in measured and calculated hemoglobin saturation suggests carbon monoxide poisoning.

c. **Electrocardiogram (ECG).** The ECG can diagnose cardiac arrhythmias and show evidence of myocardial ischemia. Metabolic and electrolyte disturbances may be suspected from the ECG before results of blood chemistry analyses are available.

d. **Lateral Cervical Spine and AP Chest Radiographs.** These are needed to exclude cervical spine injury, aspiration and pneumothorax and to check placement of endotrachial and gastric tubes.

TABLE 77–3. TYPICAL SIGNS IN COMA*

	History (Prior to Coma)	Pupils	Oculocephalic Response and Calorics	Motor	Rostal Caudal Progression	Best Test
Supratentorial mass lesions	Trauma, headache, focal signs	Unilateral enlargement with cranial nerve III dysfunction†	Deviate away from hemiplegia; calorics overcome conjugate gaze, or are absent	Focal signs present (early) or flaccid	Present	CT scan
Subtentorial mass lesions	Occipital headache,† nausea, vomiting, vertigo, diplopia, ataxia (truncal)	Commonly impaired, often asymmetric	Deviate toward hemiplegic; calorics† fail to overcome disconjugate gaze, or are absent	Signs usually symmetric or flaccid	Absent	CT scan
Diffuse toxic or metabolic	Confusion, apathy, delirium, somnolence	Preserved despite other brain stem signs†	Generally symmetric or absent	Seizures, myoclonus, possible signs usually symmetric or flaccid	Often present	Blood chemistries, LP (if infection is suspected)
Psychogenic unresponsiveness	Previous psychiatric history	Intact, normal	Absent, nystagmus with normal calorics†	Flaccid or avoidance	None	EEG (if unsure)

*Exceptions occur and differentiation may be especially difficult late in clinical course. (Adapted from Plum F, Posner J, pp. 353–362.[1])
†Most helpful in differential diagnosis.

5. *Subsequent Laboratory Tests.* Subsequent tests are determined by the results of the initial clinical and laboratory
   evaluation. These tests should be obtained as rapidly as
   possible but only with specific clinical indications.
   a. **Blood for Specific Tests**
      1). *Blood Alcohol Determination.* Additional clinical
         chemistry analysis includes a blood alcohol determi-
         nation. In certain clinical settings this may be consid-
         ered a part of the immediate laboratory evaluation.
         Alcohol remains the most common drug cause of coma,
         either singly or in combination with other agents.
      2). *Drug Screen.* Qualitative tests can be run on blood,
         urine, and gastric contents. These tests are not very
         sensitive (0.60 to 0.70), do not detect a number of
         important drugs, and wide variability exists between
         laboratory results. Newer developments in methodol-
         ogy may improve these figures somewhat. Detection of
         one or more drugs on a qualitative test does not
         guarantee that these agents are responsible for coma,
         nor does a negative drug screen exclude the diagnosis
         of drug intoxication.
      3). *Specific Drug Levels.* Levels of anticonvulsant med-
         ication and barbiturates may roughly correlate with a
         patient's clinical condition. Aspirin and acetaminophen
         levels may be helpful in subsequent management.
         Drug levels are expensive and should not be ordered
         without appropriate clinical suspicion or a positive
         drug screen.
      4). *Liver Enzymes, Prothrombin Time, and Bilirubin
         Determinations.* Elevations of these tests may sug-
         gest hepatic encephalopathy. Blood arterial ammonia
         levels have also been found to correlate roughly with
         the clinical symptoms.
      5). *Carboxyhemoglobin Level.* This test is mandatory
         for diagnosis of carbon monoxide poisoning because
         clinical signs are insensitive and nonspecific.
      6). *Serum Phosphokinase Isoenzyme (CPK BB).* Ele-
         vation of this enzyme for six hours or longer following
         cardiac arrest has been associated with severe anoxic
         brain injury.
      7). *Additional Metabolic Studies.* Additional studies
         may include thyroid function tests and adrenocortico-
         tropic hormone and cortisol levels.
      8). *Other Toxicology Tests.* These include serum iron,
         heavy metals, and methemoglobin.
   b. **Computed Tomography (CT) Scan**
      1). The CT scan is the radiographic procedure of choice
         for detecting intracranial mass lesions.
      2). Resolution depends on the generation of the scanner
         and the density of any lesion. High-density intracra-
         nial bleeds as small as a few millimeters may be

detected. CT has a sensitivity of 0.95 and a specificity of 0.90 for detecting mass lesions in the cerebral hemispheres, diencephalon, and cerebellum.

3). Lesions in the midbrain, pons, and medulla are more easily missed owing to interference from adjacent bone, although CT may still detect up to 85 per cent of these lesions. Nuclear magnetic resonance imaging may become the procedure of choice for evaluation of these areas.

4). CT detects about 60 per cent of subarachnoid hemorrhages. The lumbar puncture (LP) remains a more sensitive procedure for confirming this diagnosis.

5). Administration of contrast material prior to the initial CT scan may obscure diagnosis by CT of subarachnoid hemorrhage.

6). Subacute and chronic subdural hematomas may evolve through an isodense phase and be suspected only by their mass effects. Reexamination following administration of contrast material confirms the diagnosis.

7). CT is not useful in detecting toxic or metabolic coma, meningitis, or many cases of encephalitis. Brain contusion, small subtentorial lesions, brain stem infarction, pituitary apoplexy, and disseminated tumor may also be missed by CT.

c. **Lumbar Puncture (LP)**

1). The LP is essential in the evaluation of suspected meningitis or encephalitis and is the most sensitive test for subarachnoid hemorrhage.

2). Lumbar puncture can be hazardous with increased intracranial pressure and may precipitate herniation.

3). When an intracranial mass lesion is suspected, an emergency CT scan should be obtained prior to an LP.

4). Papilledema is a relatively late sign of increased intracranial pressure and may be absent in acute processes. Venous pulsations in the optic discs virtually assure normal pressure but are infrequently seen.

5). True blood in the cerebrospinal fluid (CSF) can be distinguished from a traumatic tap by the presence of xanthochromia, no decrease in red blood cell count between the first and last tubes, or a final sample red blood cell count of greater than 1000 per cu mm.

6). Gram's stain, india ink preparation, cultures for bacteria, fungi, and tuberculosis, cell count and differential, glucose and total protein measurements should be part of each CSF evaluation in coma.

7). CSF protein, sugar, and cell count may be normal with brain tumors or abscess, although the opening pressure is commonly elevated.

8). Specific additional studies on CSF may include glutamine (elevated in hepatic encephalopathy), creatine phosphokinase (present in anoxic encephalopathy), viral studies, fungal antigens, and so on.

9). Most complications of lumbar puncture develop within 12 hours.

d. Electroencephalogram (EEG)

1). The EEG is cumbersome and has little place in the emergent evaluation of coma of unknown cause.

2). The EEG is much less helpful than CT in discriminating structural from metabolic lesions.

3). Metabolic disease most commonly produces symmetric and diffuse slowing, although periodic lateralizing epileptiform discharges (PLEDS) can be seen.

4). The EEG is probably most helpful in distinguishing repetitive or subclinical seizure activity and in confirming brain death. Seizures rarely cause coma without overt convulsions.

5). Coma can be reliably differentiated from psychogenic unresponsiveness by the EEG. However, most cases can be distinguished on clinical grounds.

6). Severe toxic or metabolic encephalopathy and hypothermia can produce an isoelectric EEG and must be excluded prior to a diagnosis of brain death.

e. Skull Films

1). CT scanning has largely replaced skull films in the evaluation of suspected intracranial mass lesions after head trauma. The sensitivity of skull films for detecting intracranial tumors is less than 0.35.

2). Skull films can still provide valuable inferential evidence regarding the severity of head injury and are a more sensitive test for detecting skull fracture.

3). High-yield criteria have been developed for ordering skull films, of which coma, focal neurologic signs, and a decreasing mental status are the most predictive.

4). Regardless of whether skull films or a CT scan are obtained, the importance of cervical radiographs to exclude spinal injury cannot be overemphasized.

f. Brain Scan

1). The brain scan is a less sensitive (0.75) and less specific (0.85) test compared with CT for intracranial mass lesions.

2). Brain scan should be considered when CT is unavailable and an intracranial mass lesion is suspected.

3). Brain scans may detect some cases of encephalitis or meningiomas missed by CT.

g. Cerebral Angiography

1). Angiography is rarely indicated for the early evaluation of the comatose patient.

2). Angiograms are sensitive (greater than 0.95) but less specific (0.85) than CT for detecting mass lesions and much more hazardous to perform.

3). The primary utility of angiography in coma is to locate aneurysms and confirm vascular spasm, although surgery in comatose patients is of questionable value.

PROGNOSIS OF COMA

Studies on prognosis of coma have generally divided cases into two groups: traumatic and nontraumatic coma. Outcomes of anoxic brain injury and drug overdose have been considered separately. Overall mortality and degree of functional recovery of patients following the onset of coma depends on a variety of factors:

A. Type of Neurologic Insult

1. About half of patients in coma from head injury die compared with three quarters of those who are comatose following subarachnoid bleeds or other cerebrovascular accidents. About 40 per cent of patients admitted in coma following out-of-hospital cardiac arrest die, as well as 40 to 50 per cent of patients in coma resulting from tumor, infection, or metabolic insults.

2. Fewer than 10 per cent of patients in coma following drug overdose die. Mortality principally results from respiratory, infectious, and cardiovascular complications.

3. Approximately 15 to 25 per cent of survivors of coma from most causes are either severely disabled or vegetative. Almost all survivors of nonnarcotic overdose recover completely unless neurocellular damage has occurred from complications or other toxins.

B. Severity of the Insult

1. *Death and Disability.* The incidence of death and disability is higher for patients with anoxic coma following cardiac arrest if the arrest was unwitnessed, cardiopulmonary resuscitation or defibrillation was delayed, or the resuscitation attempt was prolonged.

C. Extent of Neurologic Injury

1. *Brain Stem Injury.* Brain stem injury, as indicated by loss of pupil, corneal, and oculocephalic reflexes six hours after the onset of coma, is associated with over 95 per cent mortality for both traumatic and nontraumatic coma. Drug overdose is the exception to this rule.

2. *Progressively Abnormal Motor Signs.* These are associated with a worse prognosis in traumatic coma. Extensor or flaccid responses carry a mortalilty of over 80 per cent.

3. *Fixed Pupils and Ophthalmoplegia in Coma from Drugs or Hypothermia.* Only in coma from drugs or hypothermia is the presence of fixed pupils and ophthalmoplegia compatible with complete recovery. Such patients still require aggressive general support to survive.

4. *Intact Pupils, Oculocephalic Responses, and Withdrawal from Pain.* These findings predict a good recovery in 70 per cent of patients who are comatose after cardiac arrest. However, these findings predict a good recovery for only 23 per cent of patients following nontraumatic coma from other causes.

D. Short-Term Clinical Course

1. *Length of Coma.* Prognosis worsens as coma lengthens in all cases except drug overdose.

2. *Clinical Improvement Over Time.* This pattern may be more favorable than a better initial level of function without subsequent improvement.
3. *After Four Days.* Few patients awakening from nontraumatic coma after four days recover without persistent cognitive or motor deficits.

E. Age

1. *Advanced Age in Traumatic Coma.* Older age is adversely related to outcome in traumatic coma. Survival and recovery are both much more likely in younger patients.
2. *Age in Nontraumatic Coma.* No consistent relationship between age and prognosis has been observed in nontraumatic coma.

REFERENCES

*1. Plum F, Posner J: The Diagnosis of Stupor and Coma. 3rd ed. Philadelphia, F A Davis Company, 1980.
*2. Sabin T: Coma and the acute confusional state in the emergency room. Med Clin North Am 65:15–32, 1981.
3. Sabin T: The differential diagnosis of coma. N Engl J Med 290:1062–1064, 1974.
*4. Finklestein S, Ropper A: The diagnosis of coma: Its pitfalls and limitations. Heart Lung 8:1059–1064, 1979.
*5. Gallagher J: Coma. Chap. 45. In Kraus T, Warner C (eds.): Emergency Medicine. A Comprehensive Review. Rockville, Aspen Systems Corporation, 1983.
6. Fishman R.: Brain edema. N Engl J Med 293:706–711, 1975.
7. North J, Jerrett S: Abnormal breathing patterns associated with acute brain damage. Arch Neurol 31:338–344, 1974.
*8. Holliwell M, Hampel G, Sinclair E, Huggett E, Flanagan R: Value of emergency toxicological investigations in differential diagnosis of coma. Br Med J 2:819–821, 1979.
9. Inglefinger J, Isakson G, Shine D, Costello C, Goldman P: Reliability of the toxic screen in drug overdose. Clin Pharmacol Ther 29:570–575, 1981.
10. Bell RS, Loop JW: The utility and futility of radiographic skull examinations for trauma. N Engl J Med 284:236–239, 1971.
*11. Levy D, Bates MB, Caronna J, et al.: Prognosis in nontraumatic coma. Ann Intern Med 94:293–301, 1981.
*12. Jerrett B, Teasdale G, Braakman R, et al.: Prognosis of patients with severe head injury. Neurosurgery 4:283–288, 1979.
13. Arieff A, Friedman E: Coma following non-narcotic drug overdosage: Management of 208 adult patients. Am J Med Sci 266:405–426, 1973.
*14. Longstreth W, Inui T, Cobb L, Copass M: Neurologic recovery after out of hospital cardiac arrest. Ann Intern Med 98(Part I):588–592, 1983.
15. Baker HL, Houser OW, Campbell JK: National Cancer Institute Study: Evaluation of computed tomography in the diagnosis of intracranial neoplasms. Radiology 136:91–96, 1980.

---

*"Classic" references or excellent sources.

DELIRIUM

By ARTHUR KELLERMANN, M.D., M.P.H.

DEFINITION

A. **Delirium.** Delirium is an organic mental disorder that is characterized by a generally transient but global impairment in cerebral function. The syndrome results from some widespread derangement in cerebral metabolism. Impaired consciousness of some degree is essential to the diagnosis.

B. **Criteria for Diagnosis.** The *Diagnostic & Statistical Manual of Mental Disorders* of the American Psychiatric Association lists five criteria for the diagnosis of delirium:

1. Clouding of consciousness (reduced clarity of awareness of the environment) with reduced capacity to shift, focus, and sustain attention to environmental stimuli
2. At least two of the following:
   a. Perceptual disturbance: misinterpretations, illusions, or hallucinations
   b. Speech that is at times incoherent
   c. Disturbance of sleep-wakefulness cycle, with insomnia or daytime drowsiness
   d. Increased or decreased psychomotor activity
3. Disorientation and memory impairment (if testable)
4. Clinical features that develop over a short period of time (usually hours to days) and tend to fluctuate over the course of the day
5. Documented evidence of an organic cause

C. **Clinical Subtypes.** Two major clinical subtypes have been described that differ by the level of consciousness. The hyperalert confusional state is more commonly emphasized in standard textbooks. The hypoactive somnolent variant is therefore more frequently misdiagnosed. Individuals may move from one state to the other.

D. **Delirium with an Organic Brain Syndrome.** It is not unusual to find delirium superimposed on a chronic organic brain syndrome or dementia (see Chapter 79). Such individuals are usually identified by a relatively abrupt change in awareness and cognition from a previously stable level of functional impairment.

PATHOGENESIS

A. **Level vs. Content of Consciousness.** While the level of consciousness is a function of both the cerebral cortex and the reticular activating system, the content of consciousness appears to be largely a cortical function.

B. **Causes of Delirium vs. Causes of Coma.** Since the majority of cases of delirium are related to metabolic imbalances or intoxications, there is considerable overlap between causes of delirium and causes of coma (see Table 78–1).

C. Focal Lesions. Focal lesions in the frontal and occipital lobes as well as in the distribution of the middle cerebral artery may produce acute confusional states as their only manifestation.

D. Frontal and Temporal Lobe Seizures. These seizures may cause only behavioral and cognitive changes and require an electro-encephalogram (EEG) for confirmation.

EPIDEMIOLOGY

A. Prevalence. Delirium of some degree has been estimated to occur in between 5 to 15 per cent of all patients hospitalized on general medical and surgical floors. Estimates are higher for patients on psychiatric floors (5 to 40 per cent) and in intensive care units (20 to 50 per cent).

B. Relative Risk. Elderly patients are twice as likely to develop delirium following a given physiologic stress.

C. Mortality. The one-year mortality for patients admitted with delirium has been estimated at between 30 and 50 per cent. Medically hospitalized patients with cognitive impairment have higher mortality than general medical patients, independent of underlying diagnosis.

DIFFERENTIAL DIAGNOSIS

A. Delirium vs. Functional Psychiatric Disorders. The physician must distinguish between delirium and functional psychiatric disorders (see Table 78–2).
  1. Psychiatric symptoms (agitation, apathy, psychosis, or combative or inappropriate behavior) commonly predominate in delirium and lead to inappropriate triage or premature psychiatric referral.
  2. Over 3 per cent of patients "medically cleared" for psychiatric admission have been found to have delirium.
  3. Delirium may coexist with a previously diagnosed psychiatric disorder, making evaluation even more difficult.
  4. Disorientation, clouding of consciousness, age over 40 without a previous psychiatric history, and abnormal vital signs have been suggested as screening criteria for delirium.

B. Delirium vs. Dementia in the Elderly. The physician must distinguish between delirium and dementia in the elderly.
  1. Delirium commonly has an onset of days to weeks rather than months to years, as in dementia.
  2. Alterations in consciousness, fluctuation in clinical course, and lucid intervals are characteristic of delirium.
  3. Delirium may coexist with dementia and should be considered in the event of rapid deterioration or abnormal vital signs in a previously stable patient.

TABLE 78–1. CAUSES OF DELIRIUM

DIAGNOSIS	PER CENT
Toxic	25–50
Alcohol	
Drugs (illicit, prescribed, over-the-counter)	
Inhalants (gasoline, glue, ether, liquid paper)	
Poisons (solvents, carbon monoxide, organophosphates, heavy metals, etc.)	
Infections	10–20
Systemic (sepsis, pneumonia, pyelonephritis, typhoid, legionnaires' disease, etc.)	
Intracranial (meningitis, encephalitis, abscess)	
Withdrawal syndromes (alcohol, sedative hypnotics, amphetamines)	10–15
Epilepsy (status epilepticus, postictal states)	10–15
Fluid and electrolytes	10–15
Hypo- or hypernatremia	
Hypo- or hypercalcemia	
Acidosis or alkalosis	
Hypo- or hypermagnesemia	
Metabolic	5–10
Hepatic encephalopathy	
Uremia and dialysis syndromes	
Respiratory failure (hypercarbia, hypoxia)	
Circulatory failure (hypertensive encephalopathy, shock, congestive heart failure)	
Porphyria	
Wilson's disease	

Table continued on opposite page

C. **Other Conditions Mistaken for Delirium.** Wernicke's aphasia, Korsakoff's syndrome, denial states following certain cerebrovascular accidents, mental retardation, and Ganser's syndrome ("pseudoinsanity") may be mistaken for delirium.

D. **Conditions to Be Considered in the Evaluation of Acute Confusion.** These conditions are summarized in Table 78–1 with approximate frequencies of occurrence. Delirium may be the only sign of a potentially life-threatening physiologic impairment. Delirium is a symptom, not a disease.

SIGNS OF DELIRIUM

A. **Abnormal Vital Signs.** Abnormal vital signs should not be dismissed as secondary to agitation. An associated medical condition such as infection, withdrawal, intoxication, or metastatic disturbance should be sought.

B. **Disordered Wakefulness or Sensorium.** This finding is required for the diagnosis of delirium. The level of consciousness may be either increased or decreased, but concentration is impaired and attention cannot be sustained. Insomnia is commonly seen.

TABLE 78–1. CAUSES OF DELIRIUM *Continued*

DIAGNOSIS	PER CENT
Endocrine	2–5
Hypo- or hyperglycemia	
Hypo- or hyperthyroidism	
Addison's disease or Cushing's syndrome	
Hypo- or hyperparathyroidism	
Hypopituitarism	
Trauma	2–5
Head (concussion, contusion, epi- or subdural and intracerebral hematomas)	
Systemic (burns, surgery, intensive care unit status, multiple injuries, fat embolism)	
Cerebrovascular disease	2–5
Transient ischemic attacks	
Cerebrovascular accident	
Subarachnoid hemorrhage	
Complex migraine	
Nutritional	(<3)
Deficiency (thiamine, niacin, vitamin B_{12}, pyridoxine, folate)	
Excess hypervitaminosis A and D	
Neoplastic	(<3)
Primary intracranial neoplasms	
Cerebral and meningeal metastases	
Carcinoid and paraneoplastic syndromes	
Autoimmune (lupus, polyarteritis, rheumatic fever)	(<3)
Miscellaneous	(2–5)
Hypo- or hyperthermia	
Sleep or sensory deprivation	
Hospitalization (intensive care unit and postoperative delirium)	
Toxemia of pregnancy	

TABLE 78–2. DIFFERENTIAL DIAGNOSIS OF THE "CONFUSIONAL" STATE

Delirium
Dementing disorders*
Psychiatric disorders
    Acute schizophrenia
    Acute manic and paranoid states
    Depression
    Acute grief reaction
    Hysterical psychosis
    Ganser's syndrome
    Conversation disorder
Korsakoff's syndrome
Fluent aphasia
Denial syndromes (past cerebrovascular accident)
Mental retardation

*See Chapter 79.

C. **Impaired Cognition.** Impaired cognition may be manifested as disorientation, illusions, hallucinations (most commonly visual), delusions, and defects in short-term memory and recall.

D. **Emotional Lability.** Emotional lability is characteristic and may range from apathy to fear to anger. Hallucinations are commonly perceived as foreign ("ego-dystonic") and frightening to the patient, in contrast to schizophrenia.

E. **Psychomotor Disturbance.** Psychomotor disturbance ranges from quiet apathy to gross agitation. Picking at clothes and intravenous tubing, wandering from bed or ward, and combative behavior may occur. Gross tremors, seizures, ataxia, myoclonic jerks, asterixis, and choreoathetoid movements are common manifestations of delirium.

F. **Varying Degrees of Impairment.** Fluctuation from moment to moment is common. Symptoms are generally more severe at night when organizing sensory input is decreased.

RECOMMENDED DIAGNOSTIC APPROACH

A. **Initial Stabilization.** Stabilization should precede the diagnostic approach in a manner analogous to the methods outlined in Chapter 77 for coma. If hypoglycemia is suspected, glucose and thiamine should be provided while initial laboratory tests are pending. Patients should be gently restrained to avoid injury to themselves or others.

B. **History.** A history should be obtained from all available sources. Despite confusion the patient may provide valuable clues, which should be corroborated whenever possible. A history of ingestion, substance abuse or addiction, head trauma, and associated symptoms should be carefully sought. All available pill containers should be identified, since vitually any drug can produce delirium. Coincident head trauma and intoxication demand a high level of suspicion for an intracranial process.

C. **Physical Examination.** Special emphasis should be placed on the vital signs. Fever, tachycardia, or hypertension should prompt a particularly careful evaluation for an underlying medical condition. Cardiopulmonary problems and occult infections are common causes of delirium in the elderly.

D. **Mental Status Examination.** This examination should narrow the differential diagnosis and provide an index of severity. The Mini Mental State evaluation outlined in Chapter 79 may be helpful. Fluctuation is common, and frequent reevaluation is mandatory until the diagnosis is established.

E. **Laboratory Evaluation.** The laboratory evaluation should be tiered with an initial limited battery of tests designed to screen for major physiologic derangements. Further evaluation should proceed on the basis of these preliminary tests as well as the history and physical examination.

1. *Initial Screening Tests.* These should be obtained early so that they can be processed during the subsequent examination. (Data on the sensitivity, specificity, and predictive value of these tests in evaluating delirium are not available.) The tests include:

a. Complete blood count with differential
b. Electrolytes, blood-urea nitrogen, glucose and calcium determinations
c. Electrocardiogram
d. Chest x-ray
e. Urinalysis
f. Stool for occult blood test

2. **Subsequent Confirmatory Tests.** These should be done when dictated by clinical suspicion.

a. Emergency Toxicology: qualitative toxicologic screens may have a sensitivity of only 0.5 to 0.7 and should supplement but not overrule clinical suspicion. Blood alcohol level determinations are fast, inexpensive, and generally accurate. Quantitative drug levels may be extremely important in certain clinical situations such as suspected overdoses of aspirin, acetaminophen, aminophylline, lithium, diphenylhydantoin, or digoxin but should only be ordered selectively.

b. Lumbar puncture should be performed at the slightest suspicion of meningitis and is mandatory when delirium is accompanied by fever or other signs of infection. (Discussion of risks and precautions is outlined in Chapter 77.)

c. A computed tomographic scan should be obtained immediately if an intracranial mass lesion is suspected. A history of recent head trauma or a newly focal neurologic examination is a strong indication.

d. Further laboratory tests, including arterial blood gas, liver enzymes, serum ammonia, endocrine studies, antinuclear antibody assay, serum protein electrophoresis, bromide level, cerebrospinal fluid glutamine, and urine for porphyria or heavy metals, should only be obtained when there is appropriate clinical suspicion.

e. The EEG has little place in emergent evaluation but may confirm temporal or frontal lobe status epilepticus or unusual causes of clinical delirium.

REFERENCES

*1. Lipowski ZJ: Delirium: Acute Brain Failure in Man. Springfield, Charles C Thomas, 1980.

2. Fauman MA, Fauman BJ: The differential diagnosis of organic based psychiatric disturbance in the emergency department. J Am Coll Emerg Phys 6:315–323, 1977.

*3. Varsamis J: Clinical management of delirium. Psychiatr Clin North Am 1:71–80, 1978.

*4. Khantzian EG, McKenna GJ: Acute toxic and withdrawal reactions associated with drug use and abuse. Ann Intern Med 90:361–372, 1979.

*5. Purdie F, Honigman B, Rosen P: Acute organic brain syndrome: A review of 100 cases. Ann Emerg Med 10:455–461, 1981.

*6. Rabin P, Folstein M: Delirium and dementia: Diagnostic criteria and fatality rates. Br J Psychiatr 140:149–153, 1982.

*"Best" references.

7. Liston E: Delirium in the aged. Psychiatr Clin North Am 5:49–66, 1982.
*8. Dubin WR, Weiss K, Zeccardi J: Organic brain syndrome. The psychiatric imposter. JAMA 249:60–62, 1983.
9. Massey EW, Coffey CE: Delirium: Diagnosis and treatment. South Med J 76:1147–1150, 1983.
10. American Psychiatric Association: Diagnostic & Statistical Manual of Mental Disorders (DSM-III). Washington, D.C., American Psychiatric Association, 1980.

*"Best" references.

79

DEMENTIA

By RICHARD O. CUMMINS, M.D., M.P.H.

DEFINITION

Dementia is an organic cerebral disorder that is a syndrome, not a disease characterized by one etiologic diagnosis. Consciousness is not impaired until the late stages or unless other conditions that cause delirium coexist. Dementia is primarily a global disturbance in memory, orientation, behavior, emotions, and capacity for intellectual thought.

EPIDEMIOLOGY

A. **Prevalence.** Up to 5 per cent of people over age 65 and up to 20 per cent of people over 80 are intellectually impaired to a degree that warrants the term "dementia."

CRITERIA FOR DIAGNOSIS

A. **Required Diagnostic Criteria.** The American Psychiatric Association's *Diagnostic & Statistical Manual of Mental Disorders (DSM-III)* lists five diagnostic criteria required for the diagnosis of dementia:
   1. Memory impairment
   2. Loss of intellectual abilities to a degree sufficient to interfere with social or occupational functioning
   3. Impairment in at least one of the following areas: abstract thinking, judgment, higher cortical functions (aphasia, apraxia, agnosia, and constructional difficulty), and personality
   4. Clear state of consciousness
   5. Documented or presumed evidence of organic cause

B. Quantitative Assessment of Cognitive Performance. This assessment is recommended for initial diagnosis, for following patients over time, and for monitoring therapy. The Mini Mental State evaluation in Table 79–1 is a short standardized form that requires only five to ten minutes to complete and that can be used serially.

Scores are not diagnostic. People who have "overlearned" (such as doctors, lawyers, or engineers) may have scores of over 25 and still display the signs and symptoms of dementia in its early phases. Scores of 23 or lower have a sensitivity for dementia of greater than 90 per cent; however, the false-positive rate is high (owing to deafness, language problems, education deficiencies, mental retardation, and so forth). Low scores require an explanation, not necessarily a work-up for dementia.

DIAGNOSTIC CONSIDERATIONS

In the past the concept of "reversible" versus "irreversible" dementia has dictated the diagnostic work-up of patients with clinical dementia. For subsets of demented patients, this is probably a useful concept (such as for patients younger than 60; in acute, less severe dementia; and in dementia of short duration, less than 12 months). However, the idea of a reversible-irreversible, treatable-untreatable dichotomy may have only limited value for patient care.

A. Differential Diagnosis

1. Coexistent Treatable Disorders. An elderly patient with global mental dysfunction can have various coexistent treatable disorders. The potential exists for the dementia to disappear if the associated disorder is effectively treated. Usually, however, treatment causes some improvement but not complete reversal to a normal mental status.

2. Dementia Associated with Potentially Reversible Disorders. Several studies suggest that in unscreened populations of apparently "demented" persons (with cognitive failure) 15 to 20 per cent have dementia associated with potentially reversible disorders or are not truly demented.

3. Conditions That Must Be Considered in Evaluation of Any Demented Person. These conditions are listed in Table 79–2. The estimates of expected frequency of occurrence are very rough. In practice such frequencies vary by age, sex, acuteness of the dementia, and whether the patients are hospitalized or ambulatory outpatients.

B. Distinguishing Features of Several of the Major Dementia Syndromes

1. Primary Degenerative Dementia (Formerly Called Senile Cortical Atrophy or Dementia of Alzheimer's Type [DAT])

    a. **Insidious, Gradual Onset.** This is more common in women than in men.

    b. **Course**

        1). Early. Mental and behavioral changes predominate.

        2). Middle. Disorientation, deterioration of personality,

TABLE 79–1. MINI MENTAL STATE EVALUATION

	MAXIMAL SCORE	SCORE
Orientation		
1. Time: What is the (year) (season) (date) (day) (month)?	5	_____
2. Place: Where are we (state) (county) (town) (hospital) (floor)?	5	_____
Registration		
1. Name 3 objects: allow 1 second to say each slowly and clearly. Then ask the patient to say all three after you have said them. Give one point for each correct answer.	3	_____
2. Number of trials: ____(For future comparisons; limit 6 trials)		
Attention and calculation		
1. Serial 7's: The patient must subtract 7 from 100, 93, 86, and so forth. Stop after 5 subtractions (93, 86, 79, 72, 65). Give 1 point for each correct answer. Alternatively spell "world" backwards. The score is the number of letters in the correct order (dlrow = 5; dlorw = 3).	5	_____
Recall		
1. Ask the patient for the 3 objects named earlier (Registration). Give 1 point for each correct object.	3	_____
Language		
1. Naming: show the patient a wrist watch and ask what it is. Repeat for a pencil.	2	_____
2. Repetition: ask the patient to repeat the sentence "No ifs, and, or buts." Allow 1 trial. The repetition must be completely correct.	1	_____
3. Three-stage command: give the patient a blank piece of paper and command him to "take the paper in your right hand, fold it in half, and put it on the floor." Give 1 point for each part correctly performed.	3	_____
4. Reading: write clearly on a blank sheet of paper, "Close your eyes." Ask the patient to read it and do what it says. Give 1 point if the patient actually closes his eyes.	1	_____
5. Writing: give the patient a blank piece of paper and ask him to write a sentence. The sentence must be written spontaneously and must contain a subject and verb and be sensible. Do not dictate.	1	_____
6. Copying: draw intersecting pentagons, about one inch per side; ask the patient to copy it exactly. Score 1 point if all 10 angles are present and 2 intersect.	1	_____
MAXIMAL SCORE	30	

**TABLE 79-2. CONDITIONS THAT MUST BE CONSIDERED
IN CASES OF DEMENTIA**

DIAGNOSIS	PER CENT
Probably irreversible causes	80-90
Primary degenerative dementia (Alzheimer's type)	50-70
Senile onset, up to 60%	
Presenile onset, up to 5%	
With Parkinson's disease, up to 5-10%	
Multiple infarct dementia	5-10
Alcoholic dementia	5-10
Huntington's chorea	1-4
Creutzfeldt-Jakob disease	1-2
Others (postsubarachnoid hemorrhage, postencephalitis, amyotrophic lateral sclerosis)	1
Potentially reversible causes	<15
Normal pressure hydrocephalus	
Age less than 65	4-5
Age over 65	1
Depression (pseudodementia)	4-5
Intracranial masses (depends on setting)	1-5
Drug toxicity (therapeutic drugs, alcohol, bromides, others)	2-5
Others	5-10
Metabolic-endocrine derangements	
Renal failure	
Hypo- or hypernatremia	
Hypoglycemia	
Volume depletion	
Hypo- or hyperthyroidism	
Hepatic failure	
Hypercalcemia	
Cushing's syndrome	
Addison's disease	
Hypopituitarism	
Deficiency states	
Vitamin B_{12}	
Folate (doubtful cause)	
Niacin (rare in United States)	
Thiamine (rare in United States)	
Cardiopulmonary disorders	
Congestive heart failure	
Arrhythmias	
Chronic obstructive pulmonary disease	
Infections	
Meningitis	
Neurosyphilis	
Abscess	
Tuberculosis	
Endocarditis	
Miscellaneous	
Sensory deprivation (blindness, deafness)	
Hospitalization	
Posttraumatic conditions	
Epilepsy	
Remote effects of cancer	

poor activities of living, and inability to perform self-care are characteristic.

    3). Later. Corticospinal tract signs, cortical release signs, aphasia, and agnosia are present.

    4). End. There is inanition and death.

  c. **Keys to Diagnosis.** These consist of characteristic cognitive defects (IIIA), often primitive reflexes (frontal lobe signs), lack of the motor and sensory deficits of localized cerebral lesions, and exclusion of other causes of dementia.

  d. **Diagnostic Tests**

    1). Computed Tomographic (CT) Scan. Often nonspecific and age-related findings are noted, such as enlarged cortical sulci, generous ventricles, and gaping Sylvian fissures secondary to temporal lobe atrophy. The CT scan cannot diagnose primary degenerative dementia but is used to exclude other diagnoses such as mass lesions, normal pressure hydrocephalus, and cerebrovascular accidents.

    2). Cerebrospinal Fluid. The cerebrospinal fluid is invariably normal.

    3). Electroencephalogram (EEG). The EEG shows diffuse slowing and later disorganization.

    4). Pneumoencephalogram. This is completely supplanted by CT scanning.

2. *Multi-Infarct Dementia.* This term replaces the old refuted concepts of "atherosclerotic dementia" and "cerebral atherosclerosis." Men are more commonly affected than women.

  a. **Occlusions of Cerebral Vessels.** Multi-infarct dementia follows multiple occlusions of small cerebral vessels that produce widespread cerebral softening.

  b. **Keys to Diagnosis.** Dementia is marked by:

    1). Sudden Onset

    2). Stepwise Decline in Cognitive Function

    3). Association with Hypertension or Strokes

    4). Focal Neurologic Signs. In particular these include pseudobulbar palsy, dysarthria, and bilateral corticospinal trait signs (weakness, spasticity, hyperreflexia, and gait abnormalities).

3. *Alcoholic Dementia.* In theory, alcoholic dementia occurs in patients who have not fully recovered from an episode of Korsakoff's psychosis. The residual mental state meets the criteria for dementia as defined earlier. Many patients do not have a clinical history of Korsakoff's episodes, and thus the condition is diagnosed by exclusion and by a history of heavy alcohol abuse. The syndrome is also called "alcoholic deteriorated state" or "organic brain syndrome due to alcohol."

  a. **History.** Sometimes only a careful history confirms that the patient experienced the clinical features of Wernicke's encephalopathy or Korsakoff's psychosis, both of which are parts of a single process, a vitamin B–deficiency disease.

  b. **Wernicke's Encephalopathy.** This is an acute disorder with three classic features:

    1). Ocular Disturbances. These are usually lateral and

conjugate gaze palsies and horizontal and vertical nystagmus. (Diagnosis is almost impossible without some ocular disturbances.) The disturbance often responds within hours to thiamine administration.

2). *Ataxia.* There is a wide-based uncertain gait.

3). *Mental Dysfunction.* This can be global confusion, delirium tremens or some variant thereof, or the memory disorder of Korsakoff's psychosis.

c. **Korsakoff's Psychosis.** Retentive memory is deranged out of proportion to other cognitive functions. Two variable but conjoined features are (1) retrograde amnesia (the patient cannot remember the past) and (2) antegrade amnesia (the patient cannot learn or form new memories). Confabulation often is present but is not necessary. The diagnosis requires an alert attentive patient who understands language and can solve problems.

d. **Keys to Diagnosis of Alcohol-Nutritional Dementia.** These include a history of alcohol abuse, residual gait disturbance, horizontal nystagmus, large memory gaps, and inability to sort out temporal relationships.

4. *Normal Pressure Hydrocephalus (NPH).* NPH is caused by a relative block to free cerebrospinal fluid circulation. The condition leads to ventricular dilatation and possibly to reduced cerebral blood flow.

a. **Reversibility.** NPH is not as common as was once suspected; it is a potentially reversible cause of dementia. Unfortunately, only about 50 to 65 per cent of patients with secondary NPH respond to shunting. If a gait disturbance precedes the dementia, the chances of response are increased.

b. **Dementia with Incontinence and Gait Difficulty.** The sensitivity of the well-known triad of dementia, incontinence, and gait difficulty approaches 100 per cent (almost everyone with NPH has the triad), but the predictive value of the triad is low (most people with the triad do not have NPH). This is especially true in dementia of Alzheimer's type, in which the triad is common in late stages.

c. **Keys to Diagnosis.** These consist of prominence of gait disturbance and relatively mild dementia. NPH often appears as abulic dementia with reduced speech and activity, in contrast to the more energetic patients with primary degenerative dementia.

d. **NPH Secondary to Other Causes.** Large series suggest that over 60 per cent of cases of NPH are secondary to other causes (mostly subarachnoid hemorrhage, 34 per cent; head injury, 11 per cent; after craniotomy, 5 per cent; meningitis, 4 per cent, and tumors, 4 per cent).

e. **Diagnosis of NPH.** The diagnosis is controversial.

1). *Isotope Cisternogram.* This is the major test and can show a variety of patterns. With NPH there is slowed isotope clearance from the parasagittal area and isotope reflux and stasis in the lateral and third ventricles.

2). **Lumbar Puncture.** This technique reveals high normal pressure (110 to 180 mm H_2O), which is often followed by a "favorable clinical response."

3). **CT Scan.** The CT scan is variable, but unequivocable cases display ventricular enlargement without cortical atrophy.

5. **Pseudodementia (Depression).** This term should be abandoned. This is not a true dementia syndrome. The patient's gross appearance simulates dementia, but cognitive function is spared. The condition is typically caused by an affective disorder rather than an organic central nervous system disorder. Some helpful distinguishing features include the following:

a. **Short Duration.** It is not long before families express concern.

b. **Symptoms.** There are a greater sense of distress and more complaints of cognitive and memory loss; complaints often indicate greater severity than testing indicates.

c. **Other Signs.** There are more mood disturbance, more vegetative signs of depression, and no nocturnal worsening, in contrast to dementia.

d. **Positive Response to Empiric Trial of Antidepressants**

6. **Drug Toxicity.** The increased prevalence of illness in the elderly leads to the pervasive use of many drugs. The elderly experience prolonged drug half-life, alteration in volume of distribution, low albumin concentration with increased unbound drug levels, and decreased renal clearance.

a. **Offending Pharmacologic Agents.** The worst of these are neuroleptics, hypnotics, antihypertensives, antidepressants, sedatives, and cimetidine.

b. **Drugs Causing Dementialike Conditions.** Many other drugs such as digitalis, propranolol, antihypertensive agents, and diuretics can produce cognitive derangements that are often misdiagnosed as dementia.

C. **Syndromes Confused with Dementia.** The dementia syndromes can be confused with and must be distinguished from the following conditions:

1. **Benign Senescent Forgetfulness.** This is controversial as a clinical entity. There is some slight decline in recent and remote memory that commonly occurs with age, especially the speed of recall. Forgetfulness in the elderly falls short of the devastating deficits seen in dementia; normal cognition is easily detected by the Mini Mental Status evaluation.

2. **Amnesic Syndrome.** This is an isolated inability to retain new information; in contrast to dementia, other cortical or intellectual functions are intact. This syndrome is usually seen in alcoholics but also after head trauma, encephalitis, vascular accidents, and third ventricle tumors.

3. **Delirium.** (See Chapter 78.) This is always a more acute alteration of cerebral function than dementia. Delirium is characterized by fluctuating alterations of consciousness, combined with confusion, disorientation, alterations in perception,

hallucination, increased vigilance, and excessive autonomic activity. It is usually seen in drug and alcohol withdrawal or certain types of intoxication such as from steroids or atropine. Delirium may also be caused by underlying medical illnesses in the elderly such as pneumonia, appendicitis, or urinary tract infections.

4. *Acute Confusional State.* This is the same as delirium but with reduced vigilance and normal or reduced autonomic function.

5. *Abulia.* Abulia is a state of reduced spontaneous motion and verbal activity. Responses are slow but often intact. Abulia is usually seen in frontal lobe disease (tumors, strokes, abscess, or hydrocephalus).

DIAGNOSTIC EVALUATION

A. **History.** The history should concentrate on the features noted earlier. Usually someone who knows the patient well is needed to validate information or to supply an accurate history. Inventory of prescription and over-the-counter drugs is of great importance.

B. **Physical Examination.** The physician should attempt to identify the many underlying medical conditions that may have reversible dementia as a feature. (See Table 79–2.)

C. **Mental Status Examination.** It is desirable to document in medical records some quantitative assessment of the mental status. Several are available. The authors use the Mini Mental State evaluation (Table 79–1).

D. **Laboratory Evaluation.** Most experts recommend a routine battery of tests to ensure that many reversible dementias are not missed.

1. *Screening Tests.* The Task Force sponsored by the National Institute on Aging recommended considering the following as screening tests (unfortunately, data on predictive value, sensitivity, and specificity are not available):

   a. **Complete Blood Count with Sedimentation Rate**
   b. **Urinalysis**
   c. **Stool for Occult Blood**
   d. **Electrolytes, Blood-Urea Nitrogen, and Glucose**
   e. **Calcium, Phosphorus, and Bilirubin**
   f. **Serum Vitamin B_{12} and Folate Levels**
   g. **Thyroid Function Tests**
   h. **Venereal Disease Research Laboratories (VDRL)**
   i. **Chest X-Ray**
   j. **Electrocardiogram**
   k. **Computed Tomographic (CT) Scan of the Brain.** As noted previously, this is used mainly to rule out space-occupying lesions, hydrocephalus, hemorrhage, infarction, and edema. CT scans cannot reliably diagnose primary degenerative dementia. The cortical atrophy seen on CT scans relates more to age than to the degree of dementia.

2. Other Procedures. These methods are possibly useful (if suggested by the clinical picture or results from the earlier tests):

  a. **Electroencephalogram (EEG).** The EEG provides evidence of organic disease, whether focal or diffuse, stable, resolving, or progressing.

  b. **Lumbar Puncture.** This is not performed routinely. Lumbar puncture is performed in acute confusional states, subacute course to the dementia, suspected NPH, and with a positive VDRL.

  c. **Technetium Brain Scan.** This method is used more when CT scanning is not available, when the EEG shows focal signs, or when chronic subdural hematoma is suspected.

  d. **Toxic Screens.** Bromide level, ammonia level, cerebrospinal fluid glutamine, and urinary porphobilinogen should be considered.

3. Negative Laboratory Results. Negative laboratory results do not rule out specific medical causes for a dementia and should not inhibit frequent clinical reassessment.

REFERENCES

1. Funkenstein HH: Dementia. *In* Branch WT: Office Practice of Medicine. Philadelphia, W. B. Saunders Company, 1982.

   A thorough and intelligent discussion. Written for outpatient evaluation by internists.

2. Small GA, Liston EH, Jarvik LF: Diagnosis and treatment of dementia in the aged in geriatric medicine. West J Med 135:469–481, 1981.

   An up-to-date review article with many recent references.

3. Folstein MF, Folstein SE, McHugh PR: "Mini-Mental State". A practical method for grading the cognitive state of patients for the clinician. J Psychiatr Res 12:189–198, 1975.

   Original presentation of the Mini Mental State evaluation. Merits more widespread use. Easy yet comprehensive.

4. Task Force Sponsored by the National Institute on Aging: Senility reconsidered—treatment possibilities for mental impairment in the elderly. JAMA 244:259–263, 1980.

   Recommends minimal screening of all suspected dementia patients to rule out reversible causes.

5. Beck JC, Benson DT, Scheibel AB, et al.: Dementia in the elderly: The silent epidemic. Ann Intern Med 97:231–241, 1982.

   An up-to-date review with 76 references.

6. Larson EB, Reifler BV, Featherstone HJ, English DR: Dementia in elderly outpatients: A prospective study. Ann Intern Med 100:417–423, 1984.

   Challenges emphasis on distinguishing reversible from irreversible forms of dementia. Recognition and treatment of associated medical illnesses perhaps provide a more valuable approach.

HEADACHE

By HASI M. VENKATACHALAM, M.B.B.S., M.P.H.

EPIDEMIOLOGY AND GENERAL COMMENTS

Headache is a symptom, not a disease. It is one of the ten leading reasons patients visit doctors and accounts for 1.9 per cent of all office visits. An estimated 5 to 10 per cent of the general population seeks medical help annually for headache complaints, and nearly half the United States population admits to having had at least one severe headache. Headaches contribute significantly to medical care expenditures and are a source of considerable patient morbidity.

DIFFERENTIAL DIAGNOSIS

A. **Definition.** The term "headache" commonly refers to head pain from brow level up. The Ad Hoc Committee on Classification of Headache gives a broader definition, including "both painful and unpainful discomforts of the entire head, including the face and upper nucha." The committee's classification includes the following categories:

1. Vascular headache of migraine type: classic and common migraine, cluster headache, hemiplegic and ophthalmoplegic migraine, and lower-half headache
2. Muscle-contraction headache (tension headache)
3. Combined headache: vascular and muscle-contraction
4. Headache of nasal vasomotor reaction
5. Headache of delusional, conversion, or hypochondriac states
6. Nonmigrainous vascular headaches
7. Traction headache
8. Headache caused by overt cranial inflammation
9–13. Headache caused by disease of ocular, aural, nasal and sinusal, dental, or other cranial or neck structures
14. Cranial neuritides
15. Cranial neuralgias such as trigeminal neuralgia

Around 35 per cent of ambulatory patients with headache have tension-muscle contraction headaches. Migraine accounts for 20 to 25 per cent of cases. The remainder consists mostly of the combined variety but also includes cases related to eye, ear, nose, dental problems, and other head and face pains. Less than 0.5 per cent are related to brain tumor.

B. **Key to Diagnosis.** The key is to differentiate between headaches with benign prognoses and potentially serious headaches.

HISTORY, SIGNS, AND SYMPTOMS

A well-recorded history is essential to diagnosis, and when coupled with a focused neurologic examination leads to diagnosis in over 90 per cent of patients. The headache's onset, duration, and pattern of recurrence are helpful in making the diagnosis (Fig. 80–1).

The distinguishing clinical features of the common headache syndromes are described here:

A. **Migraine**

1. *Classic Migraine.* Onset occurs by the third decade of life, rarely after age 40. There is a positive family history in 60 per cent of cases or more. The incidence is higher in males before puberty and in females after puberty. The hallmark of classic migraine is that all patients experience some prodrome, whether it is visual or auditory or consists of other sensory symptoms. A third of these cases have some very distinct visual prodrome, including photophobia, fortification spectra or teichopsia (zigzag lines of light) with scintillating scotomas (10 per cent), and unformed flashes of light or photopsia (25 per cent). Headache is mostly unilateral (two thirds or more of cases). Initially pain is dull and progresses from throbbing and severe to intense. Duration ranges from two hours to two days, but most migraine headaches last several hours. There is associated nausea (68 per cent) or vomiting and abdominal pain (20 per cent of children and 1.5 per cent of adult patients). The patient prefers to "sleep off"

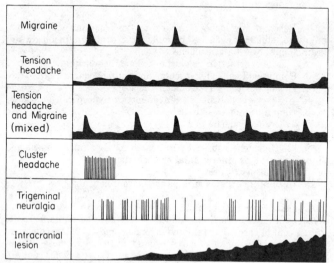

Figure 80–1. Temporal patterns of headache. (Reproduced with permission, from Lance JW: Mechanism and Management of Headache, 4th ed., London, Butterworths, 1982.)

the headache. Results of physical examination are usually normal. Precipitating factors may include diet, noise, light, or stressful stimuli.

2. **Common Migraine.** This is more common than the classic migraine and affects females more often than males. It is similar to classic migraine, but there are no visual symptoms or clear-cut prodrome.

3. **Complicated Migraine.** This category includes ophthalmoplegic and hemiplegic varieties. The prodrome is present and headache is usually unilateral. In 4 per cent of all migrainous patients there may be unilateral paresthesias with hemiparesis or dysphasia. Temporary or rarely permanent neurologic deficits outlast the headache.

4. **Facial Migraine or Lower-Half Headache.** This type is usually unilateral and may be throbbing. It involves the nostrils, cheek, gums, and teeth and may spread to the neck, ear, or eye, in which case it can be confused with cluster headache. The difference from cluster headache is (1) the absence of remissions, which usually occur between bouts of cluster headache and (2) episodes that last from four hours to several days, while cluster headaches last two hours or less.

B. **Cluster Headache (Horton's Histamine Headache; Migrainous Neuralgia).** Age of onset is usually from the fourth decade onward, with some cases occurring by the second decade. The ratio of male to female patients is about 10:1. Alcohol may precipitate headaches in susceptible individuals during a "cluster." The term "cluster" is used because the headaches occur daily, usually once a day, over a period of from one to two to four to eight weeks and then cease abruptly. The patient may remain symptom-free for years. Each headache has a sudden onset with severe, boring, throbbing, or pulsating pain that is centered over one eye and the adjacent head and face. There is associated ipsilateral erythema, sweating, lacrimation, partial Horner's syndrome with ptosis and miosis, and either ipsilateral rhinorrhea or blocked nostril. During an attack the patient is restless and pacing (in contrast to a migraineur, who prefers to lie quietly).

C. **Tension or Muscle Contraction Headache.** Pain is constant or pressing, almost always bilateral, initially episodic, and can become chronic on a daily basis. Headache is bilateral in 90 per cent of cases with a "hatband" distribution of pressing, dull, undulating pain during the day. Results of physical examination are usually normal.

D. **Mixed Headache Syndrome.** This syndrome combines muscle-contraction and migraine qualities but no single feature or group of identifying features. There is a slight preponderance of female over male patients. Results of physical examination are usually negative. A headache pattern and headache history chronicle kept by the patient may be helpful.

E. **Serious Headaches.** These cases are more likely to have neurologic findings on physical examination. The more common findings include subarachnoid hemorrhage, chronic subdural hematoma, other intracranial mass lesions, and infections as in meningitides.

RECOMMENDED DIAGNOSTIC APPROACH

A. History. The history is of paramount importance. The essential items of the headache history include:

1. Number and types of headaches present
2. Age and circumstances of onset
3. Family history
4. Characteristics of pain: location, frequency, duration, quality, and time of onset
5. Prodromal symptoms
6. Precipitating factors: environmental (external), psychologic, and internal
7. Emotional patterns: sleep pattern
8. Medical history: past illnesses, concurrent disease, trauma, surgery, and alcoholism
9. Allergies
10. Response to medication (including names, dosage, and side effects): past and present

In cases of recurring or chronic headaches, if diagnosis is inconclusive, the physician should ask the patient to keep a headache diary to ascertain patterns and symptoms.

B. Physical Examination. In addition to a directed physical examination, a neurologic examination should be included to detect underlying organic disease. Focal neurologic signs, including papilledema, altered mental status, or personality changes, especially in older or debilitated people or in people with high alcohol intake, or history of major or minor trauma should alert the physician to the possibility of intracranial mass lesions.

C. Laboratory Evaluation. This is seldom necessary, since it adds little to the history and physical examination. When underlying organic disease is suspected (because of abnormal neurologic findings), further investigations are warranted.

Tests that may be helpful in the diagnosis of headache include:

   1. Hematology. Complete blood count with differential should be done if infection is suspected, and erythrocyte sedimentation rate (ESR) should be determined if temporal arteritis is suspected (in new onset headaches occurring after age 50). The sedimentation rate is always elevated and is greater than 40 per mm per hour in 70 per cent of patients with temporal arteritis.

   2. Computed Tomography (CT) Scan. The CT scan may be useful when results of neurologic examination are abnormal and generally is not indicated with normal results. Its primary use is to rule out intracranial mass lesions. It can also demonstrate hydrocephalus or cystic lesions. Table 80–1 illustrates the frequency of abnormal CT scans even with abnormal neurologic findings.

   3. Lumbar Puncture. This is indicated in acute episodes such as with subarachnoid hemorrhage or bacterial meningitis, when

TABLE 80-1. FREQUENCY OF ABNORMAL FINDINGS IN PATIENTS WITH HEADACHES*

PROCEDURE	OVERALL ABNORMAL FINDINGS Per Cent	DIAGNOSTIC YIELD	
		Per Cent Abnormal with Abnormal Findings from Neurologic Examination	Per Cent Abnormal with Normal Findings from Neurologic Examination
Neurologic examination (n = 161)	10		
EEG (n = 161)	12	44	9
Computed tomographic scan (n = 40)	2	11	0
Cerebral angiograms (n = 7)	29	40	0
Skull roentgenograms (n = 93)	1	0	0

*Modified table reproduced with permission from JAMA 243:359–362, 1980.[6]

immediate diagnosis is urgent. Lumbar puncture is dangerous when intracranial mass lesion is suspected.
4. **Skull X-Rays.** Skull x-rays are indicated only in selected cases of posttraumatic headache on the basis of high-yield criteria. CT scanning has largely replaced plain radiography for other indications.
5. **Electroencephalogram (EEG).** The EEG is useful only if the patient has neurologic deficits or seizures or in some systemic infections such as herpes encephalitis.
6. **Cerebral Angiogram.** This can be used to confirm diagnosis of specific vascular lesions, including small aneurysms, angiomas, and other space-occupying lesions.

It is important to remember that negative laboratory results do not rule out specific medical causes of headache. Hence, appropriate clinical reassessments are essential.

REFERENCES

1. Ad Hoc Committee: Classification of Headache. JAMA 179:717–718, 1962.
2. Adams RD, Victor M: Principles of Neurology. 2nd ed. New York, McGraw-Hill, 1981.
3. Diamond S, Dalessio DJ (eds.): The Practicing Physician's Approach to Headache. 3rd ed. Baltimore, Williams & Wilkins, 1982.
4. Diehr P, Wood RW, Barr V, Wolcott B, Slay L, Tompkins RK: Acute headaches: Presenting symptoms and diagnostic rules to identify patients with tension and migraine headache. J Chron Dis 34:147–158, 1981.
5. Lance JW: Mechanism and Management of Headache. 4th ed. London, Butterworths, 1982.
6. Larson EB, Omenn GS, Lewis H: Diagnostic evaluation of headache. Impact of computerized tomography and cost-effectiveness. JAMA 243:359–362, 1980.

ALCOHOLISM

By PETER COGGAN, M.D.

DEFINITION AND CRITERIA FOR DIAGNOSIS

A. **World Health Organization Classification.** Alcoholism is a progressive illness characterized by loss of control over alcohol consumption, which may result in a wide variety of behavioral and biomedical manifestations. There is no consensus on the precise definition; variability among patients is considerable. The World Health Organization differentiates among the following states, which may or may not coexist:

1. *Alcohol Dependency Syndrome.* This is a psychic and usually physical state that is characterized by behavioral responses that always include a compulsion to take alcohol on a continuous or periodic basis to experience its psychic effects and sometimes to avoid the discomfort of its absence. Tolerance may or may not be present.

2. *Problem Drinking.* Problem drinking involves people who cause or experience mental, physical, or significant social harm associated with drinking.

3. *Heavy Drinking.* This category is normatively defined by the drinking habits of the bulk of the population to include people who drink significantly more than their peers. Dependency or harm, or both, may occur.

B. **Criteria of the American Psychiatric Association.** The *Diagnostic and Statistical Manual of Mental Disorders (DSM-III)* of the American Psychiatric Association lists criteria for the diagnosis of a *substance abuse disorder*. A patient may be said to be an alcohol abuser if alcohol:

1. Interferes with performance as a student or employee
2. Creates problems in the family
3. Causes problems in social relationships
4. Causes legal problems, such as in instances of driving while intoxicated
5. Results in medical problems (such as gastritis)

C. **Criteria of the National Council on Alcoholism.** The diagnosis of alcoholism may be made if *any* of the following criteria apply:

1. Blood alcohol concentration greater than 300 mg per dL (65 mmol per L) at any time
2. Blood alcohol concentration greater than 150 mg per dL (33 mmol per L) in an apparently unintoxicated patient
3. Blood alcohol concentration greater than 100 mg per dL (22 mmol per L) at a routine examination

D. **Working Definition.** A simple working definition for busy medical practitioners defines the alcoholic as "one who experiences repeated negative consequences of drinking."

EPIDEMIOLOGY

Approximately 10 per cent of the adult population may be defined as alcohol abusers by the criteria of the American Psychiatric Association. Estimates in the elderly population vary. Two to 10 per cent is a realistic range. Abuse among young people is very high. Eighty-seven per cent of high school students have experimented with alcohol. Published studies suggest that Irish Americans, Native Americans, Hispanics, and black youth are at increased risk of developing alcoholism, while Jewish and Italian Americans are relatively protected. There are definite genetic components to alcoholism. The risk of developing the disease if one parent is alcoholic is 2.5 times the risk of the general population. Those in the catering and brewing industries are at increased risk. Women under the age of 30, who are members of the health professions tend to be addicted to other drugs as well as alcohol.

Thirteen per cent of the health care budget is spent on the consequences of alcoholism and alcohol abuse. Twenty-five per cent of hospital admissions and 25 to 30 per cent of emergency room visits are alcohol-related.

DIFFERENTIAL DIAGNOSIS

The key is careful history-taking to distinguish between:

1. Alcoholism as the primary complaint.
2. Alcohol abuse secondary to a primary depressive disorder, bipolar depression, sociopathic drinking, or other drug abuse. The essential question is which came first, the alcohol abuse or the depression.
3. Alcoholism as the underlying cause of a multitude of medical problems.

CLINICAL MANIFESTATIONS

A. **Presentation.** Early alcoholism rarely appears as an overt problem. It is much more likely to appear as: (1) a hidden diagnosis in an apparently well patient; (2) the result of information received from a relative or another indirect source; (3) behavioral changes; (4) the diagnosis underlying the main medical complaint; (5) abnormal laboratory data.

Behavioral changes usually occur before medical problems supervene. Later, alcoholism may be obvious because of overt intoxication or the development of well-recognized medical complications. It may be 10 to 15 years before this occurs, and some individuals are remarkably resistant to long-term damage.

B. **History.** In any routine examination or when alcohol abuse is

TABLE 81–1. FACTORS THAT SHOULD BE EXAMINED IN SUSPECTED CASES OF ALCOHOL ABUSE

Drinking to relieve stress
Amount consumed
Frequency of drinking
Increasing tolerance
Attempts to cut down drinking
Morning drinking
Gulping of drinks
Guilt feelings about drinking
Criticism from others
Family, job, social, legal, and financial consequences
Previous withdrawal symptoms
Family history of alcoholism
Occupation
Smoking or other drug abuse

suspected as the underlying cause of a physical complaint, questions about alcohol consumption should be asked. Since denial, manipulation, or minimization are so characteristic of the alcoholic, any response should be carefully evaluated for verbal or nonverbal clues to problem drinking (Table 81–1). A contract to cut down on alcohol use can be helpful in breaking

TABLE 81–2. THE BRIEF MICHIGAN ALCOHOLISM SCREENING TEST*

QUESTIONS	CIRCLE CORRECT ANSWERS		POINTS
1. Do you feel you are a normal drinker?	Yes	No	N2
2. Do friends or relatives think you are a normal drinker?	Yes	No	N2
3. Have you ever attended a meeting of Alcoholics Anonymous?	Yes	No	Y5
4. Have you ever lost friends, girlfriends, or boyfriends because of drinking?	Yes	No	Y2
5. Have you ever gotten into trouble at work because of drinking?	Yes	No	Y2
6. Have you ever neglected your obligations, your family, or your work for two or more days in a row because you were drinking?	Yes	No	Y2
7. After heavy drinking, have you ever had delirium tremens (DTs), severe shaking, heard voices, or seen things that weren't there?	Yes	No	Y2
8. Have you ever gone to anyone for help about your drinking?	Yes	No	Y2
9. Have you ever been in a hospital because of drinking?	Yes	No	Y5
10. Have you ever been arrested for drunk driving or driving after drinking?	Yes	No	Y2

Score 6 = probable diagnosis of alcoholism

*From Pokorny AP, Miller BA, Kaplan HB: A paper-and-pencil questionnaire, Am J Psychiatr 129:342–345, 1972.

TABLE 81–3. CLINICAL MANIFESTATIONS OF ALCOHOLISM

	Early (in first 5 years)	Late
General appearance	Excitability, irritability, nervousness, alcoholic facies	Rosacea, unkempt appearance, jaundice,* parotid swelling
Cardiovascular system	Palpitations, hypertension, especially labile or difficult to control	Cardiomyopathy
Respiratory system		Recurrent chest infections, chronic obstructive pulmonary disease
Gastrointestinal tract	Coated tongue, alcoholic fetor by day,* dyspepsia, morning nausea and vomiting,* acute pancreatitis (sometimes),* hepatomegaly,* gastrointestinal bleeding (sometimes)	Recurrent abdominal pain, acute and chronic pancreatitis,* splenomegaly, ascites, gastrointestinal bleeding
Genitourinary tract	Polyuria, impotence	Amenorrhea
Central nervous system	Hand tremor*	Peripheral neuropathy, seizures, ataxia
Mental status or affect	Depression, poor memory for recent events	Blackouts
Musculoskeletal system		Dupuytren's contracture,* myopathy, gout
Skin		Spider nevi, seborrhea
Miscellaneous	Frequent or unusual trauma,* multiple surgical or nonsurgical scars,* frequent office visits, emergency room visits or hospitalizations, family violence or dysfunction, financial problems (unpaid medical bills), legal problems (driving while intoxicated)	

*Great diagnostic value.

TABLE 81–4. LABORATORY STUDIES

Test	Normal Values	Comment
Blood alcohol*	See Definitions	See Definitions
Red cell morphology: macrocytic indices, especially MCV,*† poikilocytosis Thrombocytopenia	MCV* 82–98 femtoliters	Poor specificity, moderate sensitivity; not folate-dependent; returns to normal after several months' abstinence
Liver enzymes		
gamma glutamyl transferase*	Male <35 u/L Female <30 u/L	Moderate specificity and sensitivity
AST (SGOT)*†	<25 u/L	Poor specificity, moderate sensitivity; returns to normal levels in 1–2 weeks provided liver damage is not extensive
ALT (SGPT)†	<30 u/L	
LDH†	<290 u/L	
Alkaline phosphatase	20–105 u/L	
Lipids		

Cholesterol*	Male 140–280 mg/dL Female 150–300 mg/dL			Poor specificity and moderate sensitivity; returns to normal by 2 weeks after alcohol is withdrawn
HDL†				
HDL-cholesterol†	Age	Female	Male	
	20–29	36–78	30–65	
	30–39	33–77	30–59	
	40–49	40–81	25–61	
	50–75	38–91	29–72	
Triglycerides	60–136 mg/dL			
Uric acid	Male 4.3–7.6 mg/dL Female 3.2–6.0 mg/dL			Poor specificity and sensitivity; returns to normal in a few days

*Most useful.
†MCV = mean corpuscular volume; AST = aspartate aminotransferase; ALT = alanine amino transferase; SGOT = serum glutamic oxaloacetic transaminase; SGPT = serum glutamic oxaloacetic transaminase; LDH = lactic dehydrogenase; HDL = high-density lipoprotein.
No single test or combination of tests is diagnostic, but the gamma GT, AST, and red cell indices are likely to be the most appropriate combination. Interpretation in conjunction with history and physical examination data is necessary.

through denial. The exact quantity and type of alcohol to be consumed each day should be specified and the patient seen in several weeks to assess compliance. This strategy can sometimes be helpful in showing the patient that control has been lost.

Questions to ask are listed in Table 81–2. Questionnaires may be helpful, such as the Michigan Alcohol Screening Test (MAST), its shorter version (SMAST; Table 81–2) or the CAGE questions (Have you ever tried to cut down? Have you ever annoyed anyone with your drinking? Do you ever feel guilty? Do you have a morning eye-opener?).

C. **Physical Examination.** Clinical signs are summarized in Table 81–3. There is enormous variability from patient to patient. Women are more susceptible to liver damage leading to cirrhosis than are men.

LABORATORY STUDIES

(Only commonly available tests are discussed.)

Several batteries or combinations of tests have been advocated. None is definitive and each must be interpreted in conjunction with historical or physical examination data. It is difficult to estimate the predictive value of laboratory tests, but some estimates are listed in Table 81–4.

RECOMMENDED DIAGNOSTIC APPROACH

A. **History.** A history of alcohol consumption should always be recorded at any routine examination or when a problem could be alcohol-related. The response should be treated with circumspection. A family history places the patient at risk. Multiple behavioral or medical consequences or a history of symptoms of withdrawal are highly suggestive.

B. **Physical Examination.** Early in the development of alcoholism there may be no physical findings. The development of signs and symptoms is quite variable.

C. **Laboratory Data.** Some tests may be helpful in conjunction with information gained from the history or physical examination, but none except the blood alcohol concentration (BAC) is diagnostic.

Pointers identified in any of these three categories (history, physical examination, or laboratory findings) should raise the physician's suspicion. When two categories are involved, there is almost certainly an alcohol-related problem.

Confrontation is always appropriate if the evidence suggests a drinking problem. Not to confront the patient does the patient a disservice. Laboratory data can be helpful in breaking down denial. A "contract to reduce drinking" may also assist. A crisis, either behavioral or medical, can be used as the focus of an "intervention" or group confrontation by family members and other concerned individuals. Sometimes family members may be willing to precipitate a crisis. Many alcohol treatment centers or private counselors are able to provide training in this technique. Alanon provides invaluable family support.

REFERENCES

1. IVth Special Report to Congress on Alcohol and Health. U.S. Department of Health and Human Services. Rockville, Maryland, NIAAA, 1981.
2. Weinberg JR: Interview techniques for diagnosing alcoholism. Am Fam Physician 3:107–115, 1974.
3. Skinner HA, Holt S, Israel Y: Early identification of alcohol abuse: 1. Critical issues and psychosocial indicators for a composite index. Can Med Assoc J 124:1141–1152, 1981.
4. Holt S, Skinner HA, Israel Y: Early identification of alcohol abuse: 2. Clinical and laboratory indications. Can Med Assoc J 124:1279–1294, 1981.
5. American Psychiatric Association: Diagnostic & Statistical Manual of Mental Disorders (DSM-III). Washington, D.C., American Psychiatric Association, 1980.
6. Pokorny AP, Miller BA, Kaplan HB: A paper-and-pencil questionnaire. Am J Psychiatr 129:342–345, 1972.

INDEX

Note: Page numbers in italics refer to illustrations; t indicates tables.

615